Cerebrospinal Fluid Disorders

Cerebrospinal Fluid Disorders

Edited by
Conor Mallucci
The Walton Centre for Neurology and Neurosurgery
Liverpool, UK
Spyros Sgouros
"Attikon" University Hospital
University of Athens
Athens, Greece

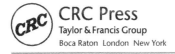
CRC Press
Taylor & Francis Group
Boca Raton London New York

CRC Press is an imprint of the
Taylor & Francis Group, an **informa** business

CRC Press
Taylor & Francis Group
6000 Broken Sound Parkway NW, Suite 300
Boca Raton, FL 33487-2742

First issued in paperback 2019

© 2010 by Taylor & Francis Group, LLC
CRC Press is an imprint of Taylor & Francis Group, an Informa business

No claim to original U.S. Government works

ISBN-13: 978-0-8247-2833-5 (hbk)
ISBN-13: 978-0-367-38461-6 (pbk)

A CIP record for this book is available from the British Library.

Library of Congress Cataloging-in-Publication Data available on application

Visit the Taylor & Francis Web site at
http://www.taylorandfrancis.com

and the CRC Press Web site at
http://www.crcpress.com

Preface

When asked what my interests are and in what age group I practice, I often reply that my interests lie in "hydrocephalus and CSF disorders from the fetus to old age."

Indeed it is hard to separate or "cut off" one's interest when a child enters adulthood still carrying these conditions, and equally, it is hard to understand how one can "limit" one's interest or "expertise" to just the brain or spine when clearly the cerebrospinal fluid dynamically affects both the compartments. The dilemma and debate continues as to whether we as neurosurgeons should limit our practice to diseases affecting children (and call ourselves pediatric neurosurgeons) or adults, but if there were ever a condition warranting a disease-specific approach as opposed to "age" specific, then it is those diseases that affect the dynamics of the cerebrospinal fluid.

This book has been conceived therefore to cover the gap in the literature on CSF disorders in a comprehensive text, which addresses the issues of disorders of the CSF pathways from birth until old age as well as to explore and manage the effects of such disorders on the brain and spine.

As neurosurgeons and health professionals, we continue to subspecialize into predominantly pediatric and adult sectors, and, in the case of neurosurgery, into those with predominantly cranial or spinal interests. In addition, healthcare delivery to children and adults often divides and segregates the two at times with poor provision to bridge the gap between the two. The result is disjointed knowledge and pockets of expertise in a variety of these areas with no unifying text to address these divisions. The losers are often the patients, stuck between the disciplines of pediatric care and adult-delivered services with little clarity on who the "experts" are to pick up their case.

In creating this book, we attempt not only to cover the understanding, diagnosis, and management of the common conditions, such as hydrocephalus, syringomyelia, and idiopathic intracranial hypertension across all ages, but also to create a reference useful to neurosurgeons and related specialties, such as neurology, pediatrics, general medicine and practice, ophthalmology, radiology, and emergency medicine, alike. We hope that the text will also provide a useful reference to nursing professionals, caregivers, and advisory bodies, as well as incorporating the patient's perspective.

With the advent of the Internet and patients' access to information, we felt it vital to create a book that will provide a reference for health professionals as well as the patients and families that we treat. Many of the conditions we treat are carried for life, and patients and families need considerable support in building up their own knowledge of their condition. We hope this text will help to guide them in attaining the understanding and support that they need.

This book is divided into four distinct sections that will be useful to different readers from many disciplines. We have invited a panel of international experts recognized in their field to share their knowledge with us. In addition to the conventional author-led chapters, you will also find "boxes" included within a chapter but written by different authors, designed to give brief updates on the literature or specific techniques and also to give different viewpoints on the subject.

The first section serves as a background to CSF disorders and diseases including the pathophysiology of the CSF pathways; a fascinating chapter on the history of the treatment of CSF pathways by Dr Jim Goodrich, including many figures from his private collection not available or seen by the general public; and chapters covering neuropsychology, imaging, and antenatal screening.

The second section focuses on disease specific discussion of all disorders that affect the brain and the spine in all ages, thus including not only the usual causes of hydrocephalus in children and adults but also conditions often missed out in books on hydrocephalus such as idiopathic intracranial hypertension, Chiari malformation, and syringomyelia.

The third section concentrates on the treatment techniques that unify all these conditions, necessary to any surgeon declaring an interest in the management of them. In particular, the focus is on the evidence and literature for the techniques and choices we need to make.

In the final section, we thought it appropriate to address topics not necessarily addressed in such texts or those of particular interest. Thus, you will see interesting chapters on fetal surgery, ethical considerations in managing CSF disorders, the management of hydrocephalus in the developing world, and the most importantly, a chapter on the patients perspective.

Finally, we would like to acknowledge and remember Dr Patrick Hanlo and Dr Tony Hockley, authors of two of the chapters, who died suddenly before the completion of this book, and hence they did not have the chance to see their work come to fruition. Dr Hockley's sudden death earlier this year has touched especially both of us, as he trained both of us in our early careers setting us on our paths. He in particular was a strong supporter of the idea behind the book, as he had recognized that these conditions, although often starting in childhood, often affect the patient and the family throughout the whole lifetime and had devoted his career in treating these patients with due compassion, care, and attention to detail so that they can enjoy a long and healthy quality of life.

The color printing of the illustrations in this book was made possible with the generous unconditional sponsorship from the following companies: Aesculap AG; BBraun Aesculap UK; Christoph Miethke GmbH und Co. KG; and Vamvas Medical Greece.

Conor Mallucci
Spyros Sgouros

Contents

Contributors

Ferdinando Aliberti   Department of Pediatric Neurosurgery, Santobono Children's Hospital, Naples, Italy

Jörg Baldauf   Department of Neurosurgery, Ernst-Moritz-Arndt University, Greifswald, Germany

Carys M. Bannister   Department of Neuroscience, University of Manchester, Manchester, U.K.

Rosemary Batchelor   Association for Spina Bifida and Hydrocephalus, Peterborough, U.K.

Rachid Bech-Azeddine   University Clinic of Neurosurgery, Neuroscience Centre, Rigshospitalet, Capital Region, Copenhagen, Denmark

R. G. J. Bloemen   Rudolf Magnus Institute of Neuroscience, Department of Neurosurgery, University Medical Center, Utrecht, The Netherlands

Hieronymus Damianus Boogaarts   Department of Neurosurgery, Radboud Universiteit Nijmegen, Medical Centre, Nijmegen, The Netherlands

Triantafyllos Bouras   Department of Neurosurgery, "Attikon" University Hospital, University of Athens, Athens, Greece

Andrew Brodbelt   The Walton Centre NHS Foundation Trust, Liverpool, U.K.

Maria Consiglio Buonocore   Department of Pediatric Neurosurgery, Santobono Children's Hospital, Naples, Italy

Sergio Cavalheiro   Department of Pediatric Neurosurgery, Federal University of São Paulo, São Paulo, Brazil

Emilio Cianciulli   Department of Pediatric Neurosurgery, Santobono Children's Hospital, Naples, Italy

Giuseppe Cinalli   Department of Pediatric Neurosurgery, Santobono Children's Hospital, Naples, Italy

Paul Chumas   Department of Neurosurgery, Leeds General Infirmary, Leeds, U.K.

Hartmut Collmann   Section of Pediatric Neurosurgery, Neurosurgical Department, University of Würzburg, Würzburg, Germany

Shlomi Constantini   Department of Pediatric Neurosurgery, Tel Aviv Medical Center, Dana Children's Hospital, Tel Aviv, Israel

Daniel Crimmins   Department of Neurosurgery, Leeds General Infirmary, Leeds, U.K.

Marek Czosnyka   Academic Neurosurgical Unit, Department of Neurosciences, Addenbrooke's Hospital, Cambridge, U.K.

Zofia Czosnyka   Academic Neurosurgical Unit, Department of Neurosciences, Addenbrooke's Hospital, Cambridge, U.K.

Mateus Dal Fabbro   Division of Neurosurgery, State University of Campinas, Campinas, Brazil

Philippe Decq   Service de Neurochirurgie, Hôpital Henri Mondor, Créteil, France

Patrick Dhellemmes   Pediatric Neurosurgery, Lille University Hospital, Lille, France

Concezio Di Rocco   Department of Pediatric Neurosurgery, Catholic University Medical School, Rome, Italy

Federico Di Rocco   Pediatric Neurosurgery, Université René Descartes Paris V, Hôpital Necker Enfants Malades, Paris, France

Mark S. Dias   Department of Neurosurgery, Section of Pediatric Neurosurgery, Penn State Milton S. Hershey Medical Center, Penn State University College of Medicine, Hershey, Pennsylvania, U.S.A.

Argirios Dinopoulos   3rd Pediatric Department of the University of Athens, "Attikon" University Hospital, Athens, Greece

Yusuf Erşahin   Division of Pediatric Neurosurgery, Ege University Faculty of Medicine, Izmir, Turkey

Igor Vilela Faquini   Department of Pediatric Neurosurgery, Federal University of São Paulo, São Paulo, Brazil

Graham Fieggen   Division of Neurosurgery, University of Cape Town, Cape Town, South Africa

Tony Figaji   Paediatric Neurosurgery Unit, Red Cross Children's Hospital and University of Cape Town, Cape Town, South Africa

Flemming Gjerris   University Clinic of Neurosurgery, Neuroscience Centre, Rigshospitalet, Capital Region, Copenhagen, Denmark

James Tait Goodrich   Division of Pediatric Neurosurgery, Children's Hospital at Montefiore, Albert Einstein College of Medicine, Bronx, New York, U.S.A.

Cathy Grant   Paediatric Psychology, Child Development Centre, Leicester Royal Infirmary, Leicester, U.K.

Gahl Greenberg   Division of Diagnostic Imaging, Chaim Sheba Medical Center, Tel Hashomer, Israel

J. André Grotenhuis   Department of Neurosurgery, Radboud University Nijmegen Medical Center, Nijmegen, The Netherlands

Daniel J. Guillaume   Department of Neurosurgery, Oregon Health & Science University, Portland, Oregon, U.S.A.

Patrick W. Hanlo[†]   Rudolf Magnus Institute of Neuroscience, Department of Neurosurgery, University Medical Center, Utrecht, The Netherlands

Caroline Hayhurst   Department of Neurosurgery, The Walton Centre for Neurology and Neurosurgery, Liverpool, U.K.

Anthony D. Hockley[†]   Department of Neurosurgery, Birmingham Children's Hospital, Birmingham, U.K.

Mark R. Iantosca   Department of Neurosurgery, Section of Pediatric Neurosurgery, Penn State Milton S. Hershey Medical Center, Penn State University College of Medicine, Hershey, Pennsylvania, U.S.A.

[†]Deceased.

Jo Iddon   Department of Medicine and Therapeutics, Chelsea and Westminster Hospital, London, U.K.

Mohammed Al Jumaily   Department of Neurosurgery, The Walton Centre for Neurology and Neurosurgery, Liverpool, U.K.

Jothy Kandaswamy   Department of Neurosurgery, The Walton Centre for Neurology and Neurosurgery, Liverpool, U.K.

Konstantina Karabatsou   Department of Neurosurgery, The Walton Centre for Neurology and Neurosurgery, Liverpool, U.K.

John Kestle   Division of Pediatric Neurosurgery, University of Utah, Salt Lake City, Utah, U.S.A.

Dorothee Koch-Wiewrodt   Neurochirurgische Klinik und Poliklinik, Bereich Pädiatrische Neurochirurgie, Johannes Gutenberg-Universität Mainz, Germany

Dimitris Kombogiorgas   Department of Neurosurgery, Birmingham Children's Hospital, Birmingham, U.K.

Jürgen Krauß   Section of Pediatric Neurosurgery, Neurosurgical Department, University of Würzburg, Würzburg, Germany

Abhaya V. Kulkarni   Department of Neurosurgery, Hospital for Sick Children, Toronto, Ontario, Canada

Conor Mallucci   Department of Neurosurgery, The Walton Centre for Neurology and Neurosurgery, Liverpool, U.K.

Paul May   Department of Neurosurgery, The Walton Centre for Neurology and Neurosurgery, Liverpool, U.K.

Arnold H. Menezes   Department of Neurosurgery, University of Iowa Hospitals and Clinics, Iowa City, Iowa, U.S.A.

Sherif Mohammed Al-Sayed Al-Kheshen   Department of Neurosurgery, Faculty of Medicine, Tanta University, Tanta, Egypt

Khaled Elsayed Mohammed   Department of Neurosurgery, Faculty of Medicine, Suez Canal University, Ismailia, Egypt

Peter Murphy   Department of Neurosurgery, The Walton Centre for Neurology and Neurosurgery, Liverpool, U.K.

Cheryl Muszinski   Department of Neurosurgery, Division of Pediatric Neurosurgery, Medical College of Wisconsin, Milwaukee, Wisconsin, U.S.A.

Toba Niazi   Department of Neurosurgery, Primary Children's Medical Center, University of Utah, Salt Lake City, Utah, U.S.A.

Jardel Mendonça Nicácio   Department of Pediatric Neurosurgery, Federal University of São Paulo, São Paulo, Brazil

Shizuo Oi   Division of Pediatric Neurosurgery, Jikei University Hospital Women's & Children's Medical Center, Tokyo, Japan

John J. Oró   The Chiari Care Center, Neurosurgery Center, The Medical Center of Aurora, Aurora, Colorado, U.S.A.

John D. Pickard   Academic Neurosurgical Unit, Department of Neurosciences, Addenbrooke's Hospital, Cambridge, U.K.

Charles Raybaud   Division of Neuroradiology, Hospital for Sick Children, University of Toronto, Toronto, Ontario, Canada

Harold L. Rekate Pediatric Neurosciences, Barrow Neurological Institute, St. Joseph's Hospital and Medical Center, Phoenix, Arizona, U.S.A.

Hugh Richards Cambridge Shunt Registry, Cambridge, U.K.

Jerard Ross Department of Paediatric Neurosurgery, The Royal Hospital for Sick Children, Edinburgh

Fiona Rowe Division of Orthoptics, University of Liverpool, Liverpool, U.K.

Alison Rowlands Department of Ophthalmology, North Cheshire NHS Trust, Warrington, U.K.

Claudio Ruggiero Department of Pediatric Neurosurgery, Santobono Children's Hospital, Naples, Italy

Christian Sainte-Rose Pediatric Neurosurgery, Université René Descartes Paris V, Hôpital Necker Enfants Malades, Paris, France

Henry W. S. Schroeder Department of Neurosurgery, Ernst-Moritz-Arndt University, Greifswald, Germany

Wan Tew Seow Neurosurgery Service, KK Women's and Children's Hospital, Singapore

Spyros Sgouros Department of Neurosurgery, "Attikon" University Hospital, University of Athens, Athens, Greece

Vit Siomin Department of Pediatric Neurosurgery, Tel Aviv Medical Center, Dana Children's Hospital, Tel Aviv, Israel

Niels Sörensen Section of Pediatric Neurosurgery, Neurosurgical Department, University of Würzburg, Würzburg, Germany

Pietro Spennato Department of Pediatric Neurosurgery, Santobono Children's Hospital, Naples, Italy

Arleta Starza-Smith Paediatric Neuropsychology Service, Regional Neurosciences Centre, Nottingham University Hospitals, Nottingham, U.K.

Marcus Stoodley The Australian School of Advanced Medicine, Macquarie University, New South Wales, Australia

Satoshi Takahashi Division of Pediatric Neurosurgery, Jikei University Hospital Women's & Children's Medical Center and Department of Neurosurgery, Keio University School of Medicine, Tokyo, Japan

Emily Talbot Paediatric Neuropsychology Service, Regional Neurosciences Centre, Nottingham University Hospitals, Nottingham, U.K.

Gianpiero Tamburrini Department of Pediatric Neurosurgery, Catholic University Medical School, Rome, Italy

Charles Teo The Centre for Minimally Invasive Neurosurgery, Prince of Wales Private Hospital, Randwick, New South Wales, Australia

Atul Tyagi Department of Neurosurgery, Leeds General Infirmary, Leeds, U.K.

W. Peter Vandertop Department of Neurosurgery, Neurosurgical Center Amsterdam, Amsterdam, The Netherlands

Kristina Vella Paediatric Neuropsychology Service, Regional Neurosciences Centre, Nottingham University Hospitals, Nottingham, U.K.

Matthieu Vinchon Pediatric Neurosurgery, Lille University Hospital, Lille, France

Wolfgang Wagner Neurochirurgische Klinik und Poliklinik, Bereich Pädiatrische Neurochirurgie, Johannes Gutenberg-Universität Mainz, Germany

Marion L. Walker Department of Neurosurgery, Primary Children's Medical Center, University of Utah, Salt Lake City, Utah, U.S.A.

Benjamin C. Warf Department of Neurosurgery, Children's Hospital Boston and Harvard Medical School, Boston, Massachusetts, U.S.A.

George Seow Heong Yeo Antenatal Monitoring Clinic and Antenatal Diagnostic Clinic, Department of Maternal Fetal Medicine, KK Women's and Children's Hospital, Singapore

1 | An Anatomical and Physiological Basis for CSF Pathway Disorders

Andrew Brodbelt
The Walton Centre NHS Foundation Trust, Liverpool, U.K.

Marcus Stoodley
The Australian School of Advanced Medicine, Macquarie University, New South Wales, Australia

INTRODUCTION

"Water, water everywhere, nor any drop to drink"
Samuel Taylor Coleridge. The Rime of the Ancient Mariner

More than 60% of the human body weight is made of water (1). Water surrounds, permeates, flows, and forms an integral component of the brain and the spinal cord. Cerebrospinal fluid (CSF) is one part of this integrated system. CSF has important mechanical and biochemical functions and is actively produced at a rate of 500 mL/day, circulates through the ventricles, subarachnoid space and parenchyma, and is reabsorbed into the venous circulation (Fig. 1). Failures of this system manifest as clinical CSF disorders. This chapter reviews current concepts of the relevant anatomy and physiology to provide a basis for understanding CSF pathway disorders, and existing and future treatment options.

Cerebral Water

Water permeates the cranial contents in the intracellular, interstitial or extracellular, and intravascular spaces, and in the CSF. This fluid system is dynamic, with careful controls limiting water and solute movement among compartments. Intracranially there are approximately 100 mL of CSF and 150 mL of blood. Interstitial fluid (ISF) has been variously estimated as being between 100 and 300 mL (up to 20% of brain volume) (1,3–8). Optimal neuronal function requires precise control of the extracellular environment. Barriers therefore exist between plasma and ISF (the blood–brain barrier or BBB), between plasma and CSF (the blood–CSF barrier or BCSFB), and between interstitial and intracellular fluids (ICF) (9). Barriers can consist of cell membranes, tight junctions between cells, and various cellular transport processes that control solute and water movement.

Water and solutes enter cerebral water from the blood vessels via active and selective transport into the interstitial and CSF spaces. ISF may also derive in part from cellular metabolism (6,9). There is only a limited barrier between the CSF and the ISF (8). Fluid leaves the system via CSF pathways (see below). Despite the control systems, problems within one part of the fluid system can impact on other parts of the cerebral water system and hence brain function. This chapter concentrates on CSF but includes the other compartments when relevant.

CSF Function

Traditionally, the major function of CSF was held as a cushion for the brain and the spinal cord. Calculations by some researchers suggest that within a CSF bath, the 1500-g brain weighs only 50 g, reducing tension on nerve roots and acting as a strong mechanical buffer (6). In addition, and perhaps of greater importance, CSF also acts like a lymphatic system by allowing movement of metabolites, toxins, and nutrients, and has roles in homeostatic hormonal and signaling mechanisms, chemical buffering, and neurodevelopment (6,8,10–13).

This chapter is an extension of an article previously published: Brodbelt A, Stoodley MA. CSF pathways: A review. Br J Neurosurg 2007; 21(5):510–520.

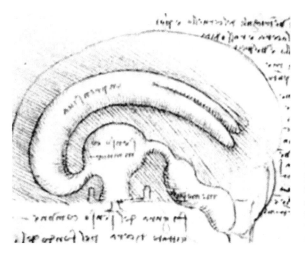

Figure 1 The cerebral ventricles. Drawing by Leonardo da Vinci (1508–1509). The third ventricle (3v) was believed to be the site of afference and elaboration of the "sensus communis" (Latin for peripheral physical sensations). *Source*: The Royal Collection © 2009 Her Majesty Queen Elizabeth II.

Composition and Amount

Cerebrospinal fluid is clear and colorless with a density of 1.003 to 1.008 g/cm^3 (13,14). There is, on average, 140 mL of CSF, divided between the ventricular system (35 mL, or 25%), the spinal canal (30–70 mL, or 20–50%), and the cranial subarachnoid space (35–75 mL, or 25–55%) (3,4,6,7,13,15). In young children, the total amount of CSF is smaller, around 70 mL, divided between the various compartments in a way similar to adults. Comparison of the contents of the CSF, extracellular fluid (ECF), intracellular fluid (ICF), and plasma is shown in Table 1. CSF has a lower concentration of protein, glucose, potassium, and higher concentration of chloride than plasma. β-2 Transferrin is the desialated isoform of the iron-binding glycoprotein transferrin and is only found in CSF, perilymph, and ocular fluids (16). When tested with a paired serum sample, the presence of β-2 transferrin in a persistent watery discharge can be used to confirm CSF leakage (16,17).

CSF PRODUCTION

Most CSF is produced by a highly vascular ingrowth through the ependymal lining of the ventricles known as the choroid plexus (Fig. 2). In addition, approximately 10% to 30% of CSF arises from the movement of ISF (6,8,25,26). Mean CSF production in humans is 0.36 mL/min (approximately 20 mL/hr, or 500 mL/day), although in young children the total daily production is smaller than in adults, possibly half (3,4,6,8,13,26–29). The choroid plexus has a blood supply 10 times that of the cortex and can produce CSF at a rate up to 0.21 mL/min/g tissue, a rate higher than any other secretory epithelium (6,8).

Table 1 Chemical Composition of Body Fluids

	Plasma	ECF/ISF	ICF	CSF
Na (mM)	135–145	138–142	5–15	135–147
K (mM)	3.4–4.7	3.8–5	135–155	2.6–3.1
pH	7.35–7.45	7.44		7.3–7.6
Cl (mM)	99–108	118	9.0	115–130
Ca (mM)	2.1–2.6			1–1.5
Prot (g/L)	50–80			0.15–0.45
Glu (mM)	3.9–6.1			2.8–4.2
Mg (mM)	0.7–1.0			1.0–2.3
Osmolality (mM)	280–296	280–296	280–296	280–296
Amino acids (g/L)	2.62			0.72
β-2 Transferrin	–			+

Source: Adapted from Refs. 1,3,10,13,18–24.

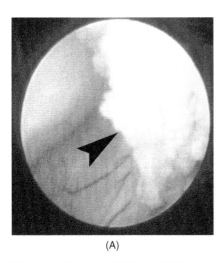
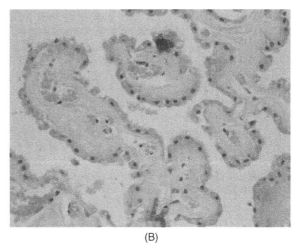

(A) (B)

Figure 2 The Choroid Plexus. (**A**) Endoscopic view of the choroid plexus (*arrowhead*) of the lateral ventricle looking into the third ventricle through the foramen of Monro. (**B**) Hematoxylin and eosin stained section of normal choroid plexus (D Crooks, Walton Centre, Liverpool).

Choroid Plexus

Development

Shortly after closure of the neural tube, the choroid plexus begins to appear as invaginations of mesenchymal-derived epithelial tissue that push into the neural tube at the sites of formation of the cerebral ventricles (6,30). Choroid plexus in the fourth ventricle appears first followed by the lateral ventricle, and finally the third ventricle (30). Carbonic anhydrase (required for secretion) is produced by the ninth week, and tight junctions (required to maintain the BCSFB) are present very early on in development, although the cells at this stage have few cilia, microvilli, or mitochondria (3,30). Choroid plexus blood flow increases considerably between the third and fourth postnatal week (3,30). Putative functions of the choroid plexus and CSF during development include producing expansion for normal brain shape and development, acting to transport protein from the blood to the brain, and having a role in the function of neurotrophic factors and neurodevelopment (30).

Anatomy

The choroid plexus arises from the roofs of the third and fourth ventricles and the wall of each lateral ventricle. The invaginated highly vascular pial stroma is covered by a choroidal epithelium similar to ventricular ependymal lining, except that the cells are joined by tight junctions, forming a watertight barrier separating the ventricular CSF from the choroidal ISF (3). The anterior choroidal (from the supraclinoid internal carotid artery) and the lateral posterior choroidal (from the posterior cerebral artery) arteries are the main supply to the lateral ventricular choroid plexus (3). The choroid plexus in the third ventricle is supplied by the paired medial posterior choroidal arteries arising from the posterior cerebral arteries. The fourth ventricle choroid plexus is supplied by the posterior interior cerebellar artery. A thin membranous structure with a free border is thus produced (3). Rich venous networks join at a thickened site in the free membranous edge, termed the glomus, and form a single large vein that continues to run anteriorly in the free border (3). The choroidal epithelium is composed of simple cuboidal cells covered in cilia and forms fine frond-like projections, consisting of a tiny villous process composed of an enclosing central core containing a capillary and a small amount of loose connective tissue (3,8,31,32). This produces a large surface area of approximately 200 cm^2 for a mass of only 2 g (6).

The microstructure of the choroid plexus is a guide to its function. The vascular endothelium within the choroid plexus is fenestrated, unlike most cerebral vessels (6,26,32). Although zonula occludens connect choroidal endothelial cells, they permit most small hydrophilic molecules to pass (8). Fluid and solute exchange is controlled by barriers at the choroid plexus epithelial cell level. A mechanical barrier between the choroid plexus epithelial cells limits pericellular movement, a metabolic barrier (peptidases are expressed on the apical brush border) degrades unwanted proteins, and a cellular barrier exists based on specific membrane and transporter proteins for transcellular movement both to and from the CSF (6,8,26,31,32).

Unlike the ventricular ependyma, which is leaky, choroid plexus epithelial cells have tightly sealed cell junctions (6,8,26,31,32). These tight junctions, present on the apical border of the cells, prevent any paracellular traffic of solutes between blood and CSF and help form the BCSFB (6,8,26,31,32). This barrier is 10 times more leaky than the blood–brain barrier and might explain the protein reabsorption and proteinase functions of the choroid plexus (8,26,32). The choroid plexus epithelial cells have abundant mitochondria, Golgi bodies, endoplasmic reticulum, ribosomes, and a vesicular network (8,26,33). Coupled with a good blood supply, fenestrated capillaries, large surface area, and extensive infolding on the basal side, the choroid plexus is a well-designed structure for secretion (8,26,33).

CSF Secretion

The main function of the choroid plexus is to secrete CSF (8). Ultrafiltration of water, ions, and solutes from plasma occurs across the leaky vascular endothelial wall to the vascular border of the choroid plexus epithelial cells (5). ATP hydrolysis is used to generate a unidirectional flux of sodium, chloride, and bicarbonate ions across the choroid plexus epithelial layer, which drives the transcellular movement of water by osmosis (8,10,33,34). This mechanism depends on the position and the presence of ion channels (Fig. 3) (6,8,10,26,34,35). Much interest has been generated regarding the transmembrane group of water channels or Aquaporins (AQP). Subtype AQP 1 is found on the apical surface of the choroid plexus epithelium, and AQP 4 is prevalent on astrocytes (6,35). AQP 1 inhibition has been proposed as a method to treat hydrocephalus by reducing CSF production; however, AQP knockouts (mice bred without the AQP 1 channel) have normal CSF production, suggesting other transmembrane mechanisms of water transport exist (6,35).

Larger molecules are transported by transcytosis, endocytosis, or specific oligopeptide transporters (26). CSF formation is influenced by enzyme inhibitors, the autonomic nervous system, and choroidal blood flow (5). Steroids, acetazolamide, diuretics, low temperatures, and changes in CSF osmolality can all reduce CSF production (5). Acute rises in intracranial pressure probably result in a reduced CSF production by reducing choroidal blood flow (5).

Other Functions of the Choroid Plexus

The choroid plexus is also involved in supply and distribution of peptides and growth factors to the brain (26,33). Growth factors and other proteins identified as produced and/or secreted from the choroid plexus include insulin-like growth factor II (IGF II), transforming growth factor β, growth hormone, fibroblast growth factor, some bone morphogenic proteins, as well as arginine vasopressin (8,26). Vasopressin has a higher concentration in CSF than that in the plasma and is under both neuronal and endocrine controls (8). CSF peptides can act on other structures including the hypothalamus and chemosensitive or satiety areas of medulla oblongata, or in an autocrine fashion on the choroid plexus (10,26). Suggested functions of vasopressin and other peptides include affecting hypothalamic or respiratory function, as an initial response to ischemia, trauma, or fluid disorders, and trophic support (8,10,26). Dual transport through both choroid plexus and across the blood–brain barrier may also help to ensure ample provision of peptides to areas of receptor presence (26).

Recent studies suggest that the choroid plexus also acts to eliminate xenobiotics (substances foreign to the body, such as antibiotics) and endogenous waste from CSF to blood, almost like a kidney in cleansing and adjusting CSF and hence brain extracellular fluid (26,31,33). There are organic anion-transporting polypeptides (OATP), organic ion transporters (OAT), peptide transporters (PEPT2 in humans), and multidrug-resistance-associated proteins on the apical (CSF) border of the choroid plexus epithelial cells (26,31). Coupled with the continuous turnover of CSF, these provide a powerful homeostatic mechanism aiding removal of products of brain metabolism (8). The importance of homeostasis of the cerebral extracellular environment, as discussed earlier, correlates with the use of ions for neuronal function and signaling (9). With increased age the height of epithelial cells is reduced by 10%, the basement membrane thickens,

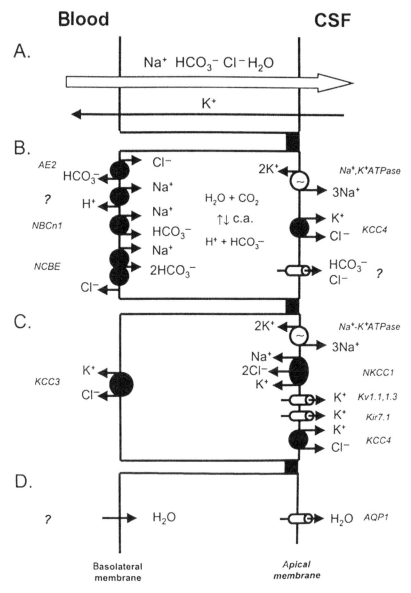

Figure 3 Distribution of ion transporters, co-transporters, and channels in the choroid plexus epithelium (10). (**A**) Major fluxes of ions across the choroid plexus epithelium. (**B**) Ion transporters involved in Na^+, HCO_3^-, and Cl^- secretion by the choroid plexus. *Abbreviation*: c.a., carbonic anhydrase. (**C**) Mechanism of K^+ absorption. (**D**) H_2O transport in the choroid plexus epithelium. Note the intercellular block to fluid and ion flow. *Source*: Taken with permission from Brown et al. Molecular mechanisms of cerebrospinal fluid production, Neuroscience 2004; 129:957–970 © Elsevier 2004.

infiltrating arteries become fragmented and thickened, there is reduced CSF production, CSF turnover takes longer, and there is a reduction in the clearance of toxic substances (33).

CSF PATHWAYS
CSF is produced mainly within the lateral, third, and fourth ventricles. Net bulk flow occurs from the lateral to the third ventricle via the foramen of Monro, on into the fourth ventricle via the aqueduct of Sylvius, and then out of the fourth ventricle via the midline foramen of Magendie, and the lateral foramina of Lushka into the cisterna magna (36; Fig. 4). Once produced, CSF circulation is limited by the cells, membranes, and junctional barriers lining the ventricular and subarachnoid spaces. The dynamics of CSF flow are in part governed by these anatomical configurations, and hence abnormalities within the system can affect the CSF flow.

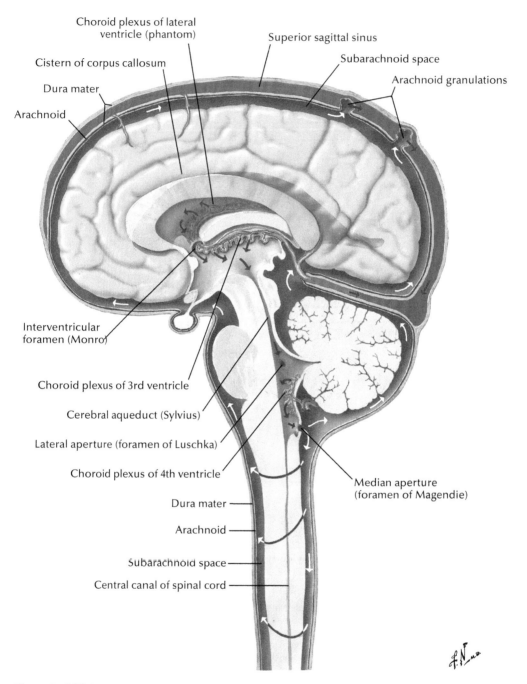

Figure 4 CSF drainage pathways. A schematic section through the brain and spinal cord showing the drainage pathways for CSF. The CSF is formed by the choroid plexuses of the lateral ventricles with a small portion derived from fluid exudate from the cerebral parenchyma. Once formed the CSF passes out via the foramina of Monro into the third ventricle, more fluid being added by the plexus in this ventricle. CSF then flows through the narrow aqueduct of Sylvius into the fourth ventricle, which has a single-sided sheet-like plexus. From there fluid exits into the various basal cisterns and then into the subarachnoid space through paired foramina of Luschka and the single foramen of Magendie. CSF flows through SAS over the surface of the cortex. A portion of the CSF drains back into the blood via the arachnoid granulations into the superior sagittal sinus, some via the spinal nerve roots, and the remainder via the olfactory tracts (not shown). Taken with permission from Netter medical illustrations used with permission of Elsevier. All rights reserved.

Ventricular Surface Structures (Ependyma, Tanycytes and Labyrinths)

The ventricles and central canal are lined by a continuous layer of ependymal cells and occasional tanycytes. The ependyma is a single-layered cuboidal to columnar ciliated epithelium derived from germinal matrix cells (38,39). In the brain, ependymal cells are connected by zonula adherens and have abundant gap junctions (39,40). They may function to regulate water movement and act as a leaky barrier between the CSF and extracellular spaces (39). Cilia are present that may contribute to the direction and quantity of CSF flow. Tanycytes are specialized forms of ependyma found in the ependymal lining or subependyma with radially directed basal processes that extend into the neuropil where they typically enwrap blood vessels (39,41–44). A significant population of tanycytes exists abutting the third ventricle and extend from CSF contact in the floor to the capillary plexus in the median eminence of the hypothalamus (42,44,45). In the third ventricle, tanycytes may regulate neuroendocrine function (42,44,45). The function of tanycytes in the spinal cord is unknown, although neuronal guidance, structural support, neuroendocrine roles, and a limited transport system from the CSF to the ECF have been suggested (39,41,43). Tanycytes have been implanted into a rat spinal cord injury model and supported the regeneration of lesioned axons (46). The functions of ependyma and tanycytes in human spinal cord may be less important than that in the brain, or in other mammals.

Directly under the ependyma and between ependymal cells there are basement membranes that form labyrinths connecting the ependymal basement membrane with perivascular basement membranes of subependymal capillaries and postcapillary veins (46,47). Morphological studies have shown similarities between human, rabbit, and rat anatomy, although human and rabbit basement membranes are stratified (46). These glycolipid and glycoprotein structures not only hold fluid by swelling, but may also function to form a pathway between the ependyma and subependymal vessels (46).

Meningeal Structures (Pia, Arachnoid, Dura, and Blood Vessels)

The meninges are made up of pia, arachnoid, and dura mater. Dura is adherent to the skull and composed of fibroblasts, dense extracellular collagen, elastic fibers, and glycoproteins (14,48,49). Collagen fibers provide strength and are arranged in a variety of directions (48,49). The outer periosteal layer and inner meningeal layer contain nerves and blood vessels and separate to form venous sinuses (48,49). The dural border cell layer abuts the arachnoid and contains elongated flattened fibroblasts, extracellular spaces, few cell junctions, and no extracellular collagen (48,49).

The arachnoid barrier cell layer is an important component of the BBB and is formed of closely packed cells, numerous cell junctions, and an internal basement membrane (14,48,49). Congenital duplication or splitting of this arachnoid layer is thought to lead to the formation of primary congenital arachnoid cysts (50).

Attached to the arachnoid barrier cell layer by desmosomes are fibroblasts and collagen, which form arachnoid trabeculae, bridge the subarachnoid space, and attach and surround traversing blood vessels (14,48,49,51). Blood vessels in the subarachnoid space lie within these trabeculae or have a leptomeningeal cell coat (51). The cerebral subarachnoid space is partitioned into cisterns by arachnoid trabeculae (Fig. 5; 52). The walls of the trabeculae consist of various sized openings, allowing free passage of CSF in the normal situation (53). However, intraoperative observations suggest that some cisternal partitions may be more complete and might retard or even direct the flow of CSF (3,52). An obstruction at the level of the cisterns would explain why some patients with postmeningitic or hemorrhagic hydrocephalus, traditionally thought of as *communicating* hydrocephalus, respond to third ventriculostomy. There are similar features in the spine. Parkinson examined 62 human spinal cords and found that trabeculae are most prevalent posteriorly, forming a spongy mass of interlacing fibrils below C5 throughout the entire posterior subarachnoid space (54). Trabeculae occur rostral to C5 as single strands or isolated septa in the posterior compartment and occasionally occur in the anterior compartment (54). Animal and human studies suggested that these do not form a barrier to CSF flow, but could slow or direct flow, or alter local compliance with potential implications for syrinx formation (3,55,56,57)

The pia is composed of a single continuous layer of flattened fibroblasts attached to the external glial limiting membrane (14,48,51,58). There are few cell junctions (48,51).

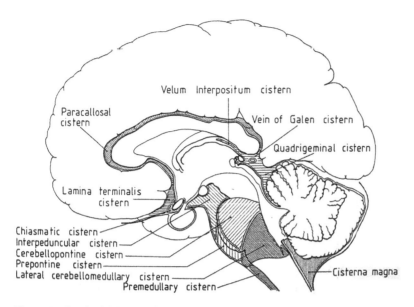

Figure 5 Arachnoid cisterns. Schematic representation of a midsagittal view of the cerebral arachnoid cisterns. Cisterns are formed from loculations within the subarachnoid space. A free and rapid intercommunicating system is not found at surgery, as the arachnoid partitions the subarachnoid space into relatively discrete chambers. Flow studies demonstrate movement of tracers between compartments, but this flow may be slow and controlled. *Source*: Taken with permission from Yasargil MG (1984). Operative Anatomy. Microsurgical anatomy of the basal cisterns and vessels of the brain. New York, Thieme Stratton.

The anatomical and functional relationships of vessels to meninges have implications for cerebral water movement. As vessels enter the brain and the spinal cord parenchyma, they lose their pial coat (Fig. 6) (51,58–61). Some authors argue that a pial coat distinct from the adventitia is discernible around arterioles and becomes fragmented at its deeper aspect (62,63). The space between the blood vessel and the brain or the spinal cord is the perivascular, or Virchow Robin, space and is continuous with subpial and interstitial spaces, providing a pathway for fluid flow from the subarachnoid space into the brain and the spinal cord (58,59,61–63). This has been demonstrated using a number of CSF tracers, including horseradish peroxidase (HRP). Once injected into rat or sheep cerebral ventricles or cisterna magna, HRP demonstrates rapid staining of perivascular spaces that continues along capillaries and in the spinal cord to the central canal (56,57,64 66). The fluid spaces of the subarachnoid space, ventricles, and central canal constitute an anatomical continuity via perivascular and interstitial spaces. Fluid may move by bulk flow (distinguishable from diffusion by its relatively slow flow independent of molecular size) along ISF pathways or along perivascular spaces at a rate estimated in the rat of 0.1 to 0.3 μL/g/min (8,9,67).

CSF Flow in the Ventricles
CSF moves in a pulsatile manner between compartments through movements of the brain and the spinal cord with each cardiac systole and respiratory inhalation and to a lesser extent because of the movement of the ependymal cilia. A number of studies have examined the speed and direction of fluid movement in the ventricles and subarachnoid spaces. Technetium-labeled albumin injected into the lateral ventricle of patients undergoing intrathecal chemotherapy for the treatment of leukemia was present within 60 minutes in the lumbar cistern, although it could take five hours to reach the superior sagittal sinus (68).

MR phase imaging, intraoperative ultrasound, and animal experimental work support a dominant role of cardiac pulsation in relation to CSF flow (65,69–74). Peak CSF velocities occur within the lower fourth ventricle, followed by the aqueduct and the foramen of Monro and implicate the movement of the cerebellum, tonsils, and choroid plexus in the initiation of CSF flow (3,70,71,73–76). Although the actual calculations are not available in the literature (they were presented at a meeting), based on postmortem measurements of the cerebral aqueduct,

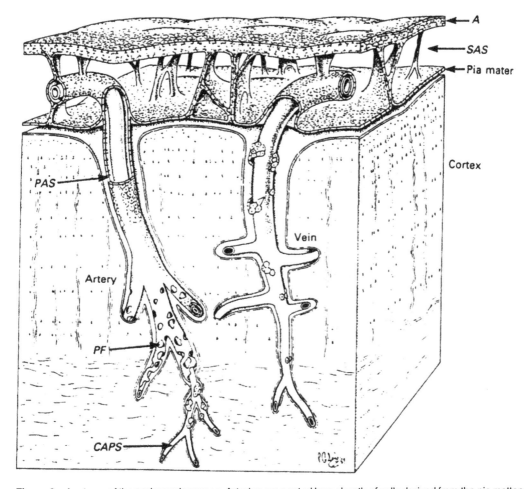

Figure 6 Anatomy of the perivascular space. Arteries are coated by a sheath of cells derived from the pia matter, which becomes perforated (PF) and incomplete as smooth muscle cells are lost from the smaller branches of the artery, eventually disappearing as perivascular spaces are obliterated around capillaries (CAPS). Perivascular spaces of vein are confluent with the subpial space and only small numbers of pial cells are associated with the vessel wall. *Abbreviations*: A, arachnoid matter; SAS, subarachnoid space; PAS, periarterial space. *Source*: Adapted from Ref. 63.

Ball and Dayan suggested that a pulse pressure of 4×10^{-5} mm Hg would be generated by intracranial pulsations forcing fluid down the central canal (77).

CSF flow is also influenced by respiratory function (69–72,78,79). During a cough or Valsalva maneuver, CSF flows cranially then caudally (79). In patients with a Chiari I malformation, Valsalva maneuvers can produce significant increases in intraspinal and intracranial pressures (80). Pressure waves in the subarachnoid space attributable to respiratory function have been demonstrated in humans and dogs (79,81).

CSF Flow in the Cranial Subarachnoid Space
Dye and isotope tracer studies indicate that CSF rapidly moves around the basal cisterns, and then moves more slowly into the subarachnoid space on the cortical convexity and to a lesser extent on the spinal subarachnoid space, until reabsorption occurs at the dural venous sinuses and around neural sheaths (3).

CSF Flow in the Spinal Subarachnoid Space
In humans, it is unlikely that the central canal has a significant role in spinal CSF flow. In two large human autopsy series, central canal stenosis or occlusion was present in 75% to 97% of cases after the third decade of life, and isolated segments occurred between stenotic regions

(82–84). Canal stenosis has been postulated as occurring because of mild ependymal injury or viral infection (39,83).

In the spinal canal, MR imaging indicates that cardiac systole initiates an anterior and caudal spinal cord movement, followed by caudal CSF flow and then a diastolic cranial return (69,71). Spinal cord movement and cord systolic expansion also produce significant local CSF flow, which is more prominent beyond the distal cervical spine (71). In recent canine investigations and human MR studies, lumbar CSF pulse waves consisted of spinal arterial pulsations (40%), venous pulsations in the lumbar canal (40%), and intracranial pulsations (20%) (71,85).

CSF Flow in Perivascular Spaces
Perivascular flow of CSF has been demonstrated in animal experiments, where a CSF tracer moves within 10 minutes from the cisterna magna to the perivascular spaces of spinal arteries and on into the central canal (47,56,57,64,86,87). Further evidence for a perivascular flow is derived from radiolabeled albumin that moves from the cortex or cerebral subarachnoid space into perivascular spaces and crosses the pial membrane (88). This process is delayed by edema and the use of larger particles, such as ink, as tracers (88,89). The speed of CSF tracer movement following injection is too rapid for diffusion and therefore must represent bulk flow (64,87,88).

The driving force for perivascular flow may be the pulsations of the arteries themselves. In sheep, fluid flows from the subarachnoid space along perivascular spaces and into the spinal central canal (65). Stoodley et al. performed partial ligation of the brachiocephalic artery to selectively maintain mean arterial pressures but abolish spinal arterial pulsations and dramatically reduced the speed and the amount of perivascular fluid flow (65,86). Biomedical engineering modeling based on an axisymmetric (single wedge into the center of a cylinder) model of the perivascular space has been created for an open-ended tube containing a vessel (90). Simulated arterial pulsations induce fluid movement in the PVS of approximately 1 μL/s in the direction of arterial wave travel into the spinal cord, even against an adverse pressure gradient of 3.6 kPa (90). Flow was influenced by alterations in local SAS compliance, suggesting a possible mechanism for syrinx formation (56,57,90–92).

CSF Flow in the Interstitial Space
As previously discussed, approximately 10% to 30% of CSF arises from bulk flow of ISF (6,8,25,26). A continuous perivascular flow into the parenchyma mandates an outflow mechanism. It is difficult to examine this experimentally. The perivenular space or periaxonal spaces may act as this conduit (9,93).

CSF REABSORPTION
Reabsorption into the systemic circulation occurs via the venous system at the arachnoid granulations in the superior sagittal sinus, the lymphatics across the cribriform plate, and the nerve root subarachnoid angles (3).

Arachnoid Granulations
Arachnoid granulations were classically thought to be the main site of CSF reabsorption. Originally described by Pacchioni in 1721, it wasn't until 1875 when Key and Retzius demonstrated a role in CSF drainage (3). An arachnoid *villus* is an invagination of the arachnoid into a venous area (Fig. 7) (3,36). They are present in the cranial venous sinuses and have also been described at arachnoid angles in spinal nerve roots. A massive dilatation of the subarachnoid space within a villus produces an arachnoid, or Pacchionian, granulation or body. Arachnoid *granulations* are usually found in humans over the age of 18 months, while arachnoid *villi* have been found in younger infants and other animals (3,94). A recent study of 100 patients used 3D MRI techniques and demonstrated 433 arachnoid granulations in 92 patients situated in the superior sagittal (54%), transverse (28%), and straight sinuses (18%) (95). Mean granulation diameters were 1.5, 4.1, and 3.8 mm for superior sagittal, transverse, and straight sinuses, respectively (95).

In an arachnoid villus, cords of arachnoid membrane penetrate the dura, often surrounding a draining vein (3,36,95). Once through the dural wall the cords become solid tissue capped by a mesothelial cover of arachnoid cells (3,36). These arachnoid cells may also form part of the villous body (3,36). The cranial subarachnoid space is continuous with the area under the outer arachnoid membrane, allowing a site for drainage (3,36).

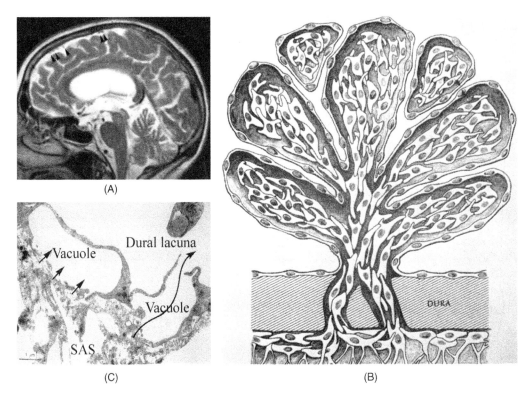

Figure 7 (**A**) T2 weighted magnetic resonance image demonstrating arachnoid granulations in the superior sagittal sinus (arrows) (T Smith, The Walton Centre, Liverpool). (**B**) Diagram illustrating structure of the arachnoid granulation based on studies of the sheep and dog. The granulation projects up into the sagittal sinus. Below the dura are the arachnoid cells with extensions passing across the subarachnoid space. Arachnoid cells are shown extending through two defects in the dura to become the stroma of the granulation. The two extensions of the arachnoid cells through the dura form the double neck of this granulation. On the upper surface of the dura is a layer of endothelial cells lining the sagittal sinus. These cells extend over the surface of the granulation and into the surface fissures and endothelium-lined tubules. Between the endothelial cells of the granulation and the stromal cells is the subendothelial space. The spaces between the arachnoid cells in the core of the granulation are termed stomal spaces which are in continuity with the subarachnoid space. *Source*: Taken with permission from Pots DG et al. Morphology of the arachnoid villi and granulations. Radiology 1972; 105:333–341. (**C**) Electron micrograph of the mesothethial cells lining an arachnoid villus showing electron-optically empty giant vacuoles. At this level of section, the vacuole on the right has both basal and apical openings. Beneath the mesothelial lining lies a labyrinth of open spaces, the subarachnoid space (SAS) filled in life with CSF, intervened by cellular and fibrous components. *Source*: Taken with permission from Tripathi BJ, Tripathi RC. Vacuolar transcellular channels as a drainage pathway for cerebrospinal fluid. J Physiol 1974; 239:195–206. © Blackwell publishing 1974.

CSF flow into the sinuses appears to be passive along a pressure gradient. Electron microscopy shows that cells form giant vacuoles that may communicate with both the subarachnoid and luminal parts of the cell simultaneously (97). The greater the pressure differential, the greater the number of vacuoles that forms, supporting an energy independent transcellular route for fluid transport (3). There does not appear to be much morphological evidence for a mechanical one-way flap valve mechanism controlling CSF flow into the venous sinuses.

Lymphatic Drainage
Lymphatics are not found within the central nervous system, although experimental observations suggest a route to extracranial lymphatics exists. Ink tracers, labeled albumin, or Microfil injected into the brain of experimental animals and human cadavers is found in the perivascular spaces, around cranial nerves, and eventually in the cervical and spinal lymph nodes, reaching a peak after 4 to 15 hours (3,98–104). In animals, obstruction of the lymphatic pathways from the head leads to raised intracranial pressure and cerebral edema (3,100,105,106). Furthermore, once

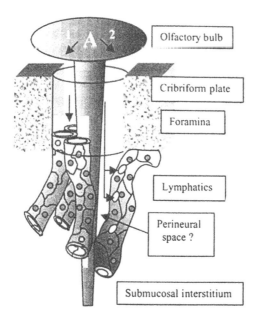

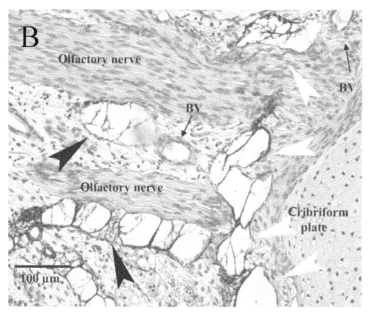

Figure 8 Potential anatomical connections between the olfactory nerve and extracranial lymphatic vessels. In schematic (**A**) the lymphatics are connected directly with the CSF space. In A1, the lymphatic vessels form a collar around the emerging olfactory nerve root with the lymphatic endothelium fusing to the perineural sheath of the nerve and the periosteum or dura associated with the cribriform plate. In effect this lymphatic collar provides a "seal" that ensures that little or no CSF enters the submucosal interstitium. In A2, the lymphatics join with the cribriform plate and nerve as above, but in this scenario, a collar of CSF follows the nerve some distance into the submucosa. This CSF collar is delimited by the lymphatic vessel. As in the scenario outlined in A1, no CSF is permitted to enter the interstitium. (**B**) Uptake of Microfil by lymphatic vessels adjacent to cribriform plate. This histological section was stained with hematoxylin and eosin. In this example, yellow Microfil was infused into the CSF space (appears dark brown in section) and blue Microfil was injected into the arterial circulation. Distended lymphatic vessels containing Microfil are especially prominent in the area surrounding the olfactory nerve roots as they emerge from the cribriform plate (*white arrowheads*). Lymphatics are also observed fused to the olfactory nerves at discrete locations away from the cribriform plate (black arrowheads). Microfil is not observed free within the interstitium of the submucosa. Regarding the relationship between cranial CSF and lymph, examples such as this would appear to support the schema illustrated in A. *Abbreviation*: BV, blood vessels. *Source*: Adapted from Ref. 103.

lymphatic pathways were obstructed, much higher CSF pressures were required to maintain a given CSF absorption rate (107). In humans, extracranial metastases from high-grade cerebral glioma are rare (about 2%) and preferentially metastasize to cervical lymph nodes and lung (108,109,110).

The cribriform plate appears to be the central region for extra-arachnoidal cranial CSF clearance (19). Animal studies in rats and sheep indicate that 50% of CSF exits the skull in this location (111,112,113). Anatomical and tracer studies suggest that there may be a direct communication between the perineural space of the olfactory neurons and lymphatics in the nasal submucosa (Fig. 8; 103).

Some authors suggest that no evidence exists for a direct communication between the subarachnoid space and extraspinal lymphatics, yet others describe anatomical evidence for spinal arachnoid villi and granulations (103,114). The existence of a spinal absorptive route is supported as studies in sheep show that approximately 25% of total CSF clearance occurs in the spine (115). Furthermore, radionucleotide testing of healthy human volunteers showed that 0.11 to 0.23 mL/min (40%–70%) could be absorbed in the spinal canal and the higher values occurred with exercise (4). Possible anatomical routes for spinal CSF reabsorption include flow out as the nerve root sheaths merge with the perineurium at the arachnoid angle, spinal arachnoid granulations, or direct movement across the dura into the epidural space to be absorbed by blind-ending spinal lymphatic vessels (103,114,115).

CONCLUSIONS

The treatment of patients with CSF pathway disorders requires an understanding of CSF pathways and the cerebral water system. Advances in MRI, new experimental approaches, and further technical developments may improve our understanding of water circulation and why disorders occur. Clinicians, scientists, and biomedical engineers need to continue to work together to comprehend the system and optimize patient care.

REFERENCES

1. Ganong WF. Review of medical physiology. London, U.K.: Prentice Hall International Inc, 1995.
2. Toni R, Roti E, et al. Endocrinology and art. Saint Onofrio. J Endocrinol Invest 2003; 26(12):1248.
3. Davson H, Segal MB. Physiology of the CSF and Blood Brain Barriers. Boca Raton, FL: CRC Press, 1996.
4. Edsbagge M, Tisell M, et al. Spinal CSF absorption in healthy individuals. Am J Physiol Regul Integr Comp Physiol 2004; 287(6):R1450–R1455.
5. Gjerris F, Borgesen SE. Pathophysiology of cerebrospinal fluid circulation. In: Crockard HA, Hayward R, Hoff JT, eds. Neurosurgery: The Scientific Basis of Clinical Practice. Oxford, U.K.: Blackwell Science Ltd., 2000:1.
6. Kimelberg HK. Water homeostasis in the brain: basic concepts. Neuroscience 2004; 129(4):851–860.
7. Kohn MI, Tanna NK, et al. Analysis of brain and cerebrospinal fluid volumes with MR imaging. Part I. Methods, reliability, and validation. Radiology 1991; 178(1):115–122.
8. Redzic ZB, Segal MB. The structure of the choroid plexus and the physiology of the choroid plexus epithelium. Adv Drug Deliv Rev 2004; 56(12):1695–1716.
9. Abbott NJ. Evidence for bulk flow of brain interstitial fluid: significance for physiology and pathology. Neurochem Int 2004; 45(4):545–552.
10. Brown PD, Davies SL, et al. Molecular mechanisms of cerebrospinal fluid production. Neuroscience 2004; 129(4):957–970.
11. Jones HC. Cerebrospinal fluid research: a new platform for dissemination of research, opinions and reviews with a common theme. Cerebrospinal Fluid Res 2004; 1(1):1.
12. Miaki K, Matsui H, et al. Nutritional supply to the cauda equina in lumbar adhesive arachnoiditis in rats. Eur Spine J 1999; 8(4): 310–316.
13. Rosenberg GA. Brain Fluids and Metabolism. Oxford, U.K.: Oxford University Press, 1990.
14. Kiernan JA. Barr's the human nervous system, an anatomical viewpoint. Philadelphia, PA: Lippincott-Raven, 1998.
15. Xenos C, Sgouros S, Natarajan K. Ventricular volume change in childhood. J Neurosurg 2002; 97: 584–590.
16. Papadea C, Schlosser RJ. Rapid method for beta2-transferrin in cerebrospinal fluid leakage using an automated immunofixation electrophoresis system. Clin Chem 2005; 51(2):464–470.

17. Sloman AJ, Kelly RH. Transferrin allelic variants may cause false positives in the detection of cerebrospinal fluid fistulae. Clin Chem 1993; 39(7):1444–1445.
18. Freeman LW, Wright TW. Experimental observations of concussion and contusion of the spinal cord. Ann Surg 1953; 137(4):433–443.
19. Kjeldsberg CR, Knight JA. Cerebrospinal fluid. Body fluids: Laboratory examination of amniotic, cerebrospinal, seminal, serous and synovial fluids: A textbook atlas. Chicago, IL: American Society of Clinical Pathologists, 1986:59.
20. Kratz A, Lewandrowski KB. Case records of the Massachusetts General Hospital. Weekly clinico-pathological exercises. Normal reference laboratory values. N Engl J Med 1998; 339(15):1063–1072.
21. Laha RK, Malik HG, et al. Post-traumatic syringomyelia. Surg Neurol 1975; 4(6):519–522.
22. Nurick S, Russell JA, et al. Cystic degeneration of the spinal cord following spinal cord injury. Brain 1970; 93(1):211–222.
23. Rossier AB, Foo D, et al. Posttraumatic cervical syringomyelia. Incidence, clinical presentation, electrophysiological studies, syrinx protein and results of conservative and operative treatment. Brain 1985; 108(Pt 2):439–461.
24. Sambrook MA. The concentration of cerebrospinal fluid potassium during systemic disturbances of acid–base metabolism. J Clin Pathol 1975; 28(5):418–420.
25. Segal MB. Transport of nutrients across the choroid plexus. Microsc Res Tech 2001; 52(1):38–48.
26. Smith DE, Johanson CE, et al. Peptide and peptide analog transport systems at the blood–CSF barrier. Adv Drug Deliv Rev 2004; 56(12):1765–1791.
27. Cutler RW, Page L, et al. Formation and absorption of cerebrospinal fluid in man. Brain 1968; 91(4): 707–720.
28. Milhorat TH, Hammock MK, et al. Cerebrospinal fluid production by the choroid plexus and brain. Science 1971; 173(994):330–332.
29. Shapiro K, Marmarou A, et al. Characterization of clinical CSF dynamics and neural axis compliance using the pressure–volume index: I. The normal pressure–volume index. Ann Neurol 1980; 7(6): 508–514.
30. Dziegielewska KM, Ek J, et al. Development of the choroid plexus. Microsc Res Tech 2001; 52(1): 5–20.
31. Kusuhara H, Sugiyama Y. Efflux transport systems for organic anions and cations at the blood–CSF barrier. Adv Drug Deliv Rev 2004; 56(12):1741–1763.
32. Vorbrodt AW, Dobrogowska DH. Molecular anatomy of interendothelial junctions in human blood–brain barrier microvessels. Folia Histochem Cytobiol 2004; 42(2):67–75.
33. Emerich DF, Skinner SJ, et al. The choroid plexus in the rise, fall and repair of the brain. Bioessays 2005; 27(3):262–274.
34. Speake T, Whitwell C, et al. Mechanisms of CSF secretion by the choroid plexus. Microsc Res Tech 2001; 52(1):49–59.
35. Gunnarson E, Zelenina M, et al. Regulation of brain aquaporins. Neuroscience 2004; 129(4):947–955.
36. Williams PL, Warwick R, Dyson M, et al., eds. Gray's Anatomy 37th Edition. London, U.K.: Churchill Livingstone, 1989.
37. Netter FH. The nervous system. In: Netter FH, eds. The Ciba Collection of Medical Illustrations. New Jersey, NJ: Ciba Pharmaceutical Products, 1953:1–44.
38. Bruni JE, Reddy K. Ependyma of the central canal of the rat spinal cord: a light and transmission electron microscopic study. J Anat 1987; 152:55–70.
39. Del Bigio MR. The ependyma: a protective barrier between brain and cerebrospinal fluid. Glia 1995; 14(1):1–13.
40. Brightman MW, Reese TS. Junctions between intimately apposed cell membranes in the vertebrate brain. J Cell Biol 1969; 40(3):648–677.
41. Bruni JE. Ependymal development, proliferation, and functions: a review. Microsc Res Tech 1998; 41(1):2–13.
42. Garcia MA, Carrasco M, et al. Elevated expression of glucose transporter-1 in hypothalamic ependymal cells not involved in the formation of the brain–cerebrospinal fluid barrier. J Cell Biochem 2001; 80(4):491–503.
43. Honda T, Yokota S, et al. Evidence for the c-ret protooncogene product (c-Ret) expression in the spinal tanycytes of adult rat. J Chem Neuroanat 1999; 17(3):163–168.
44. Wittkowski W. Tanycytes and pituicytes: morphological and functional aspects of neuroglial interaction. Microsc Res Tech 1998; 41(1):29–42.
45. Peruzzo B, Pastor FE, et al. A second look at the barriers of the medial basal hypothalamus. Exp Brain Res 2000; 132(1):10–26.
46. Leonhardt H, Desaga U. Recent observations on ependyma and subependymal basement membranes. Acta Neurochir (Wien) 1975; 31(3–4):153–159.

47. Cifuentes M, Fernandez-LLebrez P, et al. Distribution of intraventricularly injected horseradish perox-idase in cerebrospinal fluid compartments of the rat spinal cord. Cell Tissue Res 1992; 270(3):485–494.
48. Haines DE, Harkey HL, et al. The "subdural" space: a new look at an outdated concept. Neurosurgery 1993; 32(1):111–120.
49. Vandenabeele F, Creemers J, et al. Ultrastructure of the human spinal arachnoid mater and dura mater. J Anat 1996; 189(Pt 2):417–430.
50. Schachenmayr W, Friede RL. Fine structure of arachnoid cysts. J Neuropathol Exp Neurol 1978; 38:434–446.
51. Alcolado R, Weller RO, et al. The cranial arachnoid and pia mater in man: anatomical and ultrastruc-tural observations. Neuropathol Appl Neurobiol 1988; 14(1):1–17.
52. Yasargil MG. Operative Anatomy. In: Yasargil MG ed. Microsurgical Anatomy of the Basal Cis-terns and Vessels of the Brain, Diagnostic Studies, General Operative Techniques and Pathological Considerations of the Intracranial Aneurysms. New York: Thieme Stratton, 1984:1.
53. Key A, Retzius G. Studien in der anatomie des nervensystems und des Bindegewebes. Stockholm: Norstad, 1875.
54. Parkinson D. Human spinal arachnoid septa, trabeculae, and "rogue strands." Am J Anat 1991; 192(4):498–509.
55. Bilston LE, Fletcher DF, et al. Focal spinal arachnoiditis increases subarachnoid space pressure: A computational study. Clin Biomech (Bristol, Avon) 2006; 21(6):579–584.
56. Brodbelt AR, Stoodley MA, et al. Altered subarachnoid space compliance and fluid flow in a model of post-traumatic syringomyelia. Spine 2003; 28(20):E413–E419.
57. Brodbelt AR, Stoodley MA, et al. Fluid flow in an animal model of post-traumatic syringomyelia. Eur Spine J 2003; 12:300–306.
58. Hutchings M, Weller RO. Anatomical relationships of the pia mater to cerebral blood vessels in man. J Neurosurg 1986; 65(3):316–325.
59. Esiri MM, Gay D. Immunological and neuropathological significance of the Virchow-Robin space. J Neurol Sci 1990; 100(1–2):3–8.
60. Krahn V. The pia mater at the site of the entry of blood vessels into the central nervous system. Anat Embryol 1982; 164(2):257–263.
61. Nicholas DS, Weller RO. The fine anatomy of the human spinal meninges. A light and scanning electron microscopy study. J Neurosurg 1988; 69(2):276–282.
62. Adachi M, Hosoya T, et al. Dilated Virchow-Robin spaces: MRI pathological study. Neuroradiology 1998; 40(1):27–31.
63. Zhang ET, Inman CB, et al. Interrelationships of the pia mater and the perivascular (Virchow-Robin) spaces in the human cerebrum. J Anat 1990; 170:111–123.
64. Rennels ML, Blaumanis OR, et al. Rapid solute transport throughout the brain via paravascular fluid pathways. Adv Neurol 1990; 52:431–439.
65. Stoodley MA, Brown SA, et al. Arterial pulsation-dependent perivascular cerebrospinal fluid flow into the central canal in the sheep spinal cord. J Neurosurg 1997; 86(4):686–693.
66. Wagner HJ, Pilgrim C, et al. Penetration and removal of horseradish peroxidase injected into the cere-brospinal fluid: role of cerebral perivascular spaces, endothelium and microglia. Acta Neuropathol (Berl) 1974; 27(4):299–315.
67. Cserr HF, Cooper DN, et al. Efflux of radiolabeled polyethylene glycols and albumin from rat brain. Am J Physiol 1981; 240(4):F319–F328.
68. Chiro GD, Hammock MK, et al. Spinal descent of cerebrospinal fluid in man. Neurology 1976; 26(1):1–8.
69. Greitz D, Greitz T, et al. A new view on the CSF-circulation with the potential for pharmacological treatment of childhood hydrocephalus. Acta Paediatr 1997; 86(2):125–132.
70. Heiss JD, Patronas N, et al. Elucidating the pathophysiology of syringomyelia. J Neurosurg 1999; 91(4):553–562.
71. Henry-Feugeas MC, Idy-Peretti I, et al. Origin of subarachnoid cerebrospinal fluid pulsations: a phase-contrast MR analysis. Magn Reson Imaging 2000; 18(4):387–395.
72. Levy LM. MR imaging of cerebrospinal fluid flow and spinal cord motion in neurologic disorders of the spine. Magn Reson Imaging Clin N Am 1999; 7(3): 573–587.
73. Nitz WR, Bradley WG Jr., et al. Flow dynamics of cerebrospinal fluid: assessment with phase-contrast velocity MR imaging performed with retrospective cardiac gating. Radiology 1992; 183(2): 395–405.
74. Oldfield EH, Muraszko K, et al. Pathophysiology of syringomyelia associated with Chiari I malforma-tion of the cerebellar tonsils. Implications for diagnosis and treatment. J Neurosurg 1994; 80(1):3–15.
75. Bering EA. Circulation of the cerebrospinal fluid: demonstration of the choroid plexus as the generator of the force for flow of fluid and ventricular enlagement. J Neurosurg 1962; 19:405–413.

76. Gardner WJ, Angel J. The cause of Syringomyelia and its surgical treatment. Cleve Clin Q 1958; 25:4–8.
77. Ball MJ, Dayan AD. Pathogenesis of Syringomyelia. Lancet 1972, 2.799–801.
78. Carpenter PW, Berkouk K, et al. A theoretical model of pressure propagation in the human spinal CSF system. Eng Mech 1999; 6(4/5):213–228.
79. Williams B. On the pathogenesis of syringomyelia: a review. J R Soc Med 1980; 73(11):798–806.
80. Hackel M, Benes V, et al. Simultaneous cerebral and spinal fluid pressure recordings in surgical indications of the Chiari malformation without myelodysplasia. Acta Neurochir (Wien) 2001; 143(9): 909–917.
81. Hall P, Turner M, et al. Experimental syringomyelia: The relationship between intraventricular and intrasyrinx pressures. J Neurosurg 1980; 52(6):812–817.
82. Aboulker J. La syringomyelie et les liquides intra-rachidiens. Neurochirurgie 1979; 25(suppl. 1):1–44.
83. Milhorat TH, Kotzen RM, et al. Stenosis of central canal of spinal cord in man: incidence and pathological findings in 232 autopsy cases. J Neurosurg 1994; 80(4):716–722.
84. Yasui, K, Hashizume Y, et al. Age-related morphologic changes of the central canal of the human spinal cord. Acta Neuropathol 1999; 97:253–259.
85. Urayama K. Origin of lumbar cerebrospinal fluid pulse wave. Spine 1994; 19(4):441–445.
86. Rennels ML, Gregory TF, et al. Evidence for a "paravascular" fluid circulation in the mammalian central nervous system, provided by the rapid distribution of tracer protein throughout the brain from the subarachnoid space. Brain Res 1985; 326(1):47–63.
87. Stoodley MA, Jones NR, et al. Evidence for rapid fluid flow from the subarachnoid space into the spinal cord central canal in the rat. Brain Res 1996; 707(2):155–164.
88. Ichimura T, Fraser PA, et al. Distribution of extracellular tracers in perivascular spaces of the rat brain. Brain Res 1991; 545(1–2):103–113.
89. Blaumanis OR, Rennels ML, et al. Focal cerebral edema impedes convective fluid/tracer movement through paravascular pathways in cat brain. Adv Neurol 1990; 52:385–389.
90. Bilston LE, Fletcher DF, et al. Arterial pulsation-driven cerebrospinal fluid flow in the perivascular space: a computational model. Comput Methods Biomech Biomed Engin 2003; 6(4):235–241.
91. Brodbelt AR, Stoodley MA, et al. Nontraumatic syringomyelia. The Cervical Spine. The Cervical Spine Research Society Editorial Committee. Philadelphia, PA: Lippincott-Raven Publishers, 2005.
92. Stoodley MA, Jones NR, et al. Mechanisms underlying the formation and enlargement of noncommunicating syringomyelia: experimental studies. Neurosurg Focus 2000; 8(3: Article 2):1–7.
93. Brodbelt AR. Investigations in Post Traumatic Syringomyelia. Sydney, Australia: Prince of Wales Medical Research Institute, University of New South Wales, 2004:224.
94. Weed LH. The pathways of escape from the subarachnoid spaces with particular reference to the arachnoid villi. J Med Res 1914; 31:51–91.
95. Liang L, Korogi Y, et al. Normal structures in the intracranial dural sinuses: delineation with 3D contrast-enhanced magnetization prepared rapid acquisition gradient-echo imaging sequence. AJNR Am J Neuroradiol 2002; 23(10):1739–1746.
96. Potts DG, Deonarine V, et al. Perfusion studies of the cerebrospinal fluid absorptive pathways of the dog. Radiology 1972; 104:321–325.
97. Tripathi BJ, Tripathi RC. Vacuolar transcellular channels as a drainage pathway for cerebrospinal fluid. J Physiol 1974; 239(1):195–206.
98. Cserr HF, Knopf PM. Cervical lymphatics, the blood–brain barrier and the immunoreactivity of the brain: a new view. Immunol Today 1992; 13(12):507–512.
99. Foldi M. The brain and the lymphatic system revisited. Lymphology 1999; 32(2):40–44.
100. Johnston M, Papaiconomou C. Cerebrospinal fluid transport: a lymphatic perspective. News Physiol Sci 2002; 17:227–230.
101. Johnston M, Zakharov A, et al. Evidence of connections between cerebrospinal fluid and nasal lymphatic vessels in humans, non-human primates and other mammalian species. Cerebrospinal Fluid Res 2004; 1(1):2.
102. Kida S, Weller RO, et al. Anatomical pathways for lymphatic drainage of the brain and their pathological significance. Neuropathol Appl Neurobiol 1995; 21(3):181–184.
103. Koh L, Zakharov A, et al. Integration of the subarachnoid space and lymphatics: Is it time to embrace a new concept of cerebrospinal fluid absorption? Cerebrospinal Fluid Res 2005; 2(6).
104. Weller RO. Pathology of cerebrospinal fluid and interstitial fluid of the CNS: significance for Alzheimer disease, prion disorders and multiple sclerosis. J Neuropathol Exp Neurol 1998; 57(10): 885–894.
105. Foldi M, Csillik B, et al. Lymphatic drainage of the brain. Experientia 1968; 24(12):1283–1287.
106. Mollanji R, Bozanovic-Sosic R, et al. Blocking cerebrospinal fluid absorption through the cribriform plate increases resting intracranial pressure. Am J Physiol Regul Integr Comp Physiol 2002; 282(6):R1593–R1599.

107. Mollanji R, Bozanovic-Sosic R, et al. Intracranial pressure accommodation is impaired by blocking pathways leading to extracranial lymphatics. Am J Physiol Regul Integr Comp Physiol 2001; 280(5):R1573–R1581.
108. Gonzalez Campora R, Otal Salaverri C, et al. Metastatic glioblastoma multiforme in cervical lymph nodes. Report of a case with diagnosis by fine needle aspiration. Acta Cytol 1993; 37(6):938–942.
109. Hoffman HJ, Duffner PK. Extraneural metastases of central nervous system tumors. Cancer 1985; 56(suppl. 7):1778–1782.
110. Smith DR, Hardman JM, et al. Metastasizing neuroectodermal tumors of the central nervous system. J Neurosurg 1969; 31(1):50–58.
111. Boulton M, Flessner M, et al. Lymphatic drainage of the CNS: effects of lymphatic diversion/ligation on CSF protein transport to plasma. Am J Physiol 1997; 272(5 Pt 2):R1613–R1619.
112. Boulton M, Flessner M, et al. Determination of volumetric cerebrospinal fluid absorption into extracranial lymphatics in sheep. Am J Physiol 1998; 274(1 Pt 2):R88–R96.
113. Boulton M, Flessner M, et al. Contribution of extracranial lymphatics and arachnoid villi to the clearance of a CSF tracer in the rat. Am J Physiol 1999; 276(3 Pt 2):R818–R823.
114. Kido DK, Gomez DG, et al. Human spinal arachnoid villi and granulations. Neuroradiology 1976; 11(5):221–228.
115. Bozanovic-Sosic R, Mollanji R, et al. Spinal and cranial contributions to total cerebrospinal fluid transport. Am J Physiol Regul Integr Comp Physiol 2001; 281(3):R909–R916.

Embryology of CNS with Emphasis on CSF Circulation

Sergio Cavalheiro, Jardel Mendonça Nicácio, and Igor Vilela Faquini
Department of Pediatric Neurosurgery, Federal University of São Paulo, São Paulo, Brazil

GASTRULATION

Based on internal and external morphological studies that originated from Carnegie's embryos collection, the first eight weeks of evolution were divided in 23 morphological stages (Carnegie's stages). Stages 8 to 23 are relevant to the development of the central nervous system (CNS) and are marked by events like the formation of the primitive streak around the 23rd day.

After fertilization, the zygote's cleavage starts to generate cells called blastomeres. In the third day, this spherical ball of cells becomes the morula and soon appears a cavity, the blastocyst, which is the embryoblast (primordial embryo). The embryo growth begins within the embryonary disc around the third week and is divided in three main events: the appearance of primitive streak, development of notochordal plate, and differentiation of all three germinal layers. We name this period gastrulation, which is the most important of embryogenesis and is considered the birth of the CNS (1). Gastrulation's first sign consists of the formation of the primitive streak. As the primitive streak expands in caudal direction, the cranial pole proliferates and gives origin to Hense's node, which acts as an embryonic organizer. Mesenchymal cells from primitive node and primitive groove organize to form the notochordal process and notochordal canal, which folds and becomes the notochord. The notochord defines the primitive axis and induces intervertebral discs formation. In addition, it induces the neural plate growth, which will later differentiate into the neural tube.

NEURULATION

Neurulation is the neural tube formation phase that begins in stage 10 of development (22nd–23rd days). Failure during neurulation can result in serious CNS malformations. In advanced vertebrates, neurulation is divided in two phases: primary and secondary neurulation. Primary neurulation is responsible for the formation of the anterior part of the neural tube, while secondary neurulation for the posterior part.

Primary neurulation can be divided into four steps:

- Induction of neural plate by the notochord
- Thickening and modeling of neural plate
- Inclination and curvature of neural plate
- Closure of neural plate forming the neural tube

Fusion of neural folds to form the neural tube advances in the cranial and caudal direction remaining just an opening in both extremities called rostral and caudal neuropores. The rostral neuropore closes around the 25th day and the caudal neuropore two days after. In mammals, the neural tube closure starts at diverse points through the anterior–posterior axis, in a wave pattern and in both directions.

After the closure of the caudal neuropore, secondary neurulation begins exactly when from the coalescence of caudal mesenchymal cells, the neural tube amounts and forms a compact structure that posteriorly converts in a tubular framework. After the complete closure of the neural tube, just a small cavity named neurocele remains. This neurocele freely communicates with amniotic cavity rostrally and caudally.

OCCLUSION OF SPINAL NEUROCELE

Immediately after the closure of neural tube and anterior neuropore, the spinal neurocele temporarily closes and blocks the communication between central neurocele and amniotic cavity. This occlusion occurs in the cranial–caudal direction from the first to the ninth pair of somites involving almost 60% of the neuraxis. It results in a compartmentalization of the neural tube superior pole, forming a primitive ventricular cavity. The pressure inside this cavity becomes higher when compared to the amniotic one, which results in a faster embryonic brain growth. Some studies in birds' embryos demonstrated that introducing a cannula into this primitive ventricular cavity and inducing a reduction of intraluminal pressure can inhibit the ventricular and cerebral development (2).

The ventricular cavity expansion is linear unlike the exponential pattern documented in the brain parenchyma. Jelínek and Pexieder (3) working with animal embryos demonstrated that after removing a considerable quantity of CSF, the ventricular pressure returned to normal values after 2 to 2.5 hours. This rise in intraventricular pressure suggests that there is an activator system to CSF secretion.

MENINGEAL FORMATION AND DEVELOPMENT

The meninges are very important structures because they constitute a fibrous envelope protecting the CNS, acting in the blood–brain barrier and participating in the physiology of CSF circulation. They also have a trophic activity during fetal life. O'Rahilly and Muller (4) studied human meningeal embryogenesis. Early in embryonic evolution, the neural tube is surrounded by a mesenchymal cell layer and neural crest cells that evolve to a primitive meningeal layer at around the eighth week, according to Lemire et al. (5). This will form two distinct layers (pachymeningeal and leptomeningeal). The first one is the arachnoid (12th week) and the last one the dura mater (20th week).

Though several in vitro studies have demonstrated meningeal trophic activity, this has not been completely observed in vivo. In the medical literature, the study of such activity is performed in three different brain components: cerebellum, cerebral cortex, and hippocampus. In all of these experimental studies, the meningeal destruction resulted in nervous system hypoplasia, subarachnoid space neuronal heterotopy, and gyral malformations (6,7). These data allow us to confirm that meningeal cells act in CNS morphogenesis, although this is not clearly demonstrated in mammal embryos (8).

CHOROIDAL PLEXUS—FORMATION AND DIFFERENTIATION

The choroidal plexus is a structure that extends from the ependymal surface into the ventricular cavity. In the majority of reptiles, birds, and mammals, the choroidal plexus is founded in all ventricular cavities. The lateral ventricle choroidal plexus in advanced mammals is a floating formation immersed in CSF, while in the fourth ventricle it looks like a bunch of vessels (9).

It is accepted that the first evidence of this process in rats is detected around the 13th day of embryonic life regarding the lateral and fourth ventricles and around the 14th day in the third ventricle. Moreover, in humans this occurs in the seventh week in the lateral ventricles, eighth week for third ventricle, and eighth week for the fourth ventricle (10,11).

With 11 weeks of pregnancy, the choroidal plexus runs freely in the fourth ventricle. By this period, the foramens of Luschka and Magendie communicate this ventricle with the subarachnoid space. Microscopically, the choroidal plexus surface area is increased by villi composed of cuboidal epithelial cells (12).

The choroidal plexus epithelium comes from the ventricular ependymal layer and also from tela choroidea blood vessels. With active pia mater proliferation, the choroidal tela invaginates in the fourth ventricle to form the choroidal plexus. The differentiation of ependymal mesenchymal cells into choroidal epithelium happens early in embryonic life (around 41st day) and progresses until total formation around the 29th week. This event is not synchronous for all ventricles. It starts at the fourth ventricle, then lateral ventricles, and lastly at the third ventricle. Shuangshoti and Netsky (13) described the telencephalic choroidal plexus differentiation in four stages. Many functions are attributed to choroidal plexus. Besides CSF production, it regulates the access of chemical substances from the blood to CSF and the synthesis and secretion of biologically active components like growth factors and hormones (14).

ONTOGENESIS OF CSF DYNAMICS

The CSF flow development begins with the CNS neuronal maturation process. First, there is the formation of the choroidal plexus inside the primitive ventricular cavity. As previously discussed, the first evidence of choroidal differentiation is described between the 41st and the 44th days inside the fourth ventricle, in the 41st day for the lateral ventricles, and in the 57th day in the third ventricle.

When the choroidal plexus is formed around the 7th week, the ventricular cavity in embryos and fetuses is relatively big with a thin cortical layer until the growth of hemisphere's white and gray matter around the 14th week with sulci and gyri development by the 38th week. In early phases, the fourth ventricle outflow tract is obstructed by a thin membrane, but the flow is present through intercells pores. These pores become larger over time until the disappearance of the membrane and opening of the fourth ventricle (15).

The embryology of the roof of the hindbrain has been the subject of many observations and much debate. Most of the early 20th century studies on mammal embryos failed to find a metapore (foramen of Magendie) other than in anthropoids (16), and only detected lateral foramina in the later stages of development. These findings were confirmed in more recent studies (17,18). Initial observations on human fetal material suggested that the metapore appeared in the fifth month.

Further observations confirmed attenuation of the roof of the developing hindbrain in seven-week embryos in areas just rostral and caudal to the choroid plexus fold (19,20). The appearance was of deficiencies surrounded by cells staining positively with Periodic Acid Schiff (PAS) reagent. The rostral area (sometimes termed area membranacea superior) became a thick intact structure again by the eighth week, but the metapore was clearly apparent in the caudal area (area membranacea inferior) from this stage onwards.

The lateral foramina are not present until much later in human fetal development. Weed (21) stated that the roof of hindbrain opens in the eighth week immediately after the choroidal differentiation. Osaka et al. (15) pointed out that the subarachnoid space formation occurred before the fourth week in humans and was not contiguous with the fourth ventricle's opening. Therefore, they suggest that the formation of the CSF flow is not the main force that expands and creates the subarachnoid space as stated in the concept of "via major" of CSF dynamics described for adult humans. The concept of a "via major" for CSF flow is based on the classical description of the flow between ventricular cavities, cisterns, and subarachnoid space with reabsorption through granulations and villi as commented previously. The so-called "via minor" although reported as an alternative route in adults has an important role during fetal life. It is composed of the ventricular ependymal layer, perivascular spaces, and lymphatic channels with reabsorption through pia-arachnoid capillaries, leptomeninges, and choroidal plexus (22). This probably explains higher rates of failure in the treatment of obstructive hydrocephalus through endoscopic third ventriculostomy (ETV) in newborns and children younger than one year of age.

REFERENCES

1. Pinter JD, Sarnat HB. Youmans neurological surgery, 5th ed. W.B. Saunders: Philadelphia, PA, 2003.
2. Desmond ME, Jacobson AG. Embryonic brain enlargement requires cerebrospinal fluid pressure. Dev Biol 1977; 57:188–198.
3. Jelínek R, Pexieder T. Pressure of the CSF and the morphogenesis of the CNS. Folia Morphol (Praha) 1970; 18;102–110.
4. O'Rahilly R, Muller F. The embryonic human brain: An atlas of developmental stages, 2nd ed. New York, NY: Wiley-Liss, 1999.
5. Lemire JR, Loeser JD, Leach RW, et al. Normal and abnormal development of the human nervous system. Hagerstown, MD: Parper & Row, 1975:283.

6. Hartmann D, Sievers J, Pehlemann FW, et al. Destruction of meningeal cells over the medial cerebral hemisphere of newborn hamsters prevents the formation of the infrapyramidal blade of the dentate gyrus. J Comp Neurol 1992; 320;33–61.
7. Sievers J, Pehlmann FW, Gude S, et al. A time course study of the alterations in the development of the hamster cerebellar cortex after destruction of the overlying meningeal cells with 6-hydroxydopamine on the day of birth. J Neurocytol 1994; 23:117–134.
8. Catala M. Embryonic and fetal development of structures associated with the cerebro-spinal fluid in man and other species. Part I: The ventricular system, meninges and choroids plexuses. Arch Anat Cytol Pathol 1998; 46:153–169.
9. Strazielle N, Ghersi-Egea JF. Choroid plexus in the central nervous system: Biology and physiopathology. J Neuropathol Exp Neurol 2000; 59:561–571.
10. Chamberlain JG. Analysis of developing ependymal and choroidal surfaces in rat brains using scanning electron microscopy. Dev Biol 1973; 31:22–30.
11. Otani H, Tanaka O. Development of the choroids plexus anlage and supraependymal structures in the fourth ventricular roof plate of human embryos: Scanning electron microscopic observations. Am J Anat 1988; 181:53–66.
12. Gomez DG, Potts G. The surface characteristics of arachnoid granulations. A scanning electron microscopical study. Arch Neurol 1974; 31:88–93.
13. Shuangshoti S, Netsky MG. Histogenesis of choroid plexus in man. Am J Anat 1966; 118:283–316.
14. Chodobski A, Wojcik BE, Loh YP, et al. Vasopressin gene expression in rat choroids plexus. Adv Exp Med Biol 1998; 449:59–65.
15. Osaka K, Handa H, Matsumoto S, et al. Development of the cerebrospinal fluid pathway in the normal and abnormal human embryos. Childs Brain 1980; 6(1):26–38.
16. Coben LA. Absence of a foramen of Magendie in the dog, cat, rabbit and goat. Arch Neurol 1967; 141:499–512.
17. Blake JA. The roof and lateral recesses of the fourth ventricle considered morphologically and embryologically. J Comp Neurol 1900; 10:79–108.
18. Krabbe KH. Morphogenesis of the vertebrate brain. Copenhagen, Denmark: Einar Munksgaard, 1947.
19. Bartelmez GW, Dekaban AS. The early development of the human brain. Contr Embryol 1962; 37:13–32
20. Brocklehurst G. The development of the human cerebrospinal pathway with particular reference to the roof of the fourth ventricle. J Anat 1969; 105:467–475.
21. Weed LH. Studies on cerebrospinal fluid. III. The pathways of escape from the subarachnoid spaces with particular reference to the arachnoid villi. J Med Res 1914; 31:51–91.
22. Di Rocco C, Oi S. Proposal of "evolution theory in cerebrospinal fluid dynamics" and minor pathway hydrocephalus in developing immature brain. Childs Nerv Syst 2006; 22:662–669.

2 | Hydrocephalus: Historical Review of Its Treatment

James Tait Goodrich

Division of Pediatric Neurosurgery, Children's Hospital at Montefiore, Albert Einstein College of Medicine, Bronx, New York, U.S.A.

No subject or disease entity is more fundamental to a pediatric neurosurgical practice than hydrocephalus and its treatment. In 1929, the founder of our Department of Neurosurgery at the Albert Einstein College of Medicine, Leo Davidoff, MD, offered his views on dealing with hydrocephalus:

> Hardly any other pathologic condition has been accorded more determined attention on the part of the medical profession with the aim of finding a cure for it than has hydrocephalus. And in hardly a single other condition have cures been so illusive or so often wrecked on purely mechanical obstacles. Yet the outlook is certainly not hopeless. Especially during the past twenty years, during which surgery of the nervous system has improved so remarkably, frequent reports of cures by surgical means have appeared (1).

Many things have changed in the field of pediatric neurosurgery when it comes to the medical and surgical treatment of hydrocephalus. This chapter reviews the history of this subject along with contributions to the treatment of hydrocephalus. Our surgical brethrens were quite inventive and sometimes offered novel treatments—a few of which worked.

Cultures from around the world offer a great variety of artifacts showing clinical findings consistent with hydrocephalus. Prior to the introduction of the written document, there existed only figures in clay and stone (and occasionally other materials) showing representations of individuals with hydrocephalus. Meso-American cultures include a number of examples. We have provided two figures, one from the early Olmec culture showing a child with hydrocephalus, and the second from the Mexican west coast from the Colima area showing an individual with spina bifida and hydrocephalus. Many examples of these figures with various diseases are to be found throughout Meso-American cultures (Figs. 1 and 2) (2).

To Hippocrates (ca. 460–368 BC) we owe some of the earliest medical writings on hydrocephalus. Hippocrates erroneously believed that the accumulation of cerebrospinal fluid (CSF) was due to the excess "pituita" of chronic epilepsy. As a clinician he gave a clear picture of signs and symptoms associated with hydrocephalus: headache, vomiting, visual loss, diplopia, and squinting. Hippocrates also noted that outcome and prognosis of hydrocephalus were extremely poor—a theme that remained constant throughout history until the 19th century, when important corrections of this view became possible (3). When it came to treatment, Hippocrates could only offer laxatives and dietary supplements. Over the years a number of authors suggested that Hippocrates advocated trephination over the anterior fontanelle to relieve pressure in hydrocephalus. A recent examination of the Hippocratic corpus by this author failed to disclose any recommendations of surgical treatment for internal hydrocephalus. It is possible that Hippocrates might have advocated a form of trephination in a case of "external" hydrocephalus, a situation where fluid collects above the pericranium (4).

One of the great figures in the history of medicine and surgery was Galen of Pergamon (AD 130–200). This great Alexandrian anatomist and surgeon provided several early descriptions of hydrocephalus (5). To help the surgeon understand this disorder, he categorized hydrocephalus into four types according to the site of fluid accumulation: between brain and meninges, between meninges and bone, between bone and pericranium, and between pericranium and skin. Following views originating with Hippocrates, Galen argued that in cases in which fluid accumulated below the meninges, the condition was not curable. However, fluid that accumulated above the pericranium could be surgically drained.

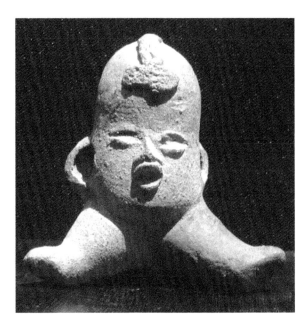

Figure 1 An early Olmec figure dating from about 1500 BC showing a child with hydrocephalus and most likely an associated spina bifida. (Author's personal collection.)

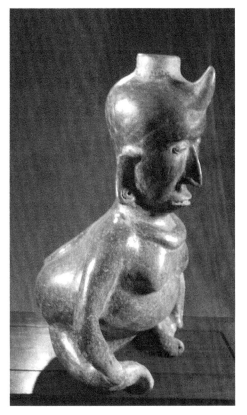

Figure 2 A terracotta figure from the west coast of Mexico (the state of Colima) showing an individual with hydrocephalus and classic findings of an associated spina bifida. (Author's personal collection.)

Galen did a number of studies on the brain and appreciated that CSF was in free communication within the ventricular system, that is, flowed freely throughout the ventricles, a concept lost and not revived until the 18th century. Galen was the first to describe what we now call the Aqueduct of Sylvius. This current eponym for this anatomical CSF pathway is erroneously attributed to Franciscus de le Boë, or Sylvius (1614–1672), a professor of medicine

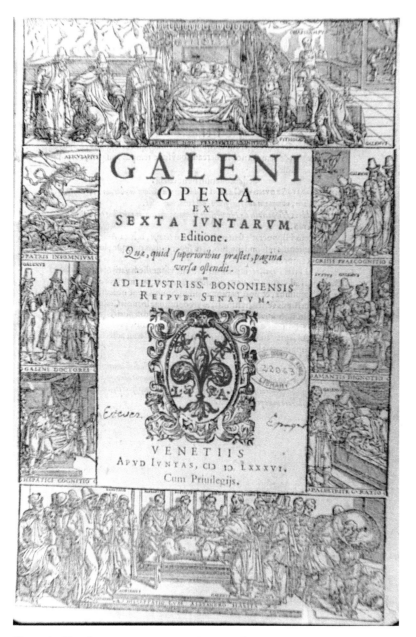

Figure 3   The allegorical title page from Galen's collected works. Venice 1576–1577 (5). In the panels surrounding the title are listed many of the famous figures of medicine and surgery. The panel at the bottom shows Galen performing a surgical transection of the recurrent laryngeal nerve in a pig. (Author's personal collection.)

at Leyden (6). Galen also provided an elegant description of what we now call the foramen of Monro, the communication between the two lateral ventricles. Alexander Monro *Secundus* (1737–1817) did not publish his comparable anatomical findings until 1783, nearly 1500 years later (7). Following up on further findings having to do with the CSF circulation, Galen provided the first anatomical description of the choroid plexus as well as its name (Fig. 3).

In attempting to understand the physiology of CSF, Galen applied his humoral theory, theorizing that the "animal spirit" was an entity residing within the ventricles. In his view, this "spirit" was purified by its passage through pores in the brain. The waste products then passed through the pituitary gland for discharge through the nose as "pituita." Following these concepts, Galen felt hydrocephalus to be caused by a defect in the formation of the "animal spirit" that results in a backup of fluid. This humoral theory remained a dominant concept and prevailing influence in medicine until well into the 16th century. The concept was not challenged until the classic work by Andreas Vesalius (1519–1564) on human anatomy, published in 1543 (8). Once Galen's "animal spirit" had been called into question, later authors characterized the contents of the ventricles as air, vacuum, vapor, or water. However, the true relationships of CSF and the brain were not developed until the 18th century, as we shall see.

Following Greco-Roman medicine came the Byzantine era and a number of important eastern medical figures. The Byzantine Empire began with Constantine the Great and his ascent to the Roman throne in AD 324. The capital of the Roman Empire now moved from Rome to a small town, Byzantium, soon renamed Constantinople (now Istanbul, Turkey). This was to remain the capital and the center of the Byzantine Empire till 1453, when the Turks conquered it.

Several important Byzantine era surgeons contributed to the study of hydrocephalus: Oribasius (4th century AD), Aetius (6th century AD), and Paul of Aegina (7th century AD). Oribasius (AD 325–403), a surgeon, classified hydrocephalus into three types: fluid collections between brain and meninges, which he deemed not operable, whereas fluid collections between bone and pericranium and pericranium and scalp could be surgically drained (9). Oribasius did make an interesting technical suggestion, namely, that the surgeon should always place the lance behind the hairline so as not to leave a visible scar (10,11).

The classification of hydrocephalus and related views on the surgical treatment of it, like those discussed above, have remained a dominant theme in the literature until recent times. An inadequate understanding of CSF physiology and the risk of surgical infection and meningitis secondary to contaminated surgical instruments lead one to understand why the outcomes of surgery on hydrocephalus were almost invariably lethal. Such outcomes led many surgeons away from any form of surgical treatment.

Aetius of Amida (AD 502–573), another of the great Byzantine physicians, wrote on hydrocephalus and offered surgical intervention as a form of treatment. Aetius studied in Alexandria and lived in Byzantium, where he was court physician to Emperor Justinian I. In his work, he described the different type of fluids seen in the ventricles (12). The causes of this condition of hydrocephalus are not always known. For a classification system, he used the same principles that Oribasius introduced, also asserting that surgery is indicated only in the external types of hydrocephalus. With regard to incisions he declared that sometimes several are needed to adequately drain the fluid. He also believed that a cause of hydrocephalus was violent handling of the head by midwives, a common theme in the writing of physicians of that era. He also recommended different medications for treatment of hydrocephalus, mostly desiccants "designed" to draw the fluid out.

Paul of Aegina (Paulus Aegineta Lt) (AD 625–690?), among the last of the great Byzantine physicians and a skilled surgeon, also followed a similar theme of treating external hydrocephalus but not operating on the internal type. He did recommend a different type of incision—which he felt offered a better solution—an "H" type of incision of his own design for the more extreme cases of hydrocephalus, reasoning that as more fluid was present in these cases a larger incision was needed (12–14).

A dominant figure in Eastern medicine was a learned Islamic Moorish Spaniard, Albucasis (Abu Al-Qasim or Al-Zahrawi; AD 936–1013). He is remembered as a great compiler, scholar, and surgeon, whose writings (some 30 volumes!) were focused mainly on surgery, dietetics, and materia medica (15). While reviewing his writings, we come upon an interesting discussion of hydrocephalus:

> On the cure of hydrocephalus: This disease occurs most commonly in infants upon delivery when the midwife grasps the child's head roughly. It also sometimes happens from some hidden and unknown cause. I have never seen this disease except in very small children; and death very quickly overtook all those that I have seen; therefore I have preferred not to undertake operation in these cases. I have seen a child whose head was filled with fluid and daily growing in size, until the child could not sit upright on account of the size of his head, and the humidity increased till he died (16).

الفصل الأوّل فى علاج الماء الذى يجتمع فى رؤوس الصبيان

إنّ هذا السقم كثيرا ما يعرض للصبيان عند الولادة او اذا ضغطت

القابلة رأس الصبّى بغير رفق وقد يعرض أيضا من علّة خفيّة لا تعرف

ولم أر هذه العلّة فى غير الصبيان وجميع من رأيت منهم أسرع اليه

٥ الموت فلذلك رأيت ترك العمل به ولقد رأيت منهم صبيّا قد امتــلأ

رأسه ماء والرأس يعظم فى كلّ يوم حتّى لم يطق الصبّى يقعد عـلى

نفسه لعظم رأسه والرطوبة تتزايد حتّى هلك، وهذا الرطوبة إمّا أن

تجتمع بين الجلد والعظم وإمّا أن تجتمع تحت العظم على الصفـاق،

والعمل فى ذلك إن كانت الرطوبة فيما بين الجلد والعظم وكان الورم

١٠ صغيرا فينبغى أن تشقّ فى وسط الرأس شقّا واحدا بالعرض ويكــون

طول الشقّ نحو عقدين حتّى تسيل الرطوبة وهذه صورة المبضع:

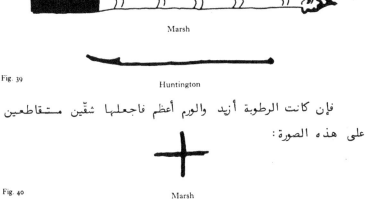

Marsh

Fig. 39

Huntington

فإن كانت الرطوبة أزيد والورم أعظم فاجعلها شقّين مــتقاطعين

على هذه الصورة:

Fig. 40

Marsh

V, او اذا صعطت AP, واذا اضغطت 2.·BP. ⟨من هذا الباب⟩.١.

H. تتولد MV, تتزيد M. 3. واذا قطعت

Figure 4 From a manuscript by Albucasis showing his specially designed instrument for the treatment of hydrocephalus (the top image). The "+" incision he designed is shown at the bottom (16). (Author's personal collection.)

Following earlier authors already discussed, Albucasis would only operate on cases of "external hydrocephalus," fluid between the scalp and the skull or the dura and the skull. An inventive surgeon, Albucasis designed a "+" type incision to drain off the "humidity," and in these cases claimed good results (17). Albucasis also designed a special surgical instrument for treatment of hydrocephalus (Fig. 4). He cautioned the surgeon against incising over an artery lest a severe hemorrhage result in the death of the patient. Before considering an operation for hydrocephalus, Albucasis would offer the child a more conservative nonsurgical treatment. He would "bind" the head with a tight constricting wrap and then place the child on a "dry diet" with fluid restrictions. Should these conservative measures fail he would offer surgical drainage of the fluid, but only, as noted, in cases of external hydrocephalus (17,18). Albucasis's surgical writings were used extensively in the schools of Salerno and Montpellier and hence had an important influence in the Middle Ages.

The Middle Ages is notable for the lack of any new insights into hydrocephalus, save that of Nicolas Massa (1485–1569), a physician and an anatomist born in Venice, Italy. Massa studied medicine at the University of Padua. It was through investigative studies by this anatomist that we have the first clear description of CSF. What is of particular interest is how rapidly this new information disappeared from the literature! After its introduction in 1535 by Massa, it disappeared until the 18th century, when it reappeared in the work of Cotugno, which will be discussed in the following texts. In Massa's *Liber Introductoris anatomiae* (19), he gave a clear and accurate description of CSF and interestingly he denied the concept that psychological function, that is, the cell doctrine theory, resides in the ventricles. The cell doctrine theory had developed from concepts put forward by Aristotle, that is to say, a cardiocentric view according to which the main functions of the body reside within the heart, with the brain merely cooling the heart. To further compound the error, the cell doctrine theory claimed that the functions of the brain resided within the ventricular system rather than in the brain parenchyma:

> Folio 84v: . . . Observe the watery superfluity in these cavities (Massa is speaking of the ventricles), sent there from the other parts of the brain and expurgated through a foramen from the cavities of the ventricles. . . . It is especially noteworthy that I have always found these cavities full or half-full of the aforementioned, watery superfluidity of the rational brain (20)—Massa continues:

> Folio 86r–86v: . . . you must understand that these ventricles are rather for the collection and expulsion of superfluidities than for the diverse operations of the mind, which are performed through different parts, since no veins or arteries are found in the last (i.e, fourth ventricle) which proceeds into the posterior cerebellum. . . (20).

With the beginnings of the Renaissance, one of the great figures, Leonardo da Vinci (1452–1519) also offered some interesting views on the anatomy of the brain and the ventricular system. Leonardo had planned on compiling a large 120-volume work on anatomy but did not live long enough to complete it (21). After his death, Leonardo's anatomical illustrations were dispersed, but fortunately the main body of these anatomical drawings still resides in England as part of the Windsor collection, property of the Queen of England (22). Within this remarkable treasure trove are several drawings dealing with the brain and the ventricles. Leonardo developed an ingenious system of injecting liquid wax into the ventricles to make a cast of the ventricular system. His drawings derived from this technique are shown in Figures 5(A–C). Leonardo unfortunately followed the "cell doctrine" theory that the function of the brain resided within the ventricles rather than in the brain parenchyma. But even though he maintained this erroneous theory, it is to Leonardo da Vinci that we owe some of the earliest reasonable illustrations of the brain and the ventricular system. Unfortunately, Leonardo's drawings disappeared after his death in 1519, only to circulate locally among artists and did not reappear until the 18th century, when they were "rediscovered" in England. The drawings surfaced in an old chest in Windsor Castle during the reign of King George III. How the drawings arrived there has never been determined. A number of these drawings have been elegantly reproduced by several publishers (21,22).

Andreas Vesalius (1519–1564) recorded an interesting clinical description of a beggar child with hydrocephalus. It appears in his *magnum opus, De Humani Corporis Fabrica,* published in Basle in 1543 (8). In Book I, a discussion of "Heads of other shape," he wrote ". . . at Genoa a small boy is carried from door to door by a beggar woman, and was put on display by actors in noble Brabant in Belgium, whose head, without any exaggeration, is larger than two normal human heads and swells out on either side" (23). In 1555, Vesalius published his second edition of this work. In it he described a second hydrocephalus case, that of a young girl whom he noted to have a head "larger than any man's" (24). Vesalius went on to discuss an important observation, namely, that the fluid had collected within the ventricles and not between the dura and the skull, and therefore a case of internal hydrocephalus. At autopsy Vesalius reported removing "nine pounds of water" from the ventricles (24,25). No surgical intervention was offered. Following the Hippocratic doctrines of internal hydrocephalus, these would not be regarded as surgical cases.

The first printed illustration of a child with hydrocephalus in a book appeared in an early work on surgical pathology by Marco Aurelia Severino (1580–1656) published in 1632 (26) (Fig. 6), which is considered the first textbook in this field. Severino was a widely known and

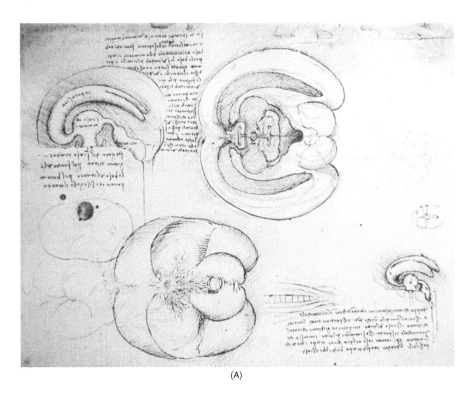

(A)

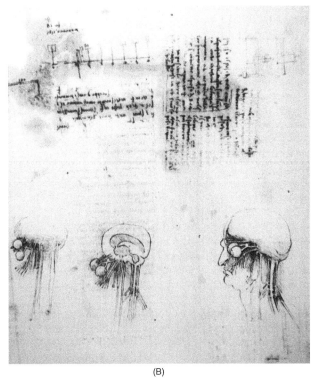

(B)

Figure 5 (**A**) The ventricular system using Leonardo da Vinci's wax casting technique. (**B**) The ventricular system illustrated along with depictions of cranial nerves. (**C**) Leonardo's view of the cell doctrine theory where brain function resides within the ventricular system as opposed to the brain parenchyma (21,22). (Author's personal collection.)

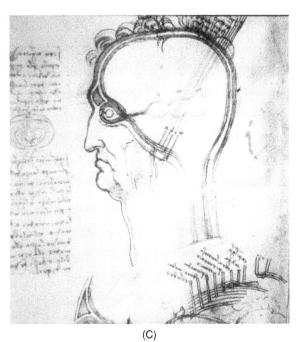

(C)

Figure 5 (*Continued*)

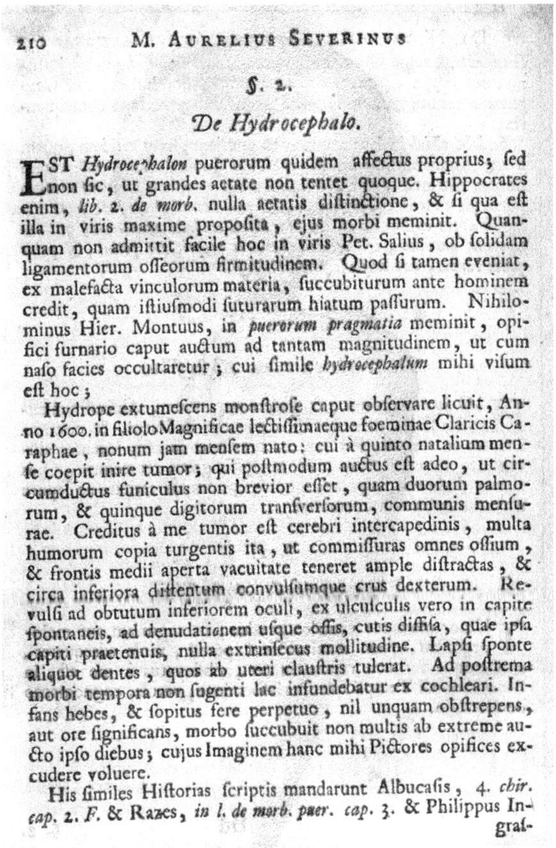

210   M. AURELIUS SEVERINUS

§. 2.

De Hydrocephalo.

EST *Hydrocephalon* puerorum quidem affectus proprius; sed non sic, ut grandes aetate non tentet quoque. Hippocrates enim, *lib. 2. de morb.* nulla aetatis distinctione, & si qua est illa in viris maxime proposita, ejus morbi meminit. Quanquam non admittit facile hoc in viris Pet. Salius, ob solidam ligamentorum osseorum firmitudinem. Quod si tamen eveniat, ex malefacta vinculorum materia, succubiturum ante hominem credit, quam istiusmodi futurarum hiatum passurum. Nihilominus Hier. Montuus, in *puerorum pragmatia* meminit, opifici furnario caput auctum ad tantam magnitudinem, ut cum naso facies occultaretur; cui simile *hydrocephalum* mihi visum est hoc;

Hydrope extumescens monstrose caput observare licuit, Anno 1600. in filiolo Magnificae lectissimaeque foeminae Claricis Caraphae, nonum jam mensem nato: cui à quinto natalium mense coepit inire tumor; qui postmodum auctus est adeo, ut circumductus funiculus non brevior esset, quam duorum palmorum, & quinque digitorum transversorum, communis mensurae. Creditus à me tumor est cerebri intercapedinis, multa humorum copia turgentis ita, ut commissuras omnes ossium, & frontis medii aperta vacuitate teneret ample distractas, & circa inferiora distentum convulsumque crus dexterum. Revulsi ad obtutum inferiorem oculi, ex ulculculis vero in capite spontaneis, ad denudationem usque ossis, cutis diffisa, quae ipsa capiti praetenuis, nulla extrinsecus mollitudine. Lapsi sponte aliquot dentes, quos ab uteri claustris tulerat. Ad postrema morbi tempora non sugenti lac infundebatur ex cochleari. Infans hebes, & sopitus fere perpetuo, nil unquam obstrepens, aut ore significans, morbo succubuit non multis ab extreme aucto ipso diebus; cujus Imaginem hanc mihi Pictores opifices excudere voluere.

His similes Historias scriptis mandarunt Albucasis, 4. *chir. cap. 2. F.* & Razes, *in l. de morb. puer. cap.* 3. & Philippus In-graf-

(A)

Figure 6 (**A**) Severino's discussion of hydrocephalus from his book of 1632 (26). (Author's personal collection.) (**B**) The earliest known printed illustration of a child with hydrocephalus, from Serverino's text of 1632 (26).

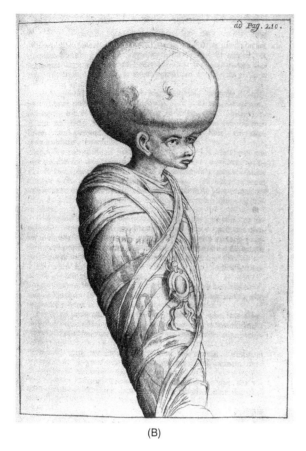

(B)

Figure 6 *(Continued)*

respected teacher in Naples, Italy. As a result of its superb illustrations and excellent clinical discussions, this textbook underwent many editions. The first appearance of an illustration showing a child with hydrocephalus appears in this book. In the section on the "obscure nature of tumors" is a remarkable collection of pathological lesions and tumors, often called "swellings." What made this work unique was that Severino often added the patient's history, and if surgery was performed, the techniques used were discussed.

Following shortly after Severino's work was another interesting book, in this instance, by Nicolaas Tulp (1593–1674) on a series of "medical observations." Included in the series was a discussion and illustration of a child with spina bifida and associated hydrocephalus (Fig. 7). This book was entitled *Observationes Medicae* and was published in 1641. It became very popular, leading to the publication of several editions (27). Tulp is best remembered from Rembrandt's painting of "The Anatomy Lesson of Dr. Tulp," painted in 1632, which was Tulp's second year in practice as an anatomical lecturer. To Nicolaas Tulp (his real name was Claes Piereszoon) we also owe the introduction of the term "spina bifida." Tulp's illustration shows a child with a large lumbosacral myelomeningocele, which he attempted to repair surgically. The child also had a clearly enlarged head consistent with hydrocephalus. The child died after surgery as a result of sepsis. Tulp did not discuss management of the enlarged head.

In the 17th and 18th centuries initial steps were finally taken, though the path was circuitous, toward an understanding of hydrocephalus. In regard to both CSF production and hydrocephalus treatment, theories were offered that contained as many errors as correct observations. An example was Thomas Willis (1621–1675), the prominent London physician and anatomist who advanced his belief in 1670, in a monograph entitled *Pathologiae Cerebri*, that the choroid plexus acted only as a "blood filterer" (28). The nature and structure of the choroid plexus led to this belief, or so he believed. Contrary to Willis' view were the writings of Contanzo Variolio [Varolius] (1543–1575), Professor of Anatomy at the University of Bologna

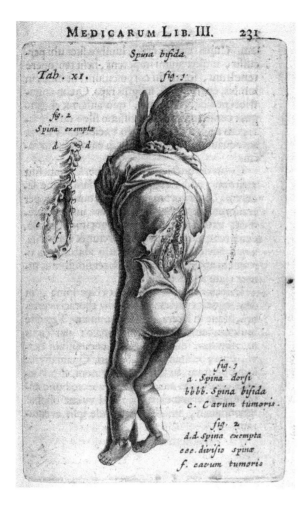

MEDICARUM LIB. III.   231

Spina bifida

Tab. XI.   fig. 1.

fig. 2
Spina exemptæ
d   d

e
f

fig. 1
a . Spina dorsi
bbbb. Spina bifida
c . Cavum tumoris .

fig. 2
d.d. Spina exempta
eee. divisio spinæ
f. cavum tumoris

Figure 7 One of the earliest known printed examples of hydrocephalus, in a child with spina bifida, from Tulp's *Observations medicae* (27). This illustration shows a patient in whom Tulp had attempted to repair a myelomeningocele. The child died shortly after surgery as a result of sepsis. The child clearly has a large head consistent with hydrocephalus, a pathological condition commonly associated with spina bifida (27). (Author's personal collection.) In the lower right legend is the first use of the term "spina bifida."

and physician to the Pope (29). Variolio believed that the choroid plexus merely absorbed ventricular fluid. Adding confusion to the picture was Jean Riolan (1580–1657), a Paris anatomist, who noted the exceptional vascularity of the choroid plexus and called its constituent vessels the *rete mirabile*, thereby reintroducing an erroneous anatomical concept first postulated by Galen in the second century AD (30,31). In the midst of all this confusion came the brilliant Dutch anatomist Frederik Ruysch (1638–1731), who suggested that the choroid plexus was actually a gland and that it formed CSF (32). A differing view was offered by Albrecht von Haller (1708–1777), a prolific writer, anatomist, physiologist, and physician and one of the intellectual giants of the 18th century. Haller had just adopted the controversial concept of the circulation of the blood (33). Haller's erroneous opinion was that the contents of the ventricles were formed by the "vapor produced by the exhalation of the arteries and its subsequent inhalation by the veins." So it would appear that the contemporary 18th century "geniuses of science" had even less success in understanding CSF and its circulation.

To Antoni Pacchioni (1665–1726), an Italian anatomist and close collaborator with Marcello Malpighi (1628–1994), we owe a bizarre sidelight into the concept of CSF circulation. In 1701, Pacchioni clearly described what we now call Pacchionian granules of the dura mater over the convexity bordering the sagittal sinus (34). But in moving adrift from the true anatomy, Pacchioni suggested that the dura matter was in reality just a layer of muscle designed to move "nervous fluid" toward the periphery of the brain. Pacchioni as it happened had no concept of the physiological role of the granules he described; this had to await the elegant 19th century writings of Key and Retzius, to be discussed in what follows (Fig. 8).

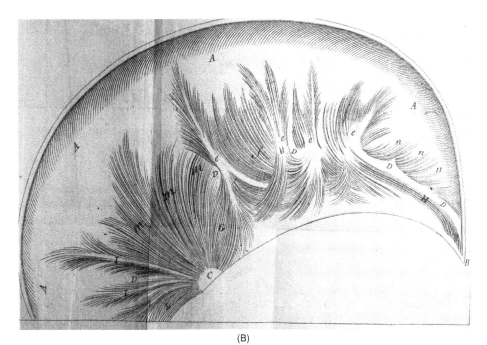

(A)

(B)

Figure 8 (**A**) The title page from Pacchioni's monograph on the meninges and dura. In this work is the first description of the Pacchionian granules (34). (Author's personal collection.) (**B**) Plate from Pacchioni's 1701 work demonstrating his erroneous view of the "muscular fibers" in the dura, used to move the CSF through the brain.

One of the best early pathological description of hydrocephalus was that of G.B. Morgagni (1682–1770), a teacher of anatomy at Padua. In his classic work of 1761 (35,36) in a section entitled "*Sermo de Hydrocephalus et de Aqueis Spinae Tumoribus*," he described a case "of the hydrocephalus and watery (sic) tumor of the spine." This clinical description appears to be the first in which hydrocephalus and spina bifida were clearly described as an associated clinical disorder. Several other cases of hydrocephalus are discussed, but since this was a book of postmortem examinations, no clinical observations or treatment recommendations were offered (Fig. 9).

> The hydrocephalus, or dropsy of the head, is either external or internal. The former has its seat in the cellular substance, between the skin and the pericranium, or between this membrane and the skull. In the internal hydrocephalus, the water is sometimes collected between the cranium and dura mater, or between this last and the pia mater; but most commonly is found in the ventricles of the brain, immediately below the corpus callosum; And this is not only the most frequent and fatal species of the hydrocephalus, but also that with which medical writers seem to have been least acquainted (37).

The above quotation comes from one of the first monographs devoted entirely to hydrocephalus. This book was published by an English physician, Robert Whytt (1714–1766). His monograph, *Observations on the Dropsy in the Brain* (37), appeared in 1768, two years after his death. This book, published in 1768, provides an extensive discussion of hydrocephalus along with a number of remarkable clinical observations including descriptions of its various clinical stages. Unfortunately, the work is rich in clinical observations, but Whytt offered little in the way of clinical treatment and actually was merely adopting the views of Jean Astruc (1684–1766) (38)—that is, the views of the "ancients"—which have been discussed above. It is Whytt's clinical findings regarding patients with hydrocephalus that we find of greater interest. These findings were divided into three stages of severity: stage 1, quickened pulse; stage 2, slow irregular pulse; stage 3, rapid pulse; and in the last stage, the pupils become dilated and are no longer responsive even "in the greatest light" (39). Whytt offered the following treatments for hydrocephalus: emetics, purging, blisters, and the like. Surgical treatment was not even an option. When it came to the late stages of hydrocephalus Whytt was quite pessimistic: "[When] so much water is accumulated as, by its pressure on the sides of the ventricles, to disturb the action of the brain, we have little to hope from medicine"—a clinical correlation that remained essentially correct for the next 150 years (39) (Fig. 10).

Following up on Whytt's work on hydrocephalus was a British physician, Henry Manning. In his book on the *Practice of Physic*, Manning offered insights on treating internal hydrocephalus (40). He began with an introduction stating that the disease was only recently well classified and documented, namely, in the recent works of Drs. Whytt, Fothergill, and Watson. All agreed that hydrocephalus is generally a fatal disease and that its origin or cause remains obscure. Its clinical course is relatively rapid, with most patients dying in a matter of weeks. Manning noted that the disorder primarily affects children but can sometimes be seen in adults. The pain reported by patients is not always well localized; the head and shoulders are the most common subjects of complaint. Very violent and severe headaches were not uncommon in this group. Lethargy and difficulty in breathing occur as the disease progresses. In more advanced cases the pulse becomes irregular and slows. As "fatal termination" approaches, the breathing becomes deep, irregular, and laborious. The pupils of the eyes are much dilated, and the patients are averse to light, avoiding the patients by going into darkened rooms. There is inability to control urine or stool. No surgical treatment options are offered. The typical contemporary purges and emetics are offered, but the clinical course is almost always fatal.

In completing the summary of the 18th-century medicine and its treatment of hydrocephalus, it is useful to look at the writings of John Fothergill (1712–1780), a prominent London physician and a medical figure well known to both Americans and English. Fothergill was raised as a Quaker and early on became a supporter and advocate of the American colonies. He initially started in medicine as an apprentice to a local apothecary. But with his skills in medicine evident early, he became a medical student at the University of Edinburgh. He returned to London in 1740 to establish what became a large and lucrative private practice. He is remembered in neurology for early and accurate descriptions of tic douloureux and migraine

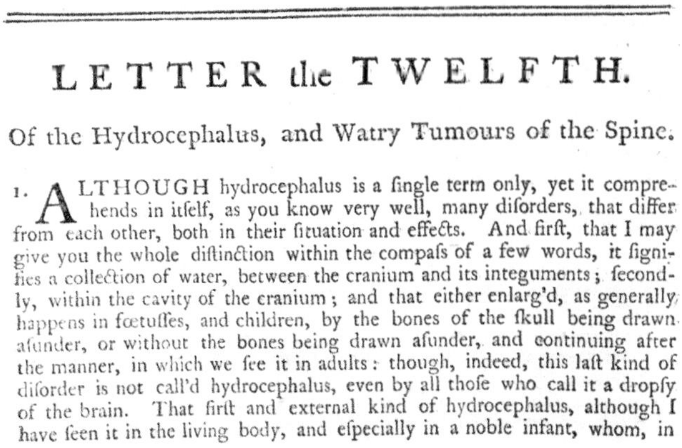

LETTER the TWELFTH.

Of the Hydrocephalus, and Watry Tumours of the Spine.

1. ALTHOUGH hydrocephalus is a fingle term only, yet it comprehends in itfelf, as you know very well, many diforders, that differ from each other, both in their fituation and effects. And firft, that I may give you the whole diftinction within the compafs of a few words, it fignifies a collection of water, between the cranium and its integuments; fecondly, within the cavity of the cranium; and that either enlarg'd, as generally happens in fœtuffes, and children, by the bones of the fkull being drawn afunder, or without the bones being drawn afunder, and continuing after the manner, in which we fee it in adults: though, indeed, this laft kind of diforder is not call'd hydrocephalus, even by all thofe who call it a dropfy of the brain. That firft and external kind of hydrocephalus, although I have feen it in the living body, and efpecially in a noble infant, whom, in

(A)

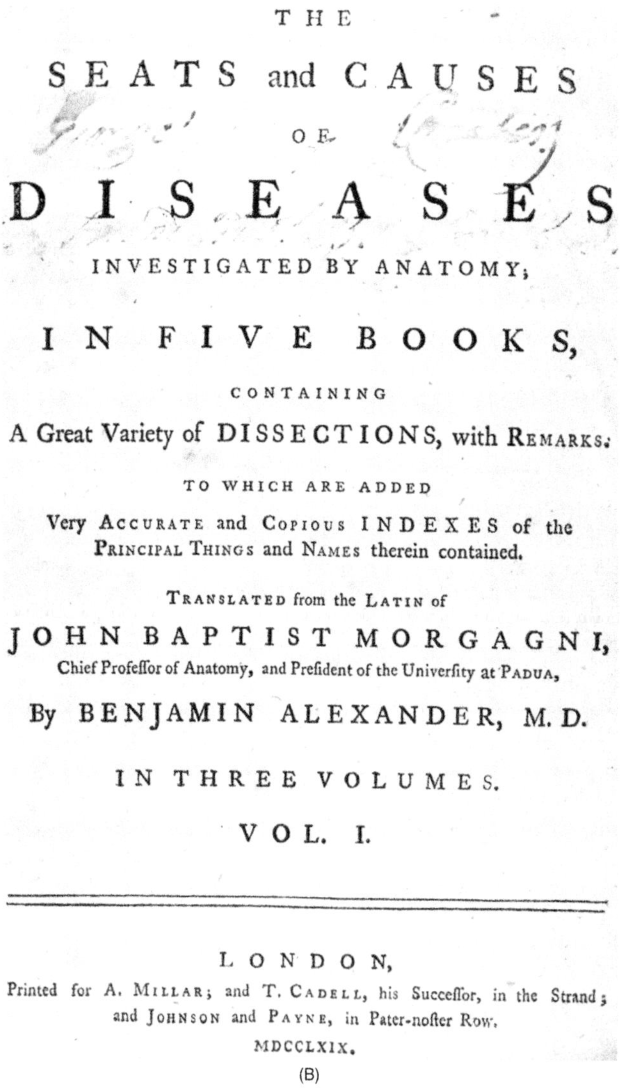

THE

SEATS and CAUSES

OF

DISEASES

INVESTIGATED BY ANATOMY;

IN FIVE BOOKS,

CONTAINING

A Great Variety of DISSECTIONS, with REMARKS.

TO WHICH ARE ADDED

Very ACCURATE and COPIOUS INDEXES of the PRINCIPAL THINGS and NAMES therein contained.

TRANSLATED from the LATIN of

JOHN BAPTIST MORGAGNI,

Chief Profeffor of Anatomy, and Prefident of the Univerfity at PADUA,

By BENJAMIN ALEXANDER, M. D.

IN THREE VOLUMES.

VOL. I.

LONDON,

Printed for A. MILLAR; and T. CADELL, his Succeffor, in the Strand; and JOHNSON and PAYNE, in Pater-nofter Row,

MDCCLXIX.

(B)

Figure 9 Morgagni's description of hydrocephalus associated with spina bifida, that is, "watry tumours of the spine" (sic) is seen in the top of figure. The title page from the English edition of this work is seen below (35). (Author's personal collection.)

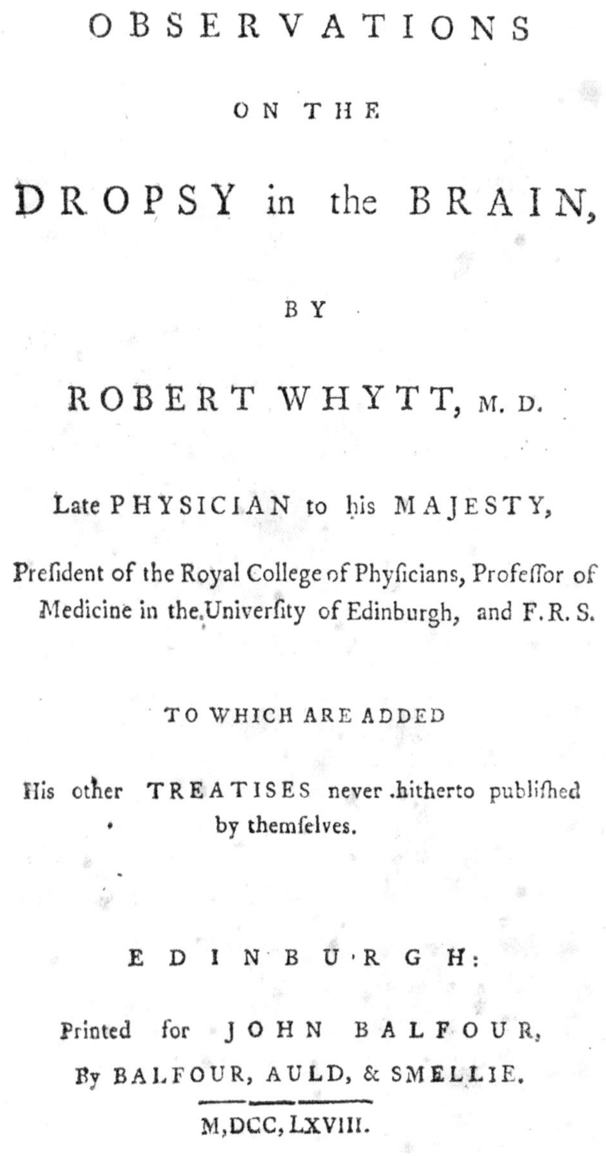

O B S E R V A T I O N S

O N   T H E

D R O P S Y in the B R A I N,

B Y

R O B E R T   W H Y T T, M. D.

Late P H Y S I C I A N to his M A J E S T Y,

Prefident of the Royal College of Phyficians, Profeffor of
Medicine in the Univerfity of Edinburgh, and F. R. S.

T O   W H I C H   A R E   A D D E D

His other T R E A T I S E S never .hitherto publifhed
by themfelves.

E D I N B U·R G H:

Printed for J O H N   B A L F O U R,

By B A L F O U R, A U L D, & S M E L L I E.

M,DCC, LXVIII.

Figure 10 The title page from Whytt's book, the first English work devoted solely to the treatment of hydrocephalus (39). (Author's personal collection.)

headaches. He also had a significant interest in hydrocephalus, a disease that he felt quite
helpless in treating. In his "Remarks on the Hydrocephalus Internus," Fothergill wrote:

> I have for a long time proposed to myself, to lay before you some account of a disease
> which occurs more frequently, I believe, than is generally apprehended, and is very often
> confounded with another, to which, in many respects, it appears not dissimilar; yet arises
> from a very different cause. At the same time, I must own to you, it is not in my power
> to suggest any probable means of curing the disease of which I treat: it has baffled all my
> attempts, both when confided in alone, and in consultation with the ablest of faculty. All
> that I pretend to do is, to exhibit such an idea of this disease as may serve to make it known
> when it occurs in practice, and to form such a prognositic of its progress and event, as may
> justify practitioners to themselves, and to the families in which such fatal occurrences may
> present themselves (41).

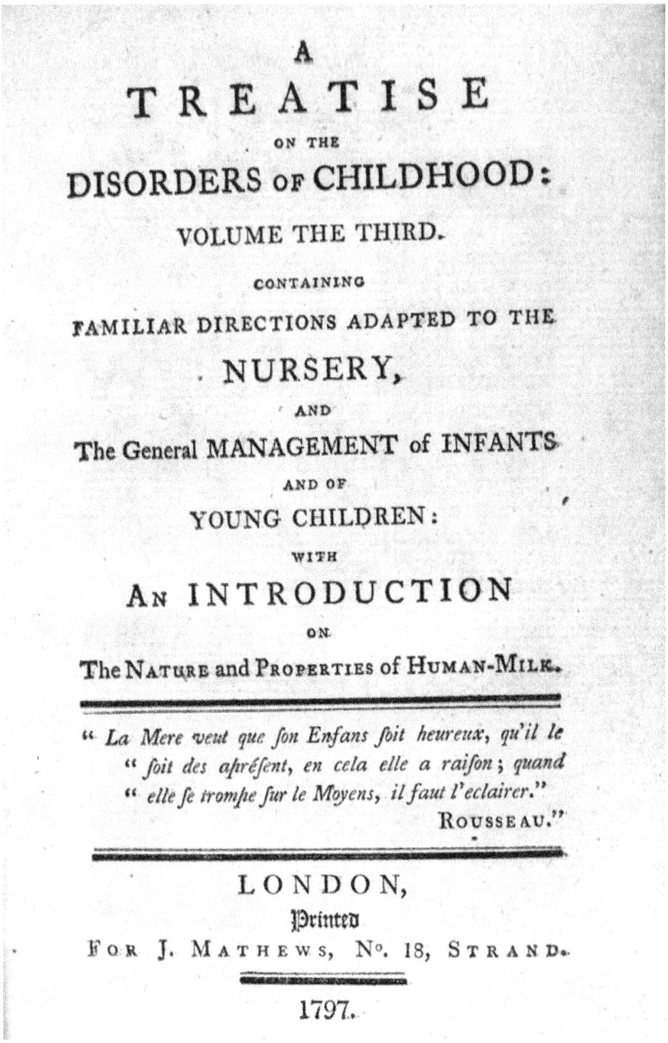

A

TREATISE

ON THE

DISORDERS OF CHILDHOOD:

VOLUME THE THIRD.

CONTAINING

FAMILIAR DIRECTIONS ADAPTED TO THE

NURSERY,

AND

The General MANAGEMENT of INFANTS

AND OF

YOUNG CHILDREN:

WITH

AN INTRODUCTION

ON

The NATURE and PROPERTIES of HUMAN-MILK.

" La Mere veut que son Enfans soit heureux, qu'il le
" soit des aprésent, en cela elle a raison; quand
" elle se trompe sur le Moyens, il faut l'eclairer."
ROUSSEAU."

LONDON,
Printed
FOR J. MATHEWS, N°. 18, STRAND.

1797.

Figure 11 Title page from one of the earliest monographs to deal with diseases of childhood (43). (Author's personal collection.)

Fothergill went on to report that he had rarely seen the disease of hydrocephalus in the child under the age of three—but most frequently in the 5- to 10-year-old age group. In several autopsies he found enlarged ventricles. He felt that because the fluid was under the corpus callosum "... it was impossible to discharge it by any medicine or operation hitherto discovered" (41). He offered the interesting but erroneous observation that hydrocephalus is often caused by infection with worms and that in those cases "anthelmintics" (sic) might be of some use. In his clinical description of the disease, he stated that the patient often presents with a severe headache: "They are generally very sick between whiles, crying out in the most affecting manner, *Oh my head! Oh, I am sick!*" (41). Along with the headache, he observed, as the condition worsened the pulse gradually became slower, the breathing then become deep, irregular, and laborious, and the pupils of the eyes "much dilated"—an interesting early observation of bradycardia associated with increased intracranial pressure. He also described "sundowning" of the eyes— "great part of the whites of the eyes are seen, and they are undisturbed by any thing but moving them" (42). Fothergill's only treatments were the usual cathartics, worm medications, and purging among other medical treatments. He offered no surgical options and pointed out that for the most part hydrocephalus is fatal.

In reviewing the history of the treatment of hydrocephalus, the author felt it is important to take account of one of the eminent treatises on childhood disorders, that by Michael Underwood (1736–1820) (43). Most historians consider Underwood to be the physician who laid the foundation of modern pediatrics. Underwood's book was written in a straightforward style with an excellent index and treatment that tended to be conservative and usually effective. Underwood, an obstetrician, served at the British Lying-In Hospital and so was not what we would call a pediatrician today. But a review of his treatise on disorders of childhood nevertheless reveals a clinician of considerable insight, one who appeared to have had significant experience in treating pediatric disorders. Most scholars now consider this work the most respected of the 18th-century monographs on pediatric disorders, making his views on both the origins and the treatment of hydrocephalus of special interest. In a section entitled "Watery Heads," he went into detail regarding the diagnosis and uniformly poor prognosis in such cases. He completed the Hippocratic exercise of differentiating external from internal hydrocephalus, pointing out that outcomes are the same, that is, poor, in both the types. He recognized that hydrocephalus is a common finding in children born with myelomeningoceles, and he described clearly the relationship between CSF in the spine and the head. Underwood gave clinical descriptions in extremis cases, in which the child's pupils are dilated and the child may have seizures and become incontinent of bowel and bladder. The treatment recommended would be considered barbaric by today's standards—bleeding and purging, with the removal of copious amount of blood being the norm. Administration of agents that cause purging of the bowels and clinical dehydration of the patient were a common practice. The use of foxglove or digitalis as a diuretic was advocated at one point but outcomes remained poor. Underwood even mentioned Dr. Benjamin Rush, a legendary American bleeder and purger, as one who might have the appropriate treatment options for treating hydrocephalus. Rush is most notorious for bleeding our first president, George Washington, to death in the treatment of a fever. To return to Underwood, he was clearly a skilled diagnostician who confined treatment to medications; in his view surgical intervention was not an option.

It seems quite remarkable that the physiological understanding of CSF did not come about until the 18th century. The mere existence of CSF was not recognized at autopsies, as CSF had typically already leaked out by the time the examiner came to the cranium and the brain. To Domenico Cotugno (1736–1822), professor of surgery and anatomy at Naples, Italy, we owe the first description and understanding of the anatomical distribution of CSF. In an elegant series of experimental studies published in 1764, Cotugno showed that CSF was a liquid, not a gas or vapor as was first proposed (44) (Fig. 11). His classic description from the English edition, published in 1775, of his monograph follows (45) (Fig. 12):

> This water, which fills the tube of the Dura Mater even to the *Os sacrum*, does not entirely enclose the spinal marrow, but even abounds in the cavity of the skull, and fills all the spaces which are between the brain and the *ambitus* of the Dura Mater. Some of these spaces are always to be met with about the basis of the brain; and it is not uncommon to find a considerable space between the *ambitus* itself of the brain, and the surrounding Dura Mater. This is principally to be found in consumptive persons, and old men (45).

Also important was Cotugno's description of the subarachnoid space through which CSF flows. Unfortunately, Albrecht Haller's vapor theory was firmly in vogue, and so years passed before Cotugno's work was accepted (33). Although Galen's view of the animal spirit had been tossed aside by this time, his view that the pituitary body was the exit portal of the ventricular contents was still strongly advocated by a number of 18th-century physicians. An interesting additional note is that Cotugno differentiated and described the respective clinical findings of arthritis from nervous sciatica in this book—the first to introduce sciatica as a separate disease entity.

From the anatomical dynasty at the University of Edinburgh came the most distinguished of three anatomists from the same family, Alexander Monro *Secundus* (1733–1817). In a book, published in 1783, on the structure and functions of the nervous system, he provided a superb anatomical diagram of what we now call the Foramen of Monro (46) (Fig. 13). Although an able anatomist, Monro lacked insight into the causes of hydrocephalus. Following the views of early ancients, Monro argued that hydrocephalus occurred with sclerosis of the pituitary

DOMINICI COTUNNII

PHIL. ET MED. DOCT.

DE

ISCHIADE

NERVOSA

COMMENTARIUS.

NEAPOLI, ET BONONIÆ

Ex Typographia Sancti Thomæ Aquinatis

MDCCLXXV.

SUPERIORUM AUCTORITATE.

Figure 12 Title page from Cotugno Latin monograph on sciatica and CSF circulation (44). In addition to his findings regarding CSF, in this work Cotugno differentiated and described the respective clinical findings of arthritis from those of nervous sciatica. Cotugno was thus the first to introduce sciatica as a separate disease entity. (Author's personal collection.)

body, a pathological condition that prevented egress of CSF, resulting in a backup of fluid and hydrocephalus (46).

John Cheyne (1777–1836) provided the first 19th-century monograph of any note on acute hydrocephalus (Fig. 14) (47). Cheyne was a pupil of Sir Charles Bell, to whom his monograph was dedicated; he is well known for his description of what is now called "Cheyne–Stokes respiration." Cheyne excelled in medicine at an early age, starting out by giving medicines to his father's poorer patients. He kept detailed clinical notes of his patients while in practice and often performed postmortem examinations—Cheyne called them necroscopic examinations—to find the cause of death. Cheyne begins his monograph on hydrocephalus with an extensive contemporary review of the literature. He cited the then important monograph on hydrocephalus by Dr. Whytt. He gave extensive clinical details on the presentations seen in children with

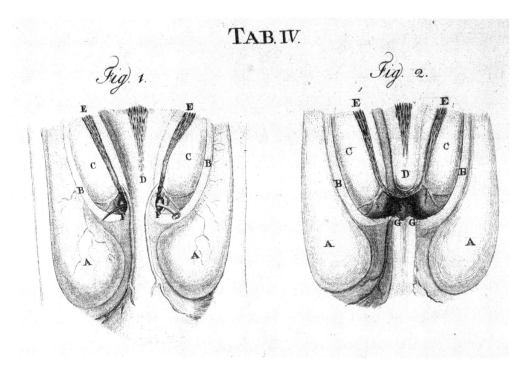

Figure 13 Table IV from Monro's work where he anatomically describes what is now called the Foramen of Monro, the foramen that allows communication between the lateral ventricles (46). (Author's personal collection.)

hydrocephalus and focused on the neurological findings of headaches, vomiting, lethargy, and the like. He noted that once lethargy sets in and the pulse begins to slow, the duration of the disease will be short (48). In a detailed case report (49), he described the case of a two-and-a-half-year-old boy with acute hydrocephalus. His treatments were a series of emetics and cathartics as well as application of blisters to the belly. He gave the details of the clinical findings over a two-week period including headache, vomiting, slow pulse, lethargy, blindness, and dilated pupils. By day 18, however, he stated: "I found this boy amusing himself, still extremely languid, but daily convalescing. His stools are quite natural" (50). Cheyne was clearly satisfied that all of his purging, blisters, and emetics had cured the child by getting his viscera in order! Cheyne's mention of surgical interventions in acute hydrocephalus is very brief. Cheyne asked the question: "What is the result of tapping the brain in chronic hydrocephalus? This operation, which has often been performed by ignorant men, is generally almost immediately productive of fatal consequences" (51). So in Cheyne's mind surgical intervention was contraindicated. What, then, was Cheyne's rationale for his own approach? "Purges have generally been given in this disease; but, when called early, what I recommend is the exhibition of the largest dose, which can with safety be prescribed, if some powerfully cathartic medicine, two, three, four times a day; and this continued for several days, or until natural stools are procured. The advantage of keeping the intestinal canal under the continued influence of a stimulus, I have, in various instances, found to be so great, that I am induced to repeat the declaration of my belief, that the happiest result may be expected from this measure." And if that fails, add blisters! Cheyne did not recommend bloodletting as Dr. Benjamin Rush proposed because it proved to be too debilitating. However, he would occasionally apply leeches in "robust constitutions" to take off a bit of blood to help the constitution (52). He presented the clinical details of 14 cases of acute hydrocephalus, in which he kept a daily diary of the medications and treatment along with symptoms. The routine was as described above with the focus always on the bowels—get them working correctly and the patient will do well. In no case was surgical intervention offered or even discussed. The final section of the book ends with a series of five autopsies done on children with acute hydrocephalus. In each case, the first focus was on the condition of the brain

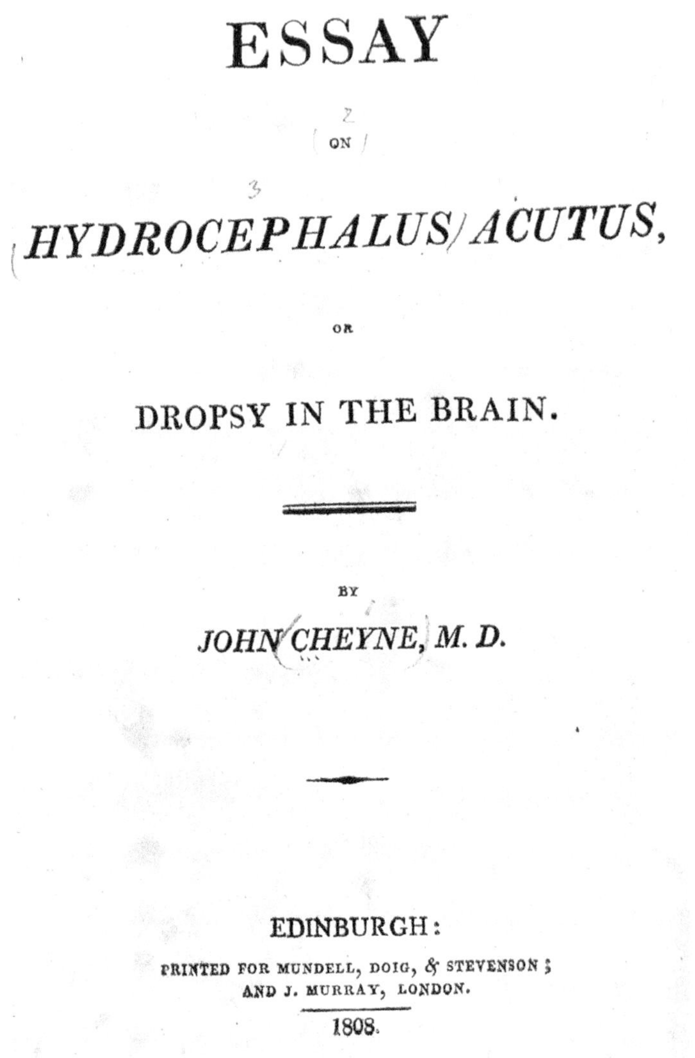

ESSAY

ON

HYDROCEPHALUS ACUTUS,

OR

DROPSY IN THE BRAIN.

———

BY

JOHN CHEYNE, M. D.

———

EDINBURGH:

PRINTED FOR MUNDELL, DOIG, & STEVENSON ;
AND J. MURRAY, LONDON.

1808.

Figure 14   Title page from Cheyne's 1808 Edinburgh edition monograph on hydrocephalus (47). (Author's personal collection.)

and the ventricle size along with the amount of water obtained. The second focus was always on the bowels and the conditions of the liver and the intestines—which were almost always diseased in some fashion.

A rare and often overlooked monograph on hydrocephalus was published in 1815 with an appendix in 1819 (53,54). These two volumes were the work of Grant David Yeats and dealt with "early symptoms of water in the brain, containing cases successfully treated." Little is known of Yeats other than that he was associated with Trinity College at Oxford, England. He was a member of the Royal College of Physicians, London, and the Royal Medical Society, Edinburgh. He was also physician to the Lunatic Asylum and Infirmary, as well as physician to his Grace the Duke of Edinburgh.

In this monograph, which is addressed to "Sir" (an individual not named or described), Yeats expressed his dismay at the lack of attention to make this diagnosis with "young sufferers being lulled into a false security" (55); hence, he felt it necessary to point out the early symptoms and preparations for treatment. Yeats felt his ". . . remarks may be considered as chiefly applicable to children, from 2 to 12 years of age." He believed that the reason that such children are not adequately treated is that symptoms are not diagnosed early and hence treatment is late, leading to bad outcomes. Yeats went to great lengths to emphasize the necessity of early diagnosis. He focused on one part of John Cheyne's monograph on hydrocephalus (47) in which Cheyne declared that the disease is not curable: "... he (Cheyne) has never been so lucky as to cure one patient, who had those symptoms (hydrocephalus) which, with, certainty, denote the 'disease'" (55). Yeats was also concerned that children with "water on the brain" are more susceptible to injury by blows to the head: even trifling blows can lead to severe consequences and should be avoided (56).

Unfortunately, Yeats followed a common theme of the period, namely, that hydrocephalus is associated with disorders of the bowels, as these children commonly had vomiting and constipation. Hence, he recommended purging to remove the "... accumulated diseased load from the intestines by several large evacuations at once" (57). The many evacuations produced by a strong purgative restored a gradual healthy action to the glands of the intestines and the alimentary tract. Yeats' treatment is based on the intestinal tract, purgatives and restoration of alimentary tract to normal function, but not in a violent way. The typical drugs used were mercury and calomel among others. He was emphatic on their use and dosage and was not above insulting those colleagues who would ignore these useful remedies. It is interesting to note at this point the similar treatment by Yeats as advocated by Cheyne above.

Yeats' emphasis on the etiologic importance of bowel dysfunction is captured in his comment on a colleague's work: "The late Dr. Warren, of Taunton, candidly states, that of the ten cases he attended all died, although mercury was used in large quantities, externally and internally; three or four grains of calomel were taken every eight hours, without producing any purgative effect. On opening the head, water was found in the ventricles; and in one case, two ounces of blood were effused on the pia mater. No account of the state of the bowels is given. I have scarcely a doubt, that the treatment of hydrocephalus in this way without the combination of purgatives with calomel, for the reasons already mentioned, would almost uniformly prove fatal" (58).

In addition to purgatives, Yeats readily used leeches or the lancet for bloodletting. In reviewing a typical treatment of hydrocephalus, Yeats described a 13-year-old child sent to him for consultation on hydrocephalus. Yeats described his treatment in the following terms: "This patient was bled from the arm with relief to the acute pain of the head; had also leeches twice to the temples and to the epigastric region, and by the use of saline medicines with mercury till the gums were affected, and the occasional exhibition of active purgatives which the very torpid state of the bowels required, completely recovered (59)."

Yeats also described a case of "an interesting and beautiful little girl of eight years of age, the only surviving child of a fond mother ... I found the little girl ... labouring under much febrile excitement ... with a visible morbid irregularity and protrusion of the vertebrae of the lumbar region and accompanied by a tottering hesitation in her gait when she attempted to walk" (60). He appeared to be describing the case of a child with myelomeningocele and hydrocephalus. He saw the child two years later when she was laboring in the end stages of hydrocephalus; his request for an autopsy was refused.

Yeats "take-home" message was that the child with hydrocephalus who was diagnosed early, properly purged, bled, could survive the disorder. Unfortunately, in his practice he often saw patients too late for adequate treatment. At no point did Yeats discuss any form of surgical intervention. To him hydrocephalus was clearly a disorder of the bowels and a healthy condition of the digestive organs would clearly clear this disease.

The "Sir" to whom Yeats addressed his work was never identified in the text, but Yeats concluded the first volume with the statement "... my recollection those years of my younger days, which I happily spent in study under her sacred and respected groves—*Inter sylvas Academi quarere verum*" I have the honour to be, Dear Sir, With great respect and esteem, Your very faithful and obedient Servant G.D. Yeats" (Figs. 15 and 16).

During this period a number of debates on anatomical studies of CSF pathways were being offered by a number of anatomists and physicians. As noted, Alexander Monro *Secundus* (1733–1817) had accurately described the Foramen of Monro (46). Interestingly although Monro denied the existence of another foramen, that of Magendie. Both Albrecht Haller and Dominco Cotugno were to confirm its existence anatomically. Monro came to his conclusion based on

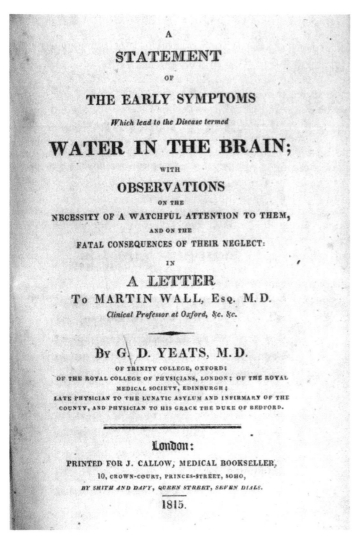

A

STATEMENT

OF

THE EARLY SYMPTOMS

Which lead to the Disease termed

WATER IN THE BRAIN;

WITH

OBSERVATIONS

ON THE

NECESSITY OF A WATCHFUL ATTENTION TO THEM,

AND ON THE

FATAL CONSEQUENCES OF THEIR NEGLECT:

IN

A LETTER

To MARTIN WALL, Esq. M.D.

Clinical Professor at Oxford, &c. &c.

By G. D. YEATS, M.D.

OF TRINITY COLLEGE, OXFORD;
OF THE ROYAL COLLEGE OF PHYSICIANS, LONDON; OF THE ROYAL
MEDICAL SOCIETY, EDINBURGH;
LATE PHYSICIAN TO THE LUNATIC ASYLUM AND INFIRMARY OF THE
COUNTY, AND PHYSICIAN TO HIS GRACE THE DUKE OF BEDFORD.

London:

PRINTED FOR J. CALLOW, MEDICAL BOOKSELLER,
10, CROWN-COURT, PRINCES-STREET, SOHO,
BY SMITH AND DAVY, QUEEN STREET, SEVEN DIALS.

1815.

Figure 15   Title page from Yeats 1815 book (53). (Author's personal collection.)

postmortem examination of a child with hydrocephalus. During the autopsy Monro noted the absence of communication between the fourth ventricle and the spinal subarachnoid space; this space was occluded by the choroid plexus. Reflection suggests that this lack of communication of CSF was the most likely etiology of the hydrocephalus.

Moving further into the 19th century, we begin to see remarkable changes in the understanding of hydrocephalus along with further insights into anatomy and potential surgical intervention. One of the finest pathological atlases on the brain was published in the 19th century and in it are remarkable illustrations and case discussions dealing with hydrocephalus (61). This work was published by Richard Bright (1789–1858), who is best remembered as the discoverer of "Bright's disease," now better known as nephritis. Bright was a physician at Guy's Hospital in London and a leading consultant. Bright's claim to a place in the history of medicine is that he was the first to integrate the clinical course of disease along with a detailed pathological examination plus laboratory testing, including postmortem findings. Bright is best remembered for his studies of kidney disorders, in particular, nephritis. By correlating symptoms with a chemical examination and postmortem findings, Bright transformed "dropsy" into "Bright's disease."

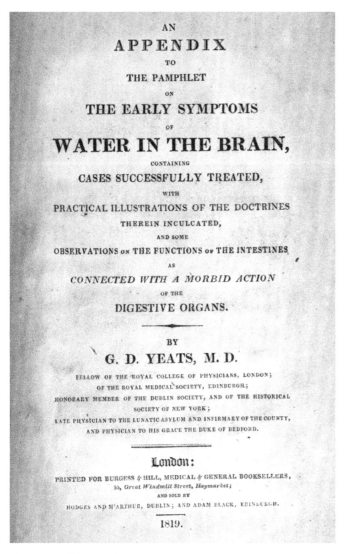

AN

APPENDIX

TO

THE PAMPHLET

ON

THE EARLY SYMPTOMS

OF

WATER IN THE BRAIN,

CONTAINING

CASES SUCCESSFULLY TREATED,

WITH

PRACTICAL ILLUSTRATIONS OF THE DOCTRINES

THEREIN INCULCATED,

AND SOME

OBSERVATIONS ON THE FUNCTIONS OF THE INTESTINES

AS

CONNECTED WITH A MORBID ACTION

OF THE

DIGESTIVE ORGANS.

BY

G. D. YEATS, M. D.

FELLOW OF THE ROYAL COLLEGE OF PHYSICIANS, LONDON;

OF THE ROYAL MEDICAL SOCIETY, EDINBURGH;

HONORARY MEMBER OF THE DUBLIN SOCIETY, AND OF THE HISTORICAL

SOCIETY OF NEW YORK;

LATE PHYSICIAN TO THE LUNATIC ASYLUM AND INFIRMARY OF THE COUNTY,

AND PHYSICIAN TO HIS GRACE THE DUKE OF BEDFORD.

London:

PRINTED FOR BURGESS & HILL, MEDICAL & GENERAL BOOKSELLERS,

55, *Great Windmill Street, Haymarket;*

AND SOLD BY

HODGES AND M'ARTHUR, DUBLIN; AND ADAM BLACK, EDINBURGH.

1819.

Figure 16   Title page from Yeats 1819 book (54). (Author's personal collection.)

Within Bright's reports are other important contributions to general pathology and, germane to this paper, discussions of neuropathology. His two-volume work covers 200 neuropathology cases with detailed descriptions and clinical histories. In his second volume he provides several excellent descriptions of both chronic and congenital hydrocephalus. Along with a clinical description of the cases Bright provided meticulously hand-colored plates showing the pathology; these plates remain some of the best examples of medical illustrations on these subjects to date. Included is a colored plate of a child with a pontine glioma and secondary hydrocephalus. In addition is the famous illustration of a boy with massive hydrocephalus included here.

In his section on "Chronic Hydrocephalus" Bright gives some interesting contemporary discussions of this disorder. He clearly recognized that this was often a prenatal disorder and that not uncommonly the child was delivered with hydrocephalus already present.

"... it not infrequently happens that at the time the foetus is arrived at the period when it should be expelled from the uterus, and even long before that period, a morbid and often a most excessive accumulation of watery fluid takes place within the ventricles of the brain: this sometimes goes to an extent which prevents the possibility of the birth of the child,

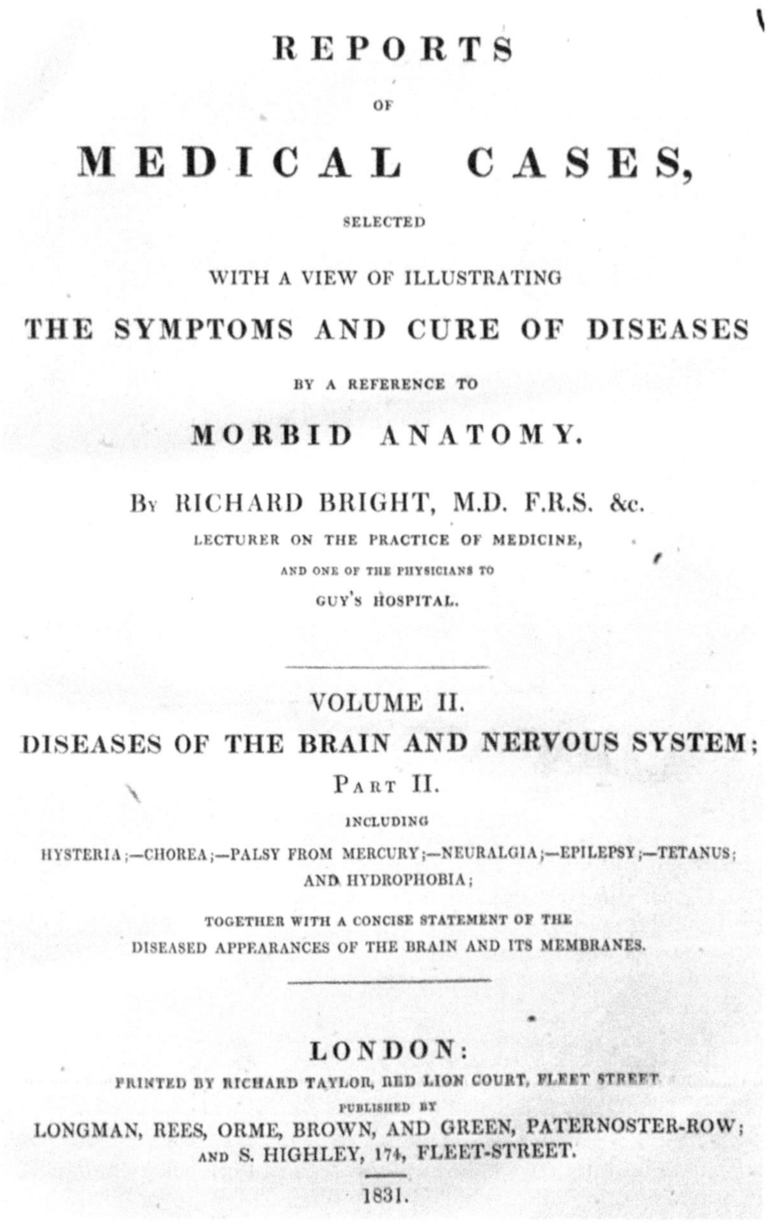

REPORTS

OF

MEDICAL CASES,

SELECTED

WITH A VIEW OF ILLUSTRATING

THE SYMPTOMS AND CURE OF DISEASES

BY A REFERENCE TO

MORBID ANATOMY.

By RICHARD BRIGHT, M.D. F.R.S. &c.

LECTURER ON THE PRACTICE OF MEDICINE,

AND ONE OF THE PHYSICIANS TO

GUY'S HOSPITAL.

VOLUME II.

DISEASES OF THE BRAIN AND NERVOUS SYSTEM;

PART II.

INCLUDING

HYSTERIA;—CHOREA;—PALSY FROM MERCURY;—NEURALGIA;—EPILEPSY;—TETANUS;
AND HYDROPHOBIA;

TOGETHER WITH A CONCISE STATEMENT OF THE
DISEASED APPEARANCES OF THE BRAIN AND ITS MEMBRANES.

LONDON:

PRINTED BY RICHARD TAYLOR, RED LION COURT, FLEET STREET.

PUBLISHED BY

LONGMAN, REES, ORME, BROWN, AND GREEN, PATERNOSTER-ROW;
AND S. HIGHLEY, 174, FLEET-STREET.

1831.

Figure 17   Title page of Volume 2 of Bright's volume on neuropathology. (Author's personal collection.)

and it becomes necessary to draw off the water before the head can pass from the pelvis. At other times the child is born with the head not at all, or very slightly, disproportioned to the body; but in a few days or weeks, perhaps not till a few months have passed, it is perceived to increase beyond the unusual ratio: it becomes deformed; the two frontal bones, instead of falling gently backward from the eyebrows, generally assume a perpendicular or even a projecting position... the head becomes distorted, and the sutures so separated, that a space of two or three inches often intervenes between the bones. Sometimes at birth, and sometimes within a few weeks after, the sight is lost, though the hearing generally remains acute . . . ."

Bright went on to describe continued detorioration with loss of mental and motor skills among other findings (62).

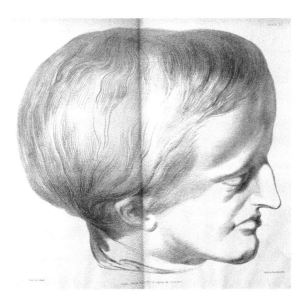

Figure 18 Bright's famous case of James Cardinal—illustrated here with his massive head and hydrocephalus. (Author's personal collection.)

Bright discussed both medical and surgical treatment of hydrocephalus. He discussed a case in the former group, that of a Dr. Traill of Liverpool (from Baillie's *Morbid Anatomy of the Human Body*) that involved cure of hydrocephalus (63). The patient was a child of 18 months with an enormous head, strabismus, and frequent convulsions. A mercurial liniment was applied to the head daily, and the bowels were purged "briskly" with calomel along with other cathartics. This was done for a month and the child was subsequently cured of his hydrocephalus—"the child was seen in perfect health of mind and body, though the head continued rather large" (64). When discussing surgical options for the treatment of hydrocephalus, the prevalent view all that was available was puncture of the ventricles. Bright commented, "One question which arises with regard to treatment is, the propriety of removing the fluid from the brain by puncture. . . .Hopeless as this appears, it is in general almost the only chance remaining; and the alternative being to suffer mental and bodily imbecility for the whole of life, or to risk a more speedy death in the hope of relief, it is plain to which side our duty and inclination would prompt us, if but a reasonable prospect of success could be established" (64). In effect computing a risk–benefit ratio here, Bright clearly held that it favored surgical treatment, although he was clear that the outcome was not always good—but then what else was there to offer!

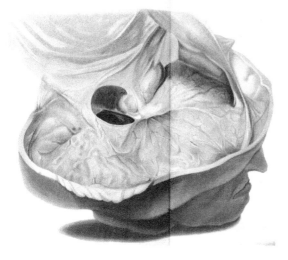

Figure 19 The postmortem examination of James Cardinal in a wonderful hand-colored illustration, showing the massive hydrocephalus found by Bright. (Author's personal collection.)

One of the most cited cases on hydrocephalus from this era was Bright's case of a boy name James Cardinal. The case was entitled: "Chronic Hydrocephalus from Childhood, in an Adult, Ossification complete, Intellect moderate." "James Cardinal, aged 29, was admitted to Guy's Hospital, under the care of Sir Astley Cooper, December 1, 1824. He was the subject of chronic hydrocephalus to a very marked degree, and had lately been in St. Thomas's Hospital for several months, under the care of Mr. Green; his case, however, admitting of little medical and no surgical aid, had been dismissed. His general appearance was very remarkable, from the extraordinary disproportion between his head and the other parts of his body; for he was well-formed, and nearly of the middle stature, but his head was at least twice the size which his spare body would lead us to expect" (65). At birth the head was normal and then rapidly started to grow and continued to do so until the child was about five years of age at which point the growth stopped. He did not begin walking until six years of age and then could not run, as he would fall. He attended school but was not a particularly good student but did learn to read and write. An interesting finding reported by Bright was the following: "If a candle was held behind his head, or the sun happened to be behind it, the cranium appeared semitransparent; and this more or less evident till he attained his fourteenth year." (66). He developed a seizure disorder around the age of 23. The bones and anterior fontanelle did not finally close and ossify until well into adulthood. At the time of admission, he was walking, cognition good, his taste perfect but he was near-sighted. His memory was tolerable but he did not remember dates or events that well. Bright commented that "There was something childish and irritable in his manner, and he was easily provoked. He was stated not to have sexual desires, but he was fond of society, and affectionate to his mother" (66). During his admission to Guy's Hospital he seemed to be doing well for a few weeks. But then he developed a cold, and febrile symptoms arose. He lost his appetite entirely, becoming increasingly feeble, and died on February 24, 1825. Figures 17 to 19 illustrates Bright's famous case of James Cardinal.

In a later section Bright provided the earliest pathological description of a pontine glioma with secondary hydrocephalus. He described a "tumour of the Pons Varolii" in which there was morbid enlargement of that Pons structure involving the third, fourth, fifth, sixth, seventh, and eighth pair of nerves, all of which were soft and somewhat indistinctly seen" (Figs. 20 and 21). In these figures he clearly showed the distorted pons with diffuse infiltration of tumor, most likely a low-grade astrocytoma. Secondary obstruction of the aqueduct leads to hydrocephalus. Bright's pathological discussion describes only gross characteristics. The concept that this might be a tumor infiltrating the pons is interestingly not entertained by Bright, nor is the additional premise that the glioma caused the hydrocephalus secondary to obstruction considered—both concepts escaped Bright but nevertheless the illustrations are most elegant and are among the best in the historical literature.

Along with elegant and accurate anatomical drawings, the 19th century gave occasion for skilled physicians and scientists to explore both the etiology of hydrocephalus and its surgical treatment. Among the leaders was François Magendie (1783–1855), one of France's finest anatomists and physiologists and the first to use the term "cerebrospinal fluid." To Magendie we owe final clarification of an important CSF anatomical pathway, that is, the foramen of Magendie.

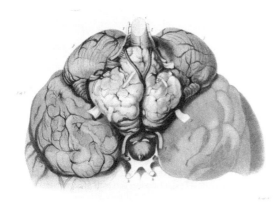

Figure 20 Bright provided elegant illustrations of a case of a pontine glioma—tumor of the Pons Varolii. Secondary obstructive hydrocephalus is also described. (Author's personal collection.)

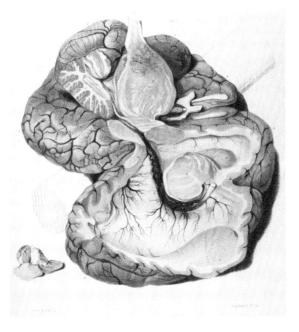

Figure 21 In this illustrations, we see Bright's tumour of the Pons Varolii—the pons has been sagittally sectioned, showing the swollen diffuse tumor, most likely a low-grade pontine glioma. (Author's personal collection.)

In a classic monograph entitled *Recherches Physiologiques et Cliniques sur le Liquide Céphalo-Rachidien ou Cérébrospinal* (Paris, 1842), Magendie brought forth a number of new and more accurate concepts of CSF circulation and its anatomical pathways (67,68). Although Magendie described the foramen that bears his name, it was Herbert von Luschka (1820–1875), Professor of Anatomy at Tübingen, who in 1854, in a series of animals studies, clearly documented its existence and named it after Magendie (69). These anatomical findings were later supported by the work of John Hilton (1804–1878), a Guy's Hospital physician who provided the first anatomical drawings of these pathways and showed that internal hydrocephalus could occur secondary to obstruction along these CSF pathways—this last a most remarkable advance in the understanding of hydrocephalus (70).

Below is Magendie's description of cerebral spinal fluid along with the anatomical description of what we now call the foramen of Magendie. Below we have reproduced 6 of the 11 observations that Magendie made on CSF (71):

Excerpt pp. 79–80
From facts and experiments reported in the three parts of this Memoir; I have deduced the following conclusions:

1. The cerebrospinal fluid is one of the natural fluids of the body and henceforth because of its uses it must be given first place in a list of these fluids.
2. It is indispensable to the free exercise of the functions of the brain and the spinal cord.
3. It protects these parts from external injuries.
4. It influences the functions of the brain and the spinal cord by the pressure that it transmits to these parts, by its temperature, and by its chemical nature.
5. At the base of the fourth ventricle opposite to the calamus scriptorius there is a constant opening which permits an easy communication between the cavities of the brain and the cerebrospinal fluid [i.e., what we now call the "foramen of Magendie"].
6. The ventricles are constantly full of this fluid. These cavities can contain two ounces of it without there being any defect of intellectual faculties; beyond that quantity there is a disturbance [of them], ordinarily a paralysis of movement and more or less decrease of intelligence.

With Magendie's studies we now have the first conclusive demonstration of CSF, its characteristics and physiological properties—a landmark advance toward the eventual treatment of hydrocephalus.

Magendie made a number of other important contributions to the understanding of the etiologies of hydrocephalus. In studies using an animal model of the condition, Magendie went onto demonstrated in living subjects that the ventricles and the subarachnoid space were filled with a watery fluid that communicates freely between the ventricles and the spinal subarachnoid space via the foramen of Magendie, an important concept in understanding obstructive hydrocephalus. Understanding this concept, Magendie described cases of hydrocephalus secondary to obstruction at the aqueduct of Sylvius and the foramen of Magendie. In an autopsy, he found a puerperal thrombosis that led to a thrombosis of the Vein of Galen and dural sinuses, all resulting in hydrocephalus. Magendie added the postulate that hydrocephalus occurred because of reduced absorption of CSF secondary to venous obstruction (67,68). However, Magendie was not always without error: he proposed that CSF is produced by the pia mater, a view that continued to be asserted by other contemporary and later authors, including Lewandowsky (72), Spina (73), and Schmorl (74), well into the 20th century. Max Lewandowsky (1876–1918) of Berlin declared that CSF was primarily a brain secretion of which only a small portion was produced by the pia. Spina argued that CSF was a transudation product of brain capillaries as well as of the pia. Georg Schmorl stated that CSF was formed both by the ventricles and by the pia. Interestingly, he believed there was no anatomic communication between the ventricles and the spinal subarachnoid space.

It was not until the publication by Walter Dandy (1886–1946) and Kenneth D. Blackfan (1883–1941) of their classic study of 1914 using a series of artificial blockages in dogs and phenolsulphonephthalein dye that the true pathways of communication were conclusively established (75). Equally important, Dandy and Blackfan demonstrated how blockage of the pathways at one or another site caused the various forms of hydrocephalus, resolving the centuries-old dispute (76).

Following on Magendie's studies came the conclusive investigations of CSF circulation by two Swedish investigators—Gustaf Magnus Retzius (1842–1919) and Axel Key (1832–1901) (77). While working at the Karolinska Institute, these authors completed one of the most complete investigations of CSF and presented it in their classic monograph of 1875–1876 (77). This massive two-volume folio set still remains one of the most beautifully executed and colored neuroanatomical atlases of any anatomical subject. Key and Retzius injected dye in a series of experiments and traced the CSF pathways within the subarachnoid membranes and cavities of the brain and the spinal cord. Through these experiments they further confirmed the anatomical existence of the foramens of Magendie and Luschka. With their dye studies they followed the CSF as it circulated and then passed into the Pacchionian bodies and subsequently into the cerebral venous sinuses. With these studies Key and Retzius provided the first scientific documentation of CSF pathways—a truly seminal investigative work (77) (Fig. 22).

Some final thoughts on the origin and nature of hydrocephalus, that is, what was the source of CSF as viewed by the 19th and early 20th-century anatomists and physiologists? The concept that it is the choroid plexus that produces CSF was recognized as early as 1854, when Ernest Faivre (1827–1879) published his findings on CSF production (78,79). However, this view was not readily accepted by all. William Mestrezat (1883–1928), as late as 1912, proposed that the choroid plexus is not a glandular structure and does not secrete CSF (80). Nevertheless, the secretory activity of the choroid plexus was finally established by the anatomical studies of Dixon and Halliburton (81), Weed (82–85), and Cushing (86,87). The further insight that CSF is produced by both glandular secretion and filtration was established by Dandy and Blackfan, who were to go on to revolutionize the concept of hydrocephalus and its surgical treatment. This concept was refined in the classic studies summarized in Cushing's Cameron Lectures given in 1925 on the "Third Circulation" (88). In this work (as well as in earlier papers), Cushing clarified the active secretion of CSF by the choroid plexus and other details of this so-called third circulation.

In reviewing the history of hydrocephalus, it is interesting and at the same time puzzling to take note of the various medical treatments introduced over the centuries. As we have seen, treating physicians applied external vesicants, leeches, aperients, cathartics, and caustics and let blood. Laxatives and medicines for the treatment of "dropsy" were also widely used (a common misconception was that hydrocephalus represented an excessive fluid collection). A popular 18th century physician, William Buchan (1729–1805), advocated the use of sneezing

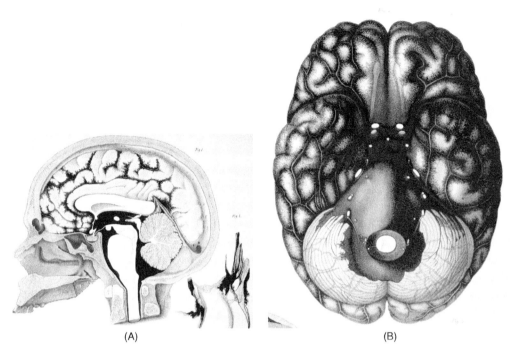

(A) (B)

Figure 22 (**A, B**) Two plates from Key and Retizus' classic work illustrating CSF circulation and foramen of Magendie. Using a blue dye they traced out the CSF pathways through the subarachnoid spaces, pathways via the ventricular system, and then reabsorption over the convexity through the sagittal sinus and the Pacchionian granulations. (Author's personal collection.)

agents (e.g., asafetida) (89). Hearty sneezing would cause the "pituita" or accumulation of fluid in the brain to be discharged through the nose—although the treatment might seem extreme, it was certainly less lethal than the surgical application of the trephine to the anterior fontanelle, a technique commonly advocated by our surgical colleagues.

Having discussed many of the ineffective medical treatments of hydrocephalus, it is time to move on to treatment by our adventurous surgical brethren.

SURGICAL TREATMENT OF HYDROCEPHALUS

> Except for cases that cure themselves, i.e., those that undergo spontaneous arrest, the outlook is almost hopeless. The majority die within the first four years of life, the first year claiming most of them . . .. At the present time, even the best-intentioned surgery can hardly serve other than to delay to some few cases the possibility of a spontaneous recovery by subjecting them to an operation and a surgical death (90).

When Paul Bucy wrote the above statement in 1932 in a textbook on pediatrics, there was virtually no effective surgical treatment of hydrocephalus. Even so it is of interest to consider what some of our surgical colleagues have attempted over the centuries in searching for a "surgical cure" of hydrocephalus. A common and standard technique for draining CSF was the use of trocars of various types introduced by a stabbing technique into the lateral ventricle via the anterior fontanelle. In a variation on this theme an adventurous Italian surgeon, Dominico Galvani (d. 1649), developed an ingenious drainage system to which he added his trocar system; this was developed in 1620. This drainage system included a device to hold the drainage tube in place and various receptacles for collecting CSF. A specially designed trocar was used to place the drain, and a cap served to prevent entry of air into the ventricles (91). Unfortunately, because of either over drainage or sepsis the outcome was death. Another trocar-type system was developed by Claude Nicholas LeCat (1700–1768) and described in the *Philosophical Transactions of the Royal Society (London)* in 1753. Mr. LeCat included an illustration of a child with severe

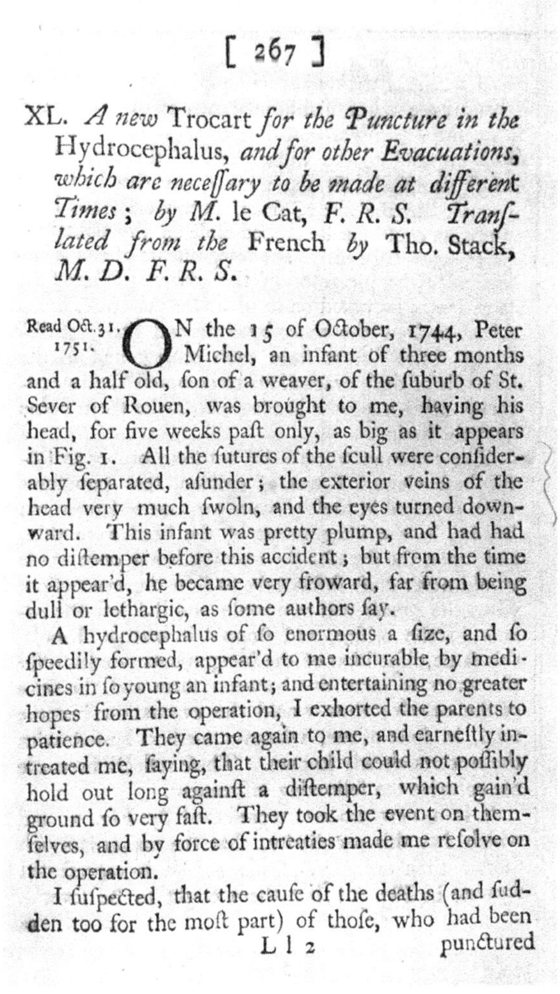

[267]

XL. *A new* Trocart *for the* Puncture *in the*
Hydrocephalus, *and for other Evacuations,*
which are necessary to be made at different
Times ; *by M.* le Cat, F. R. S. *Trans-*
lated from the French *by* Tho. Stack,
M. D. F. R. S.

Read Oct. 31, ON the 15 of October, 1744, Peter
1751. Michel, an infant of three months
and a half old, son of a weaver, of the suburb of St.
Sever of Rouen, was brought to me, having his
head, for five weeks past only, as big as it appears
in Fig. 1. All the futures of the scull were considerably separated, asunder; the exterior veins of the
head very much swoln, and the eyes turned downward. This infant was pretty plump, and had had
no distemper before this accident; but from the time
it appear'd, he became very froward, far from being
dull or lethargic, as some authors say.
    A hydrocephalus of so enormous a size, and so
speedily formed, appear'd to me incurable by medicines in so young an infant; and entertaining no greater
hopes from the operation, I exhorted the parents to
patience. They came again to me, and earnestly in-
treated me, saying, that their child could not possibly
hold out long against a distemper, which gain'd
ground so very fast. They took the event on themselves, and by force of intreaties made me resolve on
the operation.
    I suspected, that the cause of the deaths (and sud-
den too for the most part) of those, who had been
                    L l 2   punctured

Figure 23 Title page from the 1753 paper
by Mr. LeCat—a new trocar for the treatment of hydrocephalus (92). (Author's personal
collection.)

hydrocephalus (92). In the illustration are several of LeCat's trocars. He noted that his outcomes
were dismal and that the mortality rate eventually reached 100%, but nevertheless he felt this a
useful surgical design for treating hydrocephalus (Figs. 23 and 24).

In looking for surgical treatments of hydrocephalus, we reviewed the writings of Pierre
Dionis (1645–1718), a prominent 18th-century French surgeon and anatomist who practiced
in Paris. Dionis was appointed the first surgeon to Queen Maria Theresa. Later Louis XIV
established a demonstratorship in operative surgery at the Jardin in Paris and appointed Dionis
as the first holder of that position; he also became the surgeon to the King and the royal family.
Among his important publications was "A Course of Chirurgical Operations Demonstrated in
the Royal Gardens at Paris" (93), a popular and widely used 18th-century surgical handbook
eventually translated into several languages. Dionis' superb knowledge of anatomy, upon which
he heavily relied, contributed significantly to his skills as a surgeon. In an English edition of his
surgical handbook, Dionis discussed his views on hydrocephalus.

"The Etymology of the Hydrocephalum proceeds from *Hydro* Water, and *Cephale* which
signifies a Head; so that 'tis a sort of *Dropsie*, with which the Head is so full of Water; that
'tis perfectly inundated (94)." He went on to describe the two classic forms of hydrocephalus
following the ancient classification of "external" and "internal" (95; text, spelling and syntax has
been copied exactly as printed.) Dionis carried forward a common theme from antiquity, namely,
that a common cause of hydrocephalus is due to head molding by the midwives shortly after
birth, a practice which he denounced. For external hydrocephalus, Dionis suggests the surgeon

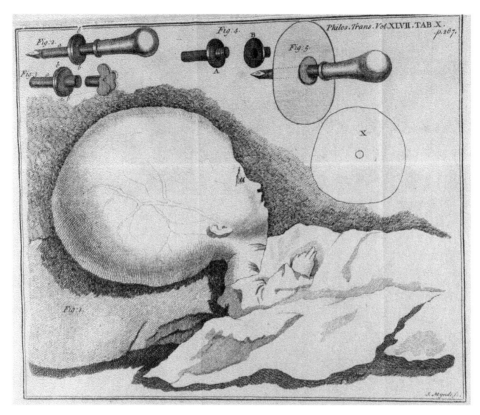

Figure 24 Illustration of the trocar system for treating hydrocephalus—by LeCat, 1753 (92). (Author's personal collection.)

make several cuts between the skin and the pericranium to relieve the fluid accumulated—but having said that, he declares that he has never seen a case of "external" hydrocephalus. As to "internal" hydrocephalus, he believes that this is a disease that is "incurable." Nevertheless, Dionis wrote that for treatment of this type, he preferred to use the trepan, the only treatment available. Included in his surgical handbook is an illustration of the instruments he used for trepanning. The surgical view of the treatment of internal hydrocephalus here reveals an ancient treatment dating back to the Greeks—little if any progress in over 2000 years (Figs. 25 and 26).

We remember Alexander Monro's *Secundus* for his remarkable works on anatomy and hydrocephalus. Not appreciated by many readers today were his surgical efforts directed toward the treatment of children with hydrocephalus. Monro was an advocate for surgical drainage of CSF through a trocar: following the earlier Hippocratic doctrine, this was only to be attempted in cases of "external hydrocephalus"; otherwise, Monro declared, the outcome was invariably lethal (95). The use of trocars often proved to be fatal, as the only outcome of such treatment would likely have been death caused by sepsis and meningitis.

With the introduction of asepsis techniques in the post-Listerian era (ca 1870s), the use of the trocar was again resurrected as a surgical treatment for hydrocephalus (Figs. 27–29). A popular advocate employing a trocar was Antoine Chipault (1866–1920), a prominent French surgeon. Interestingly, one of Chipault's surgical techniques (1894) required the trocar to be placed into the ventricle via the nose (96). Unfortunately, Chipault did not detail his outcomes, so we do not have long-term follow-ups, but one may assume the results were not good considering some of the anatomical structures that might lay in the path of that trocar. Following a different theme, Langenbeck and Hahn (97) introduced an innovative technique in which the trocar was passed through the orbital roof into the ventricle, a surgical approach later popularized in the frontal lobotomy. Despite the "improved technique" unfortunately they reported the mortality at 100%.

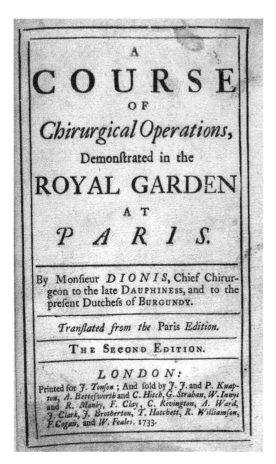

Figure 25 Title page from Dionis' textbook of surgical techniques (93). (Author's personal collection.)

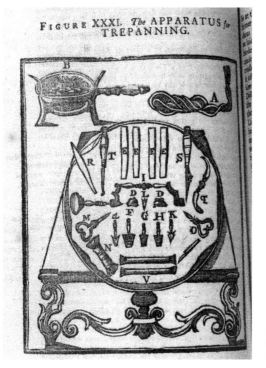

Figure 26 From Dionis' surgical textbook showing the surgical instruments he used for performing a trephination (93). (Author's personal collection.)

In the later half of the 19th century and the early part of the 20th century, a number of new approaches were devised for the surgical treatment of hydrocphalus. In 1891, Heinrich Quincke (1842–1922) introduced the lumbar puncture, thus offering one of the earliest modern methods for reducing CSF fluid accumulation, but the results were temporary at best. Quincke showed that CSF was constantly being produced, so the removed fluid was replaced in a matter of hours (98–99) (Figs. 30–31). The son of a distinguished physician, Quincke is remembered as a figure who stood straight and was always groomed to perfection. He rode his horse in a crisp, typical English style—characteristics that match his meticulous approach to science, his studies of the CNS. His personality was described by biographers as pedantic, at times obstreperous and confrontational in arguments (100). Quincke trained in medicine in Berlin and was exposed to some of the scientific giants of the period including Rudolph Virchow,

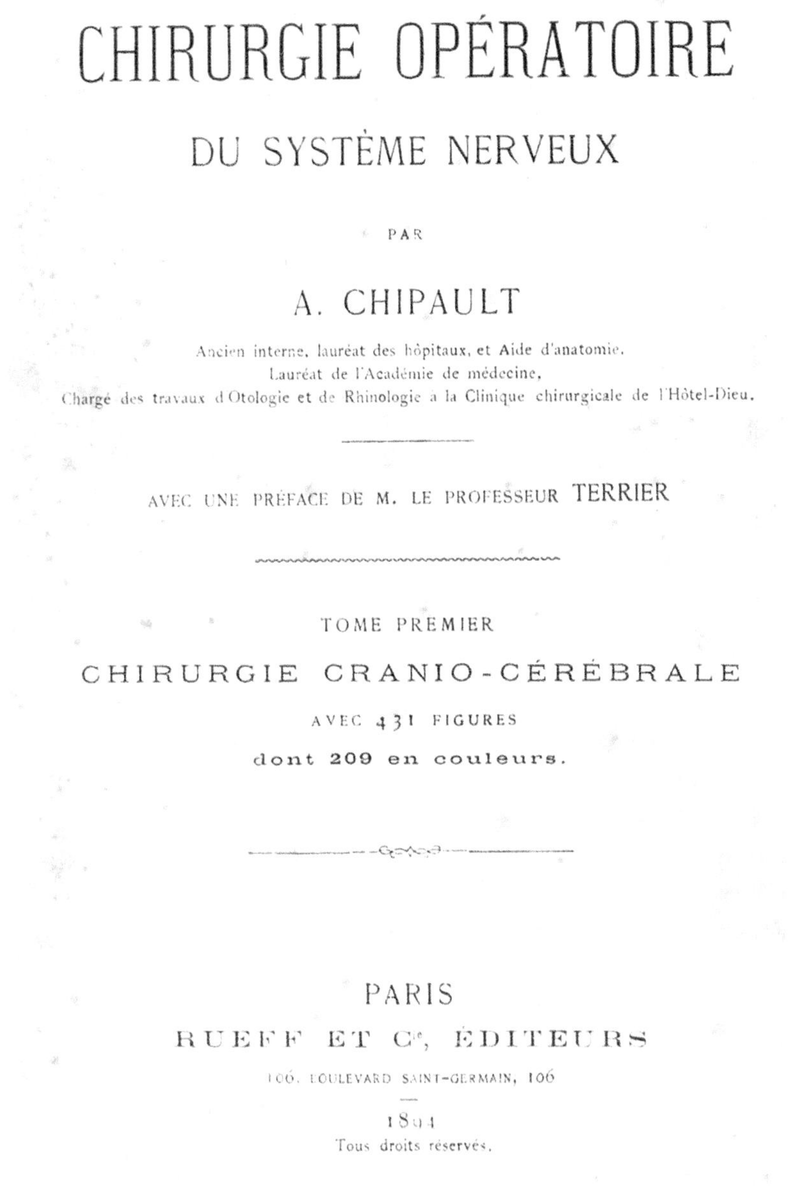

CHIRURGIE OPÉRATOIRE

DU SYSTÈME NERVEUX

PAR

A. CHIPAULT

Ancien interne, lauréat des hôpitaux, et Aide d'anatomie.
Lauréat de l'Académie de médecine,
Chargé des travaux d'Otologie et de Rhinologie à la Clinique chirurgicale de l'Hôtel-Dieu.

AVEC UNE PRÉFACE DE M. LE PROFESSEUR TERRIER

TOME PREMIER

CHIRURGIE CRANIO-CÉRÉBRALE

AVEC 431 FIGURES

dont 209 en couleurs.

PARIS

RUEFF ET Cⁱᵉ, ÉDITEURS

106, BOULEVARD SAINT-GERMAIN, 106

1894

Tous droits réservés.

Figure 27 Title page from Chipault's textbook on surgery (96). (Author's personal collection.)

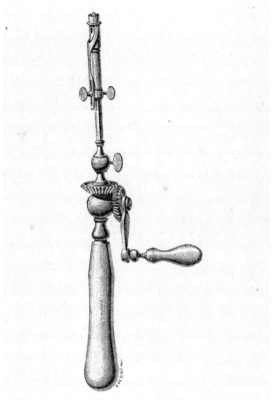

Fig. 425. — Tréphine à main, puur pratiquer la trépanation cranienne
dans l'hydrocéphalie.

Figure 28 Illustration of Chipault's hand-driven drill or trephine for the treatment of hydrocephalus (96, p. 718). (Author's personal collection.)

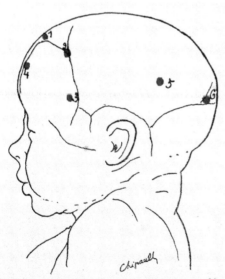

Fig. 426. — Points choisis par les divers opérateurs pour faire la ponction
ventriculaire dans l'hydrocéphalie.

Figure 29 Drawing from Chipault's textbook on surgery in which he marked out what he felt were safe points to do ventricular punctures for hydrocephalus. The instrument he designed to do the trephinations is illustrated in Figure 28. (Author's personal collection.)

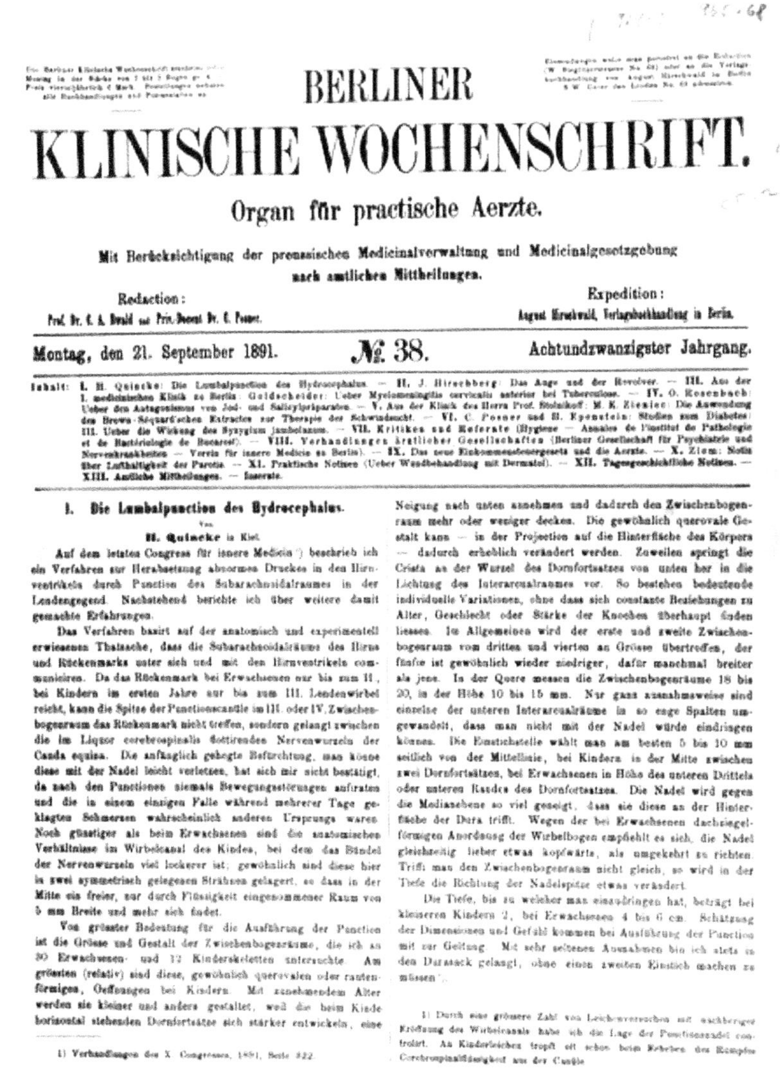

Figure 30 Quincke's paper on hydrocephalus (66). (Author's personal collection.)

Rudolph Albert von Kölliker, and Herman Helmholtz among others. Among his studies was a description of a clinical syndrome that still bears his name—angioneurotic edema. Quincke came to develop the spinal puncture while looking for the least harmful, simple way to treat hydrocephalus. He believed that part of the disease process was that the increasing pressure in hydrocephalus compressed the pacchionian granulations and blocked CSF absorption. He postulated that by removing CSF one could break the vicious cycle of overproduction and under-resorption. He began his studies using red sulfide of mercury injected into the lumbar subarachnoid space. He quickly recognized that the procedure was not only safe but could be used for both therapeutic and diagnostic purposes. He modified the technique by moving the needle back and forth in the space between the skin and the dura in an attempt to make a fistula track for CSF drainage and diversion. Quincke felt this provided for a slower and more steady absorption of CSF. He went on to withdraw CSF from the lateral ventricles in each of the two children with hydrocephalus. Interestingly, some 25 years later, Walter Dandy was to puncture the ventricle and, working with Kenneth Blackfan, developed pneumonencephalography; one wonders what influence Quincke might have had on Dandy and Blackfan (75).

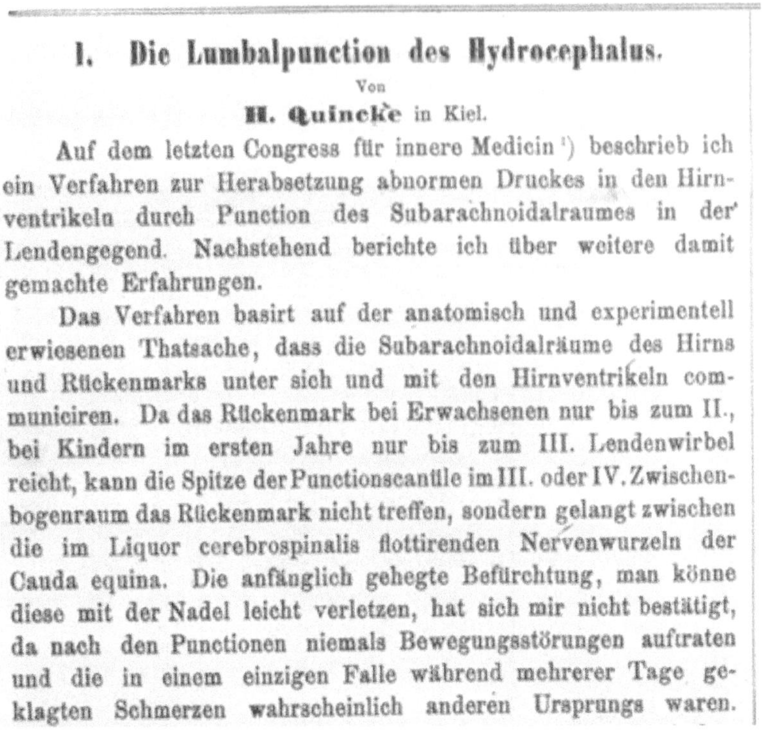

I. Die Lumbalpunction des Hydrocephalus.

Von

H. Quincke in Kiel.

Auf dem letzten Congress für innere Medicin [1]) beschrieb ich
ein Verfahren zur Herabsetzung abnormen Druckes in den Hirnventrikeln durch Punction des Subarachnoidalraumes in der'
Lendengegend. Nachstehend berichte ich über weitere damit
gemachte Erfahrungen.

Das Verfahren basirt auf der anatomisch und experimentell
erwiesenen Thatsache, dass die Subarachnoidalräume des Hirns
und Rückenmarks unter sich und mit den Hirnventrikeln com-
municiren. Da das Rückenmark bei Erwachsenen nur bis zum II.,
bei Kindern im ersten Jahre nur bis zum III. Lendenwirbel
reicht, kann die Spitze der Punctionscantüle im III. oder IV. Zwischen-
bogenraum das Rückenmark nicht treffen, sondern gelangt zwischen
die im Liquor cerebrospinalis flottirenden Nervenwurzeln der
Cauda equina. Die anfänglich gehegte Befürchtung, man könne
diese mit der Nadel leicht verletzen, hat sich mir nicht bestätigt,
da nach den Punctionen niemals Bewegungsstörungen auftraten
und die in einem einzigen Falle während mehrerer Tage ge-
klagten Schmerzen wahrscheinlich anderen Ursprungs waren.

Figure 31 Quincke's description of the lumbar puncture technique in hydrocephalus. (Author's personal collection.)

Other innovative techniques have been introduced by surgeons for the treatment of hydrocephalus. In reviewing these developments, there are two principal questions to follow: the
neurosurgical procedure to be performed on the brain, and what is to be done with excess CSF.
Addressing the latter thread first, the concept of moving CSF fluid from one anatomic space to
another was tackled by A.H. Ferguson (1853–1912) in 1898, when he described a technique for
connecting the lumbar thecal sac to the peritoneal cavity by a wire passed through a vertebral
body (101). Following on Ferguson's concept, Heile in 1908, devised a technique whereby he
anastomosed the lumbar thecal sac to the greater omentum with a vein graft (102). Kanusch
proposed a technique in 1908 for draining CSF into the subaponeurotic space of the scalp, a
technique still in use today by some surgeons (103). Presenting a variation on this last theme,
Sutherland and Cheyne published two cases of successful treatment of hydrocephalus. In two
infants with severe chronic hydrocephalus, the surgical technique involved forming a fine weave
from 16 fine strands of 2-inch long catgut. The woven catgut was placed in the ventricle on one
side with the other end in the subdural space. In both cases, they reported excellent results with
collapse of the ventricles and overriding sutures (104).

Early in the 20th century investigators proposed draining CSF from the ventricles into
neck veins as an additional form of treatment for hydrocephalus (105,106). Another diversion
scheme was devised in 1925 by Heile, namely, the lumbar ureteral shunt (107). This technique
was modified by Donald Matson in 1949 (108), who placed polyethylene tubes in the lumbar
subarachnoid space and "tunnelled" them into the peritoneal cavity. Although not commonly
used for the treatment of hydrocephalus now, this technique is still commonly used in the
treatment of pseudotumor cerebri. The literature makes it clear that virtually every potential
anatomical space has now been used for diversion of CSF from the ventricles to the chest, ureter,
fallopian tubes, mastoid cells, jejunum, various veins, gallbladder, and the like.

In an effort to find an internal technique for diverting CSF, Arne Torkildsen introduced the
ventriculocisternostomy (109). The technique, reported in 1939, was a simple one: placement

of a catheter into the lateral ventricle, followed by tunneling down to the neck, and placement into the cisterna magna or under C1. Torkildsen's technique initially proved to be effective for bypassing a stenosis of the aqueduct or a midline tumor, but as diversion shunts became more popular, it has fallen out of favor.

A number of other diversion techniques have been advocated over the years. Gardner had suggested, as early as 1895, that hydrocephalus could be treated by creating a communication between the lateral ventricle and the lymphatic or venous system (110). The concept was good one but continuous clotting of the communicating tube made it impractical. The clotting problem was finally remedied by Nulsen and Spitz in 1951 when they treated a 14-month-old child with a ball-valve-regulated subcutaneous system (111). This system was designed and further refined with the input of an engineer and a neurosurgeon. Holter, an engineer, and Spitz, a neurosurgeon, introduced the Spitz–Holter valve, a unilateral valve-regulated ventriculocaval CSF flow diversion system (112). To appreciate the importance of such diversion shunt systems, one only has to look at the results achieved with them. The systems not only worked but there was also a significant reduction in mortality, something surgeons had not been able to accomplish in the previous 3000 years. Spitz of the Children's Hospital of Philadelphia summarized his results in over 400 patients by using the Holter system (113): only 15 deaths with reduction of the shunt revision rate from a high of 37% to 22%, an incredible improvement over previous techniques.

Turning now to the first thread, the neurosurgical procedure: According to Loyal Davis, the first "plexectomy," that is, the removal of choroid plexus to treat hydrocephalus, was performed by V.L. Lespinasse in 1910 in Chicago when he introduced a small cystoscope into the ventricle and fulgurated the structure bilaterally (114). One infant died postoperatively and the other lived for five years. Regrettably these cases were reported only in the form of a presentation at a local medical society meeting and have never been published. But it is to Lespinasse that we owe the introduction of this endoscopy technique.

In understanding hydrocephalus, its various etiologies and early treatment, we must examine the fundamental studies of Dandy and his colleagues. Without these key studies, done in the early part of the 20th century, we would lack the fundamental understanding of what hydrocephalus is and even how to treat it (115–119). The anatomical and physiological results of Dandy's work are beyond the scope of this chapter, but the reader is encouraged to become familiar with the relevant literature, as it is key to understanding the modern development of neurosurgery. Following up on Lespinasse's original contribution, Dandy, Putnam, Scarff, and others initially advocated the removal of the choroid plexus by an endoscopic resection for treating of hydrocephalus (120–127). Dandy refined this technique by converting the operation into an open procedure, thereby exposing the ventricle, removing the CSF, and then fulgurating the choroid plexus (128). Dandy moved to the open technique because of the extensive debris left behind by the endoscopic approach, which not only obstructed the surgical view but also sometimes led to blockage of the foramen of Monro or the aqueduct of Sylvius.

Dandy, always progressive and looking for innovative techniques, developed several other surgical treatments for hydrocephalus. In addition to obliteration of the choroid plexus, he devised a technique for cannulation of the aqueduct of Sylvius along with the third ventriculostomy (128). Both treatments were developed in the hope of correcting newly understood abnormalities in pathways of CSF flow. By the end of the 1940s the plexectomy had become the primary treatment of choice for hydrocephalus (129).

The third ventriculostomy, popularized by Dandy in 1922, had one serious disadvantage—the sacrifice of an optic nerve when a transtemporal approach was followed. It was not until 1945 that Dandy reported his results in 92 cases: 12% mortality and 50% success in arresting hydrocephalus with follow-up ranging from 6 months to 23 years (128). In an effort to improve surgical results, Scarff and Stookey modified the third ventriculostomy by taking a transfrontal approach and puncturing the floor of the third ventricle via the lamina terminalis (127). These surgeons reported on six cases with one operative death, one failure to arrest the hydrocephalus, and four good results. The success of this technique was such that by 1951 Scarff was able to report on the follow-up of 34 cases with operative mortality of 12% and arrest of hydrocephalus in 54% (125). Putnam, another early advocate of choroid "plexectomy," also reported remarkable results: 49 operations in 26 patients with 10 operative deaths, a strikingly high number, and yet surviving patients appeared to do well and had normal mentation (121). De Martel and others reported on a single case of a subfrontal third ventriculostomy with relief of an obstructive hydrocephalus at a meeting of the Société de Neurologie de Paris in 1936 (130).

By the mid-1950s the ventriculopleural shunt was becoming the mainstay for the treatment of hydrocephalus. In 1954, Ransohoff described his experience of using it in six patients. The results of this technique were quite acceptable with no morbidity and success in diverting CSF to the pleural space (131). Ransohoff and his colleagues followed this study in 1960 with a report of 83 patients with a 4% operative mortality and 65% success rate in controlling hydrocephalus (132).

CONCLUSIONS

Hydrocephalus, this review suggests, is one of those clinical disorders that remained surgical stagnant for centuries. From the time of Hippocrates to the late 19th century, treatment of hydrocephalus remained in the hands of physicians using cathartics, purges, laxatives, and other treatments. Such treatment rarely worked and most patients so treated died either from the disease or as a result of the treatment. Our surgical brethren offered nothing better, as trepanning invariably led to the patient's death. It was not until the end of the 19th century, with the introduction of antiseptic techniques and a better understanding of the anatomy and physiology of hydrocephalus, that surgeons began to offer effective treatment. Among the first truly long-term treatments for hydrocephalus were regulated one-way valve systems. These internalized systems, allowed for the first time a truly successful treatment of a benign disease, a disease that previously had a very high morbidity and mortality. With the excellent 19th century anatomical and physiological studies of CSF, a group of inventive and adventurous surgeons led the development of successful surgical treatments for the management of hydrocephalus. As a result of their work, hydrocephalus can be considered a "benign" and "treatable" disorder.

REFERENCES

1. Davidoff LM. Treatment of hydrocephalus. Arch Surg 1929; 18:1737–1762.
2. von Winning H. Portrayal of Pathological Symptoms in Pre-Columbian Mexico. Springfield, IL: Pearson Museum, Southern Illinois University School of Medicine, 1987.
3. Hippocrates. The Genuine Works of Hippocrates. Translated from the Greek by Francis Adams with a preliminary discourse and annotations. New York: William Wood & Co.; vol. 1, 1925:353–391.
4. Hippocrates. The Genuine Works of Hippocrates. Translated from the Greek by Francis Adams with a preliminary discourse and annotations. New York: William Wood & Co.; vol 2, 1925:1–19.ibid #3 see volum2, pp. 1–19.
5. Galen of Pergamon. Omnia quae extant opera in Latinum sermonem conversa, (Quinta ed). Venice. Apud Juntas, 1576–1577.
6. Sylvius F (de le Boë). Disputationes medicarum pars prima, primatias corporis humani functiones naturales en anatomicis, practicis et chymicis experimentils deductas complectens. Amstelodami, van den Berg, 1663.
7. Monro A (Secundus). Observations of the Structure and Function of the Nervous System. Edinburgh: Creech-Johnson, 1783.
8. Vesalius A. De Humani Corporis Fabrica. Basel: Oporinus, 1543.
9. Oribasius. Opera, quae extant omnia, tribus tomis digesta. Basel: Apud Michaëlem Isingrinium, 1557.
10. Raeder I. Oribasii collectionum medicarum reiquiae Taubner, Lipsiae et Berolini; vol. E, 1931:236–259.
11. Lascaratos JG, Panourias IG, Sakas DE. Hydrocephalus according to Byzantine writers. Neurosurgery 2004; 55:214–221.
12. Aetius of Amida. Contractae ex veteribus medicinae tetrabilus. Basel: Impensis Kier. Frobenii et Nile Espicopii, 1542.
13. Paul of Aegina. Opus de re medica nunc primum integrum. Colgne: Opera et impeensa Joannis Soteris, 1534.
14. Paul of Aegina. The Seven Books of Paulus Aegineta. Translated from the Greek by Francis Adams. London: Syndenham Society, 1844–1847.
15. Albucasis [Abu Al-Quasim]. Liber theoricae necnon practicae Alsaharavii. Augsburg: Impensis Sigismundi Grimm and Marci Vuirsung, 1519.

16. Albucasis on Surgery and Instruments. A definitive edition of the Arabic text with English translation and commentary by M.S. Spink and G.L. Lewis. Berkeley, CA: UC Press, 1973:170–172. Al-Rodhan NRF, Fox JL. Al-Zahrawi and Arabian Neurosurgery, 936-1013 AD. Surg Neurol 1986; 25:92–95.
17. ibid #10.
18. ibid #10 see p. 173.
19. Massa, Niccolo (Nicholas) Liber introductorius anatmiae, sive dissectionis corporis humani. Venic: In aedibus Francisci Bindon, ac Maphei Pasini socios, 1536.
20. Clarke E, O'Malley CD. The Brain and Spinal Cord. Berkeley: University of California Press, 1982 [see page 722 of English translation].
21. Leonardo da Vinci Quaderni d'anatomia. Christiania: Jacob Dybwad, 1911–1926.
22. Leonardo da Vinci. In: Kenneth Keele and Carlo Pedretti, eds. Corpus of the Anatomical Studies in the Collection of Her Majesty the Queen at Windsor Castle. New York: Harcourt Brace, 1979.
23. Vesalius A. On the Fabric of the Human Body. Book 1: The Bones and Cartilages. A Translation of *De Humani Corporis Fabica* by William Frank Richardson in collaboration with John Burd Carman. San Francisco: Norman, 1998:48.
24. Vesalius A. De Humani Corporis Fabrica. Basel: Oporinus, 1555.
25. Ashwal S. (ed). The Founders of Child Neurology. San Francisco: Norman, 1990, 109.
26. Severino MA. De Recondita Abscessum Natura, Libri VII. Napoli, Beltranum. For an interesting historical discussion on Severino see also Lyons AE. (1995) Hydrocephalus First Illustrated. Neurosurg 1632; 37:511–513.
27. Tulpius N. Observations medicae. Amsterdam: Elzeririum, 1641.
28. Willis T. Pathologiae Cerebri, et nervosi generis specimen. Amsterdam: Apud Danielem Elzevirium, 1670.
29. Varolio C. De neruis opticis, nonullisque aliis praeter communem opinionem in humano capite obseruatis. Frankfurt: Ioannem Wechelum & Petrum Fischerum, 1591.
30. Riolan J. Opuscula anatomica nova . . .. Instauratio magna physicae & Medicinae . . .. London: Typis Milonis Flesher, 9461.
31. Riolan J. A sure guide; or The best and nearest way to physick and chyrurgery . . .. being an anatomical descrpitpion of the whole body of man, and its parts . . .. Written in Latin . . .. Englished by Nicholas Culpeper. 3rd ed. London: Printed by John Streater, 1671.
32. Ruysch F. Observationum anatomico-chirurgicarum centuria. Amsterdam: Apud Henricum & viduam Theodori Boom, 1691: 86.
33. Haller A. Elementa physiologiae corporis humani. Bern: Sumptibus Societatis Typographicae, 1757–1766.
34. Pacchioni A. De durae meningis fabrica & usu disquisitio anatomicae. Rome: D.A. Herculis, 1701.
35. Morgagni GB De Sedibus et Causis Morborum per Anatomen Indagatis. Libri quinique Venice: Ex typographia Remondinian, 1761.
36. Morgagni GB. The Seats and Causes of Diseases Investigated by Anatomy. Translated from Latin by B. Alexander. London: A. Miller, 1769. See Vol. 1 pp. 244–274 "Of hydrocephalus and water tumours of the spine."
37. Whytt R. Observations on the Dropsy in the Brain. Edinburgh: Balfour, 1768.
38. Astruc J. Tractatus pathologicus. Geneva: Apud Haer, Cramer & Fratres Philibert, 1743.
39. ibid #17. see Ashwall. pp. 87–88.
40. Manning H. Modern Improvements in the Practice of Physic. London: G. Robinson, 1780: 213–222.
41. Fothergill J. A Complete Collection of the Medical and Philosophical Works. London: John Walder, 1781:336.
42. Fothergill J. A Complete Collection of the Medical and Philosophical Works. London: John Walder, 1781: 337.
43. Underwood M. A Treatise on the Disorders of Childhood and Management of Infants from the Birth. London: J. Mathews, 1797. Later edition with the first edition in 1784.
44. Cotugno D. De Ischiade Nervosa Commentarius. Napoli: Apud Fratres simmonos, 1764.
45. Cotugno D. A Treatise on the Nervous Sciatica, or, Nervous Hip Gout. London: printed for J. Wilkie, 1775:16–17.
46. Monro A. Observations on the communication of the ventricles of the brain with each other; and on the internal hydrocephalus. Edinburgh: Adam Neil, 1797.
47. Cheyne J. An Essay on Hydrocephalus Acutus, or Dropsy in the Brain. Edinburgh: Mundell, Doig, Stevenson, 1808.
48. ibid #47 see p.23.
49. ibid #47 see p.36.
50. ibid #47 see p.40.

51. ibid #47 see p.66.
52. ibid #47 see p.93–95.
53. Yeats GD. A Statement of the early Symptoms which lead to the Disease Water in the Brain; with Observations on the Necessity of a Watchful Attention to Them, and of the Fatal Consequences of Their Neglect in a Letter to Martin Wall, Esq, M.D. London: Printed for J. Callow, 1815.
54. Yeats GD. An Appendix to the Pamphlet on the Early symptoms of Water in the Brain, containing Cases Successfully Treated. . . .London, Burgess & Hill, 1819.
55. ibid #53, see p. 2.
56. ibid #53, see p. 26.
57. ibid #53, see p. 38.
58. ibid #53, see pp. 49–50.
59. ibid #53, see pp. 66–67
60. ibid #53, see p. 102.
61. Bright R. Reports of Medical Cases, selected with a View of illustrating the symptoms and cure of Diseases by a Reference to Morbid Anatomy. London: Richard Taylor for Longman, 1827–1831.
62. ibid #61 see volume 2 p. 424.
63. Baillie M. The Morbid Anatomy of Some of the Most Important Parts of the Human Body. London: Printed for J. Johnson, 1793.
64. ibid #62 see volume 2 p. 426.
65. ibid #62 see volume 2 p. 431.
66. ibid #62 see volume 2 page 432.
67. Magendie F. Recherches Physiologiques et Cliniques sur le Liquide Céphalo-Rachidien ou Cérébrospinal. Paris: Mequignon-Marvis, 1842.
68. Magendie F. Mémoire sur un liquide qui se trouve dans le crane et le canal vertebral de l'homme et des animaux mammifères. J Physiol Exp Path Paris 1825; 5:27–87.
69. Luschka H. (1855) Zur lehre von der secretionzelle. Arch f. physiol Heilkunde. 13:1–20, 1854. See also Luschka H. Die adergeflechte des menschlichen gehirns. Berlin.
70. Hilton J. (1863) On the influence of mechanical and physiological rest in the treatment of accidents and surgical diseases, and the diagnostic value of pain. London: G. Bell and Daldy. When published in the United States this work was re-titled in the second edition as Rest and Pain. New York: Wm. Wood, 1879.
71. Magendie F. Mémoire sur un liquide qui se trouve dans le crane et le canal vertebral de l'homme et des animaux mammifères. J Physiol Exp Path Paris 1825; 5:27–87, 79–80.
72. Lewandowsky M. Zur Lehre von der Cerebrospinalflüssigkeit. Ztschr f Klin Med 1900; 40:480–490.
73. Spina A. Untersuchungen über die Resorption des Liquors bei normalen und erhalten intercraniellen Druck. Neurolog Centralbl 1901; 20:224–234.
74. Schmorl D. (1910) Liquor Cerebrospinalis und Ventrikelflüssigkeit. Erlingen, Verhandl d. Deutsch. Pathol. Gesellsch.
75. Dandy WE, Blackfan KD. Internal hydrocephalus: An experimental, clinical and pathological study. Am J Dis Child 1914; 8:406–482.
76. Dandy WE. Experimental hydrocephalus. Ann Surg 1919; 70:129–142.
77. Key A, Retzius G. Studien in der Anatomie des Nervensystems und des Bindegewebes. Stockholm, Sweden: In Commission bei Samson & Wallin, 1875–1876.
78. Faivre E. Recherches sur la structure du conarium et des plexus choroides chez l'homme et chez les animaux. Compt rend l'Acad d. sc. 1854; xxxiv:424–434.
79. Faivre E. Etude sur le conarium et les plexus choroides de l'homme et des animaux. Ann d sc nat Paris 1857; vii; 52–62.
80. Mestrezat W. Le liquide céphalo-rachidien normal et pathologique. J Physiol et de Path Gén 1912; 14:504–514.
81. Dixon WE, Halliburton WD. The cerebrospinal fluid. 1. Secretion of the fluid. J Physiol 1913; 47: 215–225.
82. Weed LH. The Cerebrospinal Fluid. Physiol Rev 1922; 2:171–182.
83. Weed LH. Studies on Cerebrospinal fluid. J Med Res 1914; 31:21–118.
84. Weed LH. The development of the cerebro spinal spaces in pig and in man. Carnegie Institute Contrib Embryol 1917; 5:1–10.
85. Weed LH. Certain anatomical and physiological aspects of the meninges and cerebrospinal fluid. Brain 1935; 58:383–397.
86. Cushing H. Studies on the cerebrospinal fluid and its pathways. J Med Res 1914; 31:1–19.
87. Cushing H. Studies in Intracranial Physiology and Surgery. The Third Circulation, The hypophysis, the gliomas. The Cameron Prize Lecture. Oxford: Oxford University Press, 1925.
88. ibid #87 see p. 15.

89. Buchan W. Domestic medicine: or, A Treatise on the prevention and cure of diseases by regimen and simple medicines. 8th ed. London: W. Strahan, et al., 1784.

90. Bucy PC. Hydrocephalus. In: Practice of Pediatrics (Brenneman). Vol 4, Chap. 3. Hagerstown, MD: W.F. Prior Co., 1932:23–27.

91. Galvani D. Della Fontanele Trattato, Diuiso in duo Libri. Padua: G. Crivellari, 1620.

92. LeCat CN. A new trocart (sic) for the puncture in the hydrocephalus, and for other evacuations, which are necessary to be made at different times. Phil Trans R Soc 1753; 47: 267–272.

93. Dionis P. A Course of Chirurgical Operations, demonstrated in Royal Garden at Paris. London: J. Tonson for J.J. and P. Knapton et.al, 1733.

94. Dionis P. A Course of Chirurgical Operations, demonstrated in Royal Garden at Paris. London: J. Tonson for J.J. and P. Knapton, 1733: 289–290.

95. Monro A. Observations on the Communication of the Ventricles of the Brain with each other; and on the internal hydrocephalus. Edinburgh: Adam Neil, 1797.

96. Chipault A. (1894–1895) Chirurgie Opératoire du Système Nerveux. Paris: Rueff. See pp. 717–717 for discusion of trocar which is illustrated on page 718.

97. Langenbeck and Hahn (As described in) Graniere, U. Il trattamento dell'idrocefalo infantile net secolo XIX. Rass Internaz Clin Ter 1969; 49:327–337.

98. Quincke H. Die lumbalpunktion des hydrocephalus. Berl Klin Wchnschr 1891; 28:929–933; 965–968.

99. Quincke H. About hydrocephaus. Verh Kong Inn Med 1901; 10:321–339.

100. Haymaker W, Schiller F. The Founders of Neurology 2nd edition, Springfield: Charles Thomas, 1970: 499–503.

101. Ferguson AH. Intraperitioneal diversion of the cerebrospinal fluid in cases of hydrocephalus. NY Med J 1898; 67:902–908.

102. Heile B. Zur Behandlung des Hydrocephalus. Deutsch Med Wochenschr 1908; 34:1468–1470.

103. Kanusch W. Die Behandlung des hydrocephalus der kleinen Kinder. Arch Klin Chir 1908; 87:709–715.

104. Sutherland GA, Cheyne WW. The treatment of hydrocephalus by intracranial drainage. Br Med J 1898, 2:1155–1187.

105. Payr E. Ueber Ventrikeldrainage bei Hydrocephalus. Verh Dtsch Ges Chir 1911; 40:515–520.

106. McClure RD Hydrocephalus treated by drainage into a vein of the neck. Johns Hopkins Hosp Bull 1909; 20:110–115.

107. Heile B. Uber neue operative Wege zur Druckentlastung bei angbornem Hydrocephalus (ureter-Dura-Anatomose). Zentralbl Chir 1925; 52:2229–2236.

108. Matson D. A new operation for the treatment of communicating hydrocephalus. Report of a case secondary to generalized meningitis. J Neurosurg 1949; 6:238–247.

109. Torkildsen A. A new palliative operation in cases of inoperable occlusion of the Sylvian aqueduct. Acta chir scand 1939; 82:117–124.

110. Gardner (1895) cited in: Pudenz, RH, Russell FE, Hurd AH, Shelden CH. Ventriculo-auriculostomy: a technique for shunting cerebrospinal fluid into the right auricle: preliminary report. J Neurosurg, 1957; 14:171–179.

111. Nulsen F. Spitz EB. Treatment of hydrocephalus by direct shunt from ventricule to jugular vein. Surg Forum 1951; 2:399–409.

112. Boockvar JA, Loudon W, Sutten SN Development of the Spitz–Holter valve in Philadelphia. J Neurosurgery 2001; 95:145–147.

113. Spitz EB. Neurosurgery in the prevention of exogenous mental retardation. Peds Clinics NA 1959; 6:1215–1235.

114. Davis L. Neurological Surgery. Philadelphia: Lea & Febiger, 1936. See p. 405 for discussion on Lespinasse and plexectomy.

115. Dandy WE. Extirpation of the choroid plexus of the lateral ventricles in communicating hydrocephalus. Ann Surg 1918; 68:569–579.

116. Dandy WE. The diagnosis and treatment of hydrocephalus resulting from strictures of the aquaduct of Sylvius. Surg Gynecol Obst 1920; 31:340–358.

117. Dandy WE. Operative procedure for hydrocephalus. Bull Johns Hopkins Hosp 1922; 33:188–190.

118. Dandy WE. The operative treatment of communicating hydrocephalus. Ann Surg 1938; 108:194–202.

119. Goodrich JT. Reprint of "The operative treatment of communicating hydrocephalus by Walter Dandy, M.D." Child Ner Sys 2000; 16:545–550.

120. Putnam TJ. Treatment of hydrocephalus by Endoscopic Coagulation of the Choroid Plexus: Description of a new Instrument and Preliminary Report of Results. New England J Med 1934; 210:1373–1376.

121. Putnam TJ. Results of the Treatment of Hydrocephalus by Endoscopic Coagulation of the Choroid Plexus. Arch Pediat 1935; 52:676–685.

122. Putnam TJ. Mentality of infants relieved of hydrocephalus by coagulation of choroid plexus. Am J Dis Child 1938; 55:990–999.

123. Putnam TJ. The surgical treatment of infantile hydrocephalus. Surg Gynec Obst 1943; 76:171–182.
124. Scarff JE. Endoscopic treatment of hydrocephalus: Description of a Ventriculoscope and Preliminary report of cases. Arch Neurol Psychiat 1936; 35:853–861.
125. Scarff JE. Treatment of obstructive hydrocephalus by puncture of the lamina terminalis and floor of the third ventricle. J Neurosurg 1951; 8:204–213.
126. Scarff JE. Treatment of hydrocephalus: an historical and critical review of methods and results. J Neurol Neurosurg Psychiatry 1963; 26:1–26.
127. Stookey B, Scarff JF. Occlusion of the aqueduct of Sylvius of neoplastic and non-neoplastic processes with a rational surgical treatment for relief of the resultant obstructive hydrocephalus. Bull Neurol Inst NY 1936; 5:348–377.
128. Dandy WE. Diagnosis and treatment of stricutres of the aqueduct of Sylvius (causing hydrocephaus). Arch Surg 1945; 51:1–14.
129. Davidoff LM. Hydrocephalus and hydrocephalus with meningocele. Their treatment with choroid plexectomy. Surgical Clinics NA 1948; 28:416–431.
130. Scarff JE. Treatment of hydrocephalus: an historical and critical review of methods and results. J Neurol Neurosurg Psychiatry 1963; 26:1–26. De Martel is discussed on page 3.
131. Ransohoff J II. Ventriculo-pleural anatomosis in reatment of midline obstructional neoplasma. J Neurosurg 1954; 11:295–298.
132. Ransohoff J, Shulman K, Fishman RA. Hydrocephalus: a review of etiology and treatment. J Pediat 1960; 56: 399–411.

Treatment of Hydrocephalus in the Modern Era (1950s–Current Date)

Paul May
Department of Neurosurgery, The Walton Centre for Neurology and Neurosurgery, Liverpool, U.K.

Spyros Sgouros
Department of Neurosurgery, "Attikon" University Hospital, University of Athens, Athens, Greece

NINETEENTH–EARLY TWENTIETH CENTURY

Since LeCat in France invented the external CSF drainage in 1744, the process of the treatment of hydrocephalus has gone through major developments. The first permanent CSF diversion was carried out by Mikulicz in 1893. He implanted a glass faser wick as a ventriculo-subarachnoid-subgaleal shunt. This was simultaneously the first intrathecal ventriculostomy and the first extrathecal CSF shunt with a drainage into an extrathecal low-pressure compartment. Other extrathecal valveless shunts drained lumboperitonael (Ferguson, 1898), from the ventricles into the peritoneal (Kausch, 1905) or pleural space (Heile, 1914), or into the veins, inaugurated by Payr in 1908.

The interventriculostomy with a tube in the aqueduct was inaugurated by Dandy, but less successful as the ventriculocisternostomy, introduced by Torkildsen in 1938.

COAGULATION OF THE CHOROID PLEXUS

The first plexectomy was possibly carried out by Lespinasse by using a cystoscope in 1913 (not confirmed). Walter Dandy made open plexectomies at the Johns Hopkins Hospital in 1920 and later Scarff tried endoscopic plexectomy.

EXTERNAL VENTRICULAR DRAIN

Ingraham invented the first closed external ventricular drain (EVD) in 1941 in Boston. Since then, the EVD has been in wide use in the temporary treatment of hydrocephalus. They are of particular use in the presence of infection, as intrathecal antibiotics could be administered. A recent development of the last decade was the introduction of the antibiotic impregnated EVD, which could be used for a considerably longer time than the conventional EVD with a lower incidence of secondary infection.

THE FIRST VALVE

In 1949, Nulsen and Spitz designed a ball-in-cone-valve, which was implanted in May 1949 in Philadelphia. It was a system including a one-way pressure regulated valve which they placed in the atrium via the jugular vein (3 implantations; published 1952). This began the modern era of hydrocephalus management.

THE IMPROVEMENT OF IMPLANTABLE MATERIAL

The breakthrough to a sufficient implant material was a spin off of the Second World War. The silicone elastomer was developed for the isolation of military airplane electrics.

The first use as implant was for a bile duct repair in 1946, shunts followed in 1956 (Holter and Spitz). In 1956, John Holter independently developed his famous valve for his own child, who had a meningomyelocele and hydrocephalus. In the summer of 1956, he started the first industrial shunt production at his garage in Bridgeport near Philadelphia.

In Los Angeles, Pudenz and Heyer made systematic animal studies with different shunt materials and designs. In 1955, they designed and implanted a Teflon distal slit valve, engineered by Ted Heyer. The German watchmaker R. Schulte joined the team and patented the first diaphragm valves in 1960.

THE FIRST EUROPEAN VALVE

The first European valve, a combined ball and distal slit valve, was implanted by Sikkens in Groningen (the Netherlands) in 1956, but was not met with wide acceptance (published 1957).

Generally, the results of all early hydrocephalus treatments before wide use of shunting were depressing: in the late 1950s, Riechert stated a good outcome in only 4% cases and a mortality in 70% cases. He compared hydrocephalus even with malignant brain tumors. Shunting converted hydrocephalus from terminal illness to a curable disease.

MODERN VALVES

Very slowly following the first generation of valves in the 1950s, a second generation of valves, designed to solve the problems of overdrainage, was introduced.

In 1969, in Switzerland, Kuffer and Strub invented and implanted the first adjustable ball valve. The adjustment required a screwdriver.

In 1973, S. Hakim was the first who proposed such autoregulation in shunts. In 1973, Hakim conceived the percutaneous magnetic adjustment of valves. The simple variation of the tension of a spring is an adjustment, not a complex regulation or programming of a computer. Well known is the Medos–Hakim adjustable valve, which is in wide use today. It is marketed as "programmable" valve, but in essence is an adjustable valve only. Less known is the Japanese MDM valve with a manual palpatoric adjustment.

To counteract the siphoning effect of the column of CSF in the peritoneal catheter, the antisiphon device (ASD) was developed by Portnoy and Schulte in 1973 in which the weight of the hanging water column was used to increase the resistance stepwise. Hakim patented the first valve with an implemented ball for the same goal in 1975 (Hakim-Lumbar).

The Orbis-Sigma valve, designed by C. Sainte-Rose, represented the French revolution in valves in 1987. CSF pressure deforms a silicone diaphragm, which moves against a fixed ruby pin, and by moving up and down it alters the diameter of the CSF passageway. Orbis-Sigma aims to keep a steady CSF flow within a pressure range, so in a sense is also controlled by pressure, similar to all other valves, although it has been marketed as "flow-regulated" valve. In general, the terms "programmable" and "flow-regulated" has been used by valve manufactures rather liberally and there is no universal agreement on their meaning.

In 1991, the gravitational valves were suggested as the best solution. The Hakim-Lumbar, designed in the 1970s, was one of the first gravitational valves. The resistance curve of this valve increases parallel to the angle of verticalization. Surprisingly, the Hakim-Lumbar played no substantial role in neurosurgical practice and there are no publications, despite an excellent technical quality and breakthrough-technology. An implantation corresponding to the body axis is the precondition for correct function. Unfortunately, the Hakim-Lumbar has a round valve body with a strong tendency to rotate in the lumbar fat leading to dysfunction. Additional problems were created by the thin lumbar catheter, which was at risk of kinking. The indications for lumbar shunts are limited (therapy-resistant CSF-fistula, pseudotumor cerebri, ca. 1% of shunts only). As a result of these factors, this type of valve was not explored for two decades. In the early 1990s, Chhabra in India independently constructed a valve body for thoracal implantation (Chhabra Z-Flow, 1993) and Affeld and Miethke conceived a three-level gravitational (g) valve, which was a precursor of the later two-level Miethke Dual-Switch (1993–1994) and its derivatives. It is argued that the gravitational ball valves (Cordis GCA, Miethke valves) show the closest relation to physiological flow requirements, but so far this has not been translated to superior clinical performance.

ANTIBIOTIC IMPREGNATED SHUNT TUBING

The idea of using antibiotic impregnated tubing in hydrocephalus shunts was explored by Bayston who studied the effects of various factors on the antibacterial activity of gentamicin-impregnated Silastic, which was shown that it is unaffected by autoclaving and storage. It was also shown that this activity persists for long periods under crudely simulated in-use conditions. His later work demonstrated that the bacteria causing shunt infection, mainly staphylococci, gain access to the shunt at operation and colonize the shunt tubing. This leads to biofilm development requiring shunt removal. The antimicrobial material incorporated into the shunt did not reduce bacterial adherence. However, 100% of attached bacteria were killed in 48 to 52 hours, even in the presence of a conditioning film. Thus, impregnated antimicrobial material is likely to reduce shunt infection rates significantly without the risks and side effects of systemic antibiotics. These developments have been incorporated in commercially available catheters. Clinical studies have not confirmed this advantage conclusively as yet, and large prospective trials are in consideration.

ENDOSCOPY

Third ventriculostomy was initiated by Dandy in 1922 in an attempt to bypass a blockage in the CSF pathways. He performed it through an open craniotomy, which required primarily the resection of one optic nerve. Scarff and Stookey improved the procedure by using the lamina terminalis.

In the 1990s, there has been a renaissance of endoscopic third ventriculostomy, which is widely accepted as the method of choice in children with congenital aqueduct stenosis and adult patients with acquired or late-onset, occlusive hydrocephalus. Other indications are discussed elsewhere in this book.

Manwaring introduced the endoscopic aqueductoplasty and interventriculostomy for the treatment of isolated fourth ventricle in children. Endoscopic aqueductoplasty or inter-ventriculostomy presents an effective, minimally invasive, and safe procedure for the treatment of isolated fourth ventricle in pediatric patients. Compared with suboccipital craniotomy and microsurgical fenestration, endoscopic aqueductoplasty is less invasive, and compared with fourth ventricle shunts, it is more reliable and effective. Aqueductoplasty performed endoscopically through a tailored craniocervical approach was introduced by Perneczky. A new endoscopic approach was suggested to perform aqueductoplasty through the fourth ventricle. Caudal endoscopic aqueductoplasty is a safe and effective method of treatment in the management of a caudally located membranous obstruction of the sylvian aqueduct. This should be considered as an alternative endoscopic method when other endoscopic solutions are not suitable.

Endoscopic third ventriculostomy has been shown to be an alternative to shunt revision for malfunctioning and infected ventriculoperitoneal shunts with few complications and a high success rate. Endoscopy is also effective in the management of pineal region tumors and of posterior fossa tumor-related hydrocephalus. Gradually, neuroendoscopy found itself a wide spectrum of indications to treat patients with various forms of hydrocephalus with specific pathophysiology. Oi in his works has included many forms of hydrocephalus, which can be treated by endoscopy such as long-standing overt ventriculomegaly in adulthood (LOVA), isolated unilateral hydrocephalus (IUH), isolated IV ventricle (IFV), disproportionately large IV ventricle (DLFV), isolated rhombencephalic ventricle (IRV), isolated quarto-ventriculomegaly (IQV), dorsal sac in holoprosencephaly (DS), and loculated ventricle (LV).

3 | Imaging (Normal and Abnormal)

Charles Raybaud

Division of Neuroradiology, Hospital for Sick Children, University of Toronto, Toronto, Ontario, Canada

Gahl Greenberg

Division of Diagnostic Imaging, Chaim Sheba Medical Center, Tel Hashomer, Israel

INTRODUCTION

Hydrocephalus is a condition in which imbalance of formation, flow, or reabsorption of cerebrospinal fluid (CSF) leads to excess CSF volume/pressure, which then compresses the brain substance and impairs its development and function. Based on its underlying mechanism, hydrocephalus can be classified into noncommunicating (obstructive) and communicating. All this sounds simple, but it is not, and any clinical approach (including clinical imaging) should be humble, as no universal model of hydrocephalus can explain all aspects of this condition (1). This chapter tries to state a few facts and a few concepts that are useful for interpreting the morphological patterns and the causal mechanisms of hydrocephalus, without any dogmatism. Hydrocephalus certainly is a different disease in a child with a medulloblastoma and in a demented elderly patient. Within the pediatric population, it is also very diverse, depending (among other things) on the etiology and on the way the brain responds, which itself depends on the nature and evolutivity of the pathology and on the age/plasticity of the brain.

ANATOMY

CSF surrounds the brain and spinal cord. It is contained within the ventricles and the arachnoid. It serves as a cushion for the brain and protects the neural structures from mechanical damage. The immersion of the brain reduces its weight substantially (~97%), and by doing so, dampens the effects of both intracranial and extracranial forces. CSF also serves as a transport vehicle for different neurotransmitters and other metabolites to and from the brain (sink effect).

The Container

1. The skull comprises the vault and the base. Although the base is traversed by many nervous and vascular foramina, the mature skull may be considered as a closed box except for the foramen magnum that leads to the spinal canal. The skull is lined with the dura. Dural folds projecting into the cranial cavity form the falx cerebri in the sagittal plane and the tentorium cerebelli that covers the posterior fossa. Within the insertions of the falx and tentorium on the calvarial dura, triangular dural channels form the dural superior sagittal, transverse and sigmoid venous sinuses that convey the blood from the brain into the internal jugular veins through the jugular foramina. Within the insertion of the falx on the tentorium, the triangular-shaped straight sinus conveys the venous blood from the vein of Galen to the transverse sinuses, the confluent of the three sinuses forming the torcular Herophili. On the sides of the sella turcica, the quadrangular intradural cavernous sinuses carry venous blood between the orbits and the inferior petrosal sinuses, toward the facial veins, the jugular foramina, and the pterygoid plexuses.

   While the mature skull is rigid, the fetal and infantile skulls are elastic—the cranial squamae being separated by the cartilaginous sutures and fontanelles. Relative to the volume of the spinal canal, the volume of the cranial cavity is much larger in fetuses and infants than it is in adults.

2. The spinal canal is contained between the vertebral bodies and the neural arches, from the foramen magnum to the sacral canal. Unlike in the skull, the dura is not attached to the bone but is separated from it by the epidural fat and the epidural veins; more, it forms 29 to 31 pairs of nerve sheaths around the 29 to 31 pairs of spinal nerves emerging through the intervertebral foramina. This anatomy allows for the flexibility and motion of the spine

relative to the nervous system, but it also confers enough elasticity to the meningeal sac to accommodate the pulsatile intradural influx of arterial blood at each cardiac stroke.

The CSF-Filled Cavities

The Ventricular System

It comprises the lateral (hemispheric, VL), the third (median, diencephalic, V3), and the fourth (median, rhombencephalic, V4) ventricles. The foramina of Monro lead from each lateral ventricle to the 3rd ventricle. The cerebral aqueduct (of Sylvius) is truly the mesencephalic ventricle; it is the narrowest portion of the ventricular system.

The frontal horn, body, and atrium of the *lateral ventricle* circumscribe the dorsal and posterior aspects of the caudate and thalamus; they are limited superiorly by the corpus callosum and forceps, and laterally, by the hemispheric white matter between the caudate and thalamus below and the corpus callosum above. The *occipital horn* is surrounded by white matter, except where the calcarine fissure encroaches on its lumen (calcar avis); it is usually only virtual in normal children. The *temporal horn* is limited by the hippocampus medially, the parahippocampal white matter inferiorly, and the deep temporal white matter superiorly. The lateral ventricle is closed medially by the septum pellucidum and fornix and by the tela choroidea in the choroid fissure. The latter appears weaker posteromedially, where it may expand and form a diverticulum in case of chronic hydrocephalus. The lateral ventricle normally is narrow, with roughly parallel walls and one acute lateral angle.

The median, slit-like *3rd ventricle* is limited laterally by the thalami (and traversed by their median adhesion, the massa intermedia) and anteroinferiorly by the hypothalamus. The anterior part of its floor is the tuber cinereum, the posterior part is the cap of the midbrain; the tuber cinereum may dilate and bulge significantly in case of obstructive hydrocephalus. The anterior wall is the lamina terminalis that contains the optic chiasm inferiorly and the anterior commissure superiorly. The supraoptic and the infundibular recesses are apparent above and behind (base of the pituitary stalk) the optic chiasm, respectively; they dilate in case of hydrocephalus. The aditus of the aqueduct lies below the posterior commissure, above which are the pineal recess (at the base of the pineal gland) and the suprapineal recess. The roof of the 3rd ventricle is the tela choroidea that contains the internal cerebral veins and posteromedial choroidal arteries; it is continuous laterally with the choroid fissures of the lateral ventricles. The 3rd ventricle contains three circumventricular organs: the anterior vascular organ of the lamina terminalis, the superior lateral subfornical organ, and the posterior subcommissural organ.

The *cerebral aqueduct* curves gently caudally through the midbrain between the 3rd and the 4th ventricles. In adults, it measures about 15 mm in length; its diameter varies from 0.5 to 2.8 mm, with two strictures corresponding to the anterior and posterior colliculi and an ampulla in between (2). It is surrounded by the gray matter of the oculomotor nuclei and lies subjacent to the tectal plate.

The *4th ventricle* lies on the dorsal aspect of the brainstem. It has a rhomboid shape with a rostral half that is pontine and a caudal half that is medullary. It is limited laterally by the anterior, middle, and posterior cerebellar peduncles. The vermis forms the roof of the rostral part; the vermian nodulus encroaches caudally upon the ventricular lumen, giving it a triangular shape on a midline sagittal plane; the dorsal apex of the triangle is the fastigium. The caudal part of the ventricle is open posteriorly into the cisterna magna. Developmentally, this opening results from the dorsal expansion of the embryonic tela choroidea (Blake's pouch) into the subvermian space. The tela choroidea then lines the inferior aspect of the vermis and cerebellar hemispheres and attaches to the posterior occipital dura, so forming the cisterna magna, which communicates with the cisterns of the posterior fossa (3). The attachment of the tela choroidea with the dura forms a transverse membrane (described by Liliequist) that separates the cisterna magna from the retrovermian cistern (3). Conventionally, the dorsal aperture is called the foramen of Magendie and its lateral extensions toward the cerebellopontine angles, the foramina of Luschka. The choroid plexus is attached transversely along the ependymal–cortical junction of the inferior cerebellum, above the ventricular outlet. The caudal apex of the 4th ventricle is continuous with the (usually virtual) central canal of the spinal cord and is covered by the obex; it is where the area postrema (most caudal of the circumventricular organs) lies.

The CSF Spaces Over the Convexity

They are intra-arachnoid, or subarachnoid, located between the dura and the hemispheric cortex and within the sulci. They are wide in fetuses, in which the cortex does not abut the calvarium. They progressively attenuate in normal infants and become hardly visible on CT during childhood and adolescence: indeed in that period the brain imprints its gyri on the inner table and forms the gyriform (or digitiform) markings. In adulthood, the spaces over the convexity tend to enlarge again, typically mostly over the parietal lobes.

The Cisterns

These are widening of CSF-containing spaces interposed between brain structures (e.g., inter-hemispheric cistern) or between the brain and the base of the skull (e.g., suprasellar cistern). They are named according to their location: suprasellar, ambient (or supratectal), interpeduncular, pontine, medullary, cerebellopontine cisterns, and cisterna magna. They are typically traversed by crossing nerves, arteries, and veins. Except for the cisterna magna (an expansion of the 4th ventricle), they contain arachnoid septations that may become inflamed and fibrotic, preventing the normal circulation of the CSF.

The Intraspinal CSF Spaces

These may be considered a single cistern. Rostrally, they communicate widely through the foramen magnum with the cisterna magna and the perimedullary cistern. They surround the cord and are crossed by the anterior and posterior roots (which form the cauda equina in the lumbosacral segment) and the accompanying arteries and veins. They also contain the arachnoid dentate "ligaments" laterally, the septum posticum posteromedially, and the filum terminale. Laterally, they extend through the vertebral foramina toward the spinal sensory ganglions to form the nerve sheaths, usually more prominent in the lumbar spine than in the more rostral segments. Besides providing elasticity to the meninges and sliding motion to the spinal nerves, these nerve sheath diverticula seem to be important sites of CSF reabsorption.

The Vessels and Choroid Plexuses

The *cerebral arteries* originate from the internal carotid and the vertebral arteries. They are organized with multiple levels of anatomosis (basilar artery, circle of Willis in their cisternal, intra-arachnoid segment, pial anastomoses at the pial level) and form a network on the surface of the brain from which numerous perforators enter the brain from the periphery toward the ventricular wall. The only exceptions to this rule are the choroidal arteries that supply the intraventricular choroid plexuses. Arterioles are much more numerous in the gray matter, especially the cortex, than in the white matter.

The arterioles resolve into the *capillary bed*. Whereas the cerebral blood flow is extremely high (CBF = 50 mL/100 g/min in the adult, lower in neonates but twice as much in infants), the cerebral blood volume is small (CBV = 4 mL/100 g of tissue). This means that the cerebral circulation is extremely fast, systolo-diastolic, and the brain (which has no energetic reserve) is vulnerable to anoxo-ischemic events. Both the CSF and the cellular compartments being incompressible, the capillary bed is the most vulnerable compartment in case of increasing ventricular/intracranial pressure.

The *cerebral veins* are organized in two drainage systems, a superficial one that drains the cortex and adjacent white matter mostly toward the pial surface (cortical veins), and a deep one that drains the deep white matter and central gray matter mostly toward the ventricles (subependymal veins). The superficial cortical veins gather into meningeal collectors that cross the CSF spaces (bridging veins) to join the dural venous sinuses. The deep subependymal veins gather to form the internal cerebral veins and the vein of Galen, toward the straight sinus; as it crosses the ambient cistern, the vein of Galen also is a bridging vein.

The *choroid plexuses* are made of multilobulated pio-ependymal aggregates containing numerous capillaries. They are found along the choroid fissures of the lateral ventricles, especially in the ventricular atria, and on the roofs of the 3rd and 4th ventricles. They secrete CSF, but may also contribute to its dynamics by producing intraventricular pulsations. In the early fetal brain not yet vascularized, the choroid plexuses are loaded with glycogen and probably participate significantly in the nutrition of the brain (4).

CSF PRODUCTION, REABSORPTION, AND DYNAMICS

Hydrocephalus describes the morphological and pathophysiological effects of the CSF pressure on the brain, as well as the changes in the physiology and the dynamics of the CSF. Modern imaging has proved itself to be able to apprehend at least in part the morphological changes, the transmission of the CSF motion, and the interplay between both, so that imaging cannot be understood without a clear view of the anatomy of the CSF spaces, of the structures that secrete and reabsorb it, and of the structures that underlay the action of the CSF forces on the brain.

CSF Volume and Location

The total volume of CSF is classically assumed to be 40 to 60 mL in infants, 60 to 100 mL in children, and approximately 150 mL in adults (5). The volume of the adult ventricles is considered to be 25 mL [much less in infants, likely less in normal children as well (6)]. However, in the last 15 years, studies using MR imaging to quantify the CSF volume seem to point to much higher values [see Ref. (5) for review). According to these, the intracranial, extracerebral CSF itself may amount to about 150 mL and the spinal CSF to 100 to 120 mL (5). The central canal of the spinal cord is normally virtual and does not count. In the diagnosis of hydrocephalus, shape and size of the ventricles and effacement of the pericerebral spaces are used, rather than the absolute CSF-space volume.

CSF Production

To quote Greitz (7), "*CSF is produced everywhere in the CNS,*" that is, although the main production of CSF occurs in the choroid plexuses, there is everywhere continuity between the CSF and interstitial fluid (5). Rapid diffusion and mixing of both fluid compartments occur across the thin pial membrane covering the outer brain surface. Total volume of interstitial fluid is approximately twice that of the CSF, and homeostasis is maintained by permanent exchange: despite their different origins, the two elements are practically inseparable and both demonstrate a similar chemical composition (low protein concentration). In fact, it is assumed that interstitial fluid may adequately substitute the CSF in the subarachnoid space, in cases of intraventricular CSF obstructions.

Quantitatively, the CSF production has been evaluated at 600 mL/day, which is both huge (the ventricular volume is 25 mL) and small (0.35 mL/min, against a blood flow of 750 mL/min): the production of CSF cannot be individually measured with clinically acceptable means. The turnover time of CSF is approximately 5 to 7 hours, which means that the total CSF volume is renewed about four times a day. About 60% to 70% of the CSF is secreted by the choroid plexuses; 30% to 40% comes from interstitial fluid exsudated through the pia (slightly more from metabolism than from vessels) (5). Participation from the cord is negligible. The level of secretion is somewhat dependent on the blood perfusion pressure, therefore on the intracranial pressure: in case of increasing ICP, the production of CSF decreases.

CSF Reabsorption

By definition in normal conditions, the reabsorption equals the secretion. Experimental studies have shown that increasing significantly the CSF volume by intrathecal fluid infusion does not result in hydrocephalus, because reabsorption increases accordingly. Also, it increases when intracranial pressure increases (5). It is clear that it occurs mostly within cranial sites (85%–90%); it is much less but still significant in the spine (10%–15% to 25%) (5,8 10). There is much controversy concerning the structure through which this reabsorption actually happens. Radioactively labeled albumin appears in blood within minutes after injection into the lumbar CSF (6) and most (80%–90%) of the injected radioisotope is absorbed in the spinal canal (11–14). Because there is a permanent exchange and a full physiological continuity between the interstitial fluid and the CSF, it is logical and safe to assume that part of the reabsorption occurs through the parenchymal veins (7). This is exemplified by cases of chronic hydrocephalus with aqueductal stenosis in which the ventricular dilation may remain practically stable. Fluid exchange across the wall of the brain capillaries is well documented. The brain capillary system actively absorbs the macromolecules and plasma proteins present in the CSF as well as regulates and maintains fluid homeostasis at a slightly positive intracranial pressure.

The most widely accepted mechanism, however, involves the arachnoid Pacchionian granulations (villi). The idea that Pacchionian granulations could act as mechanical valves originates back in the 1960s following reports by Welch and Friedman (15). Di Chiro using radionuclide cisternography demonstrated radioisotope accumulation over the convexity around the Pacchionian granulations and this was felt to support this concept (16). However, to dispute this convention, to date no experimental evidence really proves that fluid is transported across these structures. As early as 1914, Dandy and Blackfan in their experiments realized that obstruction at the Pacchionian granulations would not dilate the ventricles but rather the subarachnoid space immediately upstream (17). (This is the pattern of the external hydrocephalus.) In addition, Pacchionian granulations are not developed in children until after the closure of the fontanelles (18), and infants suffering from aqueductal stenosis have other compensatory mechanism for absorbing the fluid.

Alternate pathways have been considered for CSF reabsorption. The route of the cribriform plate, nasal mucosa, and lymphatic system toward the cervical lymphatic chain has been extensively studied in animals (19–24) and in humans (24), and convincing anatomic and physiological evidence suggests that it is indeed a major route of reabsorption (25). Dural "clefts" into the dura conveying the CSF to the venous sinuses independently from, or alternatively in association with the arachnoid granulations have been suggested as well (9,26–28).

CSF Dynamics

The Bulk Flow of CSF

In the face of nearly a century of studies on CSF physiology, starting from the days of Dandy and Blackfan (17) and Cushing (29), our understanding of CSF hydrodynamics remains at best deficient (1). The classic theory of CSF dynamics claims that CSF is primarily formed in the choroid plexus, then transported by bulk flow through the ventricular system and exits the 4th ventricle outlets into the subarachnoid space to be absorbed in the venous sinuses through diverse reabsorption sites. The driving force of such bulk flow requires that CSF pressure at the production site would be in slight excess of the pressure at the reabsorption site. The most widely utilized concept holds that there is a pressure gradient driving the CSF from the choroid plexuses to the ventricles to the cisterns and the convexity, and from there to the venous sinuses; any obstacle along this path, or any loss of the gradient, would result in fluid accumulation upstream, that is, in hydrocephalus: Dandy and Blackfan (17) in their pioneering work showed that plugging the aqueduct in dogs results in dilation of the ventricles proximal to the obstruction, which was taken as evidence that CSF is produced in the ventricles and that CSF production exceeds its absorption in the ventricles. Yet it did not explain why an occlusion of the foramen magnum would generate hydrocephalus, nor provide a hydrodynamically convincing explanation for communicating hydrocephalus: an obstruction at the granulation site should result in a dilatation of the CSF pool upstream closest to the obstruction, that is, the subarachnoid space.

Pulsatile Forces in the CSF

CSF pulsations have been observed from the early times of neuroimaging (30,31). The arterial pulsation occurring in a rigid skull with incompressible CSF and brain tissue necessarily displaces blood toward the venous sinuses and CSF toward the more elastic, compliant dural theca. The CSF displacement is prominent at the craniovertebral junction where it has been evaluated at 6 mm per stroke in normal individual, and at 3 mm in communicating hydrocephalus (5). If the pressure wave cannot be dampened by the compliant spinal theca (for example, because of an obstructed foramen magnum, or because the spinal meninges have lost their elasticity), it exerts its force against the brain tissue, and this by definition produces hydrocephalus (7). This leads to three main conclusions:

• Even if nothing opposes the bulk flow of CSF (communicating hydrocephalus), hydrocephalus may develop because the craniospinal meningeal compliance is lost.
• Even in case of obstruction of the bulk flow pathway (obstructive hydrocephalus), part of the problem comes from the fact that the obstruction restricts the compliance of the system by not allowing the pressure waves to reach the spinal theca.

- Even without obstruction of the ventricles, increased pulsation waves within the ventricles (e.g., choroid plexus papilloma, choroid plexus hyperplasia) may overcome the compliance of the system and generate hydrocephalus. Such a situation was recreated experimentally by Di Rocco et al. in 1978 (32).

Normal volume and elasticity of the spinal theca are needed for the equilibrium of the system. In the first months of life, the volume of the spinal meninges is small in relation to the volume of the cranium. From the point of view of compliance, this is compensated for by the elasticity allowed to the skull by the sutures and fontanelles. Things may be the same in the fetuses, although the situation is compounded by the surrounding amniotic fluid with its own pressure and by a mode of systemic blood circulation that is different from the postnatal one.

Proper CSF hydrodynamics are important for a proper blood perfusion of the brain. Greitz by using dynamic MR imaging (7) has demonstrated that the pulse pressure wave, in a normal individual with normally compliant meninges, travels at 5 m/sec in the CSF. It reaches the outlets of the bridging veins in 30 msec, while in the more elastic vascular system it reaches this outlet in only 3.5 seconds. In the time interval, the CSF-mediated compression of the venous outlet results in a backward pressure increase and dilation of the venules and capillaries, while the slower incoming arterial blood pressure wave produces a forward pressure increase and a dilation of the arteriolo-capillary bed. Through a "bagpipe effect," this process of vascular dilation maintains a continuous systolo-diastolic flow, lowers the vascular resistance (thus improving the perfusion), while the pressure facilitates the exchanges through the capillary walls. Modifications of this regimen in relation with hydrocephalus may well impair the conditions of an optimal brain perfusion.

While the bulk flow cannot be detected by noninvasive means, MR phase-contrast imaging has the ability to evaluate and measure CSF motion, speed, and flow. Quantitative data in healthy adult individuals have been measured (7). Assuming a CBF of 60 mL/100 g/min, and a 60 beats/min heart rate, the volume of the arterial stroke is 15 mL for a 1500-g brain. Of this, 90% flows directly through the vascular bed to the veins and 1.5 mL (10%) correspond to the expansion of the intracranial arteries. This equals the sum of the systolic stroke volume of CSF displaced at the foramen magnum (0.8 mL) and blood in the venous sinuses (0.7 mL). The systolic expansion of the brain capillaries is minimal (0.03 mL, only 2% of the arterial expansion) but real; it is transmitted inwards to the ventricles and to the aqueduct where the displaced volume of CSF is correspondingly of 0.03 mL/beat (7). Given the small section of the aqueduct, this results in a measurable peak systolic CSF velocity. In another report, the MR-measured peak systolic velocity has been evaluated at 3.4 to 4.1 cm/sec in normal volunteers, corresponding to a mean CSF flow of 0.02 to 0.03 mL/sec (33). Using a similar MR phase-contrast-imaging-based method in groups of volunteers, Huang et al. could measure the CSF production rate and found 0.305 ± 0.145 mL/min, which is in good agreement with the data obtained with more invasive methods (34).

IMAGING HYDROCEPHALUS

Classification and Overview

Even though the pathogenesis of hydrocephalus is complex, and a clear distinction is hard to make clinically between obstructive and communicating hydrocephalus, such a classification, however, is helpful from a clinical and therapeutic point of view and should be maintained (Table 1).

Table 1 Clinical Classification of Obstructive Hydrocephalus

	Timing	Vascular bed	Ventricular size	Interstitial edema	Skull	Outcome
Hyper-acute	Sudden	↓	=	No	=	Arrest
Progressive	Weeks Months	=	↑	Yes	= / ↑	Decompensates
Chronic	Years	=	↑	No	↑	Slow ↑
Arrested	Years	=	↑	No	↑ / =	Stable?

Obstructive Hydrocephalus
Hyperacute obstructive hydrocephalus

This develops in hours from a sudden occlusion of the CSF pathways, with steep increase of the intraventricular pressure. The brain parenchyma has no time to accommodate by loss of tissue, so the ventricles are rounded but hardly increased in size. This may occur after severe head trauma, shunt obstruction, or rarely meningitis. As neither the parenchyma nor the CSF is instantaneously compressible, the only sector to give way is the vascular bed. This is made more severe by the fact that any expansion of the brain, even slight, compresses the cortical draining veins against the calvarium, while the subependymal veins are compressed by the intraventricular pressure, with further increase of intracranial (hence CSF) pressure. This vicious circle leads to a circulatory arrest. Only tapping the ventricles may allow relief of the ventricular tamponade.

Progressively acute obstructive hydrocephalus

This typically develops over weeks or months, usually from the growth of an intraventricular tumor. CSF outflow is progressively impeded, and the restricted ventricular space does not allow dampening of the CSF waves any more (loss of compliance). As this develops progressively, the ventricles are allowed to enlarge: if the head enlarges as well, the brain volume is preserved; if not, the ventricular enlargement corresponds to a brain tissue loss: this depends on the age of the patient and on the rapidity of installation of hydrocephalus. The increased ventricular pressure compresses the subependymal veins; this in turn prevents the normal absorption of interstitial fluid of the white matter and results in an accumulated periventricular interstitial edema. If not treated, progressively acute hydrocephalus will decompensate with brain herniation and/or circulatory arrest.

Chronic obstructive hydrocephalus

This may result from various causes, such as chronic aqueductal stenosis or leptomeningitis. In this chronic condition, there is no or only mild clinical signs of increased intracranial pressure, no periventricular interstitial edema, as assumedly the secretion of CSF is compensated by sufficient tissular fluid reabsorption. However, the ventricles, and typically the skull, slowly enlarge and brain volume loss over the years slowly develops, without or with a late decompensation. The term "arrested" hydrocephalus is used when no progression can be detected clinically as well as by imaging over long periods of time. This may happen but at best, uncommonly.

External hydrocephalus

This is observed in infants, usually from a few to 18 months [also called extraventricular obstructive hydrocephalus (EVOH), or benign infantile arachnoid collections]. It is characterized by the chronic accumulation of subarachnoid CSF over the anterior frontotemporal convexity with a corresponding craniomegaly. It is often assumed to be related to an immaturity of the arachnoid granulations, but this is only speculative. It is usually benign and resolves spontaneously; generally idiopathic, it may be familial. However, it may also result from increased venous pressure in various pathological conditions such as venous thrombosis (35), stenosis of the venous outlets at the jugular foramina, or intracranial, arteriovenous fistulae (AVF).

Fetal and true congenital hydrocephalus

This may be severe when evolving over several months, but may be mild and respond well to CSF diversion when developing late in gestation. It may compromise parenchymal development by affecting the germinal matrix and the vascular bed. It should not be confused with fetal ventriculomegalies of other causes, which may be destructive, malformative, or idiopathic (36–38). The term may also be a misnomer: the so-called "X-linked hydrocephalus" in reality is more a failure of white matter to form appropriately because of a L1CAM gene defect (CRASH syndrome) (39), rather than a real CSF/brain imbalance.

Communicating Hydrocephalus
This entity describes cases in which no clear obstruction can explain the development of an active progressive ventricular dilation with clinical symptoms and response to CSF diversion. Instead, when identified (symptomatic chronic communicating hydrocephalus), the causal

mechanism seems to be exclusively related to a decreased meningeal compliance (7): hypothetic subarachnoid adhesions/fibrosis when a previous history of meningeal infection or bleed, or of brain trauma, is found; segmental restriction of the meningeal space may be observed in adults with significant spinal degenerative changes; obstruction of the foramen magnum by a Chiari 1 deformity may not only be considered a CSF pathway obstruction, but also primarily a loss of compliance. If nothing is found, the term of idiopathic chronic communicating hydrocephalus is to be used. Greitz and others have hypothesized that primary vascular factors such as arteriosclerosis, both by increasing the amplitude of the arterial pressure wave and decreasing the conductivity of the vascular bed, could result in hydrocephalus as well (7,40). In any case, the term of "normal" pressure hydrocephalus might be dropped, as many physiological studies using pressure recording as well as cine-MR have shown that the amplitude of the arterial-CSF pulsation pressure wave is characteristically increased (41). Either secondary or idiopathic, chronic communicating hydrocephalus manifests itself with a clinical syndrome characterized by ataxia, dementia, and incontinence.

The Tools

Magnetic Resonance Imaging (MR Imaging)
Protocol
MR imaging is by far the best tool to investigate hydrocephalus, its causes, and its consequences. The *imaging protocol* must be adapted to the patient, but typically, thin T1 and T2 sagittal slicing to show the midline, coronal T2 for the morphology of the lateral ventricles, especially the temporal horns, and axial FLAIR to show the parenchyma make up the basic protocol (Fig. 1). FLAIR clearly shows a periventricular interstitial edema and any other lesion.

Flow voids appear nicely on FSE T2; they express patency of channels such as the aqueduct or a 3rd ventriculocisternostomy; they should be read according to the context, however, as they only reflect the velocity of the CSF: a narrowing without occlusion of the aqueduct, or a decreased compliance with increased arterial pulse amplitude, are in keeping with hydrocephalus but are expressed by a prominent flow void [Figs. 1(B) and 2 (A)]. Cine-Phase Contrast imaging is another way of demonstrating the flow, ant potentially to quantify it [Fig. 2(B–C)]. However, the CSF stroke through the aqueduct or at the foramen magnum depends on many physiological factors such as the arterial stroke (related to blood pressure, perfusion pressure), the distal vascular compliance (i.e., vascular health, Po_2, Pco_2), the meningeal compliance, the CSF pressure, the individual anatomy, etc., so that the quantification in individual patients is of little use.

High-definition T2 CISS/FIESTA demonstrates stenosis of the aqueduct, cysts, and abnormal intraventricular or arachnoid membranes much better than conventional sequences [Fig. 1(E)]. It must be part of the routine protocol.

Contrast administration would better depict tumor tissue or infection, when applicable, and may be used for perfusion studies. Intracisternal contrast has been suggested and is considered safe (42), but it has failed to gain real acceptance as the trend in brain imaging now is toward minimal invasiveness. Magnetic susceptibility T2* imaging may demonstrate blood and blood residue. MR arteriography and/or venography (MRA, MRV) would demonstrate vascular compromise better; they may be useful in specific indications but are not part of the usual protocol.

Diffusion imaging (DWI) is of limited use in the assessment of hydrocephalus, but may help to demonstrate acute ischemic changes; it is suggested to differentiate epidermoids from encysted CSF, but FLAIR can do that as well. Diffusion tensor imaging (DTI) informs on microstructural changes (mean diffusivity, MD; fractional anisotropy, FA) and may demonstrate compression of the white matter tracts (43). ^{1}H MR spectroscopy can also be used to identify changes in the energy metabolism (44). To investigate the vascular bed, MR perfusion might be used rather than the more invasive radionuclide studies.

Infants and Fetuses

Because MR imaging reflects the composition of brain tissue, sequence design must be adapted to the age of the patient. In the young child and infant, sedation/general anesthesia should be administered because of the specific way MR produces images; this means that imaging is not fully innocuous. In fetuses, imaging is done with abdominal coils, usually without sedation.

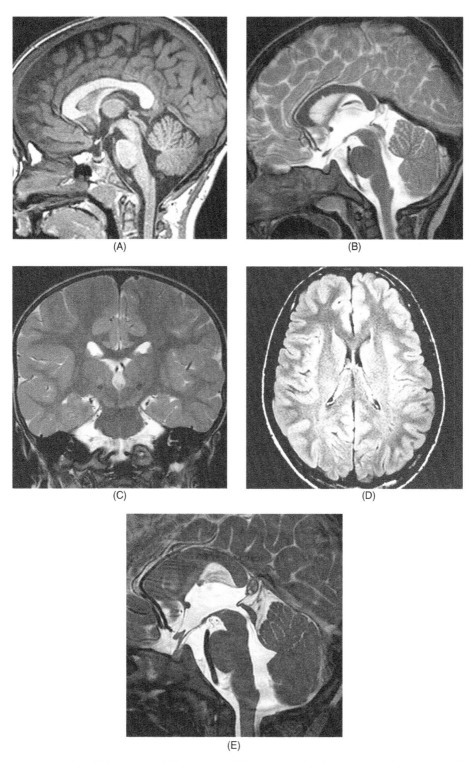

Figure 1 Normal MR imaging. Thin (1 mm) T1WI (**A**) and thin (3 mm) conventional FSE T2WI (**B**) midline sagittal cuts demonstrate the midline structures: 3rd ventricle (with its recesses and tuber cinereum), aqueduct, 4th ventricle, cisterna magna, medullary, pontine, interpeduncular and suprasellar cisterns, and foramen magnum; note in part (**B**), the flow void through the aqueduct. Coronal T2WI showing the bodies of the lateral ventricles (closed inferomedially by the transverse, nearly horizontal hippocampal commissure), the 3rd ventricle and the slit-like temporal horns (**C**). Axial FLAIR through the lateral ventricular bodies (**D**). High-definition (0.5 mm) sagittal T2 image depicts the anatomy exquisitely, without the flow void artifacts (**E**).

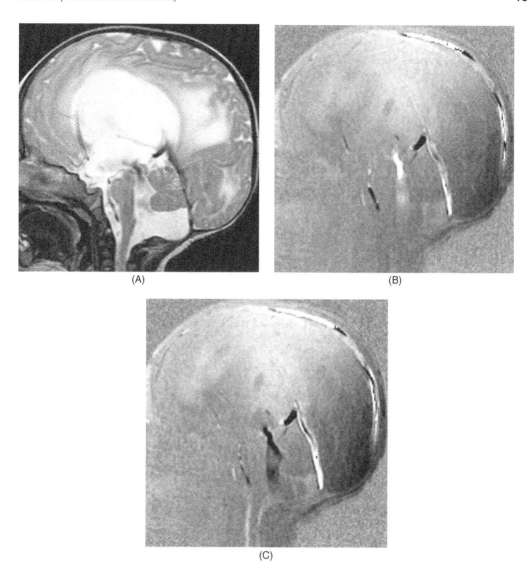

(A)

(B)

(C)

Figure 2 Flow void artifacts and cine phase-contrast imaging. Prominent aqueductal flow void in a communicating hydrocephalus (**A**) [compare with Fig. 1(B)]. Cine phase-contrast imaging: systolic (**B**) and diastolic (**C**) CSF displacement through the aqueduct.

Because of the size of the fetal brain and the dispersion of energy in the maternal abdomen, MR imaging cannot be practically done before 18 weeks of gestation at the earliest. Fat saturation can be applied to improve the signal, but leads to more energy deposition. Because the young fetus is almost continuously moving, repeated short, single shot sequences, and ultrafast T2W sequences (~1.0 seconds per slice), which are good for anatomy, should be used to create each slice and be carried out right after localizing scout images have been obtained. This can be done with appropriate equipments. Short multislice T1W sequences (~30 seconds) are useful to depict blood and calcifications, but are poor for anatomy. Complementary sequences such as MR angiography (for vascular pathologies) or cine imaging (for a "neurological" evaluation) are useful. Other approaches using DWI, ^{1}H MRS or DTI are still in a preclinical stage.

Follow-up
MR ideally can be used not only for the primary assessment of hydrocephalus, but also for the follow-up. The need for sedation in young children and the often limited access to MR, however, have resulted in CT being used more commonly for follow-up. In this context, "fast"

MR-scanning (using single-shot, ultrafast imaging sequences such as those used in fetal imaging) has been suggested, as it could, in theory, avoid both the need for sedation/anesthesia and the repetition of significant ionizing radiation exposition (45). Those heavily weighted T2 sequences, however, are adequate for assessing the ventricular or cisternal size and morphology but have a poor sensitivity and specificity for the changes in the parenchyma or in the intracranial fluids. For various reasons (not-so-easy to implement technique, limited diagnostic yield, lack of sensitivity/specificity, limited access to MR among others), it has failed to gain wide acceptance.

Spinal imaging
It should be mentioned that in some cases, hydrocephalus may have an intraspinal cause (tumor, malformation mostly) rather than an intracranial one; hydrosyringomyelia may be associated with hydrocephalus; spinal imaging may be needed in case of spinal CSF diversion. Spinal MR therefore may need to be added to the MR diagnostic evaluation of hydrocephalus. The protocol typically will include sagittal T2 sequences of the whole spine and axial T2, sagittal T1, and possibly contrast-enhanced T1 sequences on the region of interest. T2 fat saturated may be added for better recognition of soft tissue mass, fluid, or blood.

CT scanning
CT, together with MR imaging, is the most commonly used modality to evaluate hydrocephalus. Modern CT technology allows good quality reformats in any plane, so that the ventricular morphology (including that of the aqueduct on axial and midsagittal planes) and the cisternal morphology can be nicely depicted. Periventricular interstitial edema is readily apparent on CT, and subarachnoid blood may appear better on CT than on MR. Mass effects responsible for the hydrocephalus can be recognized and iodine-contrast helps in the characterization of the pathology. On the other hand, the diagnostic yield and the versatility of CT are much less than those of MR and CT typically is used for initial screening and follow-up assessment only. In addition, modern CTs expose to significant irradiation and their use in children should be limited to a necessary minimum.

Ultrasonography (US)
Head ultrasound is the primary modality of choice for the screening of infants suspected of having hydrocephalus, as well as obviously in fetal imaging. It is noninvasive, can be performed at the bedside, and the information it yields is precious: good evaluation of the ventricular size and morphology of course, sensitivity (if not specificity) to the parenchymal changes, efficient functional assessment of the vascularity. Its use, however, is limited to the first months of life when the fontanelles are open, and obviously as an imaging modality it cannot replace MR in the presurgical assessment of hydrocephalus.

Skull Plain X-Ray
Plain films of the skull are now basically useless in the assessment of hydrocephalus. They would show the craniomegaly, the splayed sutures and fontanelles in an infant and the digital marking and sellar erosions in an older child or adult. These informations are either useless or readily obtained with MR (or CT), which are needed anyway to treat the patient.

Functional imaging
Before the advent of modern, essentially MR imaging, hydrocephalus, and especially the para-doxical "normal pressure" hydrocephalus, have been extensively studied using CBF studies (by intracarotid ^{133}Xe and external detectors, SPECT, PET), perfusion studies (stable Xe CT), and metabolic studies (PET). Today, MR imaging, in an essentially noninvasive way, with or without injection of gadolinium contrast media, is able to provide the major physiological data on CSF dynamics (cine phase-contrast imaging mostly), brain metabolism (^{1}H MR spectroscopy, mono-, or multivoxel), and brain perfusion using either arterial spin-labeling perfusion imaging (ASL) or dynamic susceptibility contrast perfusion imaging (DSC) for cerebral blood volume (CBV), cerebral blood transit time, and cerebral blood flow (CBF). Such functional methods, however, are not typically used for individual diagnosis but only for protocols studying groups of subjects or patients.

Imaging Findings

The characteristic triad of hydrocephalus on imaging is the ventricular rounding and dilation, effacement of the pericerebral spaces over the convexity, and at least in children macrocephaly.

The Ventricular System

Normal *lateral ventricles* are typically narrow, encroached upon by the heads of the caudates, the thalami, the hippocampi, and the collateral eminences. In hydrocephalus, they are dilated (Fig. 3) and present a rounded appearance on the axial and mostly on the coronal images, notably of the lateral angle [Fig. 3(C)]. For the frontal horns, bodies, and atria, widening and rounding are

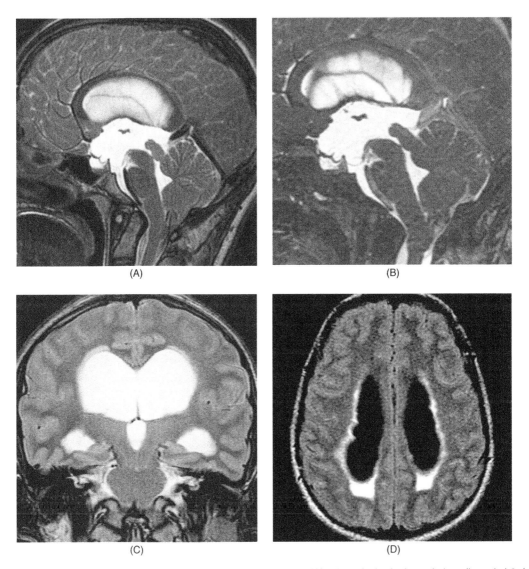

(A)

(B)

(C)

(D)

Figure 3 Obstructive hydrocephalus. FSE T2 midline sagittal (**A**): triventricular hydrocephalus, distended 3rd ventricle, arched corpus callosum, stretched septum pellucidum/hippocampal commissure; no flow void in the apparently occluded aqueduct. High-definition T2, same structures (**B**): the anatomy of the 3rd ventricle and aqueduct is better depicted. Coronal FSE T2 (**C**) shows the rounded lateral ventricles (notably the temporal horns, with compressed hippocampi) and the verticalization and stretching of the hippocampal commissure. FLAIR axial (**D**): significant widening of the lateral ventricles, interstitial edema of the periventricular white matter limited to the territory of the subependymal venous system; note the subependymal veins encroaching upon the ventricular lumen.

not really specific, as they can be observed to be similar in atrophy as well. But for the temporal horns, the pattern is quite specific: in atrophy, the roof and the floor of the horn remain roughly parallel; in hydrocephalus this is lost, the horn is rounded and the hippocampus is displaced medially [Fig. 3(C)]. Rounding may be the single feature in hyperacute hydrocephalus (within hours), when the volume of brain tissue is still preserved, or even swollen.

The dilation and tension of the lateral ventricles modifies the appearance of the midline. As the lateral ventricles are more dilated than the 3rd ventricle, the latter is pushed downward [Fig. 3(A) and (C)]. The corpus callosum is stretched, thinned, arched upward, more than the columns of the fornix, so that the distance in-between increases and the septum pellucidum is stretched (it may even be torn) [Fig. 3(A)]. The part of the fornix that forms the hippocampal commissure (the psalterium), normally transverse, becomes verticalized on each side of the midline [Fig. 3(C)]: this explains why on the midline sagittal cut, the posterior part of the fornix seems to be detached from the undersurface of the corpus callosum [Fig. 3(A) and (B)]. Depending on the specific etiological context, parenchymal paraventricular cavities (schizencephaly, porencephaly, destructive ischemic, or infectious cavitation) may be added to the ventricle and modify its morphology. In rare cases of chronic obstructive hydrocephalus (usually aqueductal stenosis), the ventricular anatomy may be compounded by a ventricular diverticulum that corresponds to the posterior inferior expansion of the medial wall of the ventricular atrium through the choroid fissure behind the thalamus (46–48) (Fig. 4). If not treated, this diverticulum, by

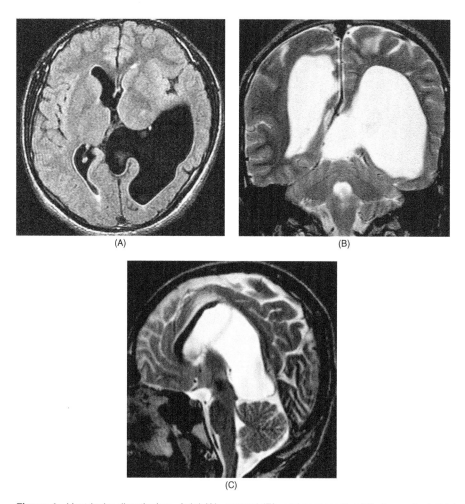

(A)   (B)

(C)

Figure 4   Ventricular diverticulum. Axial (**A**), coronal (**B**), and parasagittal (**C**) views of a left lateral ventricular diverticulum herniating through the tentorium into the quadrigeminal cistern.

extending through the lateral part of the tentorial incisura, compresses the upper brainstem with the risk of significant neurological complications.

The *3rd ventricle* is normally slit-like. It is enlarged in both atrophy and hydrocephalus, but in hydrocephalus it commonly presents with rounded recesses—anteriorly the supraoptic and infundibular recesses, posteriorly the suprapineal recess [Fig. 3(A) and (B)]. When the aqueduct or the lumen or the outlets of the 4th ventricle are occluded, the tuber cinereum is characteristically dilated and bulges into the interpeduncular cistern [Figs. 3(A) and (B)], sometimes around the head of the basilar artery. The anterior dilation of the 3rd ventricle may be so huge as to erode the dorsum sellae and widen the opening of the sellar cavity. Dilation of the suprapineal recess fills the ambient cistern and compresses the tectal plate. Because of the transverse widening of the 3rd ventricular lumen, the adhesio interthalamica (massa intermedia) usually attenuates and may be effaced. It is important to note that even with a significant ventricular enlargement, the lateral walls of the 3rd ventricle (i.e., the thalami) remain parallel to each other [Fig. 3(C)]; a rounded, circular 3rd ventricular lumen indicates the presence of a cyst, usually a suprasellar cyst with intraventricular expansion [Fig. 5(B–C)].

The *aqueduct of the midbrain* is a narrow craniocaudal curved channel with a middle ampulla limited by the encroachments of the anterior and posterior colliculi. It may be stenotic or dilated. When narrowed or occluded, it is logically the cause of hydrocephalus (aqueductal stenosis) (Fig. 2). The occlusion may be focal at any level, or global. It may be intrinsic (ependymal), usually postinflammatory, or extrinsic, then generated by a tegmental or a tectal mass lesion, or by an outside compression of the midbrain. It has been suggested that at some instances at least, aqueductal stenosis could even result from a compression by the expanded temporal lobes, rather than being the cause of the hydrocephalus. On the other hand, the aqueduct typically is dilated when the 4th ventricle is obstructed; this may be not only due to the force exerted by the CSF pressure (Fig. 6), but also due to the mechanical effect of a mass expanding the ventricular lumen (Fig. 7). Because of the increased velocity of the CSF through the normal aqueductal strictures, a striking *flow void* is observed there on the sagittal midline T2 image, extending from the posterior 3rd ventricle to the superior 4th ventricle (49). This flow void disappears if the aqueduct is occluded, but its presence does not exclude a stenosis: its intensity is increased if the aqueductal diameter is diminished, as the CSF velocity is increased. It is increased as well in case of decreased meningeal compliance (e.g., in communicating hydrocephalus) even when the aqueduct is patent or large, because the amplitude of the CSF pulsations is increased (Fig. 6).

The *4th ventricle* in hydrocephalus may be normal, mildly or markedly dilated. It is normal in *obstructive* hydrocephalus when the obstruction is located above it (Figs. 3 and 5]. It may be normal in *communicating* hydrocephalus as well, and it must be remembered that a triventricular hydrocephalic dilation does not necessary mean aqueductal stenosis (Fig. 8). In most cases of communicating hydrocephalus, the 4th ventricle is mildly dilated however (Fig. 6). If high, the CSF pressure tends to globally decrease the volume of the brain, so that all ventricles and cisterns are large; when both the 4th ventricle and the cisterna magna are involved, a posterior rotation of the vermis may occur, which does not relate to any variant of Dandy–Walker malformation but just to hydrocephalus: things go back to normal after shunt placement. Finally, the 4th ventricle may be hugely dilated when it is occupied by a tumor, or when its outlets are occluded. It may be hugely dilated in shunted hydrocephalus as well when it forms a cavity isolated between an aqueductal stenosis and a fibrotic occlusion of its outlets (Fig. 9). In that case, it tends to become spheric with ampullar dilation of both lateral recesses on each side of the brainstem at the cerebellopontine angles and massive compression of the brainstem and the surrounding cerebellum.

Appearances of the ventricular system usually define the type of an obstructive hydrocephalus:

- Univentricular hydrocephalus when the obstruction sits at a foramen of Monro: SEGA in Tuberous Sclerosis, rarely inflammatory thickening of the choroid plexus there. The affected lateral ventricle is dilated and rounded, and the septum pellucidum bulges toward the normal side.

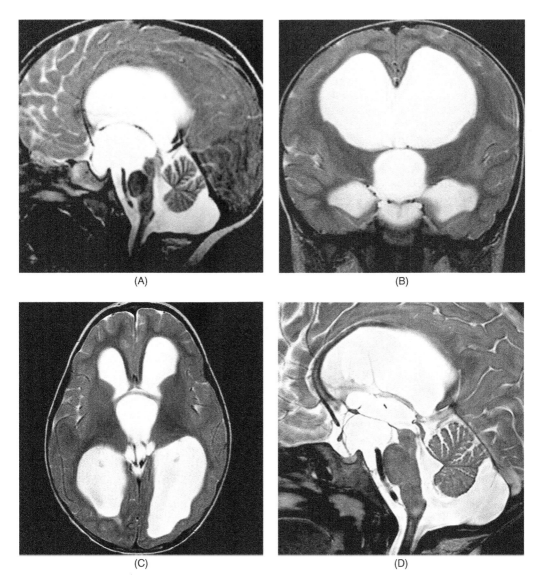

(A)   (B)

(C)   (D)

Figure 5   Suprasellar cyst. Rounded dilation of the 3rd ventricle (**A–C**), reflecting the morphology of the tense cyst herniating toward the 3rd ventricle. After drainage (**D**) the membrane of the cyst is better seen below the 3rd ventricular floor (high-definition T2).

- Biventricular hydrocephalus when the obstruction compromises both foramina of Monro: bilateral SEGA, colloid cyst of the tela choroidea, anterior 3rd ventricular tumor. Both lateral ventricles are dilated, but not the 3rd ventricle.
- Triventricular hydrocephalus, typically when the occlusion sits below the 3rd ventricle (aqueductal stenosis), but also when the lumen of the 3rd ventricle is occupied by a cyst, or a tumor (notably hypothalamic glioma or craniopharyngioma).
- Quadri-ventricular hydrocephalus when the four ventricles are dilated, either because a mass occupies the 4th ventricle or because the obstruction compromises the 4th ventricular outlets. A variant of this is when the outlets of the cisterna magna are occluded (e.g., fibrous arachnoiditis of the posterior fossa cisterns), resulting in a cisterna magna dilated together with the four ventricles.

Septations in the ventricles, often associated with cavitations in the brain, form the anatomic substrate of the complex *multicystic hydrocephalus* (usually postinfectious) in which

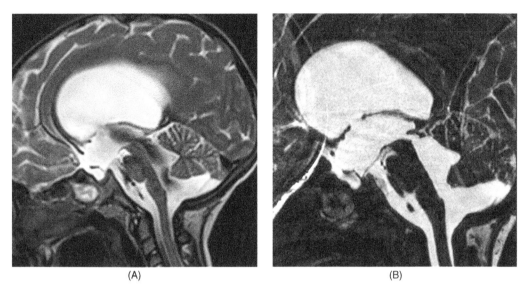

(A)   (B)

Figure 6 Dilated aqueduct and increased CSF waves in communicating hydrocephalus. Conventional FSE T2 (**A**) shows a prominent flow void (decreased craniospinal compliance), while high-definition T2 (**B**) shows the absence of ventricular or cisternal obstruction.

multiple, noncommunicating cavities accumulate CSF/interstitial fluid. Draining one of them just allows the other ones to expand, so that this type of hydrocephalus is one of the most difficult to deal with.

The Cisterns

In hydrocephalus, the cisterns may be effaced or dilated, depending on the specific anatomic/ hydrodynamic conditions in each patient.

When the obstruction is *intraventricular*, the cisterns surrounding the portion of the brain that is hydrocephalic tend to be effaced. In case of aqueductal occlusion, the supratentorial cisterns are effaced, including the suprasellar and ambient cisterns, the interhemispheric cistern as well as the arachnoid space over the convexity. In case of 4th ventricular occlusion, the

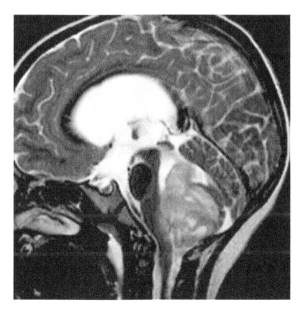

Figure 7 Mechanically dilated aqueduct asso-ciated with a 4th ventricular tumor.

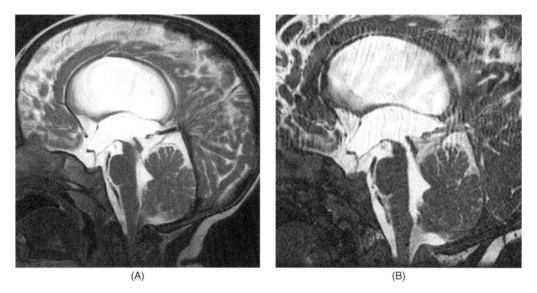

(A)   (B)

Figure 8   Triventricular hydrocephalus with clear flow void (**A**) and anatomically patent aqueduct (**B**).

posterior fossa cisterns (cisterna magna, cisterns around the brainstem and midbrain) are effaced as well.

When the occlusion is *cisternal*, the cisterns located between the occlusion and the ventricular outlets are dilated and the cisterns located between the occlusion and the main reabsorption sites are effaced (Fig. 10). However, cisternal obstructions often result from diffuse arachnoid fibrosis with multiple occlusive arachnoid adhesions, so that the cisterns often are multiloculated and sometimes really multicystic.

In case of chronic communicating hydrocephalus, all basal cisterns tend to be dilated together with the ventricles, including the insular and pericallosal cisterns, in contrast, however, with the arachnoid spaces over the convexity, which are effaced as a result of the expansion of the lateral ventricles.

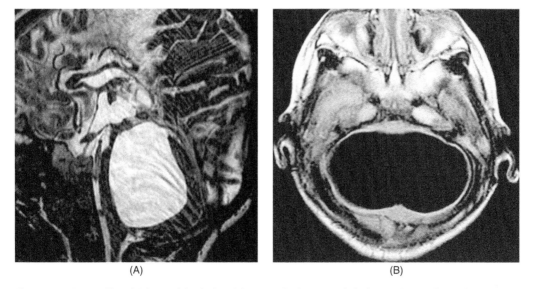

(A)   (B)

Figure 9   Hugely dilated 4th ventricle, isolated between both the occluded aqueduct and ventricular outlets (sagittal high-definition T2) (**A**); remainder of the ventricles are efficiently drained. Axial view (**B**) showing compression and stretching of cerebellum and brainstem.

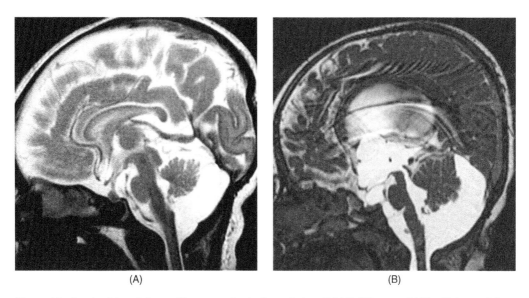

(A)   (B)

Figure 10 Arachnoid septations with progressive hydrocephalus. At birth (**A**), normal MR with large cisterna magna only in an infant presenting with neonatal seizures. At 17 months (**B**) hydrocephalus is obvious, and high-definition T2 image shows transverse prepontine septations.

Finally, there is one instance in which the arachnoid spaces over the convexity are dilated: this is called external hydrocephalus [or alternatively extraventricular obstructive hydrocephalus (EVOH), benign congenital enlargement of subarachnoid spaces, etc.). This pattern is found in infants only. It is characterized by an extracerebral accumulation of fluid with macrocephaly and without loss of brain volume (Fig. 11). This distribution fits what physics would predict in case of obstruction of the reabsorption sites over the frontotemporal convexity: dilatation of the fluid spaces located immediately upstream to the obstruction. It has been tentatively explained by an immaturity of the arachnoid granulations, but it could be immaturity of any reabsorption structure as well, such as the intradural dural clefts, or the nasal mucosal-lymphatic

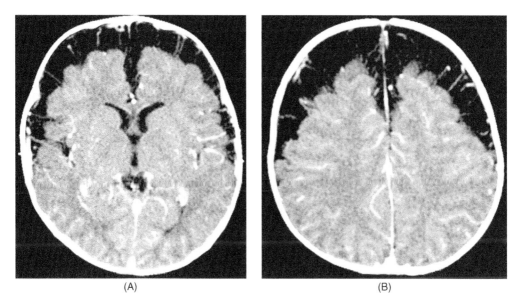

(A)   (B)

Figure 11 External idiopathic benign hydrocephalus. CT with contrast. Macrocephaly with markedly enlarged CSF spaces anteriorly, traversed by the enhanced bridging veins (**A–B**).

pathway underlying the cribriform plate (19–29). The fact that this pattern may be found in association with high venous pressure lends credence to this tentative explanation. In most cases, however, external hydrocephalus is idiopathic, and sometimes familial.

Acute Parenchymal Changes
Circulatory arrest

Because both CSF and fluid-filled parenchyma are not compressible, the main complication of a steep increase of intraventricular/intracranial pressure is the vascular compression: of the subependymal veins in the ventricles, of the cortical veins against the vault, and of the engorged intracerebral capillary bed in between. The resulting increased capillary pressure results in brain edema, herniations that obliterate the tentorial incisura and/or the foramen magnum (further increasing the pressure), and leads to circulatory arrest. This may occur early in hyperacute hydrocephalus, or as the end-complication of progressive hydrocephalus. In hyperacute hydrocephalus the ventricles remain small but rounded [Fig. 12(A–B)]. In both, the pericerebral spaces are occluded, the parenchyma becomes edematous with loss of grey–white matter contrast [Fig. 12(C)] and if administered, intravenous contrast pools in the surface vessels.

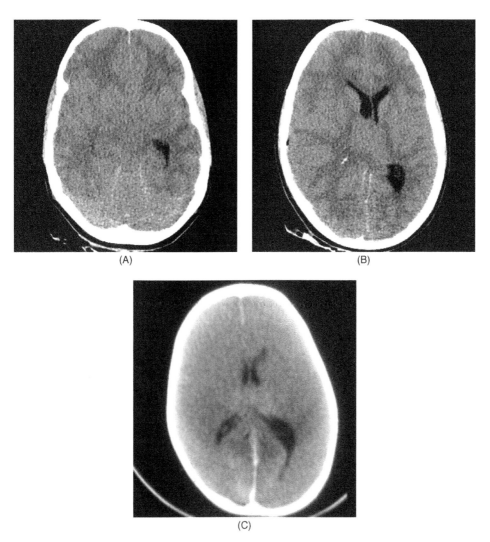

(A)   (B)

(C)

Figure 12   Severe head trauma with acute epidural bleed (not shown), demonstrating mildly dilated and rounded lateral ventricles (**A–B**); the gray–white contrast is maintained. In another patient (**C**) in similar circumstances, loss of the gray–white contrast reflecting a circulatory arrest.

Herniation

An increased ventricular pressure in the supratentorial space with ventricular dilation leads to downward herniation of the mesial temporal structures along the free edge of the tentorium toward the posterior fossa. In the process, the midbrain and the aqueduct are compressed, and the vessels are stretched with superadded focal ischemia. If the hindbrain is affected, the herniation may develop upward through the tentorial incisura and downward through the foramen magnum, with similar effects on the midbrain and medulla. Beside, the occlusion of the outlets of the cranium results in a steep, tamponade-like increase of the intracranial pressure.

Periventricular interstitial edema

Acute hydrocephalus is characterized by a periventricular band of low density on CT, low T1, and high T2/FLAIR on MR, which reflects what is described as a periventricular interstitial edema [Fig. 3(D)]. Rather than an outflow of fluid from the ventricle to the parenchyma (which could in some way relieve the ventricular pressure), this appearance is felt to represent a failure of the drainage of the parenchyma toward the ventricle/subependymal veins (50). The compression of the subependymal veins prevents the normal absorption of the interstitial fluid in the periventricular white matter, resulting in an interstitial edema that is added to, and is a complication of, hydrocephalus. It may probably be associated with other structural changes such as demyelination and astrocytosis (50). As a general rule, the topography of this periventricular interstitial edema reflects the distribution of the drainage territory of the subependymal veins [Fig. 3(D)]. For some unclear reason, however, it often extends to the cortex in acutely hydrocephalic infants.

Structural parenchymal changes

Besides the periventricular edema, various structural changes develop in the acute hydrocephalic brain. The ependymocytes are generally assumed not to proliferate beyond midgestation. With the expansion of the ventricular surface, ependymal cells flatten to maintain the lining, but the stretching possibilities are limited and the ependyma becomes rapidly disrupted, especially over the white matter and the septum pellucidum (50). The circumventricular organs have been shown to be altered in animals, but the effect of this is not known (50). Choroid plexuses also degenerate and become sclerotic, possibly with decreased secretory activity (50). Multiple experimental and animal studies have demonstrated that cerebral blood flow is compromised in hydrocephalus and may improve after shunt placement (50–52); an evaluation of this phenomenon is possible using MR technology (52). Impaired energy metabolism has been demonstrated by ^{31}P MRS and ^{1}H MRS in experimental hydrocephalus (53), but the same group could not show similar changes with ^{1}H MRS in human hydrocephalus (44). Finally, the white matter bundles ought to be affected in acute hydrocephalus; on imaging, the ventricular enlargement implies stretching of the corpus callosum, the septum pellucidum (which contains the fibers that connect the septal cortex to the cingulate cortex), the longitudinal and transverse (hippocampal commissure) fibers of the fornix, as well as lateral to the ventricles, the occipitofrontal, inferior longitudinal, and corticospinal bundles, and the optic radiations. Histologically, this stretching has been shown to be associated with axonal degeneration (50). MR imaging with DTI has been used and demonstrated microstructural changes reflecting the compression of the tracts in the white matter lateral to the ventricles (increased FA, increased longitudinal diffusivity but unchanged ADC) but not in the corpus callosum (decreased FA with increased ADC) (43).

Chronic Parenchymal Changes

Although much of the acute changes (interstitial edema, chronic demyelination, vascular compromise, and axonal loss) noted in progressive hydrocephalus appear to be reversible if shunting is performed in a timely fashion, ependymal damage, gliosis, and abnormal myelination, including aberrant myelination of glial cells, may persist (50). Demyelination typically is easily demonstrated on MR imaging as a ribbon of bright T2/FLAIR signal in the paraventricular white matter (Fig. 13). The subependymal fibrosis and sclerosis are apparent at autopsy (54); it may appear in young infants on T2-weighted MR images, as a dark line of the ventricular wall interposed between the bright CSF and the bright white matter (Fig. 14). The axonal

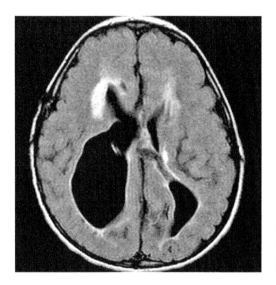

Figure 13 Periventricular white matter demyelination, fibrosis, and sclerosis appearing as a bright subependymal signal on FLAIR in a patient without increased intracranial pressure [Figure 15(**B**) as well].

degeneration is reflected by the loss of brain substance that may persist after the relief of the hydrocephalus; this is amplified by the fact that the lack of axons is accompanied by a corresponding lack of myelin and supporting tissue (Fig. 15). In chronic hydrocephalus with very slowly enlarging ventricles, there may be a threshold beyond which the neurological disorders become irreversible (54). Axonal degeneration, however, does not necessarily imply neuronal loss (55), and as long as the brain tissue still provides the cues necessary to the axonal regrowth, return to a brain shape close to normal is possible. This may be particularly spectacular in infants whose posterior cerebral mantle may sometimes be only a few millimeters thick before shunting (Fig. 16).

A rare late complication of chronic hydrocephalus is the local rupture of the ventricular wall and the development of a CSF-filled cleft that dissociates the hemispheric white matter ("ventricular disruption") (Fig. 17). Similar changes have been reported in human fetal hydrocephalus (pseudo-schizencephalies) (56) and in hydrocephalic dogs (57) and rats (58).

CSF Flow Assessment
Because it allows quantification of the CSF velocity, cine phase-contrast imaging has been used to analyze the dynamics of the CSF in health (7,11–13,33,34,59–61) and disease (62), especially

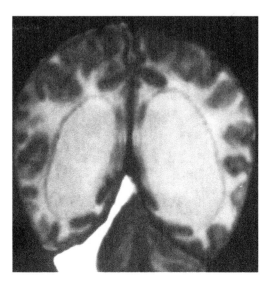

Figure 14 Neonate with hydrocephalus related to a chronic subdural collection in the posterior fossa. Note the dark T2 signal of the ventricular wall against both the CSF and the unmyelinated parenchyma, reflecting the ventricular wall fibrosis/sclerosis.

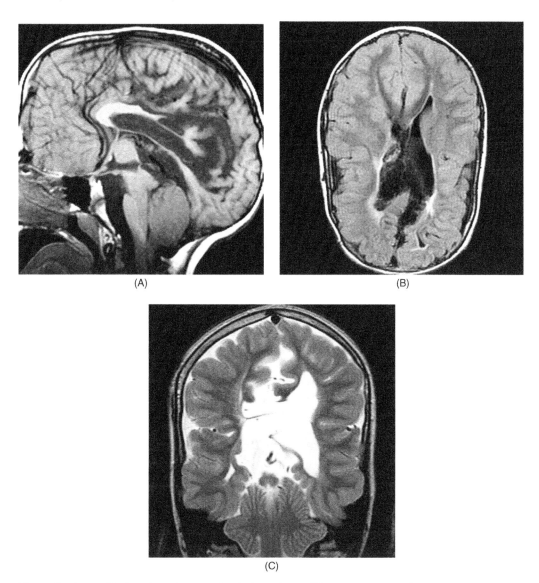

(A)							(B)

(C)

Figure 15 Loss of brain volume, longstanding hydrocephalus (Chiari 2, 18 years old). Note the prominence of the CSF spaces due to the lack of expansion of the parenchyma despite the ventricular drainage (**A–B**).

in chronic adult hydrocephalus (41,62,63–65) and Chiari I (66–68); it has been proposed to assess 3rd ventriculocisternostomy patency as well (69,70). This approach has proven to be extremely productive to understand the physiology and the pathophysiology of various types of hydrocephalus, notably the chronic communicating adult hydrocephalus (normal pressure hydrocephalus). However, as noted above, because of the many parameters involved, the quantification in individual patients is of little use. All the quantitative studies reported have been done by comparing homogeneous groups of patients with controls and in resting situation. From a practical point of view, for individual patients in a clinical setting, the qualitative assessment of the flow voids, as they are demonstrated on T2 FSE imaging, is considered as sensitive as cine phase-contrast in most instances, notably in ventriculocisternostomies (69).

Etiology and Morphologic Patterns of Hydrocephalus

Most CNS pathologies may cause hydrocephalus: malformations (notably, but not only Chiari II and Dandy–Walker malformations) and midline cysts, tumors, acute and chronic inflammation

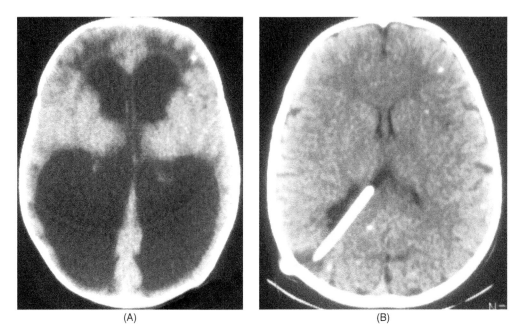

(A)   (B)

Figure 16 Good cerebral resilience. A 2.5-month-old presents with extensive hydrocephalus due to fetal toxoplasmosis (**A**); note the thinness of the cerebral mantle posteriorly. Same child at 11 months after successful
ventricular drainage (**B**): significant restoration of the cerebral mantle.

related to infection or hemorrhage, and trauma. Each specific pathology tends to create specific
conditions, and hydrocephalus can be morphologically classified in broad groups that are
relatively consistent.

Tumoral Hydrocephalus
This is the most characteristic example of progressive obstructive hydrocephalus. In children, approximately 80% of tumors develop along the midline in the anterior 3rd ventricle (e.g., optic/hypothalamic JPA, craniopharyngioma), the pineal region (e.g., germ cell
tumors, pinealoblastoma, glioma), and the posterior fossa (e.g., medulloblastoma, cerebellar
JPA, ependymoma). Hydrocephalus typically is mild to moderate at the time of diagnosis. The
ventricles are markedly rounded. A significant periventricular interstitial edema is almost constantly associated. Because the veins are more resistant to stretching than the white matter, they
encroach on the ventricular lumen [Fig. 3(D)]. When the compression is in the pineal region or
in the posterior fossa the anterior 3rd ventricle is markedly dilated. This high-pressure hydrocephalus obviously is explained by the progressive obstruction of the ventricular pathway,
but may be made worse by the resulting loss of ventricular compliance (pressure waves are
not dampened) and the added intraventricular pulsatility of the tumor (the amplitude of the
pulsatile pressure wave is increased).

Hydrocephalus associated with the choroid plexus papilloma is particular. Although the
tumor may be large, it is often seen floating in the ventricular atrium without obstructing it: yet,
the ventricles are dilated bilaterally (Fig. 18). This is commonly explained by the fact that the
choroid plexus papilloma secretes CSF in excess, and that this overproduction would overcome
that capacity of the system to reabsorb the fluid. This has been controversial however, and
it has been proposed that some obstructive effect and hyperproteinic CSF might contribute to
hydrocephalus. Another contribution may be that the papilloma is pulsating into the ventricular
lumen, and therefore increases the amplitude of the pressure wave in a way similar to what
was done experimentally by Di Rocco et al. in 1978 (32). A similar type of hydrocephalus is
uncommonly observed is association with choroid plexus hyperplasia (Fig. 19).

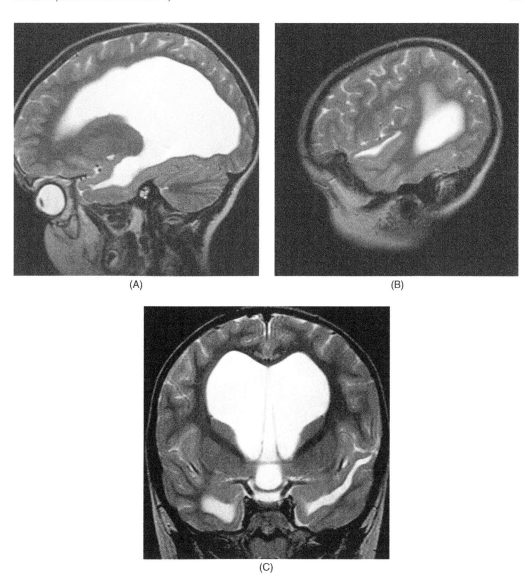

(A)

(B)

(C)

Figure 17 Ventricular disruption. In a chronic hydrocephalus, dissection cleft in the white matter because of CSF that penetrates the parenchyma through the ventricular wall at the anterior end of the left temporal horn (**A, C**) and extends along the white matter of the superior temporal gyrus (**B, C**). On repeated imaging 5 years later, the cleft had extended to the angular gyrus.

Infectious Hydrocephalus

Infectious hydrocephalus that develops in case of septic meningitis (including tuberculous meningitis) may develop early or late. Similar changes may occur in case of massive tumor seeding or massive hemorrhage. Intense meningeal inflammation obstructs the basal cisterns and leads to acute hydrocephalus that may go unrecognized, as the rounded ventricles are often not clearly enlarged because of the rapidity of the process and because of the associated brain edema. The blockage of CSF flow facilitates the penetration of infection into the ventricles, the development of a ventriculitis, which compromises the function of the choroid plexuses, and the diffusion of the germs along the inflamed veins into the parenchyma where they develop to form abscesses. If not treated quickly and efficiently, the suppuration results in loculated cisternal and ventricular spaces, communicating or not with the cavities of the abscesses (Fig. 20). This results in the severe chronic multicystic hydrocephalus. Intraventricular membrane formation results

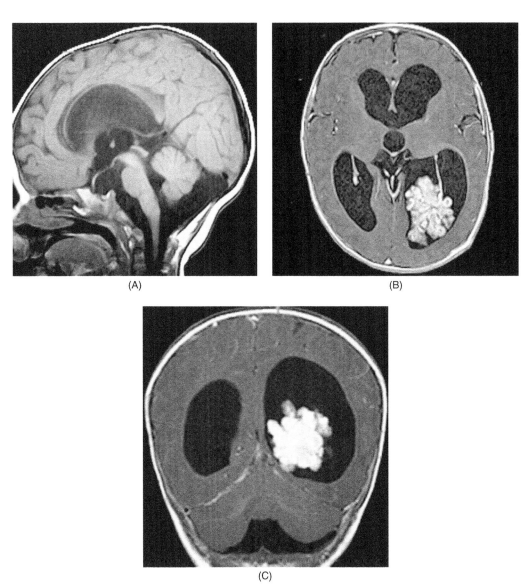

Figure 18 Choroid plexus papilloma. Communicating hydrocephalus (**A**) with a large, floating multiloculated mass in the left atrium (**B, C**) in a 4-month-old infant. Hydrocephalus is assumed to be caused by hyperproduction of CSF, but the fact that hydrocephalus is asymmetrical suggests that the pulsatility of the tumor plays a role as well.

in septation, and parts of the ventricles may become isolated (trapped), especially (but not only) the temporal horns and the 4th ventricle. Treatment is made more difficult by the lack of communication, as draining one cavity favors the expansion (and the compressive effects) of another one. Even in more benign forms, arachnoid fibrosis prevents a free circulation of CSF in the cisterns, obstructing the reabsorption pathway while decreasing the craniospinal compliance as well, with chronic "communicating" (more exactly: extraventricular) hydrocephalus as a consequence (Fig. 10). Even with minor sequelae, the loss of craniospinal compliance may explain the delayed development of adult chronic secondary communicating hydrocephalus.

Subarachnoid Blood
Subarachnoid blood may also result in both acute and chronic communicating hydrocephalus. Whatever be its origin (usually perinatal injury in the preterm and vascular malformation or

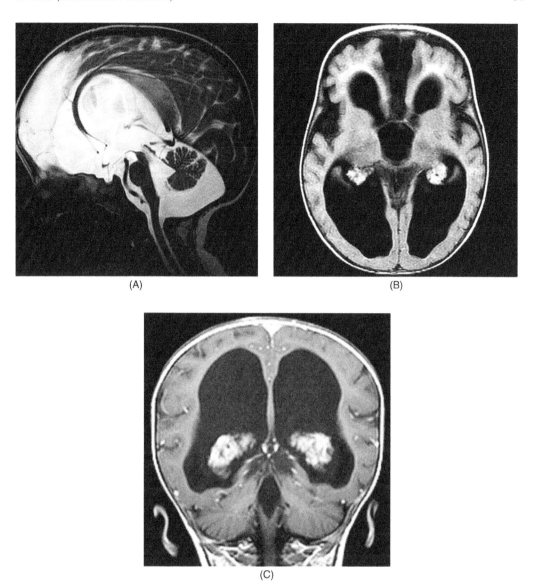

(A)   (B)

(C)

Figure 19   Choroid plexus bilateral hyperplasia. Large symmetrical communicating hydrocephalus (**A–C**). The significant enlargement of the anterior interhemispheric fissure (**A, B**) supports the hypothesis that hypersecretion is important as a cause for hydrocephalus in this 11-month infant.

trauma later in life), the accumulation of blood in the meninges blocks the CSF turnover. This may results in acute obstructive hydrocephalus, often with near-normal or mildly dilated ventricles and cerebral edema related the arterial spasm and ischemia. After washout of the blood cells, permanent inflammatory changes may affect the ependymal lining, induce arachnoid septations, and result in obstructive (usually aqueductal stenosis) or communicating (by loss of craniospinal compliance) hydrocephalus (Fig. 21).

Aqueductal Stenosis
In most cases, the term aqueductal "stenosis" describes a complete occlusion. It may be congenital, acquired in the evolution of a meningitis or ventricular hemorrhage (Fig. 22), associated with an apparently dormant tectal mass (Fig. 23), idiopathic and discovered late in adolescence

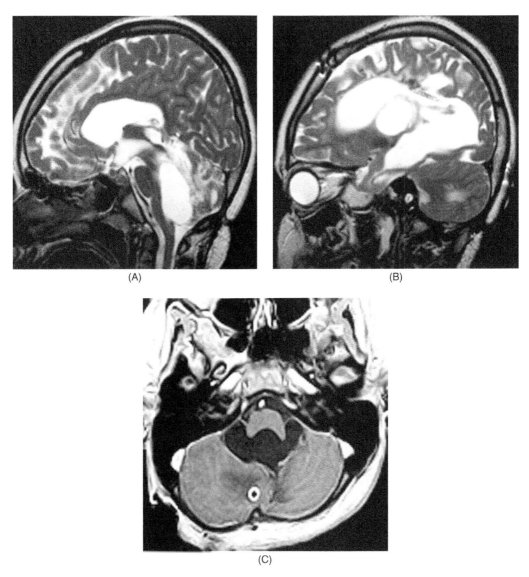

(A)   (B)

(C)

Figure 20 Previous preterm with intraventricular hemorrhage and meningitis. Multicystic, loculated hydro-cephalus with isolated 4th ventricle (**A, C**) and dilated parenchymal cavities (**B**); note the bulging of the lateral recesses of the 4th ventricle (**C**).

or in adulthood, and rarely genetic. The term aqueductal stenosis is usually not used when the compression results from an extrinsic, evolutive mass (such as an arachnoid cyst or a pineal region tumor). Although the occlusion typically appears complete, it may be well tolerated and present as a chronic, even arrested hydrocephalus, in a child with longstanding macrocephaly. But in other patients, often young infants with a similar lesion, it may present more acutely, with signs of increased intracranial pressure and even periventricular interstitial edema. The latter may be compared to progressive obstructive hydrocephalus (e.g., tumoral). The former raises the questions of why and how reabsorption of the CSF through the parenchyma apparently compensates the ventricular CSF secretion successfully over a long period of time. Even though the ventriculomegaly usually increases slowly over time (with occasional development of ventricular diverticula), some rare cases may be considered as truly arrested. Usual treatment now consists of a 3rd ventriculocisternostomy.

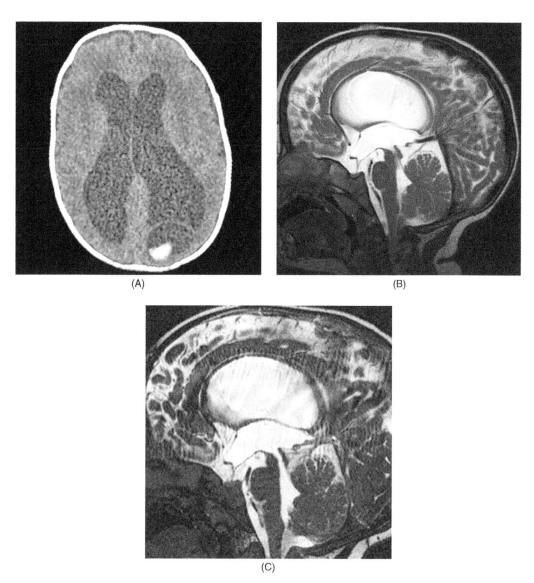

Figure 21   Preterm, intraventricular hemorrhage (**A**). MR at 10 months demonstrates communicating hydro-cephalus with good flow void through the aqueduct and 4th ventricular outlets (**B**), without any evidence of obstruction (**C**).

Compressive Midline Arachnoid Cysts

Suprasellar arachnoid cysts expand upward, displacing and stretching the floor of the 3rd ventricle toward the foramina of Monro, and typically result in a triventricular hydrocephalus in which the 3rd ventricle appears rounded and the axial transverse slices (Fig. 5). Arachnoid cysts of the ambient cistern also result in a triventricular hydrocephalus; the diagnosis rests upon the image of the tectal plate and aqueduct being displaced and compressed by a cisternal CSF-like fluid-filled mass, which should not be confused with a dilated suprapineal recess however. Retrocerebellar arachnoid cysts result in triventricular hydrocephalus as well; they also compress the cerebellum and obstruct the 4th ventricle, and occasionally the aqueduct as well.

Malformative Hydrocephalus

Malformative hydrocephalus is identified by the anatomical features specific for each malforma-tion. It concerns not only myelomeningocele/Chiari II and (true) Dandy–Walker mostly, but

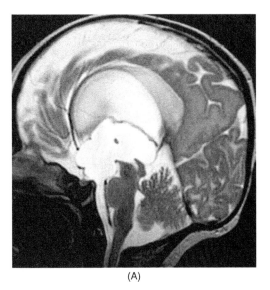 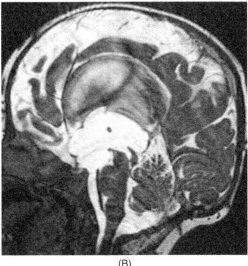

(A)   (B)

Figure 22 Congenital hydrocephalus. The aqueductal stenosis is well shown with the absence of flow void on conventional TSE T2 (**A**). High-definition T2, however, better demonstrated that the obstruction is double (**B**).

also other malformations of cortical development (e.g., cobblestone cortex) or of the white mater (e.g., X-linked hydrocephalus). It is usually recognized in utero or at birth.

Communicating Hydrocephalus

The purest form of *communicating hydrocephalus* is seen in the elderly adult. It is called idiopathic when no cause is found; however, it is suspected that a remote cause such as a minimal bleed or some infection could have caused it. Because of the common association with arterial disease, it has been suggested that an arteriopathic loss of compliance of the vascular bed in the brain tissue, in addition with the loss of elasticity of the main arterial feeders, results in an increased amplitude of the arterial pulsations. This in turn would overcome the craniospinal meningeal compliance, and therefore result in hydrocephalus (7). Radiologically, the main features are, in the absence of any obstruction in the ventricles or the cisterns, a diffuse ventricular enlargement out of proportion with the cortical atrophy, bowing of the corpus callosum, prominence of the basal cisterns, especially of the insular/sylvian cisterns (71), and an enlarged head that may suggest an old-standing process (72). There is no periventricular interstitial edema (as the

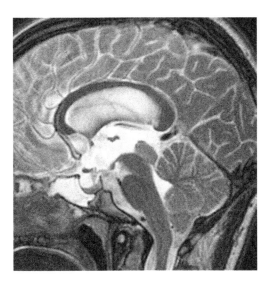

Figure 23 Aqueductal stenosis. Dormant tumor of the tectal plate.

ventricular pressure is not high enough to compress the subependymal veins), but white matter abnormalities such as leukoaraiosis may be present because of an associated arterial disease. Because of the loss of thecal compliance, the amplitude of the CSF pulsations across the aqueduct is significantly increased; this can be quantified using cine phase-contrast imaging and related methods (41,63). It can be qualitatively appreciated as it appears on T2 imaging as a markedly increased flow-void (73).

Benign Idiopathic External Infantile Hydrocephalus

Benign idiopathic external infantile hydrocephalus [extraventricular obstructive hydrocephalus (EVOH), benign enlargement of the subarachnoid spaces in infants]. The widening of the *sub-arachnoid* spaces extends over the frontal and anterior temporal convexities, together with an enlargement of the anterior part of the lateral ventricles (Fig. 11). It can be differentiated from atrophy by the presence of a concomitant macrocephaly and from subdural collections by the fact that the bridging veins traverse the widened spaces normally (Fig. 11), and are not displaced toward the brain surface as in a subdural fluid accumulation. Although the density may appear similar on CT, subdural collection always have a different signal from CSF on MR using T1, T2, and FLAIR sequences (as the protein concentration is always different in inflammatory effusions, traumatic hygromas, or evolving hematomas). Normally, external hydrocephalus resolves spontaneously by about 18 months of age and is therefore considered benign. (Whether it predisposes to subdural hemorrhages in case of minor, noninflicted trauma is still the subject of controversies) (74). However, external hydrocephalus may also be generated by any pathology that causes an increase of the venous pressure (arteriovenous malformation of fistula, venous thrombosis, bony stenosis of the venous outlets in bone dysplasia, etc.) (Figs. 24 and 25); in that case it is not benign and is considered the infantile equivalent of the later-occurring pseudotumor cerebri.

Fetal and Congenital Hydrocephalus

Fetal hydrocephalus describes hydrocephalus recognized in utero (with the help of US, possibly complemented by single-shot, ultrafast T2-weighted MR) and congenital hydrocephalus describes hydrocephalus recognized at birth; the two obviously concern the same pathologies diagnosed in different circumstances. Using MR, the diagnosis of hydrocephalus from ventriculomegaly rests on the ventricular morphology (more global dilatation, rounding of the ventricles in hydrocephalus), the effacement of the normally prominent fetal subarachnoid spaces, and the demonstration of a cause for hydrocephalus (36). The fetal head may or may not be enlarged (Fig. 26). In large hydrocephalus, the cerebral mantle is markedly thinned (Fig. 26) and the septum pellucidum may be dehiscent. If the cerebral mantle is preserved and if hydrocephalus is purely mechanical, the normal parenchymal layers can usually be recognized [Figs. 27(B) and 28(B)]. By contrast in secondary destructive nonhydrocephalic ventriculomegaly, the hemispheres are not expanded and the hemispheric multilayered pattern is usually lost (36). Infectious or hemorrhagic causes may obviously lead to hydrocephalus together with brain destruction however. In malformative hydrocephalus, the features of the malformation may be recognized: myelomeningocele, small posterior fossa with herniated cerebellum, dilated ventricles with *small head*, and effaced arachnoid spaces in Chiari II malformation (Fig. 27); high tentorium and cystic posterior fossa in Dandy–Walker spectrum (75) (Fig. 28). The so-called colpocephaly in callosal agenesis reflects a lack of white matter, not hydrocephalus (75). Identification is more difficult when the malformation associates a white matter defect and aqueductal stenosis, like in X-linked hydrocephalus (part of CRASH syndrome: Callosal agenesis, Retardation, Abducted thumbs, Spasticity, and Hydrocephalus). Other cases of aqueductal stenosis may be genetic (76,77) or acquired, mostly postinflammatory (e.g., mumps, toxoplasmosis). Vascular malformations such as a vein of Galen aneurysm, tumors, extracerebral cyst, etc., may cause fetal hydrocephalus as well. The ventricular dilation is variable, but usually more significant and associated with more brain volume loss in early than in late hydrocephalus. Depending on the etiology, it may be associated with focal mantle destruction and porencephaly. Mantle disruption may also occur as a complication of hydrocephalus (78) (Fig. 29).

Sequential ultrasonography and MR imaging help in the prognostic assessment of fetal or congenital hydrocephalus, which seems to depend on three main factors: the etiology of

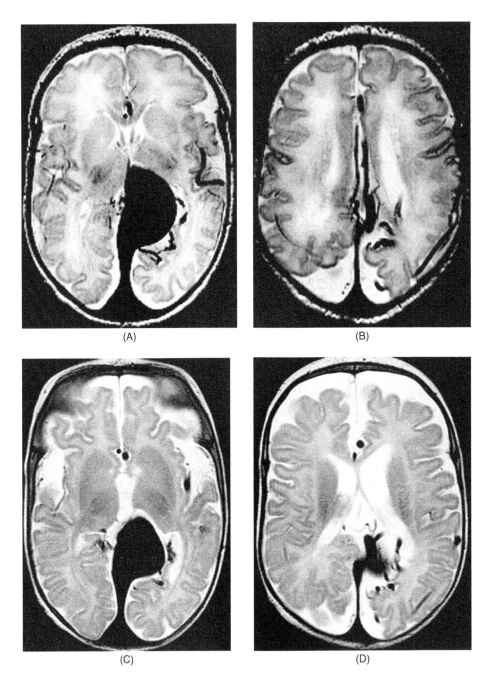

(A)   (B)

(C)   (D)

Figure 24 Hydrocephalus and vein of Galen aneurysm. Imaging in the neonatal period show the vascular malformation but no ventricular dilation (**A, B**). At 3 months, both the ventricular system and the pericerebral spaces are dilated (**C, D**).

hydrocephalus, the time in gestation of its development (the earlier the hydrocephalus, the poorer the prognosis), and the degree of the ventricular dilation (78,79).

INTRACRANIAL HYPOTENSION
Although abnormal CSF hydrodynamics usually consist of increased volume/pressure, therefore hydrocephalus, another clinical–radiological syndrome of CSF–brain interaction impairment is related to a decrease of the CSF pressure. This syndrome may be secondary to various

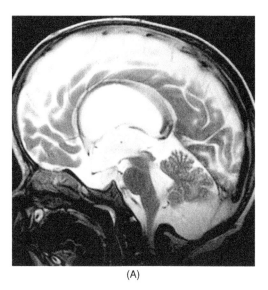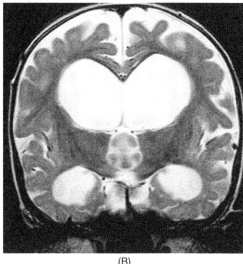

(A) (B)

Figure 25 Hurler disease. Massive communicating hydrocephalus (**A, B**), presumably related to stenosis/obstruction of the venous outlets across the cranial base.

conditions such as connective diseases (e.g., Marfan disease) or medical intervention (lumbar puncture, spinal surgery as well as CSF diversion devices); it may also be idiopathic. The main symptom is a postural headache exacerbated by standing and relieved by reclining. Other non-specific neurological manifestations may be observed, including coma. CSF leak in the spinal canal can be treated by the epidural injection of the patients' blood (blood patches).

Head MR imaging is diagnostic, showing a characteristic constellation of nonspecific abnormalities (80). The most typical findings are a diffuse pachymeningeal (dural) enhancement and thickening (PME/PMT; 100%), and the venous distension sign (VDS; 100%), which expresses the venous engorgement related to the low intracranial pressure (80; Fig. 30). PMT may be seen without contrast administration on FLAIR images; VDS may be recognized on T1 imaging without contrast as well, from the suggestive convexity of the sinus walls (80); it is the first anomaly to resolve after normalization of the intracranial pressure (80). Other abnormalities include subdural hygromas or hematomas, crowding of the cisterns, downward brain herniation with Chiari I deformity [Fig. 30(A)]. An increased height of the pituitary gland with

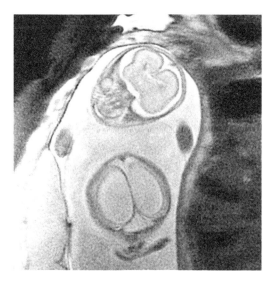

Figure 26 Twin pregnancy, with twin 1 hydrocephalic. Note that despite the massive ventricular dilation of twin 1, the head sizes are similar.

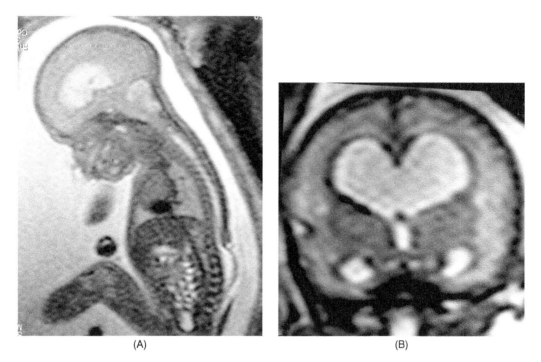

         (A)   (B)

Figure 27   Myelomeningocele and Chiari 2 (**A**). Note the absence of clear macrocrania (**A**), as well as the effacement of the pericerebral spaces (compare with normal fetus in Fig. 26). Layering in the cerebral mantle is preserved (**B**).

convex upper border is commonly observed as well (80). When the cause is a spontaneous or iatrogenic CSF leak, spine imaging, using T2W sequences with fat saturation, may show the location of the CSF leak in the peridural fat and help directing the placement of the blood patch.

FOLLOW-UP IMAGING IN HYDROCEPHALUS
Beyond the natural history of its causal disease, hydrocephalus itself is an evolutive condition. Close clinical follow-up therefore is needed, complemented by imaging. US is much helpful, but only during the first months of life. Typically, follow-up is done using CT, because it brings most of the useful information, can be done quickly without sedation, and is cheaper than MR. Repeating CT in young children, however, is concerning for irradiation, and fast single shot imaging has been recommended as an alternative, although the quality of imaging with those fast sequences is not as good as with the more classical ones, and even with CT.

The Therapeutic Options
The best treatment of hydrocephalus is to relieve its cause, whenever it is possible. This is the most common approach in case of progressive obstructive tumoral hydrocephalus, when hydrocephalus is cured by the resection of the tumor. Follow-up imaging in this case addresses the long-term resolution of the hydrocephalus, together with the follow-up of the tumor.

    In case of hyperacute hydrocephalus, *ventricular tapping* with *external ventricular drainage* (EVD) relieves the ventricular tamponade and prevents the circulatory arrest related to the compression of the vascular bed. Follow-up imaging, typically restricted to the acute period, addresses the ventricular size, the morphological features associated with high intraventricular pressure, and the related condition of the parenchyma.

    More classically however, and for decades, hydrocephalus has been not only treated with *permanent ventricular shunt placement*, typically ventriculoperitoneal shunt (VPS), but also ventriculoatrial or ventriculopleural, or cystoperitoneal or lumboperitoneal shunts. Follow-up imaging obviously addresses the brain response and checks for complications related to the

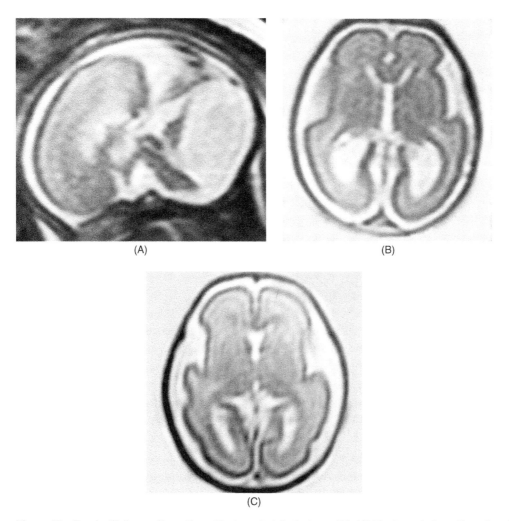

Figure 28 Dandy–Walker malformation with characteristic features (**A**). Mild hydrocephalus with pericerebral spaces hardly effaced and parenchymal layering preserved (**B**). Compare with appearance in fetus of same age 25 weeks (**C**).

shunt insertion, or to under- or overdrainage. Because the shunt is a chronic foreign body, follow-up should also check for complications—disconnection, breakage, infection, and peritoneal complications—specific for this type of material.

Modern trend is toward *endoscopic 3rd ventriculocisternostomy* (ETV). It avoids the placement of a foreign body and allows for CSF diversion when the obstruction sits between the 3rd ventricle and the suprasellar cisterns; in addition, it also alleviates the effects of hydrocephalus by increasing the craniospinal compliance. For neuroradiologists, ETV is special because it needs a precise preoperative assessment of the anterior 3rd ventricle and suprasellar cisterns, and a postoperative evaluation of the ventriculocisternostomy patency. Sagittal high-definition 3D-T2 thin slicing (0.5 mm, CISS/FIESTA sequence) provides an exquisite anatomy of the ventricular floor and surrounding structures and shows the endoscopic opening well; sagittal thin T2 FSE sequence (3 mm) nicely demonstrates the flow void across the ventriculostomy opening. Cine phase-contrast imaging has been reported as a tool to assess the ventriculostomy patency (70), but other reports and clinical practice seem to demonstrate that visual appreciation of the flow void is simpler and correlates well with clinical success (69,81) (Fig. 31).

Surgical cannulation of the aqueduct had been proposed in the 1970s–1980s for treating aqueductal stenosis (82,83), but did not get much support. A modern version of the same

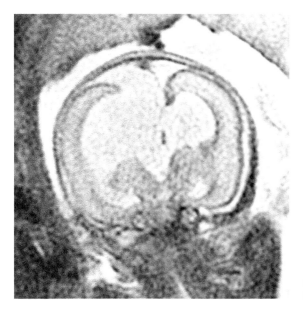

Figure 29 Fetal hydrocephalus. Note the superior disruption/diverticulum on the right.

strategy with *endoscopic aqueductoplasty* without or with stenting has been proposed as well (84,85), but again does not appear to be widely used either.

Immediate Complications of Surgery

Immediate complications of shunt placement or ETV are uncommon. Minimal hemorrhagic changes along the transmantle track may occur, but are not significant. Shunts are usually placed in the ventricular body; their location may sometimes appear unusual (cisterns, basal ganglia, centrum semi-ovale, etc.), but the efficacy of the drainage/restoration of compliance is generally maintained, even when sometimes they seem to have no connection with the CSF-filled spaces. Another early minimal complication may be the leaking of CSF along the track of the shunt or of the endoscope to the scalp and even under the skin. When a catheter needs to be withdrawn to be replaced, intraventricular bleeding may occur because of choroid plexus attachment to the old shunt; this complication as a rule is also benign (Fig. 32).

More severe, but very exceptional, is a vascular tear with massive bleeding during the endoscopic approach across the ventricles or during the ventriculostomy through the 3rd ventricular floor. The radiological picture is that of a significant ventricular or cisternal bleed delineating the surrounding anatomy.

Efficacy of the CSF Diversion

The straightforward approach is the evaluation of the ventricular size, or conversely, the cerebral mantle thickness. Ventricular size may decrease immediately after ventricular tapping, which salvages the vascular bed, or shortly afterward, when hydrocephalus was of short duration without significant alterations of the brain parenchyma. On the other hand, the ventricles may never decrease in size, either because the procedure is not efficient ("underdrainage") or because the cerebral mantle fails to regrow. Underdrainage is suspected when the ventricles remain tense, rounded, and the subarachnoid spaces effaced. Sometimes, CSF may force its way across the brain along the shunt forming CSF-filled cysts, without or with surrounding edema, that persist or even grow over time. Exceptionally, clefts may even develop into the white matter and atrial diverticula may expand medially into the ambient cistern toward the posterior fossa.

The parenchyma is said to be nonresilient when it does not recover from the loss of axons, myelin, and supporting tissues despite an appropriate CSF diversion. The ventricles become smaller but the extracerebral CSF spaces enlarge. Over the years, the brain fails to grow to compensate the collapsing ventricles, and fusion of the sutures and endocranial ossification develop that results in a sometimes major thickening of the calcarium and expansion of the paranasal, mostly frontal and sphenoid, sinuses with decreased intracranial space (Fig. 33).

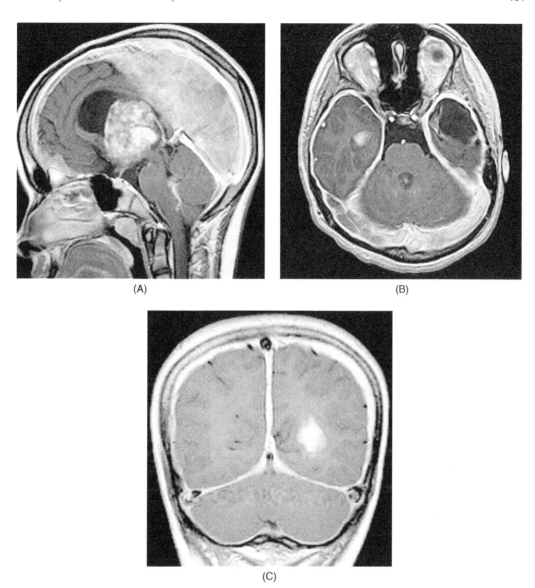

(A)   (B)

(C)

Figure 30   Intracranial hypotension in a child with recurring 3rd ventricular tumor. Contrast-enhanced MR. Note the prominence of the enhanced dura (**A–C**) (pachymeningeal thickening), the effacement of the pericerebral spaces with the Chiari 1 deformity (**A**), and the dilation and rounding of the venous sinuses (venous distension sign) (**B, C**).

This typically happens, to various degrees, when hydrocephalus has been longstanding and the thickness of the cerebral mantle significantly decreased. In infants, however, apparent major tissue loss may recover spectacularly presumably because the tissues still retain the ability to promote axonal growth, cellular multiplication, and myelination.

When in the course of the years, the patients present with new headaches or psychointellectual or neurological deterioration, loss of CSF shunt patency is suspected. New ventricular dilation, even slight, should be appreciated and quantified (frontal or atrial diameter). Effacement of the pericerebral spaces is also an important finding. Rounding of small ventricles would indicate a hyperacute hydrocephalus; periventricular edema would point to a severe increase of the ventricular pressure.

After a 3rd ventriculostomy, even in the case of a classic aqueductal stenosis, the ventricles become smaller than preoperatively but still remain larger than they would be expected to

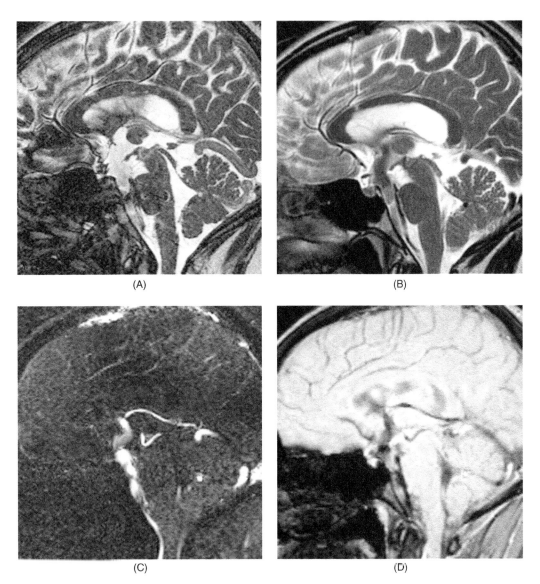

Figure 31 Successful endoscopic 3rd ventriculocisternostomy. High-definition T2 demonstrated a large opening through the tuber cinereum. TSE T2 imaging demonstrates prominent flow void across the stoma (**B**). Cine phase-contrast imaging shows the same, in the systolic (**C**) and diastolic (**D**) phases, but not more convincingly than FSE T2.

be in normal conditions, as well as after the shunt placement. The ventricular size stabilizes after several months at this relatively high level: this suggests that *"successful ETV produces a state of compensated communicating hydrocephalus"* (86). Also, ETV may fail to efficiently correct hydrocephalus in young infants and neonates, possibly because the opening in the ventricular floor tends to close at that age (87).

"Overdrainage" of the CSF
Too much depletion of the ventricles may lead to three types of complications: early development of subdural collections, delayed "slit ventricle," and progressive development of the imaging features of intracranial hypotension.

Subdural collections are uncommon. They develop in the weeks or months following the treatment of the hydrocephalus. It is hard to tell if they develop directly as subdural blood

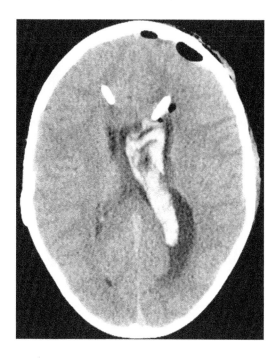

Figure 32 Ventricular hemorrhage after shunt replacement.

collections or primarily as simple hygromas, which may themselves become hemorrhagic (Fig. 34). It is difficult to understand why the ventricular collapse would result in a subdural collection. The pericerebral spaces typically become mildly dilated, and one would expect effacement of (noncommunicating) ventricles without brain restoration to be accompanied by a simple expansion of the subarachnoid spaces. A possibility is that the arachnoid septations do not have enough time to adapt and therefore are pulling the inner dural cellular layers inward, inducing the inner dural vessels to bleed. In the case of a hygroma, interstitial fluid would accumulate instead of blood. Then, like during the evolution of posttraumatic hygromas (88), neoangiogenesis could take place in the inner membrane of the collection and secondarily bleed. Whatever be their mechanism, these collections tend to attenuate and characteristically disappear spontaneously. Rarely, they may become chronic; they have been suspected of being the origin of the occasionally observed fibrous meningeal thickening, but the pathophysiology could be that of the chronic intracranial hypotension (see above).

A late, unusual complication of shunted hydrocephalus is the *slit-ventricle syndrome* (89,90). The patient presents with bout of symptoms, mostly headaches, relating to acute increase of intracranial pressure, but radiologically the ventricles are slit-like; there is nothing specific in that, as patients with slit ventricles do not necessarily present with clinical symptoms (Fig. 35). Typically, the intracranial volume is also decreased and it is assumed that this combination—small ventricle, small cranium—results in a decrease of the buffering capacity in case the shunt intermittently becomes occluded in the narrow ventricular lumen crowded with the choroid plexus.

Another delayed complication of overdrainage is the *complicated acquired Chiari I malformation* (91). CSF diversion produces a major reduction of the skull capacity because of thickening of the calvarium, a possible induced premature closure of the sutures, and expansion of the basal sinuses. Secondarily, this craniocerebral disproportion may be complicated by the development of an intracranial hypertension with tonsillar herniation that can be relieved by a decompressive supratentorial craniotomy only (91). The radiological picture includes a small posterior fossa with tonsillar herniation through the foramen magnum, small ventricles, markedly reduced pericerebral CSF spaces, and prominent thickening of the calvarium (91). As in intracranial hypotension, there may be a pachymeningeal thickening as well, avidly enhancing after contrast administration, and prominent widening of the dural venous sinuses. Clinical features suggest intracranial hypertension with symptoms pointing to the lower brainstem (91).

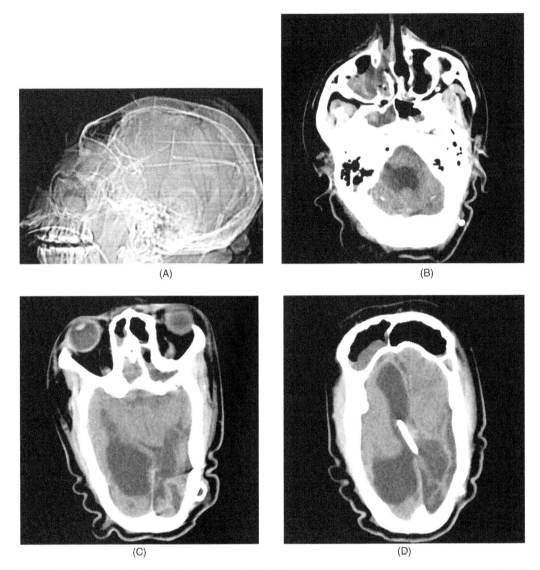

Figure 33 Considerable loss of brain volume with microcrania (**A**), and hypertrophy of the skull base (**B**), vault (**C**), and frontal sinuses (**D**).

Another variety of acquired Chiari I malformation has been described as a fairly common complication in the context of lumboperitoneal shunting (92). It is generally assumed to be caused by the CSF pressure imbalance between the cranium and the spine, but this explanation has been challenged (93).

Problems Concerning to the Shunt Tubing Itself

A shunt is essentially a mechanical device that can become disjoined, calcified, and fractured. Because it is often placed when the patients are very young, the relationships of the shunt with the ventricle and with the peritoneum may change and lead to complications such as the peritoneal cysts. Infection may develop, in the peritoneum, along the tract and in the ventricles. Fluid may sip along the subcutaneous tract of the tubing. Skin erosion may appear on the pressure points. All this may lead to intracranial complication and therefore occasionally involve neuroradiology.

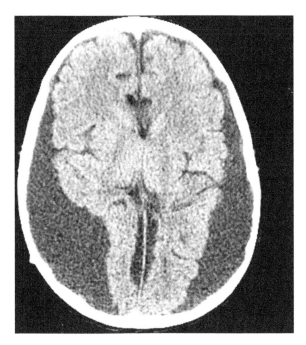

Figure 34 Bilateral subdural collections, denser than CSF.

CONCLUSION

Hydrocephalus is common at all ages, especially in children and in particular in infants. Hydrocephalus has causes that may be life threatening and devastating to the brain. It has its own natural history as well, which often continues far beyond the causal disease. This natural history, a century after the pioneer studies of Dandy and Blackfan, is still poorly understood and therefore, controversial. Not-so-recent concepts concerning the anatomy of the CSF pathways and its physiology (with the interplay between the CSF and the vascular bed and blood flow) have been recently reemphasized and they help understand MR imaging findings better: apparently both bulk flow and pulsatile flow play in association in health and disease, and this interaction has to be understood in each individual case if a proper interpretation of the imaging findings is to be done.

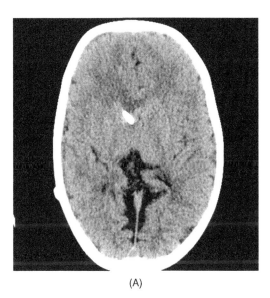
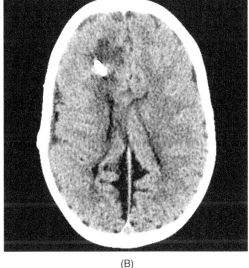

(A) (B)

Figure 35 Slit ventricles in a child without the clinical features of a slit ventricle syndrome (**A–B**).

REFERENCES

1. Bergsneider M, Egnor MR, Johnston M, et al. What we don't (but should) know about hydrocephalus. J Neurosurg (suppl. 3) 2006; 104:157–159.
2. Longatti P, Fiorindi A, Perin A, et al. Endoscopic anatomy of the cerebral aqueduct. Neurosurgery 2007; 61(suppl. 1):1–7.
3. Raybaud C. Cystic malformations of the posterior fossa. Abnormalities of the development of the roof of the 4th ventricle and adjacent meningeal structures. J Neuroradiol 1982; 9:103–133.
4. Klosovskii BN. In: Haight B, ed. The Development of the Brain and Its Disturbance by Harmful Factors. London, U.K.: Pergamon Press, 1963.
5. Artru AA. Spinal cerebrospinal fluid chemistry and physiology. In: Yaksh TL, ed. Spinal Drug Delivery. Amsterdam: Elsevier, 1999:177–238.
6. Xenos C, Sgouros S, Natarajan K. Ventricular volume change in childhood. J Neurosurg 2002; 97: 584–590.
7. Greitz D. Radiological assessment of hydrocephalus: new theories and implications for therapy. Neurosurg Rev 2004; 27:145–165.
8. Zenker W, Bankoul S, Braun JS. Morphological indications for considerable diffuse reabsorption of cerebrospinal fluid in spinal meninges particularly in the areas of meningeal funnels. Anat Embryol 1994; 189:243–258.
9. Bosanovic-Sosic R, Mollanji R, Johnston MG. Spinal and cranial contribution to total cerebrospinal fluid transport. Am J Physiol Regul Integr Comp Physiol 2001; 281:R909–R916.
10. Edsbagge M, Tisell M, Jacobsson L, et al. Spinal CSF absorption in healthy individuals. Am J Physiol Regul Integr Comp Physiol 2004; 287:R1450–R1455.
11. Greitz D. Cerebrospinal fluid circulation and associated intracranial dynamics. A radiologic investigation using MR imaging and radionuclide cisternography. Acta Radiol 1993; 34:1–23.
12. Greitz D, Jan Hannerz J. A proposed model of cerebrospinal fluid circulation: observations with radionuclide cisternography. Am J Neuroradiol 1996; 17:431–438.
13. Greitz D, Greitz T, Hindmarsh TV. A new view on the CSF-circulation with the potential for pharmacological treatment of childhood hydrocephalus. Acta Paediatr 1997; 86:125–132.
14. Greitz D, Greitz T. The pathogenesis and hemodynamics of hydrocephalus. A proposal for a new understanding. Int J Neuroradiol 1997; 3:367–375.
15. Welch K, Friedman V. The cerebrospinal fluid valves. Brain 1960; 83:454–469.
16. Di Chiro G. Observation on the circulation of the cerebrospinal fluid. Acta Radiol Diagn 1966; 5:988–1002.
17. Dandy WE, Blackfan KD. Internal hydrocephalus. An experimental, clinical and pathological study. Am J Dis Child 1914; 8:406–481.
18. Osaka K, Handa H, Matsumoto S, et al. Development of the cerebrospinal fluid pathway in the normal and abnormal human embryo. Childs Brain 1980; 6:26–38.
19. Silver I, Szalai J, Johnston M. Relationship between intracranial pressure and cervical lymphatic pressure and flow rates in sheep. Am J Physiol Regul Integr Comp Physiol 1999; 277:R1712–R1717.
20. Mollanji R, Papaiconomou C, Boulton M, et al. Comparison of cerebrospinal fluid transport in fetal and adult sheep. Am J Physiol Regul Integr Comp Physiol 2001; 281:R1215–R1223.
21. Johnston M, Zakharov A, Koh L, et al. Subarachnoid injection of Microfil reveals connections between cerebrospinal fluid and nasal lymphatics in the non-human primates. Neuropathol Appl Neurobiol 2005; 31:632–640.
22. Koh L, Zakharov A, Nagra G, et al. Development of cerebrospinal fluid absorption sites in the pig and rat: Connections between the subarachnoid space and lymphatic vessels in the olfactory turbinates. Anat Embryol 2006; 211:335–344.
23. Walter BA, Valera VA, Takahashi S, et al. The olfactory route for cerebrospinal fluid drainage into the peripheral lymphatic system. Neuropathol Appl Neurobiol 2006; 32:388–396.
24. Johnston M, Zakharov A, Papaiconomou C, et al. Evidence of connections between cerebrospinal fluid and nasal lymphatic vessels in humans, non-human primates and other mammalian species. Cerebrospinal Fluid Res 2004; 1:2.
25. Koh L, Zakharov A, Johnston M. Integration of the subarachnoid space and lymphatics: Is it time to embrace a new concept of cerebrospinal fluid absorption? Cerebrospinal Fluid Res 2005; 2:6.
26. Papaiconomou C, Zakharov A, Azizi N, et al. Reassessment of the pathways responsible for cerebrospinal fluid absorption in the neonates. Childs Nerv Syst 2004; 20:29–36.
27. Johnston M, Armstrong D, Koh L. Possible role of cavernous sinus veins in cerebrospinal fluid absorption. Cerebrospinal Fluid Res 2007; 4:3.
28. Fox RJ, Walji AH, Mielke B, et al. Anatomic details of intradural channels in the parasagittal dura: A possible pathway for flow of cerebrospinal fluid. Neurosurgery 1996, 39:84–91.
29. Cushing H. Studies on the cerebrospinal fluid. J Med Res 1914; 31:1–19.

30. Du Boulay GH. Pulsatile movements in the CSF pathways. Br J Radiol 1966; 39:255–262.
31. Du Boulay G, O'Connell J, Currie J, et al. Further investigations on pulsatile movements in the cerebrospinal fluid pathways. Acta Radiol Diagn (Stockh) 1972; 13:496–523.
32. Di Rocco C, Pettorossi VE, Caldarelli M, et al. Communicating hydrocephalus induced by mechanically increased amplitude of the intraventricular cerebrospinal fluid pressure: Experimental studies. Exp Neurol 1978; 58:40–52.
33. Lee JH, Lee HK, Kim JK, et al. CSF flow quantification of the cerebral aqueduct in normal volunteers using phase contrast cine MR imaging. Korean J Radiol 2004; 5:81–86.
34. Huang TY, Chung HW, Chen MY, et al. Supratentorial cerebrospinal fluid production rate in healthy adults: Quantification with two-dimensional cine phase-contrast MR imaging with high temporal and spatial resolution. Radiology 2004; 233:603–608.
35. Karmazyn B, Dagan O, Vidne BA, et al. Neuroimaging findings in neonates and infants from superior vena cava obstruction after cardiac operation. Pediatr Radiol 2002; 32:806–810.
36. Girard N, Gire C, Sigaudy S, et al. MR imaging of acquired fetal disorders. Childs Nerv Syst 2003; 19:490–500.
37. Oi S. Diagnosis, outcome and management of fetal abnormalities: Fetal hydrocephalus. Childs Nerv Syst 2003; 19:508–516.
38. Garel C, Luton D, Oury JF, et al. Ventricular dilatations. Childs Nerv Syst 2003; 19:517–523.
39. Fransen E, Lemmon V, van Camp G, et al. CRASH syndrome: Clinical spectrum of corpus callosum hypoplasia, retardation, adducted thumbs, spastic paraparesis and hydrocephalus due to mutation of a single gene L1. Eur J Hum Genet 1995; 3:273–284.
40. Stivaros SM, Jackson A. Changing concepts of cerebrospinal fluid hydrodynamics: Role of phase-contrast magnetic resonance imaging and implication for cerebral microvascular disease. Neurotherapeutics 2007; 4:511–522.
41. Luetner PH, Huston J, Friedman JA, et al. Measurement of cerebrospinal fluid flow at the cerebral aqueduct by use of phase-contrast magnetic resonance imaging: Technique validation and utility in diagnosing idiopathic normal pressure hydrocephalus. Neurosurgery 2002; 50:534–543.
42. Muñoz A, Hinojosa J, Esparza J. Cisternography and ventriculography gadopentetate dimeglumine-enhanced MR imaging in pediatric patients: Preliminary report. AJNR Am J Neuroradiol 2007; 28: 889–894.
43. Assaf Y, Ben-Sira L, Constantini S, et al. Diffusion tensor imaging in hydrocephalus: Initial experience. AJNR Am J Neuroradiol 2006; 27:1717–1724.
44. Braun KPJ, Gooskens RHJM, Vandertop WP, et al. [1]H magnetic resonance spectroscopy in human hydrocephalus. J Magn Reson Imaging 2003; 17:291–299.
45. Iskandar BJ, Sansone JM, Medow J, et al. The use of quick-brain magnetic resonance imaging in the evaluation of shunt-treated hydrocephalus. J Neurosurg 2004; 101(suppl. 2):147–151.
46. Childe AE, McNaughton FL. Diverticula of the lateral ventricles extending in the posterior fossa. Arch Neurol Psychiatr 1942; 47:768–778.
47. Naidich TP, McLone DG, Hahn YS. Atrial diverticula in severe hydrocephalus. AJNR Am J Neuroradiol 1982; 3:257–266.
48. Osuka S, Takano S, Enomoto T, et al. Endoscopic observation of pathophysiology of ventricular diverticulum. Childs Nerv Syst 2007; 23:897–900.
49. Bradley WG, Kortman KE, Burgoyne B. Flowing cerebrospinal fluid in normal and hydrocephalic states: Appearance on MR images. Radiology 1986; 159:611–616.
50. Del Bigio MR. Neuropathological changes caused by hydrocephalus. Acta Neuropathol 1993; 85: 573–585.
51. da Silva MC, Michwicz S, Drake JM, et al. Reduced local cerebral blood flow in periventricular white matter in experimental neonatal hydrocephalus—Restoration with CSF shunting. J Cereb Blood Flow Metab 1995; 15:1057–1065.
52. Leliefeld PH, Gooskens RHJM, Vincken Kl, et al. Magnetic resonance imaging for quantitative flow measurement in infants with hydrocephalus: A prospective study. J Neurosurg Pediatr 2008; 2: 163–170.
53. Braun KPJ, Dijkhuizen RM, de Graaf RA, et al. Cerebral ischemia and white matter edema in experimental hydrocephalus: A combined in vivo MRI and MRS study. Brain Res 1997; 757:295–298.
54. Del Bigio MR, Wilson MJ, Enno T. Chronic hydrocephalus in rats and humans: White matter loss and behavior changes. Ann Neurol 2003; 53:337–346.
55. Ding Y, McAllister JP, Yao B, et al. Neuron tolerance during hydrocephalus. Neuroscience 2001; 106:659–667.
56. Humphreys P, Muzumdar DP, Sly LE, et al. Focal cerebral mantle disruption in fetal hydrocephalus. Pediatr Neurol 2007; 36:236–243.
57. Wünschmann A, Oglesbee M. Periventricular changes associated with spontaneous canine hydrocephalus. Vet Pathol 2001; 38:67–73.

58. Yoshida Y, Koya G, Tamayama K, et al. Histopathology of cystic cavities in the cerebral white matter of HTX rats with inherited hydrocephalus. Neurol Med Chir (Tokyo) 1990; 30:229–233.

59. Levy LM, Di Chiro G. MR phase imaging and cerebrospinal fluid flow in the head and spine. Neuroradiology 1990; 32:399–406.

60. Kolbitsch C, Schoke M, Lorenz IH, et al. Phase-contrast MRI measurement of systolic cerebrospinal fluid peak velocity in the aqueduct of Sylvius: A noninvasive tool for measurement of cerebral capacity. Anesthesiology 1999; 90:1546–1550.

61. de Marco G, Idy-Peretti I, Didon-Poncelet A, et al. Intracranial fluid dynamics in normal and hydrocephalic states. J Comput Assist Tomogr 2004; 28:247–254.

62. Curless RG, Quencer RM, Katz DA, et al. Magnetic resonance demonstration of intracranial CSF flow in children. Neurology 1992; 42:377–381.

63. Mase M, Yamada K, Banno T, et al. Quantitative analysis of CSF flow dynamics using MRI in normal pressure hydrocephalus. Acta Neurochir Suppl 1998; 71:350–353.

64. Tsunoda A, Mitsuoka H, Bandai H, et al. Intracranial cerebrospinal fluid measurement studies in suspected idiopathic normal pressure hydrocephalus, secondary normal pressure hydrocephalus, and brain atrophy. J Neurol Neurosurg Psychiatry 2002; 73:552–555.

65. Stoquart-Elsankari S, Balédent O, Gondry-Jouet C, et al. Aging effects on cerebral blood and cerebrospinal fluid flows. J Cereb Blood Flow Metab 2007; 27:1563–1572.

66. Haughton VM, Korosec FR, Medow JE, et al. Peak systolic and diastolic velocity in the foramen magnum in adult patients with Chiari I malformations and in normal control participants. AJNR Am J Neuroradiol 2003; 24:169–176.

67. Iskandar BJ, Quigley M, Haughton VM. Foramen magnum cerebrospinal fluid flow characteristics in children with Chiari I malformation before and after craniocervical decompression. J Neurosurg 2004; 101(suppl. 2):169–178.

68. Hofkes SK, Iskandar BJ, Turski PA, et al. Differentiation between symptomatic Chiari I malformation and asymptomatic tonsillar ectopia by using cerebrospinal flow imaging: initial estimate of imaging accuracy. Radiology 2007; 245:532–540.

69. Fischbein NJ, Ciricillo SF, Barr RM, et al. Endoscopic third ventriculostomy: MR assessment of patency with 2-D cine phase-contrast versus T2-weighted fast spin echo technique. Pediatr Neurosurg 1998; 28:70–78.

70. Bargalló N, Olondo L, Garcia AI, et al. Functional analysis of third ventriculostomy patency by quantification of CSF stroke volume by using cine phase-contrast MR imaging. AJNR Am J Neuroradiol 2005; 26:2514–2521.

71. Kitagaki H, Mori E, Yamaji S, et al. CSF spaces in idiopathic normal pressure hydrocephalus: Morphology and volumetry. AJNR Am J Neuroradiol 1998, 19:1277–1284.

72. Bradley WG, Safar FG, Hurtado C, et al. Increased intracranial volume: A cue to the etiology of idiopathic normal pressure hydrocephalus. AJNR Am J Neuroradiol 2004; 25:1479–1484.

73. Bradley WG, Whittemore AR, Kortman KE, et al. Marked cerebrospinal fluid void: Indicator of successful shunt in patients with suspected normal-pressure hydrocephalus. Radiology 1991; 178: 459–466.

74. Hymel KP, Jenny C, Block RW. Intracranial hemorrhage and rebleeding in suspected victims of abusive head trauma: Addressing the forensic controversies. Child Maltreat 2002; 7:329–348.

75. Raybaud C, Levrier O, Brunel H, et al. MR imaging of fetal brain malformations. Childs Nerv Syst 2003; 19:455–470.

76. Schrander-Stumpel C, Fryns JP. Congenital hydrocephalus: Nosology and guidelines for clinical approach and genetic counseling. Eur J Pediatr 1998; 157:355–362.

77. Haverkamp F, Wolfle J, Aretz M, et al. Congenital hydrocephalus internus and aqueduct stenosis: Aetiology and implications for genetic counseling. Eur J Pediatr 1999; 158:474–478.

78. Oi S, Honda Y, Hidaka M, et al. Intrauterine high-resolution magnetic resonance imaging in fetal hydrocephalus and prenatal estimation of postnatal outcomes with "perspective classification". J Neurosurg 1998; 88:685–694.

79. Futagi Y, Suzuki Y, Toribe Y, et al. Neurodevelopmental outcome in children with fetal hydrocephalus. Pediatr Neurol 2002; 27:111–116.

80. Forghani R, Farb RI. Diagnosis and temporal evolution of signs of intracranial hypotension on MRI of the brain. Neuroradiology 2008; 50:1025–1034.

81. Kulkarni AV, Drake JM, Armstrong DC, et al. Imaging correlates of successful endoscopic third ventriculostomy. J Neurosurg 2000, 92:915–919.

82. Crosby RM, Henderson CM, Paul RL. Catheterization of the cerebral aqueduct for obstructive hydrocephalus in infants. J Neurosurg 1973, 38:596–601.

83. Lapras C, Bret P, Patet JD, et al. Hydrocephalus and aqueductal stenosis. Direct surgical treatment by interventriculostomy (aqueduct cannulation). J Neurosurg Sci 1986; 30:47–53.

84. Miki T, Nakajima N, Wada J, et al. Indications for neuroendoscopic aqueductoplasty without stenting for obstructive hydrocephalus due to aqueductal stenosis. Minim Invasive Neurosurg 2005; 48:136–141.
85. Erşahin Y. Endoscopic aqueductoplasty. Childs Nerv Syst 2007; 23:143–150.
86. St. George E, Natarajan K, Sgouros S. Changes in ventricular volume in hydrocephalic children following successful endoscopic third ventriculostomy. Childs Nerv Syst 2004; 20:834–848.
87. Drake JM.; Canadian Pediatric Neurosurgery Study Group. Endoscopic third ventriculostomy in pediatric patients: The Canadian experience. Neurosurgery 2007; 60:881–886.
88. Lee KS, Bae WK, Bae HG, et al. The fate of traumatic subdural hygroma in serial computed tomography scans. J Korean Med Sci 2000; 15:560–568.
89. Epstein F, Lapras C, Wisoff JH. Slit ventricle syndrome. Etiology and treatment. Pediatr Neurosci 1988; 14:5–10.
90. Rekate HL. Shunt-related headaches: The slit ventricle syndromes. Childs Nerv Syst 2008; 24:423–430.
91. Caldarelli M, Novegno F, Di Rocco C. A late complication of CSF shunting: Acquired Chiari I malformation. Childs Nerv Syst 2009; 25:443–452.
92. Chumas PD, Armstrong DC, Drake JM, et al. Tonsillar herniation: The rule rather than the exception after lumboperitoneal shunting in the pediatric population. J Neurosurg 1993; 78:568–573.
93. Di Rocco C, Velardi F. Acquired Chiari I malformation managed by supratentorial enlargement. Childs Nerv Syst 2003; 19:800–807.

4 Invasive Measurements of Cerebrospinal Fluid Pressure

Marek Czosnyka, Zofia Czosnyka, and John D. Pickard
Academic Neurosurgical Unit, Department of Neurosciences, Addenbrooke's Hospital, Cambridge, U.K.

INTRODUCTION

Monitoring of CSF (cerebrospinal fluid) pressure and testing of CSF dynamics in patients with suspected or confirmed hydrocephalus, although invasive, may help with the decision about surgery, either shunting or third ventriculostomy. It also provides a reference data for further management of shunted patients when complications, such as shunt blockage, under- and over-drainage, arise. In such cases, physiological measurement may aid the decision about revision of the shunt or prevent unnecessary surgery. This chapter provides synopsis of 25 years of experience with physiological measurements in patients suffering from hydrocephalus.

MONITORING OF ICP

Patients presenting with clinical symptoms of hydrocephalus, solely or overlapping other CNS diseases, and various degrees of ventricular enlargement on brain CT/MRI scans may have normal or increased intracranial pressure (ICP), therefore they may not always develop symptoms of intracranial hypertension.

Intracranial pressure is not a number; it contains different components carrying potentially useful information. Therefore, instant measurement using lumbar puncture manometer is useless—readings may easily miss periods of pathologically elevated ICP or pain, and muscular tension during lumbar puncture (LP) may artificially elevate readings.

Mean ICP can be assessed by minimum 30 minutes of monitoring and time averaging. Even then it may happen that the recorded mean ICP is normal and increases to clearly pathological values during limited time period, usually during the night (Fig. 1). Therefore, overnight computer-assisted monitoring by using intraparenchymal transducer seems to be most conclusive.

Apart from the mean value, dynamics of ICP should be examined carefully. Of particular clinical significance is how high ICP may rise during vasogenic waves. Peaks above 25 mm Hg not associated with coughing, straining, or movements are clearly pathological.

According to classical standards (1), when so-called "B waves" were presented for more than 80% of time of ICP monitoring, shunting was recommended. "B waves" are slow waves of ICP of periods from 20 seconds to 2 minutes. But, using computer detection, "B waves" are almost universally present, probably even in healthy volunteers. There is no data derived from normal subjects. "B waves" seen in ICP are correlated with fluctuations of cerebral blood flow velocity (2). Newer studies do not confirm obvious link between the presence of "B waves" and conditions of disturbed CSF circulation, neither their prognostic value (3). Some recent studies on pulse amplitude of CSF pressure explore the possible significance of greater pulse amplitude as indicator of clinical improvement after shunting. The significance of "B waves" requires wider prospective clinical studies.

Cerebrospinal pressure–volume compensatory reserve can be assessed using correlation coefficient [R] between the pulse amplitude [A] and the mean ICP [P], the so-called RAP index. Theoretically, it indicates the relationship between ICP and changes in intracerebral volume, classically expressed by the pressure–volume curve. A RAP coefficient close to 0 indicates a good pressure–volume compensatory reserve at low ICP. When the pressure–volume curve starts to increase exponentially, pulse amplitude covaries directly with ICP and consequently RAP rises to +1. This indicates a low compensatory reserve, which is the common occurrence in patients with disturbed CSF circulation.

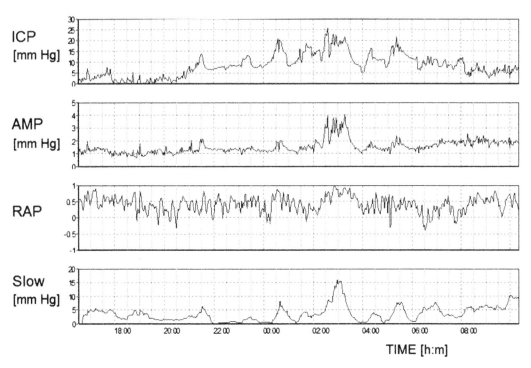

Figure 1 Example of overnight monitoring of ICP (using Camino bolt), revealing slightly increased CSF dynamics. Slow-magnitude of slow waves (B waves) is elevated. RAP: correlation coefficient between mean ICP and pulse amplitude (AMP). Patient was asleep starting from 21:00. Baseline pressure was normal (10–12 mm Hg) with episodes of vasogenic activity driving pressure up to 25 mm Hg with RAP > 0.6, indicating loss of compensatory reserve in these periods and visible synchronization from pulse amplitude. Vasogenic episodes are also visible in magnitude of ICP slow waves. They are typically equally spread in 1 to 2 hours intervals and most probably associated with REM phase of sleep.

Results of overnight ICP monitoring should be interpreted individually. Mean ICP from the period of sleep is an important index. Its value is usually greater than the mean ICP when the patient is awake. Values above 15 mm Hg indicate moderate elevation in mean ICP and above 20 mm Hg indicate intracranial hypertension. Dynamics of ICP, increases caused by vasogenic or other episodes, should also be considered. Average amplitude of slow waves has only a hypothetical clinical value. Averaged value of RAP coefficient can be taken as an index of cerebrospinal compensatory reserve (when RAP is above 0.6).

INFUSION STUDY

The aim of CSF infusion study is to measure the resistance to CSF outflow (R_{csf}) along with other compensatory parameters and consider whether the cerebrospinal circulation is disturbed and can be improved surgically.

Almost all authors agree that in hydrocephalus the drainage of CSF is disturbed. This may be expressed quantitatively by an elevated resistance to CSF outflow. The limit for elevated resistance is reported to range from above 13 to 18 mm Hg/(mL/min).

The computerized infusion test is a modification of the traditional constant rate infusion as described by Katzman and Hussey (4). The method requires a fluid infusion to be made into any accessible CSF compartment. A lumbar infusion, even if it has understandable limitations such as contraindication for lumbar puncture, possible CSF leak around the needle, need to stay flat for few hours after puncture, is less invasive than ventricular infusion. Intraventricular infusion into a subcutaneously positioned reservoir, connected to an intraventricular catheter or infusion into shunt antechamber, is quick and accurate, although it requires prior surgery.

During the infusion, the computer calculates and presents mean pressure and pulse amplitude with time along the x-axis (Fig. 2). The resistance to CSF outflow can be estimated, using

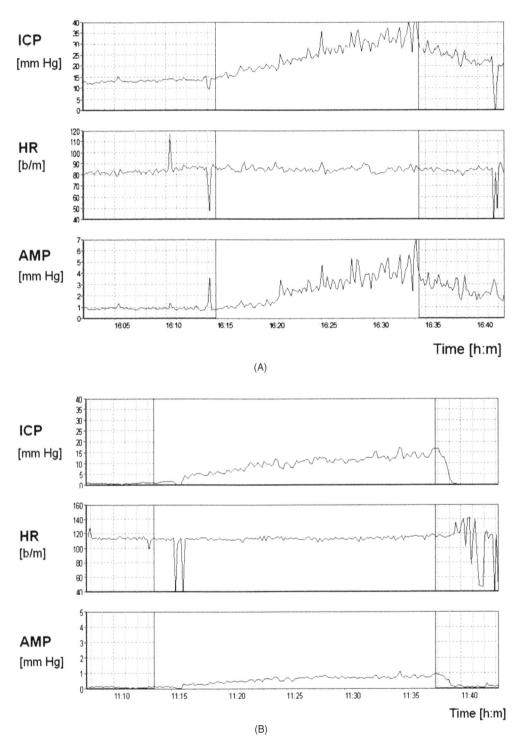

(A)

(B)

Figure 2 Examples of constant rate infusion test. ICP, mean ICP (10-second averages), HR, heart rate, and AMP, pulse amplitude of ICP. Vertical lines mark the beginning and the end of infusion of Hartman solution with the rate of 1.5 mL/min. (**A**) In patient suffering from normal pressure hydrocephalus (NPH). Baseline pressure was normal, resistance to CSF outflow increased (15.6 mm Hg/(mL/min)), there are plenty of vasogenic waves, and changes in pulse amplitude are very well correlated with changes in mean ICP. (**B**) Cerebral atrophy. Baseline pressure is also low, resistance to CSF outflow is in normal (8 mm Hg/(mL/min)), there are no vasogenic waves and pulse amplitude responds to changes in mean ICP slowly.

simple arithmetic, as the difference between the value of the plateau pressure during infusion and the resting pressure divided by the infusion rate. However, in many cases strong vasogenic waves or an excessive elevation of the pressure above the safe limit of 40 mm Hg do not allow the precise measurement of the final pressure plateau. Computerized analysis produces results even in difficult cases when the infusion is terminated prematurely (i.e., without reaching the end plateau). The algorithm utilizes a time-series analysis for volume–pressure curve retrieval, the least-mean-square model fitting, and an examination of the relationship between the pulse amplitude and the mean CSF pressure. The elastance coefficient or pressure–volume index, cerebrospinal compliance, CSF formation rate, and the pulse wave amplitude of CSF pressure are estimated. Full waveform analysis of CSF pressure at baseline and during infusion is also of potential clinical value (see section, monitoring of ICP).

However, not all patients presenting with abnormal CSF circulation may improve after shunting. Positive predictive power of infusion study is usually reported as satisfactory, but some patients with apparently normal profile of CSF circulation may still get better after surgery. Therefore, infusion test does not offer a definite indication for the management of hydrocephalus. It should be always interpreted in conjunction with other forms of investigations such as neuropsychological, brain imaging, gait analysis, CSF tap test or diagnostic drainage, vascular reactivity, and biochemical composition of CSF.

In patients with clinical symptoms of normal pressure hydrocephalus (NPH), resistance to CSF outflow is associated with severity of symptoms. There is no agreement about the threshold of abnormal resistance to CSF outflow. Values above 13 mm Hg/(mL/min) (1) or 18 mm Hg/(mL/min) (5) are given by various authors. Resistance to CSF outflow increases and estimated CSF formation rate decreases with age (6).

Vasogenic waves of ICP (i.e., pulse amplitude, slow waves, and respiratory waves measured at baseline and during infusion) are positively correlated with the resistance to CSF outflow. Baseline ICP measured after the test is usually greater than the value measured before the test. This phenomenon can be described as hysteresis of the pressure–volume curve. The width of hysteresis seems to be positively associated with the width of ventricles. Cerebral autoregulation assessed using transcranial Doppler ultrasonography or correlation between waves in arterial pressure and ICP during the test, correlate with resistance to CSF outflow in a manner suggesting worse autoregulation in those having lower resistance to CSF outflow (7).

ASSESSMENT OF SHUNT FUNCTION IN VIVO

Shunts used for the treatment of hydrocephalus drain excess CSF from the brain to elsewhere in the body according to a pressure difference between inlet (ventricles) and outlet (peritoneal or atrial) compartments. Ideally, the resistance of an open shunt taken together with the natural CSF outflow resistance, usually increased in hydrocephalus, should be close to the normal resistance to CSF outflow, that is, 6 to 10 mm Hg/(mL/min) (8). The flow through the shunt should not depend on the body posture or be affected by body temperature, external pressure within the physiological range for subcutaneous pressure, or the pulsatile component of CSF pressure.

After shunting, the model of CSF space (9) should be supplemented by the branch representing the property of the shunt. The most sensitive indicator of the shunt partial blockage is the steady state level achieved during the test. With known value of the shunt pressure–flow curve, the opening pressure and its hydrodynamic resistance where the curve is quasi-linear, the critical threshold may be evaluated for each individual type of the shunt by the formula:

$$5\ \text{mm Hg} + \text{shunt opening pressure} + \text{infusion rate} \times \text{hydrodynamic resistance of shunt}$$

Properly functioning shunt limits pressure increase during infusion. Opening pressure should be below the shunt's operating pressure plus reasonable credit for abdominal pressure. Pulse amplitude of ICP also decreases with properly functioning shunt, below 2 mm Hg, and vasogenic waves recorded during infusion usually disappear. Examples of the tests revealing properly functioning shunt and the blocked shunt are presented in Figure 3.

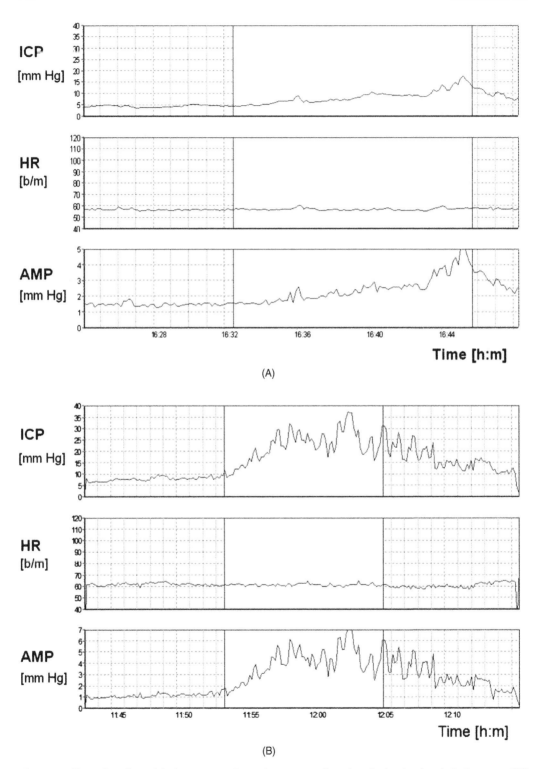

Figure 3 Examples of two infusion tests performed to assess shunt-functioning in vivo. In both cases, ICP increased in response to infusion. (**A**) Response was lower than the threshold level for the used valve (Strata, level 1.5), and there was additional pressure increase when siphon-control device was compressed, around 16:44. Shunt was patent. (**B**) Baseline pressure was low, but the response of ICP during the test exceeded the critical threshold level. Valve was blocked (Strata, level 1.0).

REFERENCES

1. Borgesen SE, Gjerris F. The predictive value of conductance to outflow of CSF in normal pressure hydrocephalus. Brain 1982; 105:65–86.
2. Droste DW, Krauss JK. Oscillations of cerebrospinal fluid pressure in nonhydrocephalic persons. Neurol Res 1997; 19(2):135–138.
3. Stephensen H, Andersson N, Eklund A, et al. Objective B wave analysis in 55 patients with non-communicating and communicating hydrocephalus. J Neurol Neurosurg Psychiatry 2005; 76(7): 965–970.
4. Katzman R, Hussey F. A simple constant infusion manometric test for measurement of CSF absorption. Neurology (Minneap) 1970; 20:534–544.
5. Boon AJ, Tans JT, Delwel EJ, et al. Dutch normal-pressure hydrocephalus study: prediction of outcome after shunting by resistance to outflow of cerebrospinal fluid. J Neurosurg 1997; 87(5):687–693.
6. Czosnyka M, Czosnyka ZH, Whitfield PC, et al. Age dependence of cerebrospinal pressure–volume compensation in patients with hydrocephalus. J Neurosurg 2001; 94(3):482–486.
7. Czosnyka Z, Czosnyka M, Whitfield PC, et al. Cerebral autoregulation among patients with symptoms of hydrocephalus. Neurosurgery 2002; 50(3):526–532.
8. Ekstedt J. CSF hydrodynamic studies in man. Normal hydrodynamic variables related to CSF pressure and flow. J Neurolog Neurosurg Psychiatry 1978; 41:345–353.
9. Marmarou A, Shulman K, Rosende RM. A non-linear analysis of CSF system and intracranial pressure dynamics. J Neurosurg 1978; 48:332–344.

Intracranial Pressure (ICP) Sensors and Surgical Technique of ICP Bolt Insertion

Federico Di Rocco

Pediatric Neurosurgery, Université René Descartes Paris V, Hôpital Necker Enfants Malades, Paris, France

INTRODUCTION

Since the pioneering studies of Nils Lundberg in the late 1950s, the monitoring of intracranial pressure (ICP) has gained a progressively wide use in neurointensive care. Nowadays such a monitoring is considered a routine procedure in most centers, the use of which has favoured the development of miniaturized sensors.

Currently, several types of devices are available based on catheter tip fiberoptic transducers (Camino®), solid-state strain-gauge sensors (Codman®), or air-filled catheter (Spiegelberg®).

The ICP can be monitored at different sites: epidurally, subdurally, intraparenchymally, or intraventricularly. In the clinical practice, the "gold standard" remains the intraventricular ICP recording through an external ventricular drainage (1) because of the reliability of the measured values, the ability to recalibrate as often as required, and the possibility of removing cerebrospinal fluid (CSF) to control abnormally increased intracranial pressures. In fact, a progressive decrease in intraparenchymal pulse ICP values has been experimentally demonstrated when increasing the distance of the sensor from the ventricular system (2).

Several authors have found a good correlation in ICP comparing these different systems (3,4,1). However, when used in the same patient, two intraparenchymal sensors may show different pressure values (5,6) due to the different drift in pressure between the two captors or due to the local effect of focal space occupying intracranial lesions.

The intraparenchymal ICP monitoring devices have some advantages compared to external ventricular drainage, namely, the ease of insertion, which is not relevant to how severely cerebral ventricles are reduced in size, the minor risk of secondary bacterial contamination, and the easier management of the patient for nursing or for the patient's transportation to carry out radiological examinations.

The impossibility to drain CSF in cases of severe intracranial hypertension, the high cost, the fragility of the system, and its sensitivity to magnetic fields as well as the impossibility to verify in situ the calibration or to recalibrate the device in case of drift constitutes the main disadvantages of nonintraventricular ICP monitoring. Differently from other sensors, the Spiegelberg® transducer, however, performs a calibration of the device in situ every hour.

Description of Devices

An ICP monitoring system consists essentially of a pressure sensor connected to a measuring/reading unit (MU) by a cable. The pressure data recorded by the sensor are transformed into variations of electric voltage or light and then transferred to the MU for direct visualization and/or storage.

The Camino® device (Camino OLM ICP Monitor, Camino Laboratories, San Diego, CA) is based on a pressure-sensitive diaphragm that transforms the changes in pressure into light variations, which are then transmitted to the MU by a fiberoptic catheter.

The Codman® microsensor (Johnson & Johnson Professional Inc, Raynham, MA) transforms the pressure changes in electric voltage variations. This device uses a strain-gauge microchip encapsulated in a titanium case within a nylon catheter.

The Spiegelberg® system (Spiegelberg GmbH & Co. KG, Hamburg, Germany) senses the pressure changes through an air pouch and transmits them along the catheter to a pressure transducer located within the MU itself.

Surgical Technique for Placing an ICP Monitoring Device

The site and side of insertion may vary according to the patient's condition and surgeon's preference. Generally, the frontal lobe is preferred for both intraparenchymal and intraventricular locations. In case of head trauma and skin lacerations or compounded fractures, the injured area is usually avoided because of increased risk of infection. Moreover, some authors have suggested to place the sensor close to the region of maximal brain damage (7).

After standard skin preparation, a 1.5-cm linear scalp incision is usually sufficient to perform a burr hole in the skull. The dura is coagulated, and the catheter is implanted through the bolt kit or tunneled subcutaneously and connected to the MU for calibration. A precise calibration (zeroing) is essential for the correct interpretation of the ICP values. The 0-mm Hg reference can be obtained by submerging the tip in a warm saline for Codman sensor or to air for Camino sensor.

Usually, a depth of 2 cm is sufficient for a reliable intraparenchymal placement.

A good fixation of the catheter by using its specific housing bolts or by fixing the catheter firmly to the patient's skin prevents any dislocation caused by abrupt movements or transportation of the patient (Figs. 1–4).

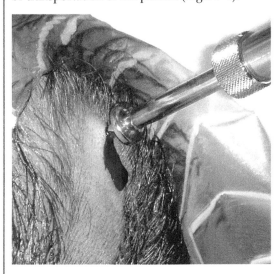

Figure 1 A small burr hole is sufficient to insert the device.

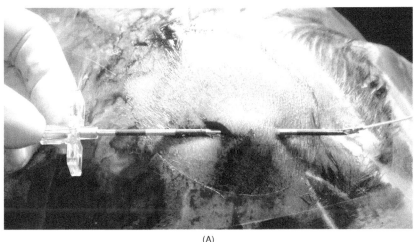

(A)

Figure 2 Subcutaneous tunnelization (**A**) of a Codman® pressure device. The catheter tip (**B**) is pushed to the level of the burr hole. The other end is plugged to the monitor.

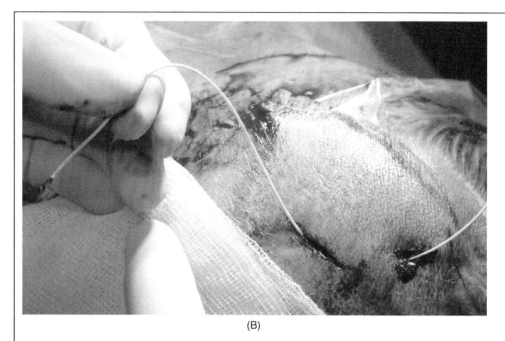

(B)

Figure 2   (*Continued*)

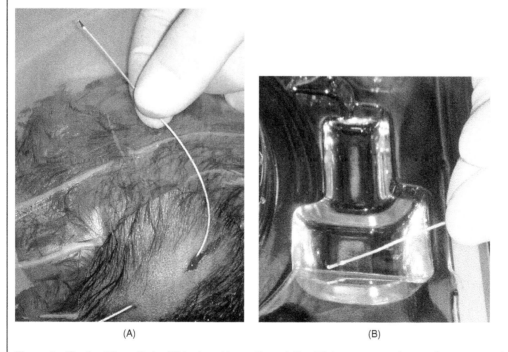

(A)   (B)

Figure 3   The tip of the catheter (**A**) is placed in a saline solution (**B**) for pressure reference (zero pressure). Avoid placement of the tip too deep in the solution.

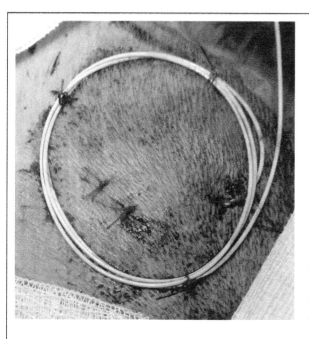

Figure 4 The device should be tightly secured. Several ways are possible to ensure a good fixation. In this occasion several nonresorbable stitches have been used. The skin incision is sutured with a resorbable stitch.

Complications

Infection, which is considered the main complication of intraventricular ICP recording coupled with external CSF drainage, occurs rarely in case of intraparenchymal ICP monitoring [0.3% in Pople et al. series (8), 0.5% in Shapiro et al. report (7)].

Table 1 Comparison of Devices

	Experimental studies			Clinical studies	
	Zero drift	Temperature drift 27–40°C	MR compatibility	Zero drift at removal of the probe	Difference with ventricular pressure
Camino®	<0.8 mm Hg (12)	0.27 mm Hg/°C (12)	Substantial artefacts movement of the probe (13)	<2 mm Hg in most patients (8) 3.5 ± 3.1 mm Hg (9)	+2.5 mm Hg (8)
Codman®	<0.8 mm Hg (12)	0.026 mm Hg/°C (12)	MR safe up to 0.5 T (13)	±2 mm Hg in 79% of the patients 0 mm Hg drift in 25% of the cases (1)	"−1.2 mm Hg" (1)
Opiegelberg®	Adjusted to 0 automatically every hour	Adjusted to 0 automatically every hour		Adjusted to 0 automatically every hour	< or − 2 mm Hg in 44% of the cases, and < or = 5 mm Hg in 87% (5)

Other rare complications include epidural [one case in Stendel et al. series (9)] or intracerebral hemorrhages [about 0.3% in Koskinen and Olivecrona (1) and Pople et al. series (8)], usually self-limited without clinical implications (10) with the exception of patients with coagulation disorders (7).

Mechanical complications are relatively more common, although, in most cases, without clinical relevance, and are represented by fracture of the device [1% Pople et al. (8), 17% in Shapiro et al. series (7)] and its accidental displacement [1% Pople et al. (8), 14% in Stendel et al. series (9)].

Noninvasive Methods

ICP can also be monitored indirectly by using ultrasonographic technology. This methodology is based on the relationship between ultrasound propagation through the brain parenchyma, cerebrovascular resistance, cerebral perfusion, and ICP. A good correlation between ultrasound data and invasive ICP recording has been found in patients with severe head injury (11).

REFERENCES

1. Koskinen LO and Olivecrona M. Clinical experience with intraparenchymal intracranial pressure monitoring Codman microsensor system. Neurosurgery 2005; 56:639–698.
2. Di Rocco C, Pettorossi VE, Caldarelli M, et al. On the source of CSF pulse, Monogr Paediat 1982; 15:33–37.
3. Gopinath SP, Robertson CS, Contant CF, et al. Clinical evaluation of a miniature strain-gauge transducer for monitoring intracranial pressure. Neurosurgery 1995; 36:1137–1140.
4. Gray WP, Palmer JD, Gill J, et al. A clinical study of parenchymal and subdural miniature strain-gauge transducers for monitoring intracranial pressure. Neurosurgery 1996; 39:927–931.
5. Chambers IR, Siddique MS, Banister K, et al. Clinical comparison of the Spiegelberg parenchymal transducer and ventricular fluid pressure. J Neurol Neurosurg Psychiatry 2001; 71:383–385.
6. Eide PK. Comparison of simultaneous continuous intracranial pressure (ICP) signals from a Codman and a Camino ICP sensor. Med Eng Phys 2006; 28:542–549.
7. Shapiro S, Bowman R, Callahan J, et al. The fiberoptic intraparenchymal cerebral pressure monitor in 244 patients. Surg Neurol 1996; 45:278–282.
8. Pople IK, Muhlbauer MS, Sanford RA, et al. Results and complications of intracranial pressure monitoring in 303 children. Ped Neurosurg 1995; 23:64–67.
9. Stendel R, Heidenreich J, Schilling A, et al. Clinical evaluation of a new intracranial pressure monitoring device. Acta Neurochir 2003; 145:185–193.
10. Anderson RC, Kan P, Klimo P, et al. Complications of intracranial pressure monitoring in children with head trauma. J Neurosurg 2004; 101(1S):53–58.
11. Fountas KN, Sitkauskas A, Feltes CH, et al. Is non-invasive monitoring of intracranial pressure waveform analysis possible? Preliminary results of a comparative study of non-invasive vs invasive intracranial slow-wave wave from analysis monitoring in patients with traumatic brain injury. Med Sci Monitor 2005; 11:CR58–CR63.
12. Czosnyka M, Czosnyka Z, Pickard J. Laboratory testing of three intracranial pressure microtransducers: technical report. Neurosurgery 1996; 38:219–224.
13. Williams EJ, Bunch CS, Carpenter TA, et al. Magnetic resonance imaging compatibility testing of intracranial pressure probes. Technical note. J Neurosurg 1999; 91:706–709.

5 | The Neuropsychological Consequences of Hydrocephalus

Cathy Grant
Paediatric Psychology, Child Development Centre, Leicester Royal Infirmary, Leicester, U.K.

Jo Iddon
Department of Medicine and Therapeutics, Chelsea and Westminster Hospital, London, U.K.

Emily Talbot, Kristina Vella, and Arleta Starza-Smith
Paediatric Neuropsychology Service, Regional Neurosciences Centre, Nottingham University Hospitals, Nottingham, U.K.

INTRODUCTION

Shunts have significantly improved the prognosis of people with hydrocephalus, and recently third ventriculostomy has increasingly become a preferred successful treatment for an increasing number of cases of obstructive hydrocephalus. Nevertheless, even with surgical treatment, this remains a lifelong condition, which in many cases is associated with a variety of cognitive deficits (1). Hydrocephalus can have a significant impact upon the developing brain, resulting in the distortion and tearing of blood vessels and neural fibers, displacement of adjacent brain structures, a disruption to myelination (2), and tissue damage and swelling within the periventricular white matter during the acute stages (3). Motor and visual impairments are strongly associated with hydrocephalus, as enlarged ventricles damage the nearby optic nerves and motor pathways (see chap. 1).

Hydrocephalus has an impact upon development in several important areas including cognitive, social and emotional developments. Developments in cognitive, social and emotional domains are interlinked, and the psychosocial environment has a further impact upon development in these areas. The focus of this chapter is on the cognitive implications of hydrocephalus. An overview of findings relating to intelligence, language, visuospatial skills, memory, attention, executive function, and processing speed in childhood is presented and then the impact of hydrocephalus into adulthood is explored.

HYDROCEPHALUS IN CHILDHOOD

Intelligence is one of the most commonly studied outcome measures in children with hydrocephalus [see Ref. (4) for review]. In more recent years, research effort has focused upon the specific cognitive deficits associated with hydrocephalus (e.g., visuoperceptual and visuomotor function, executive function, and discourse). However, much remains unknown about the developmental sequelae of neuropsychological functioning in children with hydrocephalus.

Children with hydrocephalus commonly experience academic difficulties and under achievement at school (5). As children with hydrocephalus perform well in areas of rote memory, rote reading and spelling skills (6), typically these children perform adequately during the first few years at school. However, as academic requirements become more complex, children with hydrocephalus begin to fall behind their peers (7,8). Schools are not identifying the performance drop-off as a neurologically based learning difficulty; instead children are mislabeled as "lazy" or unmotivated (9). Consequently, the child's developmental needs are commonly not identified until later on in the child's school career. It is important that children with hydrocephalus have access to neuropsychological evaluation from an early age so that individualized development plans can be put into practice to support the child in the home and school (10).

Intelligence

Children with hydrocephalus perform more poorly on tests of intelligence than typically developing children or children with the same medical condition but without associated hydrocephalus (11,12). Performance on tests of intelligence (IQ) is typically within the low-average range of ability (13–16). Moreover, children with hydrocephalus have a slower rate of cognitive development than typically developing children. For example, Jacobs et al. (15) studied 19 children with myelomeningocele, a form of spina bifida and hydrocephalus, from infancy to late childhood and found a decline in IQ scores.

Many studies have reported that nonverbal intelligence (PIQ) is less developed than verbal intelligence (VIQ) (13,16–18). However, it is unclear if this finding reflects deficits in higher order motor planning and spatial problem-solving skills or whether other factors are responsible. One difficulty is that PIQ tests are sensitive to motor and visual abnormalities as well as to slow speed of processing, because such tests are timed and place demands upon visual and motor skills (13). A discrepancy between PIQ and VIQ has been found across all etiological groups, although congenital hydrocephalus (e.g., spina bifida, aqueduct stenosis) is reported to be associated with greater PIQ–VIQ discrepancies than acquired hydrocephalus (e.g., brain hemorrhage, infection) (13). It is important to note, however, that not all studies have found a PIQ-VIQ discrepancy. A recent study (19) confirmed the findings that children with hydrocephalus perform approximately 1 standard deviation lower than controls on tests of general intelligence. However, their findings showed no statistically significant difference between their VIQ and PIQ scores. The researchers postulated that the selectivity of their sample (i.e., that they only included children who had congenital hydrocephalus requiring shunting) possibly accounted for their findings.

Several studies have examined the relationship between pathophysiology and intellectual functioning, in particular the effect of ventricle size, gray matter volumes, myelination, and corpus callosum size on IQ. The findings relating to ventricle size and IQ have been inconsistent, with some studies finding moderate negative correlations between ventricular size and IQ (18,20,21) and other studies finding only low correlations (22,23). Children with hydrocephalus who have a thin cortical mantle can have IQ scores within the normal range (24,25), although group studies demonstrate a positive association between cortical mantle size and intellectual functioning (5,21,26). Myelination is strongly associated with intellectual functioning in infants with hydrocephalus (27), but this becomes less strongly related to intelligence as children mature (28). Corpus callosum size has been reported as correlating more strongly with tests of PIQ than that of the ventricle size (18). Shunt failure and shunt revision have been reported in several studies to impact negatively on intellectual ability (8). Interestingly, Nejat and his colleagues (29) carried out a study to evaluate IQ in children with meningomyeloceles and they found no significant difference between children who had a shunt (with or without complications) and those who did not. However, these results should be interpreted with caution because a comprehensive measure (such as the WISC-IV) of intelligence was not used.

Functionally the discrepancy between PIQ and VIQ in children with hydrocephalus can have a major impact, especially within school. Children with hydrocephalus often present themselves as being verbally able and are likely to be misjudged by teachers as being at least of average ability. Consequently, it is not uncommon to find that the expectations that teachers have of these children often exceed their true intellectual ability. This mismatch can give rise to a lack of appropriate support for the child in the classroom, disruptive behavior, the development of low self-esteem in the child and ultimately school failure.

Language

Despite verbal skills being more preserved than performance skills in children with hydrocephalus on tests of intelligence, disturbances of language functioning, especially at the level of pragmatics and discourse, have been reported (30). Compared with age-matched controls, children with hydrocephalus perform poorly on tests that require inferences to be made and they had difficulty understanding ambiguous sentences and idioms (32). In contrast, several language skills are adequately developed in children with hydrocephalus including vocabulary and grammar (30). Functionally, children with hydrocephalus have difficulties with comprehension of both oral and written languages (31,32). These difficulties are likely to stem from deficits in the ability to make inferences, which is an important component of oral and written language comprehension (33). The inability to construct meaning from context is considered by Dennis and colleagues (1,34) to be a core deficit for children with hydrocephalus, because this deficit is demonstrable even in children with hydrocephalus who have IQ scores within the average to superior range.

Language in children with hydrocephalus has been associated with the "cocktail party syndrome," which is characterized by a tendency to extreme verbosity and a superficial conversational content. Tew and Laurence (35) studied this in children with spina bifida and hydrocephalus and reported that 48% of girls and 32% of boys met their definition of "cocktail party syndrome." While these children displayed intact vocabulary and syntactical skills, spontaneous speech was marked by instances of tangential language irrelevant to the conversation, excessive use of stereotypic social phrases, over-familiarity of manner, and verbal perseveration. Similar findings were presented by Dennis et al. (36) who reported that the narratives of children with hydrocephalus were verbose, lacked semantic content, and were imprecise. However, Dennis et al. (30) argued that the "cocktail party" language is more associated with depressed intelligence than with hydrocephalus.

The discrepancy between the adequate vocabulary and grammar that is typically associated with hydrocephalus and the impairment in higher order language skills becomes more of an issue as the child progresses through school. As the child progresses, success in school relates less to the literal meaning of language and more to understanding the subtleties of language. Moreover, the emphasis has shifted from learning to read, which children with hydrocephalus do adequately, to reading to learn, which taps the ability to make inferences and understand ambiguity, skills which are known to be a relative weakness (31). Children with hydrocephalus become aware of their academic difficulties and the widening gap between their academic performance and those of their peers. The likely negative impact this has on self-esteem is added to by the social difficulties that these children are likely to face. Children who process language literally are likely to experience difficulties understanding the sarcasm and jokes that typically characterize adolescent communication (37).

Motor and Visuospatial Skills

Nonverbal skills, involving visuospatial and perceptual–motor skills, are found to be less preserved than verbal skills in children with hydrocephalus, demonstrated in a commonly identified reduced PIQ versus VIQ in these children (38,39). Qualitative observations are indicative of difficulties with spatial awareness, for example, difficulties with jigsaws and puzzles and difficulties with route finding.

Children with hydrocephalus and spina bifida do commonly demonstrate motor and visual difficulties (39) that may impede performance on tests of visuospatial and perceptual–motor abilities. For example, many children with spina bifida and hydrocephalus have eye-movement disorders that have been associated with poor visual-perceptual and nonverbal skills (7,13). Moreover, hydrocephalus frequently involves brain regions that are implicated in motor control (e.g., cerebellum), and children with spina bifida and hydrocephalus often experience impaired upper limb function (40,41). In particular, children with spina bifida and hydrocephalus with higher-level lesions are likely to have more restricted mobility and therefore less opportunity for visual spatial and visuomotor learning (42).

Children with hydrocephalus have impaired fine motor function (11,13). Deficits in fine motor skill are more severe in children with shunts than in children who have unshunted, arrested hydrocephalus (14). The motor deficits associated with hydrocephalus negatively impact upon skills that require visuomotor integration, such as design copying and handwriting (14,43–45).

Efforts have been made to investigate performance on perceptual ability tests that control for motor difficulties in children with hydrocephalus, and on such tests, school-aged children with hydrocephalus have been shown to continue to demonstrate impairment on motor-free tests of perceptual ability (43). Children with shunted hydrocephalus have also been shown to perform worse than children with unshunted, arrested hydrocephalus on visuoperceptual tasks (44).

Neuroanatomical features of hydrocephalus can go some way to explaining the observed deficits in perceptual ability. For example, Baron and Goldberger (46) identify that enlargement of the ventricles can cause specific damage to optic nerves and motor pathways, and an increase in CSF and a decrease in gray matter in the posterior regions of the brain have been associated with impairment of visuospatial and visuomotor abilities (20,47).

Memory

The expansion of the ventricles associated with hydrocephalus can lead to damage to the temporal lobes, hippocampus, and other subcortical structures implicated in memory (see chap. 1). Although the pathophysiology associated with hydrocephalus would suggest memory deficits, the handful of memory studies undertaken in children with hydrocephalus have yielded inconsistent results. Some studies have reported verbal and visual memory impairments (18), whereas others have found performance to be within normal limits (17). Early studies of memory in children with hydrocephalus suffered from methodological limitations such as small sample size, lack of comparison groups (17), and samples that included a narrow age range (18).

In an attempt to address the shortcomings in existing studies, Scott et al. (48) employed a relatively large sample of children with hydrocephalus to assess verbal and nonverbal memory using recall and recognition of material. Scott et al. (48) found that children with shunted hydrocephalus performed poorly on both verbal and nonverbal memory measures. They reported weaknesses on serial learning, recognition memory, delayed story recall, and visuoconstructive memory. In order to examine the possibility that the children with hydrocephalus performed poorly on tests of nonverbal memory because such measures are confounded with visuomotor and fine motor problems, visuomotor and fine motor tasks were used to measure performance deficits. There was no significant correlation between visuomotor and fine motor task performances and nonverbal memory, suggesting that the poor performance on nonverbal memory could not be explained by fine motor or visual problems.

In contrast to the difficulties, children with hydrocephalus display on serial learning and delayed spontaneous retrieval of information, immediate recall of meaningful material such as sentences appears to be unaffected (17,18,48). There is also evidence that children with hydrocephalus benefit from cued recall. Yeates et al. (49) found that children with shunted hydrocephalus showed greater improvement on recognition tasks than that of comparison groups. This suggests that children with hydrocephalus are able to encode information but have difficulties retrieving information without cues.

Attention

The ability to sustain, focus, and shift attention is important for engaging in many tasks, and impairment in these areas can impact upon other cognitive functions. In clinical settings, parents of children with hydrocephalus commonly report difficulties with attention. Surprisingly, there are relatively few studies of attention in children with hydrocephalus. Early studies of attention in children with hydrocephalus reported deficits in attention and distractibility (e.g., 50,51). However, early studies suffered from methodological limitations that hampered the interpretability of the results (e.g., grouping both shunted and unshunted children, use of tests requiring rapid motor responses).

In a comprehensive study of attention in children with hydrocephalus, Fletcher et al. (28) reported deficits in selective and focused attention. These authors also included measures of executive function and argued that the poor performance on executive tasks could be explained in terms of attentional deficits mediated by posterior white matter regions of the brain.

Brewer et al. (52) compared the performance of children with shunted hydrocephalus, children with ADHD (attention deficit/hyperactivity disorder), and typically developing children on tests of focused attention, sustained attention, and attention shifting and reported findings similar to those of Fletcher et al. (28). They showed that the children with hydrocephalus performed poorly on tests of focused attention and attention shifting and interpreted this as evidence implicating an attention system within the posterior brain. Importantly, the attention tests employed by Brewer et al. (52) minimized motor demands, thus separating out the effect of motor deficits upon test performance. Of note is that the children with hydrocephalus did not show deficits on sustained attention, which is the ability to maintain alertness to a task over time. In contrast to focused attention, which has been linked to neuroanatomical structures within the posterior brain encompassing the inferior parietal, superior temporal, and striatal regions, the sustained attention system is related to rostral midbrain structures, the reticular formation, and the thalamus (53). This pattern of findings is consistent with the known patterns of damage that occur in hydrocephalus, in particular, the likelihood of damage occurring to the posterior regions of the brain.

Executive Functions

Children with hydrocephalus are often found to have specific deficits in executive functioning. Executive function is a cognitive system that is thought to manage and control various other cognitive processes, such as attention and memory, and is involved in processes such as planning, cognitive flexibility, self-regulation, and abstract thinking. Setting goals and sequencing the steps to achieve these goals involve executive functioning and are important for children to develop in order to function independently at school and home.

Children with shunted hydrocephalus have been shown to perform worse on the Tower of London Test (TOL), a planning test, when asked to solve complex problems (28), and have been shown to make more perseverative errors than controls on studies using the Wisconsin Card Sorting Test (54,55), although this has not been consistently found (28,52).

The ongoing development of the frontal lobes and executive functions throughout childhood and adolescence and its close relationship to other cognitive domains such as attention and memory have made primary assessment of executive function difficult in children, particularly those of preschool age. However, in recent years, there has been a rise in the number of relevant tests available for use with children, for example, Dellis-Kaplan Executive Functions System (D-KEFS), Tower of Hanoi Test, Tower of London Test, Wisconsin Card Sort Test (WCST), and consequently further research and literature is being conducted.

Dysfunction of the posterior regions of the brain has been offered as an explanation for the executive function impairments shown in children with hydrocephalus (4,20). However, some research findings have challenged this (56,57).

While executive dysfunction in adults is commonly associated with damage directly to the frontal lobes, the frontal lobes of children develop throughout childhood and further systems or connections are involved (4). Deficits in executive function of children with hydrocephalus may be caused by damage of the white matter tracts carrying information to and from the prefrontal cortex (28). A longitudinal case study of spina bifida and hydrocephalus, with serial neuropsychological assessment and shunt revision at 11 years old, demonstrated impaired executive function on inhibitory control and verbal retrieval. This was suggested to be due to shunt failure interfering with executive function development or due to shunt failure occurring at a time of rapid myelination in the frontal lobes (58).

Lindquist et al. (59) have carried out research exploring learning, memory, and executive functions in children with hydrocephalus. They found that these children have difficulties in all three areas of cognitive functioning except recognition and registration skills, which are relative areas of strength. Intelligence was strongly correlated with poor short-term memory and executive functions. Their results were homogeneous across all etiologies of infantile hydrocephalus, implying that the cognitive problems were caused by the consequence of the hydrocephalus and its effect on brain structures.

While the majority of documented studies have used cognitive batteries such as the D-KEFS to measure executive functioning in children and adolescents with hydrocephalus, a recent study by Reem et al. (60) used the BRIEF (Behavior Rating Inventory of Executive Function), which is a proxy measure of executive functioning completed by parents. Their findings showed an age-related improvement in the control group's executive control behaviors. However, the children and adolescents with myelomeningocele and shunted hydrocephalus failed to show the same age-related improvement in executive control, with their behavior remaining static. This highlights the importance of appropriate interventions to help these children achieve functional independence both at school and at home.

Processing Speed

Given that hydrocephalus is associated with disrupted myelination, slowed processing speed is likely to be a characteristic of this condition. Few studies have specifically addressed processing speed in children with hydrocephalus, although several studies have reported a slow response speed on timed tasks [e.g., Word-finding (13), Stroop (28), Attention (52)]. A recent study by Jacobs et al. (15) reported a significantly slower speed of processing in children with spina bifida and hydrocephalus compared to typically developing children on a Processing Speed Domain, which consisted of scores on Coding and Copying the Rey Complex Figure. Interpretation of this finding is limited because both of these tests are sensitive to visual and motor abilities as well as to processing speed. However, in the same group, there was also evidence of slowed speed of processing on the Controlled Oral Word Association Test, which does not impose a motor or visual demand.

In a comprehensive study of processing speed in children with spina bifida and hydrocephalus, Boyer et al. (61) used a children's version of the Paced Auditory Serial Addition Test. This test makes no demands upon visual or motor skill, thus removing confounds that had been present in previous studies. They reported that children with spina bifida and hydrocephalus had marked deficits in processing speed. Importantly, this deficit was not accounted for by other task demands such as arithmetic skills.

HYDROCEPHALUS INTO ADULTHOOD

Despite the improvements in the surgical treatment of hydrocephalus, it remains a life-long condition and anecdotal evidence suggests that cognitive difficulties persist into adult life. Indeed it is often when these individuals reach adulthood and try to lead a more independent life and seek employment that the true extent of their cognitive difficulties emerge and exhibit themselves as a significant problem. This will result in many difficulties within the workplace, for example, particularly in busy jobs where multitasking may be necessary and complex tasks need to be carried out.

A number of studies have assessed cognitive function in adults with hydrocephalus, and these have started to explain the difficulties reported by individuals and their relatives. Iddon et al. (62,63) assessed the intellectual and cognitive functioning of subgroups of young adults with hydrocephalus who had average verbal intellectual function and average social/emotional functioning. While there was a range of cognitive test results, scores were not normally distributed and significantly more scores fell within the low average range or below. A close review of the data suggested that some types of function were impaired in the majority of individuals with hydrocephalus, that is, particularly those assessing immediate and delayed memory recall, learning of new material, and in different aspects of frontal lobe executive functioning such as verbal fluency, spatial working memory, attentional set-shifting, and psychomotor speed on complex tasks involving sequencing (62,63). Poor performance was often associated with an inability to generate an effective strategy to complete the task. In contrast, other types of function involving less effortful processing and requiring less need for strategies were relatively spared, for example, semantic fluency, recognition memory, and spatial memory span (63). Individuals with spina bifida with no concomitant hydrocephalus did not show the same pattern of cognitive impairment, tending to perform in the average range or above (62,63). This is important because hydrocephalus is approximately 80% concomitant with spina bifida and often the difficulties in cognitive functioning are attributed to this rather than the hydrocephalus.

These findings are supported by other large cross-sectional studies; Barf et al. (65; $N = 168$) and Verhoef et al. (66; $N = 179$) showed that most medical problems and secondary impairments, including cognitive dysfunction, were found in patients with higher level lesions, that is, those with spina bifida and hydrocephalus as compared to patients with lower level lesions, that is, spina bifida without hydrocephalus whose cognitive status was similar to that in healthy controls. However, the authors acknowledged that all subgroups suffered from different types of health problems. Other psychological factors can also have an impact on education and subsequent intellectual and cognitive developments such as poor self-esteem in individuals with spina bifida (66–69).

Other studies have shown that hydrocephalus affects the development of basic skills such as reading, writing, and maths. Barnes et al. (70) demonstrated reading and writing deficiencies in a group of 31 young adults with spina bifida and hydrocephalus who like children with hydrocephalus were better at word decoding than reading comprehension and have lower scores on tests of writing fluency compared to population means. The route of these difficulties can be traced back to childhood because individuals with hydrocephalus have difficulties suppressing contextually irrelevant meaning and integrating information using context, affecting the development of comprehension (71). Dennis and Barnes (72) also assessed maths skills in the same group, reporting poorer computation accuracy, computation speed, problem solving, and functional numeracy. This clearly has implications for educational attainments and social, personal, and community independence.

In clinical settings, people with hydrocephalus often report being clumsy. Indeed, performance on measures of fine motor skills and persistent motor control is reported to be significantly below average in adults with hydrocephalus. For example, Hetherington and Dennis (40) gave tests of motor control, strength, balance, gait, posture, and fine motor skills to a group of hydrocephalus patients and showed them to be impaired in balance, gait, and posture and strength. Functionally cognitive and motor difficulties are exhibited as difficulties in acquiring everyday skills. For example, Simms (42) assessed the development of driving skills in 32 young people with hydrocephalus. She found that as a group they did have significant difficulties and needed a lengthy period of driving tuition to pass their tests, although approximately 50% achieved their goal after two years. The modern driving test, which includes memorizing and learning information for a written theory test poses an increasing challenge to this group.

Despite the clear results of these studies, there are a number of studies suggesting that hydrocephalus does not have a detrimental impact on cognitive functioning. For example, Hommet et al. (73,74) reported that properly shunted congenital hydrocephalus is not characterized by nonverbal learning difficulties. However, the group numbers in this study were very small ($N = 11$) and the conclusions were drawn from administering the Wechsler Adult Intelligence Scale—Revised version, which may be insensitive to some of the more subtle cognitive deficits. Other studies suggest that the degree of cognitive impairment depends on the physical phenotype, for example, level of spinal lesion (62–65,75) and number of shunt revisions, which influences cognitive and functional outcomes (75). Another study does not support the detrimental impact of multiple shunt revisions but rather suggests that epileptic seizures may account for the observed variance in scores in cognition (76).

CONCLUSION

In reality, clinical observation of individuals with hydrocephalus makes it clear that the effects of hydrocephalus on intellectual and cognitive ability do vary considerably. This is a complex group to study and there are many factors that complicate the interpretation of cognitive test results in congenital or early acquired hydrocephalus. For example, the patient group is heterogeneous with a wide variety of causes (prematurity, meningitis, hemorrhage, spinal dysraphism, Dandy–Walker Syndrome, tuberous sclerosis, Meckel Syndrome, Smith-Lemli-Opitz syndrome, etc.) and varying degrees of physical disability. There is a high incidence of epilepsy (40%), albeit usually mild. Medications and approaches to treatment vary; for example, some patients are shunted (using a wide variety of devices) very early on, while others appear to "arrest" spontaneously, but remain at risk of sudden and sometimes lethal deterioration. The number of shunt revisions individuals have undergone will also vary considerably. Some patients are treated by ventriculostomy, which may be a one off procedure, while others may undergo ventriculostomy plus a variety of other treatments (see chaps. 21 and 27).

In the normally developing human brain, improvements in cognitive functioning, such as basic memory capacities, use of memory strategies (e.g., organization, rehearsal, and elaboration) and declarative memory emerge and improve throughout childhood. Executive functions also gradually develop allowing better control over the allocation of attention and inhibitory, planning, and increased mental flexibility generally. Any neurological condition which impacts on brain development at this critical time can have long-term, sometimes devastating consequences for many aspects of cognitive function. Many individuals with congenital hydrocephalus have never developed normal cognitive function (1). This is likely to be due to the build up of CSF fluid and subsequent pressure causing irreversible damage to the frontal lobes and associated developing subcortical neural circuits that appears not to be compensated for by the developing brain (e.g., 63,77–79). It is also almost certainly the case that the normal process of myelination is disrupted (2) and that tissue damage and swelling has been caused, for example, to the periventricular white matter during the acute stages (3). However, informed and sensitive approaches to educational provision can have a marked impact on developmental progress (10).

　　　In summary, the clinical, behavioral, and cognitive difficulties associated with hydrocephalus are being increasingly understood. It is now important to widen access to neuropsychological screening in this group in order to identify particular cognitive difficulties and restrictions that many individuals with hydrocephalus will face throughout their lives. The development of behavioral and pharmacological treatment strategies, as well as rehabilitation through the educational system to help children overcome such difficulties, is of paramount importance.

REFERENCES

1. Dennis M, Barnes MA, Hetherington CR. Congenital hydrocephalus as a model of neuro-developmental disorder. In: Tager-Flusberg H, ed. Neuro-Developmental Disorders: Contribution to a New Perspective from the Cognitive Neurosciences. Cambridge, MS: MIT Press, 1999:505–532.
2. Sobkowiak CA. Effect of hydrocephalus on neuronal migration and maturation. Eur J Pediatr Surg 1992; 2(suppl 1):7–11.
3. Weller RO, Kida S, Harding BN. Aetiology and pathology of hydrocephalus. In: Schurr PH, Polket CE, eds. Hydrocephalus. New York: Oxford University Press, 1993:48–99.
4. Erickson K, Baron IS, Fantie BD. Neuropsychological functioning in early hydrocephalus: review from a developmental perspective. Child Neuropsychol 2001; 7(4): 199–229.
5. Hoppe-Hirsch E, Laroussinie F, Brunet L, et al. Late outcome of the surgical treatment of hydrocephalus. Childs Nerv Syst 1998; 14;97–99.
6. Lollar DJ. Learning patterns among spina bifida children. Z Kinderchir 1990; 45(suppl 1):39.
7. Wills KE, Holmbeck GN, Dillon K, et al. Intelligence and achievement in children with myelomeningocele. J Pediatr Psychol 1990; 15:161–176.
8. Holler KA, Fennell EB, Crosson B, et al. Neuropsychological and adaptive functioning in younger versus older children shunted for early hydrocephalus. Child Neuropsychol 1995; 1:63–73.
9. Vachha B, Adams R. Parent and school perceptions of language abilities in children with spina bifida and shunted hydrocephalus. Eur J Pediatr Surg 2002; 12:31–32.
10. Walker S, Wicks B. Educating Children with Acquired Brain Injury. London, U.K.: David Fulton Publishers, 2005.
11. Brookshire B, Copeland DR, Moore BD, et al. Pre-treatment neuropsychological status and factors in children with primary brain tumors. Neurosurgery 1990; 27:887–891.
12. Mirzai H, Ersahin Y, Mutluer S, et al. Outcome of patients with meningomyelocele: the Ege University experience. Childs Nerv Syst 1998; 14;120–123.
13. Dennis MA, Fitz CR, Netley CT, et al. The intelligence of hydrocephalic children. Arch Neurol 1981; 38:607–615.
14. Fletcher JM, Landry SH, Bohan TP, et al. Effects of intraventricular hemorrhage and hydrocephalus on the long-term neurobehavioural development of preterm very low-birthweight infants. Dev Med Child Neurol 1997; 39:596–606.
15. Jacobs R, Northam E, Anderson V. Cognitive outcome in children with myelomeningocele and perinatal hydrocephalus: a longitudinal perspective. J Phys Dev Disabil 2001; 13:389–404.
16. Lindquist B, Carlsson G, Persson E-K, et al. Learning disabilities in a population-based group of children with hydrocephalus. Acta Paediatr 2005; 94(7):878–883.
17. Donders J, Rourke BP, Canady AI. Neuropsychological functioning of hydrocephalic children. J Clin Exp Neuropsychol 1991; 13:607–613.
18. Fletcher JM, Bohan TP, Brandt ME, et al. Cerebral white matter and cognition in hydrocephalic children. Arch Neurol 1992; 49:818–824.
19. Lacey M, Pyykkonen BA, Hunter, SJ. Intellectual functioning in children with early shunted posthemorrhagic hydrocephalus. Pediatric Neurosurgery 2008; 44(5):376–381.
20. Fletcher JM, McCauley SR, Brandt ME, et al. Regional brain tissue composition with hydrocephalus. Relationships with cognitive development. Arch Neurol 1996b; 53:549–557.
21. Thompson MG, Eisenberg HM, Levin HS. Hydrocephalic infants: developmental assessment and computerised tomography. Childs Brain 1982; 9:400–410.
22. Bottcher J, Jacobsen S, Gyldensted C, et al. Intellectual development and brain size in 13 shunted hydrocephalic children. Neuropaeditrie 1978; 9:369–377.

23. Reiner D, Sainte-Rose C, Pierre-Kahn A, et al. Prenatal hydrocephalus: outcome and prognosis. Childs Nerv Syst 1988; 4:213–222.

24. Lonton AP, Barrington NA, Lorber J. Lacunar skull deformity related to intelligence in children with myelomeningocele and hydrocephalus. Dev Med Child Neurol 1975; 35:58.

25. Lorber J. Is your brain really necessary? Science 1980; 210:1232–1234.

26. Choudhury AR. Infantile hydrocephalus: management using CT assessment. Childs Nerv Syst 1995; 11:220–226.

27. Hanlo PW, Gooskens RJ, van Schooneveld M, et al. The effect of intracranial pressure on myelination and the relationship with neurodevelopment in infantile hydrocephalus. Dev Med Child Neurol 1997; 39:286–291.

28. Fletcher JM, Brookshire BL, Landry SH, et al. Attentional skills and executive functions in children with early hydrocephalus. Dev Neuropsychol 1996a; 12:53–76.

29. Nejat F, Kazmi SS, Habibi Z, et al. Intelligence quotient in children with meningomyeloceles: a case-control study. J Neurosurg 2007; (2 Suppl Pediatrics):106–110.

30. Dennis M, Hendrick EB, Hoffman HJ, et al. Language of hydrocephalic children and adolescents. J Clin Exp Neuropsychol 1987; 9:593–621.

31. Barnes M, Dennis M. Reading in children and adolescents after early onset hydrocephalus and in normally developing age peers. Phonological analysis, word recognition and passage comprehension skills. J Pediatr Psychol 1992; 17:445–466.

32. Dennis M, Barnes MA. Oral discourse after early-onset hydrocephalus: linguistic ambiguity, figurative language, speech-acts and script-based inferences. J Pediatr Psychol 1993; 18:639–652.

33. Oakhill J, Garnham A. Becoming a skilled reader. Oxford, UK: Basil Blackwell, 1988.

34. Barnes MA, Dennis M. Reading comprehension deficits arise from diverse sources: evidence from readers with and without developmental brain pathology. In: Cornoldi C, Oakhill JA, eds. Reading Comprehension Difficulties: Processes and Intervention. Hillsdale, NJ: Erlbaum, 1996:251–278.

35. Tew B, Laurance KM. The clinical characteristics of children with "cocktail party" syndrome. Z Kinderchir Grenzgeb 1979; 28;360–367.

36. Dennis M, Jacennik B, Barnes MA. The content of narrative discourse in children and adolescents after early-onset hydrocephalus and in normally developing age peers. Brain Lang 1994; 46: 129–165.

37. Vachha B, Adams R. Language differences in young children with myelomeningocele and shunted hydrocephalus. Pediatr Neurosurg 2003; 39:184–189.

38. Fletcher JM, Brookshire BL, Landry SH, et al. Behavioural adjustment of children with hydrocephalus: Relationships with etiology, neurological, and family status. J Pediatr Psychol 1995b; 20:109–125.

39. Wills K. Neuropsychological functioning in children with spina bifida and/or hydrocephalus. J Clin Child Psychol 1993; 22:247–265.

40. Hetherington R, Dennis M. Motor function profile in children with early onset hydrocephalus. Dev Neuropsychol 1999; 15:25–51.

41. Minns RA, Sobkowiak CA, Skardoutsou A, et al. Upper limb function in spina bifida. Z Kinderchir 1977; 22(4):493–506.

42. Simms B. A 3-year follow-up of the driving status of 32 young adults with spina bifida. Int Disabil Stud 1987; 9:177–180.

43. Fletcher JM, Brookshire BL, Bohan TP, et al. Early hydrocephalus. In: Rourke BP, ed. Syndrome of Nonverbal Learning Disabilities: Neurodevelopmental Manifestations. New York: Guilford Press, 1995a.

44. Brookshire BL, Fletcher JM, Bohan TP, et al. Verbal and nonverbal skill discrepancies in children with hydrocephalus: A five year follow-up. J Pediatr Psychol 1995; 20:785–800.

45. Pearson AM, Carr J, Hallwell MD. The handwriting of children with spina bifida. Z Kinderchir 1988; 43:40–42.

46. Baron IS, Goldberger E. Neuropsychological disturbance of hydrocephalic children with implications for special education and rehabilitation. Neuropsychol Rehabil 1993; 3:389–410.

47. Ito J, Saijo H, Araki A, et al. Neuroradiological assessment of visuoperceptual disturbance in children with spina bifida and hydrocephalus. Dev Med Child Neurolo 1997; 39:385–392.

48. Scott M, Fletcher JM, Brookshire BL, et al. Memory functions in children with early hydrocephalus. Neuropsychology 1998; 12:578–589.

49. Yeates KO, Enrile BG, Loss N, et al. Verbal learning and memory in children with myelomeningocele. J Pediatr Psychol 1995; 20;801–815.

50. Horn DG, Lorch EP, Lorch RF Jr., et al. Distractibility and vocabulary deficits in children with spina bifida and hydrocephalus. Dev Med Child Neurol 1985; 27:713–720.

51. Tew B, Laurance K, Richards A. Inattention among children with hydrocephalus and spina bifida. Zeitschrift fur Kindercirurgie 1980; 29:381–385.

52. Brewer VR, Fletcher JM, Hiscock M, et al. Attention processes in children with shunted hydrocephalus versus attention deficit/ hyperactivity disorder. Neuropsychology 2001; 15:185–198.

53. Mirsky AF, Anthony BJ, Duncan CC, et al. Analysis of the elements of attention: a neuropsychological approach. Neuropsychol Rev 1991; 2:109–145.

54. Hurley AD, Dorman C, Laatsch L, et al. Cognitive functioning in patients with spina bifida, hydrocephalus and the "cocktail party" syndrome. Dev Neuropsychol 1990; 6:151–172.

55. Loss N, Yeates KO, Enrile BG. Attention in children with myelomeningocele. Child Neuropsychol 1998; 4:7–20.

56. Dise JE, Lohr ME. Examination of deficits in conceptual reasoning abilities associated with spina bifida. Am J Phys Med Rehabil 1998; 77:247–251.

57. Snow JH, Prince M, Souheaver G, et al. Neuropsychological patterns of adolescents and young adults with spina bifida. Arch Clin Neuropsychol 1994; 9:277–287.

58. Matson MA, Mahone EM, Zabel TA. Serial Neuropsychological assessment and evidence of shunt malfunction in spina bifida: a longitudinal case study. Child Neuropsychol 2005; 11:315–332.

59. Lindquist B, Persson E-K, Uverbrant P, et al. Learning, memory and executive functions in children with hydrocephalus. Acta Paediatr 2008; 97:595–601.

60. Reem TA, Zabel AT, Mahone ME. Age-related differences in executive function among children with spina bifida/hydrocephalus based on parent behaviour ratings. Clin Neuropsychol 2008; 22 (4):585–602.

61. Boyer KM, Yeates KO, Enrile BG. Working memory and information processing speed in children with myelomeningocele and shunted hydrocephalus: analysis of the Children's Paced Auditory Serial Addition Test. J Int Neuropsychol Soc 2006; 12:305–313.

62. Iddon JL, Morgan DJR, Ahmed R, et al. Memory and learning in young adults with hydrocephalus and spina bifida: specific cognitive profiles. Eur J Pediatr Surg 2003; 13:32–35.

63. Iddon JL, Morgan DJR, Ahmed R, et al. Neuropsychological profile of young adults with spina bifida with or without hydrocephalus. J Neurol Neurosurg Psychiatry 2004; 75:1112–1118.

64. Barf HA, Verhoef M, Jennekens-Schinkel A, et al. Cognitive status of young adults with spina bifida. Dev Med Child Neurol 2003; 45:813–820.

65. Verhoef M, Barf HA, Post MW, et al. Secondary impairments in young adults with hydrocephalus. Dev Med Child Neurol 2004; 46:420–427.

66. Appleton PL, Ellis MC, Minchom PE, et al. Depressive symptoms and self-concept in young people with spina bifida. J Pediatr Psychol 1997; 22:707–722.

67. Appleton PL, Minchom PE, Ellis NC, et al. The self-concept of young people with spina bifida: a population-based study. Dev Med Child Neurol 1994; 36:198–215.

68. Hazlett RA. Self-perceptions of preschool children with spina bifida. J Paediatr Nurs 1997; 12:130–131.

69. Minchom PE, Ellis NC, Appleton PL, et al. Impact of functional severity on self-concept in young people with spina bifida. Arch Dis Child 1995; 73:48–52.

70. Barnes M, Dennis M, Hetherington R. Reading and writing skills in young adults with spina bifida and hydrocephalus. J Int Neuropsychol Soc 2004b; 10:655–663.

71. Barnes MA, Faulkner H, Wilkinson M, et al. Meaning construction and integration in children with hydrocephalus. Brain Lang 2004a; 89:47–56.

72. Dennis M, Barnes M. Math and numeracy in young adults with spina bifida and hydrocephalus. Dev Neuropsychol 2002; 21:141–155.

73. Hommet C, Billard C, Gillet P, et al. Neuropsychologic and adaptive functioning in adolescents and young adults shunted for congenital hydrocephalus. J Child Neurol 1999; 14:144–150.

74. Hommet C, Cottier JP, Billard C, et al. MRI morphometric study and correlation with cognitive functions in young adults shunted for congenital hydrocephalus related to spina bifida. Eur Neurol 2002; 47:169–174.

75. Hetherington R, Dennis M, Barnes M, et al. Functional outcome in young adults with spina bifida and hydrocephalus. Childs Nerv Syst 2006; 22:117–124.

76. Ralph K, Moylan P, Canady A, et al. The effects of multiple shunt revisions on neuropsychological functioning and memory. Neurol Res 2000; 22:131–136.

77. Fishman R. Normal pressure hydrocephalus and arthritis. N Engl J Med 1985; 312:1255–1256.

78. Hendy J, Anderson V. Development, pathology and the frontal lobes. J Int Neuropsychol Soc 1994; 1:199.

79. Iddon JL. Cognitive dysfunction in hydrocephalus. In: Harrison J, Owen AM, eds. Cognitive Profiles of Neuropsychiatric Disorders. London: Martin Dunitz, 2002.

6 | Antenatal Screening and Management of Hydrocephalus

Wan Tew Seow

Neurosurgery Service, KK Women's and Children's Hospital, Singapore

George Seow Heong Yeo

Antenatal Monitoring Clinic and Antenatal Diagnostic Clinic, Department of Maternal Fetal Medicine, KK Women's and Children's Hospital, Singapore

WHAT IS ANTENATAL SCREENING?

Antenatal screening is a process to assess the risk of an unborn baby (the fetus) having a congenital abnormality. Screening for neural tube defects was one of the initial routines in antenatal screening. Today, screening involves an array of biochemical and ultrasound tests, resulting in an increasing plethora of conditions that can be detected during early pregnancy. These conditions include Down's syndrome, spina bifida, sickle cell anemia, thalassemia, HIV, and hepatitis B. A diagnostic test, usually invasive, such as amniocentesis or chorionic villus sampling, is in order when the risk is assessed to be above a predefined value. Noninvasive prenatal determination of fetal Rh and sex status using cell-free fetal DNA in maternal blood is now available in some countries (1). Prenatal diagnosis of single gene disorders using cell free fetal DNA obtained from maternal blood will be available in the near future (2,3).

The screening tests include

Blood tests: These are usually carried out during the second trimester, from 14 to 20 weeks. Maternal serum alpha-feto-protein (AFP), originally used to detect neural tube defects, is a component of the double, triple, and quadruple serum test [testing for unconjugated estriol (uE3), human chorionic gonadotropin (hCG), and inhibin-A] for Down's syndrome (4,5). AFP is elevated when an open neural tube defect is present. Despite this, Down's syndrome screening during the first trimester is now done using blood tests without the AFP component, as the diagnostic accuracy of ultrasound for detection of neural tube defects is better than serum AFP (6). Maternal blood is also used to test for inherited blood diseases such as thalassemia and sickle cell anemia.

Fetal anomaly screening: This uses ultrasound scanning. Ultrasound scanning is usually carried out at 18 to 20 weeks and is used to identify heart abnormalities, cleft lip, as well as for confirmation of spina bifida and other structural abnormalities. The diagnostic accuracy for ultrasound screening of open neural tube defects has improved to the extent that it has replaced AFP assays in many centers (6).

It is possible to detect ventriculomegaly on ultrasound scanning; the role of fetal ultrasound in the antenatal diagnosis of fetal hydrocephalus is described below.

AMNIOCENTESIS

Amniocentesis is the most common diagnostic test to assess for fetal abnormality such as chromosomal conditions, which include Down's syndrome, Edward's syndrome, and Patau's syndrome. Amniocentesis is an invasive procedure and thus carries a small risk of miscarriage.

Amniocentesis may be offered in the following situations:

- if there is a previous pregnancy with a chromosomal defect;
- if there is a family history of a detectable abnormality; and
- if blood test shows high AFP, suggesting a neural tube defect or Down's syndrome screening showing an increased risk of the condition.

A definitive diagnosis made via amniocentesis will give parents a choice as to whether continue with the pregnancy or terminate the pregnancy at an early stage. Amniocentesis is usually performed between 16 and 20 weeks of pregnancy (7). Amniocentesis earlier than 15 weeks should not be carried out, as there is a higher risk of causing miscarriage. The risk of miscarriage has been variously reported from 0.3% to 1%.

During amniocentesis, a small sample of amniotic fluid is removed for testing in a laboratory. Ultrasonic guidance is used to identify a safe place for introduction of the needle. The amniotic fluid contains fetal cells and is analyzed for chromosomal and other genetic disorders, such as Down's syndrome and Edward's syndrome. Fluorescence in situ hybridization (FISH) is commonly done to detect chromosome 22q deletions in fetuses with congenital heart abnormalities to exclude Di George's syndrome.

CHORIONIC VILLUS SAMPLING

If a diagnostic test is needed in early pregnancy, chorionic villus sampling (CVS) is preferred as it can be carried out slightly earlier than amniocentesis—from about 10 weeks. A small sample of the chorionic villi (the part of the placenta that attaches to the uterus and which has the same genetic makeup as the fetus) is obtained by either percutaneous puncture through the wall of the abdomen or through the vagina and the cervix. The procedure is done under ultrasonic guidance. CVS can result in a spontaneous abortion in about 0.5% to 2% of cases. The risk of induced miscarriage is higher if the amniotic sac is punctured during the procedure. Other complications from CVS include infection, abdominal cramps, and uterine bleeding occurring during the procedure. Rarely, damage to the fetus during the procedure can result in a slightly increased risk for limb abnormalities in the fetus (such as missing or short fingers and toes).

Many fetal disorders can be detected by testing the placental (hence fetal) tissue obtained by CVS. These include Down's syndrome and other chromosomal conditions, genetic disorders such as cystic fibrosis, Duchenne muscular dystrophy, thalassemia, sickle cell anemia, and metabolic disorders such as antitrypsin deficiency and phenylketonuria (8).

FETAL ULTRASONOGRAPHY

The standard technique in the evaluation and detection of fetal CNS abnormalities is fetal ultrasonography (9). The basic ultrasonic examination to evaluate the fetal brain is usually performed around 20 weeks of gestation. The fetal head and spine are evaluated during this setting. A satisfactory evaluation of the fetal CNS can usually be obtained in the second and early third trimesters of pregnancy, although some fetal abnormalities may already be visible in the first and early second trimesters. Hence, familiarity with normal CNS appearances at different gestational ages is a prerequisite. In the later part of pregnancy, the ossification of the calvarium makes visualization of the intracranial contents more difficult.

The basic examination is usually performed using a 3- to 5-MHz transabdominal ultrasound transducer with gray-scale bidimensional ultrasound. Two axial planes are used to visualize the cerebral structures: the *transventricular plane* and the *transcerebellar plane* (10) (Fig. 1). A third plane, the *transthalamic plane* is typically described for biometry purposes (11). *The transventricular plane* cuts through the anterior and posterior parts of the lateral ventricles. In this plane, the anterior part of the lateral ventricles (the frontal horns) appears as two short straight lines in the classical axial plane and as two comma-shaped fluid filled structures when insonated from the frontal approach (Fig. 2). The lateral walls of the lateral ventricles are fairly well defined.

The centrally placed rectangular structure behind both frontal horns is the *cavum septum pellucidum* (CSP). The CSP is visible at around 16 weeks of gestation and becomes obliterated as the fetus nears term. On transabdominal ultrasonography, the CSP should always be visualized between 18 and 37 weeks (12).

The posterior part of the lateral ventricles (the occipital horns) is formed by the atrium of the lateral ventricle as it continues posteriorly and inferiorly into the occipital horn. These structures are visible at about 16 weeks of gestation. At this level, the glomus of the choroid plexus, which is brightly echogenic, fills up the atrium, while the occipital horn is filled with CSF, as the choroid plexus is not present there. During the second trimester, the medial and lateral walls of each lateral ventricle are parallel to the midline and show up on ultrasound as

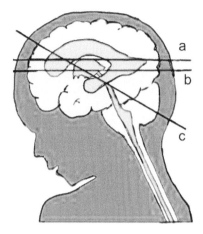

Figure 1 Axial planes for visualization of the fetal cranium on ultrasound scanning: a, transventricular plane; b, transthalamic plane; c, transcerebellar plane.

bright lines. At the level of the atrium, a small amount of fluid may be present between the medial wall and the choroid plexus, although in most instances, the atrium is completely filled up by the choroid plexus.

The transcerebellar plane is obtained at a level slightly lower than that of the transventricular plane with a slight tilt posteriorly (Fig. 3). In this plane, the frontal horns of the lateral ventricles, CSP, thalami, cerebellum, and cisterna magna are visualized. The cerebellum represents the main structure in the posterior fossa that is visualized in this plane. It appears as a butterfly-shaped structure formed by the two round cerebellar hemispheres attached in the middle by the slightly more echogenic cerebellar vermis. The cisterna magna is a fluid filled space posterior to the cerebellum.

The third plane, the transthalamic plane or biparietal diameter plane, is obtained at an intermediate level between the transventricular and transcerebellar planes (Fig. 4). From anterior to posterior, the anatomic landmarks include the frontal horns of the lateral ventricles, the cavum sepum pellucidum, the thalami, and both hippocampal gyri. The transthalamic plane does not add much more anatomical information to that obtained from ultrasonographing the other two planes. Its main use is for biometry of the fetal head. Biometry is an essential part of the sonographic examination of the fetal head because the biparietal diameter and head circumference measurements are commonly used to assess fetal age and growth. These measurements are also useful in identifying some cerebral anomalies, and a standard examination done during the second trimester and third trimester will usually include measuring the biparietal diameter, head circumference, and internal diameter of the atrium.

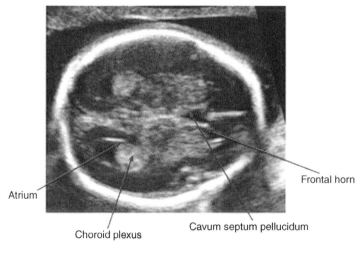

Figure 2 Transventricular plane.

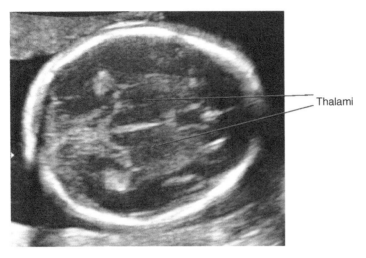

Figure 3 Transcerebellar plane.

FETAL ULTRASONOGRAPHY IN THE DIAGNOSIS OF FETAL HYDROCEPHALUS

Measurement of the ventricular atrium is important in the assessment of the ventricular system, as ventriculomegaly is a central feature of fetal hydrocephalus as well as a frequent marker of abnormal cerebral development (13). Atrial measurement is obtained at the level of the glomus of the choroid plexus, perpendicular to the ventricular cavity. To measure the atrial diameter, the calipers are positioned inside the echoes generated by the lateral walls. This measurement remains fairly constant in the second and early third trimesters, with a mean diameter of 6 to 8 mm (14). The ventricular size is considered normal when the atrium is less than 10 mm (15). Many fetal abnormalities associated with hydrocephalus such as Dandy–Walker malformations and Chiari II malformations can usually be visualized on the basic examination with the transcerebellar plane.

Hydrocephalus from spina bifida usually presents differently with head signs described as lemon-shaped head and banana-shaped cerebellum on ultrasonography performed during the second trimester (16). The head size is typically not increased at the prenatal stage and is thought to be caused by a drop in CSF pressure consequent to CSF loss through the open neural tube defect. Recently, the standard midsaggital view of the face has been used routinely to screen for chromosomal abnormalities during the first trimester. In this view, the fourth ventricle is easily identified as an intracranial translucency in the posterior cranial fossa. In fetuses with an open

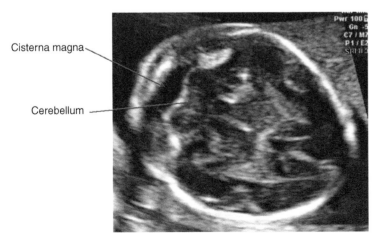

Figure 4 Transthalamic plane.

neural tube defect, the fourth ventricle is not visible because of displacement by the associated Chiari II malformation, and hence there is loss of the normal intracranial translucency. This "intracranial translucency" sign may be used for the early detection of open neural tube defects during the first trimester (17).

FETAL NEUROSONOGRAM

A fetal neurosonogram or dedicated fetal neurosonography is done when the basic ultrasonic examination suggests a fetal cranial abnormality (9). It is used for the evaluation of complex intracranial malformations and is obtained by aligning the transducer with the sutures and fontanelles of the fetal head to obtain multiplanar views of the fetal head, similar to the postnatal ultrasonic examination of the neonatal head (18). When the fetus being examined is in vertex presentation, scanning is done via a transabdominal/transvaginal approach. If the fetus is in breech presentation, a transfundal approach by positioning the ultrasound probe parallel instead of perpendicular to the abdomen is used. Vaginal probes provide better definition of anatomical details as they operate at higher frequencies than abdominal probes.

Aside from providing the standard measurements like the biparietal diameter, head circumference, and the atrium of the lateral ventricles, the neurosonographic examination allows a systematic evaluation of the fetal brain by visualizing four coronal and three sagittal planes of the fetal brain. The coronal planes used are the transfrontal plane (obtained through the anterior fontanel), which depicts the midline interhemispheric fissure and the anterior horns of the lateral ventricle on each side; the transcaudate plane (at the level of the caudate nuclei and genu of the corpus callosum); the transthalamic plane (depicting both thalami and the third ventricle and atrium of both lateral ventricles); and the transcerebellar plane (obtained through the posterior fontanel), enabling visualization of the posterior interhemispheric fissure, both occipital horns of the lateral ventricles, and the cerebellar hemisphere and vermis. The three sagittal planes studied are the midsagittal plane, which allows visualization of the midline sagittal views of the corpus callosum and the brainstem (Fig. 5), and two parasagittal planes, each lateral to the midsaggital plane, which show the entire lateral ventricle, the choroid plexus, the periventricular tissue, and the surrounding cortex. It is possible to visualize the anterior cerebral artery, the pericallosal arteries, and the vein of Galen in the midsaggital plane using color Doppler.

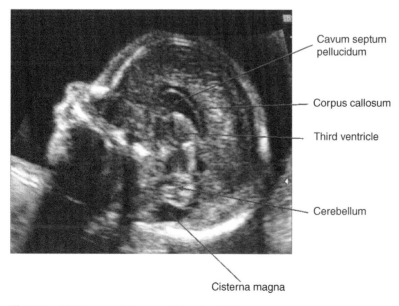

Figure 5 Midline saggital plane obtained on fetal neurosonogram.

When an abnormality is suspected, neurosonography can also be used to evaluate the convolutions of the fetal brain. The normal parietooccipital sulcus becomes visible as early as 18 weeks. As the gestation of the fetus progresses, more sulci become visible.

FETAL MAGNETIC RESONANCE IMAGING

Fetal magnetic resonance imaging (MRI) is now available in many fetal diagnostic centers. MRI does not use ionizing radiation and produces standardized and easily reproducible images with excellent tissue contrast of the fetus. MRI is able to provide more detailed anatomical information on CNS anomalies such as cortical gyral abnormalities, cortical clefts, partial or complete genesis of the corpus callosum and the septum pellucidum, midbrain dysgenesis, cerebellar hypoplasia, myelomeningocele, vermian cysts, and also hemorrhage compared to ultrasound (19,20). With the use of ultrafast MR sequences and techniques available today, there is no longer a need to sedate the fetus to reduce fetal movement during the procedure (21). This has added to the increasing use of this imaging modality.

The main uses for fetal MRI are for further morphological analysis when the fetal ultrasound suggests an abnormal lesion, or when the ultrasonographic examination is inconclusive or in doubt (22). This makes it an important adjunct for prenatal counseling. It also plays an important role in surgical planning if fetal surgery of the lesion is proposed.

In the context of fetal hydrocephalus, the progress of hydrocephalus can easily be followed on maternal ultrasound, so fetal MRI is useful mainly to identify the cause of hydrocephalus (especially for aqueductal stenosis) as well as to determine the presence of other CNS abnormalities associated with hydrocephalus (Fig. 6) (23). MRI can also be used to assess cortical development in fetuses; cortical development is delayed in fetuses with isolated ventriculomegaly and those with other CNS anomalies compared to normal fetuses (24). Fetal MRI can also be used to measure and quantify ventricular and parenchymal volumes, which may in future help prognosticate the outcomes of fetuses with ventriculomegaly.

GENETIC TESTING FOR HYDROCEPHALUS

Prenatal diagnosis of X-linked hydrocephalus can be determined by genetic testing. The disorder is transmitted from mother to sons, and it has been estimated that 25% of males with aqueductal stenosis have X-linked hydrocephalus (25,26). The gene is located at Xq28 (27,28), but it has now been established that mutations in L1CAM, the neural cell adhesion molecule (also localized to Xq28), is responsible for the CRASH syndrome, which includes **C**orpus callosum hypoplasia/agenesis, mental **R**etardation, **A**dducted thumbs, **S**pastic paraplegia, and **H**ydrocephalus, with X-linked hydrocephalus being a variation of the syndrome. Another variation is the MASA syndrome, which includes **M**ental retardation, **A**phasia, **S**huffling gait, and

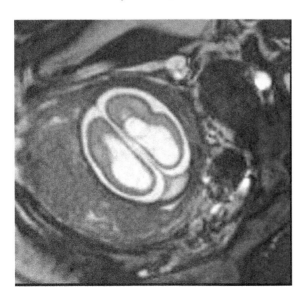

Figure 6 Fetal MRI showing ventriculomegaly in a male fetus with X-linked hydrocephalus.

Adducted thumbs. Significant phenotypic variability of L1CAM gene can occur within families; hence some males are severely affected and are readily diagnosed during pregnancy, while some affected males may not present with macrocephaly at all. Approximately 74% to 90% males with hydrocephalus, a positive family history, and at least one other feature of L1CAM disease will show mutations of the L1CAM gene.

Mutations of the L1CAM gene are identified by complete sequence analysis of the entire coding region of the gene from the DNA of the mother. It should be noted that molecular genetic analysis of the whole gene as part of prenatal workup is difficult because of the large size of the gene, which comprises 28 exons over 15 KB of genomic DNA (29,30), and hence is not readily available in many countries. Complete gene analysis can also be done for fetal samples obtained by CVS in suspected fetuses, if these are available.

CAUSES AND MANAGEMENT OF FETAL HYDROCEPHALUS

There is a wide spectrum of causes and diseases that may result in ventriculomegaly (31). The intracranial appearance of hydrocephalus on imaging is similar to ex vacuo ventriculomegaly secondary to brain insults. Hydrocephalus itself results from the obstruction of flow of cerebrospinal fluid (CSF) or poor absorption of CSF. Hydrocephalus may be caused by aqueduct stenosis and can be confirmed on fetal MRI scans. In hydrocephalus associated with spina bifida, the ventricular and corresponding head size may not increase until much later. Hydrocephalus may be seen with anomalies of the posterior fossa, such as in the Dandy–Walker malformation where there is upward displacement of the tentorium, rotation, and significant hypoplasia of the cerebellar vermis.

Ventriculomegaly can occur as a result of abnormal cerebral development, which includes structural anomalies such as agenesis of the corpus callosum or from disordered cortical development. It can also result from vascular or infective insults to the fetal brain. Definitive causes of ventriculomegaly include encephalomalacia and migrational disorders, which are often attributed to vascular, hypoxic, viral, or genetic causes. Fetal anemia from red blood cell alloimmunization, fetomaternal bleeding, and viral infection, can lead to brain injury and ex vacuo ventriculomegaly. Umbilical cord and placental disorders can lead to hypoxic insults and similar damage. A surviving monochorionic twin with single demise can develop hypoxic brain damage. It is not surprising then that ventriculomegaly is associated with an increase in fetal and neonatal morbidity and mortality. The increased morbidity and mortality is due to the associated abnormalities rather than the ventriculomegaly itself.

SURGICAL MANAGEMENT OF ANTENATAL HYDROCEPHALUS

Experimental prenatal surgical treatment of confirmed fetal hydrocephalus was performed in the early 1980s, but the poor outcome resulted in a voluntary moratorium on surgical treatment of fetal hydrocephalus in 1986 (32). In the MRI era, surgical treatment of fetal hydrocephalus should be considered still experimental (33), although it has been performed in countries where abortions are banned, such as Brazil (34). It should be considered only if the relevant expertise is available and requires a multidisciplinary team in a tertiary medical center with expertise in fetal medicine and surgery. Treatment options for treatment of fetal hydrocephalus include multiple percutaneous ventricular taps, cephalocentesis, and ventriculoamniotic shunting. The majority of patients who had undergone fetal surgery for hydrocephalus reported in the literature still required insertion of a ventriculoperitoneal shunt after birth.

ABORTION AND ABORTION LAWS

Abortion is a highly contentious topic, which has provoked both ethical and legal debates dating back to the time of the Greek philosophers and probably earlier. Consequently, the availability of abortions differs across countries depending on societal values. In some countries like the United States and Singapore, a woman can request for an abortion on demand. In the United States, the right of a woman to have an abortion is regarded as a constitutional right (35). In the United Kingdom (but not in Northern Ireland) and Australia, lawful abortions are readily available, although there is still a law against unlawful abortion. In the United Kingdom, termination of pregnancy is legal up to the 24th week of pregnancy. For the abortion to be lawful, a pregnant woman must meet one or more of the grounds specified in the *Abortion Act 1967 (UK)*, but in most instances, these grounds are loosely interpreted and it is not difficult for a woman to obtain a lawful abortion. Termination has to be authorized by two medical practitioners.

In most of the South American countries, abortion is illegal. In many countries where abortions are illegal, an abortion can still be legally performed if continuing the pregnancy would endanger the life of the mother (the double effect argument). However, even in countries where an abortion can be obtained on demand, an abortion may not be freely available once the pregnancy is more than 24 weeks. In the United Kingdom, after the 24th week of pregnancy, termination is only permitted if the mother's health is in danger, or if a "severe abnormality" in the fetus is detected; what a "severe abnormality" is, is not defined in the legislation but would presumably include severe conditions such as anencephaly, which is incompatible with life.

In the context of fetal hydrocephalus, the hydrocephalus is unlikely to endanger the life of the mother and hence aborting a hydrocephalic fetus would be illegal in those countries where all abortions are illegal except if there is danger to the mother (unless it can be argued that knowing that she has a hydrocephalic child may cause mental harm to a mother who would kill herself rather than proceed with the pregnancy). However, a hydrocephalic fetus would be one of the grounds for a lawful abortion in countries like the United Kingdom and Australia.

Neurosurgeons counseling women with congenital anomalies must have an understanding of the abortion laws in their countries so that they can counsel their patients properly and legally. In countries where abortions are illegal, it is wise not to discuss terminating the pregnancy but to focus on the postnatal management of the fetus. In countries where abortions are lawful, there will be neurosurgeons who for moral or religious reasons are conscientious objectors to abortions. In these countries, while the neurosurgeon can legitimately refuse to assist in an abortion, it is not possible to counsel a woman with a hydrocephalic fetus without discussing about termination of the pregnancy. In such a situation, the neurosurgeon should not counsel such patients but should refer the patient to another doctor who is not a conscientious objector (36).

ANTENATAL COUNSELING

In counseling with regards to the neurosurgical aspects of hydrocephalus, it is necessary to discuss the spectrum of the disease, which part of the spectrum the fetus is likely to fall into, the treatment(s) available at that part of the disease spectrum, and to suggest a treatment plan for the fetus once it is born. Outlining a treatment plan will connect the parents to the treating neurosurgeon and this is important for family support, especially in countries where termination of pregnancy is not an option or for those families who wish to continue on with the pregnancy.

When discussing the spectrum of the disease, it is important to differentiate hydrocephalus from ventriculomegaly, as no surgical treatment will be necessary for the latter. In terms of prognosis, fetuses with isolated, borderline ventriculomegaly, but without other abnormalities, generally have a good neurological outcome, particularly when the ventriculomegaly is unilateral. However, even mild isolated ventriculomegaly is known to have a 5% to 10% association with developmental delay of varied severity (37). It should be noted that hydrocephalus can manifest some weeks or even months after birth in the setting of what may be considered to be ventriculomegaly without raised intracranial pressure. For example, hydrocephalus from aqueductal stenosis may manifest a few months after birth. At that time, a better surgical option would be a third ventriculostomy instead of shunting.

On the other hand, if a diagnosis of hydrocephalus is confirmed, the prognosis is poorer, especially if hydrocephalus is diagnosed before 30 to 32 weeks (38). It is also important to discuss the outcome of hydrocephalus not only in terms of developmental milestones and the possibility of severe physical and mental disabilities but also to discuss the surgical outcome in terms of shunt failure, infection, and possibility of lifelong complications of a shunt. This will allow the family to have better understanding of the condition and treatment outcomes, and this information will be needed for families considering termination of pregnancy in countries where this is available.

REFERENCES

1. Hahn S, Chitty LS. Noninvasive prenatal diagnosis: Current practice and future perspectives. Curr Opin Obstet Gynecol 2008; 20:146–151.
2. Norbury G, Nobury CJ. Non-invasive prenatal diagnosis of single gene disorders: How close are we? Semin Fetal Neonatal Med 2008; 13:76–83.
3. Ndume FM, Navti O, Chilaka VN, et al. Prenatal diagnosis in the first trimester of pregnancy. Obstet Gynecol 2008; 63:317–328.
4. Wald NJ, Cuckle HS, Densem JW, et al. Maternal serum screening for Down's syndrome in early pregnancy. BMJ 1988; 297:883–887.
5. Benn PA, Fang M, Egan FFX, et al. Incorporation of inhibin-A in second trimester screening of Down syndrome. Obstet Gynecol 2003; 101:451–454.
6. Kooper AJA, de Bruijn D, van Ravenwaaij-Arts CMA, et al. Fetal anomaly scan potentially will replace routine AFAFP assays for the detection of neural tube defects. Prenat Diagn 2007; 27:29–33.
7. Evans MI, Andrioles S. Chorionic villus sampling and amniocentesis in 2008. Curr Opin Obstet Gynecol 2008; 20:164–168.
8. Norton ME. Genetic screening and counseling. Curr Opin Obstet Gynecol 2008; 20:157–163.
9. International Society of Ultrasound in Obstetrics & Gynecology. Sonographic examination of the fetal central nervous system: guidelines for performing the 'basic examination' and the 'fetal neurosonogram'. Ultrasound Obstet Gynecol 2007; 29:109–116.
10. Filly RA, Cardoza JD, Goldstein RB, et al. Detection of fetal central nervous system anomalies: A practical level of effort for a routine sonogram. Radiology 1989; 172:403–408.
11. Shepard M, Filly RA. A standardized plane for biparietal diameter measurement. J Ultrasound Med 1982; 1:145–150.
12. Falco P, Gabrielli S, Visentin A, et al. Transabdominal sonography of the cavum septum pellucidum in normal fetuses in the second and third trimesters of pregnancy. Ultrasound Obstet Gynecol 2000; 16:549–553.
13. Mehta TS, Levine D. Imaging of fetal cerebral ventriculomegaly: A guide to management and outcome. Semin Fetal Neonatal Med 2005; 10:421–428.
14. Cardoza JD, Goldstein RB, Filly RA. Exclusion of fetal ventriculomegaly with a single measurement: the width of the lateral ventricular atrium. Radiology 1988; 169:711–714.
15. Pilu G, Falco P, Gabrielli S, et al. The clinical significance of fetal isolated cerebral borderline ventriculomegaly: Report of 31 cases and review of the literature. Ultrasound Obstet Gynecol 1999; 14:320–326.
16. Sebire NJ, Noble PL, Thrope-Beeston JG, et al. Presence of the 'lemon' sign in fetuses with spina bifida at the 10–14 week scan. Ultrasound Obstet Gynecol 1997; 10:403–405.
17. Chaoui R, Benoit B, Mitkowska H, et al. Assessment of intracranial translucency (IT) in the detection of spina bifida at the 11–13 week scan. Ultrasound Obstet Gynecol 2009; 3:249–252.
18. Timor-Tritsch IE, Monteagudo A. Transvaginal fetal neurosonography: Standardization of the planes and sections by anatomic landmarks. Ultrasound Obstet Gynecol 1996; 8:42–47.
19. Levine D, Barnes PD, Madsen JR, et al. Fetal central nervous system anomalies: MR imaging augments sonographic diagnosis. Radiology 1997; 204:635–642.
20. Papadias A, Miller C, Martin WL, et al. Comparison of prenatal and postnatal MRI findings in the evaluation of intrauterine CNS anomalies requiring postnatal neurosurgical treatment. Childs Nerv Syst 2008; 24:185–192.
21. Levine D, Hatabu H, Gaa J, et al. Fetal anatomy revealed with fast MR sequences. AJR Am J Roentgenol 1996; 167:905–908.
22. Simin EM, Goldstein RB, Coakley FV, et al. Fast MR Imaging of fetal CNS anomalies in utero. Am J Neuroradiol 2000; 21:1688–1698.
23. Zimmerman RA, Bilaniuk LT. Magnetic resonance evaluation of fetal ventriculomegaly-associated congenital malformations and lesions. Semin Fetal Neonat Med 2005; 10:429–443.
24. Levine D, Barnes PD, Madsen JR, et al. Central nervous system abnormalities assessed with prenatal magnetic resonance imaging. Obstet Gynecol 1999; 94:1011–1009.
25. Burton BK. Recurrent risk for congenital hydrocephalus. Clin Genet 1979; 16:47–53.
26. Halliday J, Chow CW, Wallace D, et al. X linked hydrocephalus: A survey of a 20 year period in Victoria, Australia. J Med Genet 1986; 23:23–31.
27. Willems PJ, Dijkstra I, Van der Auwera BJ, et al. Assignment of X-linked hydrocephalus to Xq28 by linkage analysis. Genomics 1990; 8:367–370.
28. Jouet M, Feldman M, Yates J, et al. Refining the genetic location of the gene for X linked hydrocephalus within Xq28. J Med Genet 1993; 30:214–217.
29. Fransen E, Vits L, Van Camp G, et al. The clinical spectrum of mutations in L1, a neuronal cell adhesion molecule. Am J Med Genet 1996; 64:73–77.

30. Finckh U, Schroder J, Ressler B, et al. Spectrum and detection rate of L1CAM mutations in isolated and familial cases with clinically suspected L1-disease. Am J Med Genet 2000; 92:40–46.
31. Filly RA, Glidstein RB, Callen PW. Fetal ventricle: importance in routine obstetric sonography. Radiology 1991; 181:1–7.
32. Manning FA, Harrison MR, Rodeck C; Members of the International Fetal Medicine and Surgery Society. Catheter shunts for fetal hydronephrosis and hydrocephalus: Report of the international fetal surgery registry. N Engl J Med 1986; 315:336–340.
33. Von Koch CS, Gupta N, Sutton LN, et al. In utero surgery for hydrocephalus. Childs Nerv Syst 2003; 19:574–586.
34. Cavalheiro S, Moron AF, Zymberg ST, et al. Fetal hydrocephalus—Prenatal treatment. Childs Nerv Syst 2003; 19:561–573.
35. Roe v Wade, 410 U.S. 113 (1973).
36. Barr v Matthews (2000) 52 BMLR 217.
37. Vergani P, Locatelli A, Strobelt N, et al. Clinical outcome of mild fetal ventriculomegaly. Am J Obstet Gynecol 1998; 178:218–222.
38. Oi S. Diagnosis, outcome and management of fetal abnormalities: Fetal hydrocephalus. Childs Nerv Syst 2003:19:508–516.

7 | Posthemorrhagic Hydrocephalus

Cheryl Muszinski

Department of Neurosurgery, Division of Pediatric Neurosurgery, Medical College of Wisconsin, Milwaukee, Wisconsin, U.S.A.

INTRODUCTION

When infants are born prematurely, they are essentially arrested at a gestational stage during which the development of the highly vascularized germinal matrix in the brain is ongoing. Because the capillary network of this structure is still anatomically immature in these infants, the vessels are especially fragile and susceptible to rupture in the face of fluctuating cerebral blood flow or cerebral venous pressure, both common in premature babies, especially during periods of respiratory distress. If these vessels rupture, it can result in bleeding into the germinal matrix and subsequently into the ventricles of the brain (1), a condition known as intraventricular hemorrhage (IVH; also known as periventricular–intraventricular hemorrhage or PIVH). IVH is one of the most serious complications in premature infants and an important cause of mortality and long-term neurological sequelae in this group.

The acute vulnerability of preterm infants to IVH reflects a combination of anatomical and physiological factors that prevail at the end of the second trimester of gestational development (1–5). IVH begins as a hemorrhagic lesion in the germinal matrix, a richly vascularized, highly proliferative, and metabolically active structure that lies under the ependymal lining of the lateral ventricles. A temporary structure during gestation, the germinal matrix is most pronounced in the six- to eight-month-old fetus (1,6), thins markedly by week 32 and almost completely involutes by term (7). Cerebral neuronal precursors and glial precursors of oligodendroglia and astrocytes all originate from this structure, though at different stages of gestational development (8). During its period of rapid cell division, the germinal matrix requires a rich blood supply. However, because it is a temporary structure, the blood vessels are poorly supported by connective tissue (9,10), thus rendering them fragile and especially vulnerable to sudden hemodynamic changes, which may cause them to rupture through the ependyma into the ventricular cavity (11,12). In fact, IVH occurs in approximately 80% of cases with germinal matrix bleeding (13). If the hemorrhage is large, it may even extend into adjacent parenchymal tissue (6), where the degree of injury dramatically impacts on the neurological outcome.

The correlation between the development of IVH and the actual gestational age at birth is thus dependent upon the stage of anatomical development of the germinal matrix, with the occurrence of IVH relatively uncommon after week 32. Estimated frequencies of germinal matrix bleeding and IVH range from 50% to 75% for infants born at less than 26 weeks, decline sharply after the 30th week of gestation, and decrease to less than 5% among unselected full-term infants (14).

Grading System for IVH

IVH is characterized by a spectrum of lesions amenable to classification by grade of severity. The first classification scheme, proposed by Papile et al. (6), was based on computerized tomography (CT) scan findings of the extent of bleeding and recognizes the following four grades of IVH that are cumulative and numbered from mild to severe:

- Grade I: germinal matrix hemorrhage (GMH) only
- Grade II: GMH + IVH with no ventricular distension
- Grade III: GMH + IVH + ventricular distension
- Grade IV: GMH + IVH + intraparenchymal hemorrhage

Mild IVH (grades I and II) is generally benign (15), while grade III and particularly grade IV may be related to early complications, such as posthemorrhagic hydrocephalus (PHH) (16) with concomitant neurodevelopmental disabilities and high mortality. Grades II and III include

IVHs of variable severity as judged by the percentage of ventricle that contains blood or by the presence or absence of ventricular enlargement. Although a classification system proposed by Volpe (13) is similar in scope, it does not include a grade IV hemorrhage but rather regards it as a neuropathological consequence of IVH. In the context of the IVH grading system, PHH is considered a post-IVH complication. In general, the more severe the hemorrhage, the greater the risk for developing PHH.

Papile's classification scheme has been used extensively to predict the outcome of IVH and to establish an appropriate regimen of therapy. While this grading system is still used in most neonatology units, the brains of preterm infants are now imaged primarily by ultrasound rather than by CT scans (11).

Posthemorrhagic Hydrocephalus as a Complication of IVH

Of all the neurological sequelae that may follow IVH, the most serious is posthemorrhagic hydrocephalus (PHH), characterized by high mortality rates and associated long-term neurodevelopmental disorders (17,18). The term posthemorrhagic hydrocephalus is generally applied when there is progressive accumulation of cerebral spinal fluid (CSF) under pressure with ventricular ballooning (ventriculomegaly or VM) and accompanying enlargement of the head (1,9). VM typically develops one to three weeks following the initial intraventricular bleed (19,20) in 55% to 80% of the IVH population, with 26% to 85% of these cases progressing to PHH (13,21–23). The risk for progression of IVH to PHH depends primarily on the quantity of intraventricular blood present and increases with increasing grade of IVH (13,24). For example, VM incidence rates as high as 70% to 80% have been reported in the grade IV IVH group (1,25). On average, the incidence of VM in the entire IVH population is 40% to 50% (16). Although VM and PHH are not common in GMH and grade I IVH, VM can develop in grade II bleeds but usually requires no treatment (16).

Of those infants who do progress on to PHH, mortality is high and shunt dependence is common (26). Neurodevelopmental disabilities, including motor dysfunction and cognitive impairment (17,27,28), are largely attributed to periventricular white matter damage (13). However, some of these disabilities may also result from a prolonged period of increased intracranial pressure (ICP) prior to shunt insertion or from complications associated with treatment, such as shunt blockage and infections (29).

Epidemiology

Developed countries are currently at an all-time high for preterm births. In the United States alone, there are approximately 55,000 very low–birth-weight (<1500 g) infants born each year (13). Although technology can now keep more of these infants alive (9,30,31), at the same time, it has created something of a paradox—their survival puts them at high risk for developing IVH and all the complications associated with it. Even so, the proportion of at-risk infants who actually develop IVH has declined over the past 20 years, largely because of research efforts focused on its etiology and prevention. For example, in the early 1980s, 35% to 50% of very low-birth-weight infants developed IVH, but by the late 1990s, the proportion had declined to about 15% (32,33). The incidence still remains above 20% in infants weighing under 1000 g (1,34,35). Although IVH can often be prevented, management of the hydrocephalus that can follow IVH remains a challenge. Of those infants with IVH who progress on to PHH, over half will become shunt-dependent or die (26). Those infants who do survive ultimately will experience a high frequency of neurodevelopmental disabilities.

PATHOGENESIS AND PATHOLOGY OF PHH

PHH is defined strictly as progressive VM caused by disturbances in CSF flow or resorption (36). The hydrocephalus is usually ascribed to fibrosing obliterative arachnoiditis in the posterior fossa, meningeal fibrosis, and subependymal gliosis, which impair flow and resorption of CSF (1). The sequence of events leading to PHH is initiated by the formation of multiple small blood clots throughout the ventricular and CSF spaces (9). Their presence thickens the CSF, thus impeding its circulation and resorption via either arachnoid villi that project into the blood-filled cranial venous sinuses or across the ependyma into small blood vessels within the central nervous system (37). Studies also suggest that release of transforming growth factor β1 (TGFβ1)—virtually undetectable in normal neonatal CSF—into the CSF following IVH upregulates genes for synthesis of extracellular matrix proteins, including fibronectin and laminin

(38,39). If their deposition around the brain stem and in the subarachnoid space is extensive, it can effectively block the CSF channels, resulting in CSF accumulation under pressure and progressive ventricular dilatation. High levels of the carboxyterminal propeptide of type I procollagen have also been observed in the CSF of very low-birth-weight infants with PHH, three to four weeks after IVH, suggesting that cerebral bleeding may induce local collagen synthesis and trigger meningeal fibrosis (40). Damage to the periventricular white matter occurs in response to the increased ICP, ischemia, and inflammation (1,41). This damage may be exacerbated by oxidative stress caused by generation of free radicals (42,43) and by the actions of inflammatory cytokines, such as tumor necrosis factor-α, interleukin-1β, interleukin-6, interleukin-8, and interferon-γ, that are significantly elevated in the CSF of infants with PHH (9,44,45).

The major factors that determine an abnormal neurological outcome in infants with IVH and PHH are concomitant hemorrhagic and hypoxic-ischemic parenchymal injury (36). Infants with PHH, especially those who require shunting, are at a high risk for major neurological sequelae. Although their prognosis may be correlated in part to shunt-related complications, such as infection, septicemia, and shunt obstruction (36,46), there is increasing evidence from neuropathologic, neurophysiologic, and biochemical studies that shows potential deleterious effects of progressive PHH itself. For example, neuropathologic studies of hydrocephalus in experimental animals and humans have shown axonal stretching, swelling, and disruption resulting in gliosis. Disruption of the ventricular ependyma by progressive PHH may permit infusion of CSF into periventricular white matter causing vascular attenuation, edema, and ischemic cerebral injury. Data from animal models of hydrocephalus also suggest that there may be significant alterations in cortical neurons and disturbances in the development of neurotransmitters and synaptogenesis, which may affect the organizational development of the cerebral cortex and which may be reversible with early correction of the hydrocephalus (36). Thus, a major reason for the disabilities associated with PHH is the high frequency of associated periventricular white matter damage (13).

CLINICAL PRESENTATIONS

PHH should be suspected whenever IVH of grade II or higher is diagnosed. IVH may be accompanied by signs of hypotonia, pupillary dilation, sunsetting, ophthalmoplegia, seizures, vomiting, metabolic acidosis, bradycardia, bulging fontanel, rapidly increasing head size, or hematocrit reduction. PHH typically presents with symptoms of rising ICP, including apnea, vomiting, and abnormal posture, as well as rapidly increasing head circumference that crosses over the initial percentile or enlarges over 1.5 cm per week, a bulging anterior fontanel, and separation of the cranial sutures. However, the measurement of an enlarged head circumference is not sufficiently sensitive to aid in the diagnosis of hydrocephalus in the premature infant because ventricular dilatation can occur days to weeks prior to a detectable increase in the rate of head growth (47).

Many cases of IVH that ultimately lead to PHH are clinically silent, and early detection requires the use of intracranial imaging using either serial CT scans or portable real-time cranial ultrasounds (21,48). Cranial ultrasonography is a noninvasive, nonradiation-based procedure that can be performed at the bedside, without sedation. Because it is highly sensitive and accurate (49–53), it is an ideal method for detection and follow-up of IVH/PHH and facilitates a prompt diagnosis even in asymptomatic cases (54,55). While there are more limiting factors associated with the use of CT scans (48,56), they provide nevertheless a good alternative method for detection. Figures 1 and 2 show typical images obtained using both these technologies.

Cranial ultrasound scans (USs) are carried out via the anterior fontanel in standard coronal and parasagittal views, with IVH subsequently classified as grades I through IV, according to Volpe's classification (6). Ultrasonographic surveillance can be used to identify and confirm suspected hydrocephalus, monitor its progression, and differentiate between transient and static VM. Quantitative measurements of ventricular enlargement are recorded using a very standardized protocol. The width of the anterior horn of the lateral ventricles is measured in a coronal view, with the plane of the scan at the level of the foramina of Monro (just anterior to the choroid plexus in the third ventricle). The width is measured on each side as the distance between the medial wall and the floor of the lateral ventricle at the widest point (26). Measurement of the ventricular index (distance from the falx to the lateral-most aspect of the lateral ventricle) can then be compared with gestationally appropriate standards (57).

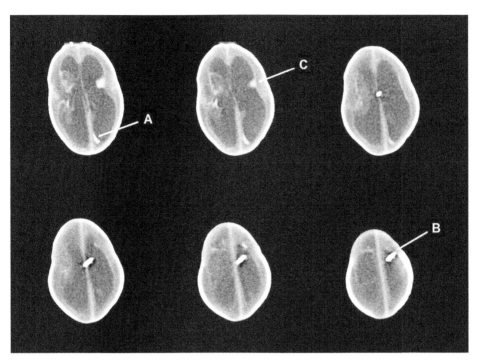

Figure 1   Noncontrast axial head CT (at corrected age of 29 weeks) demonstrates the presence of a small amount of intraventricular hemorrhage (layering posteriorly within the occipital horn of the left lateral ventricle) (**A**), hydrocephalus, and the left frontal ventricular catheter portion of a ventricular catheter reservoir (**B**). Small regions of thrombus are present within the lateral ventricles (**C**).

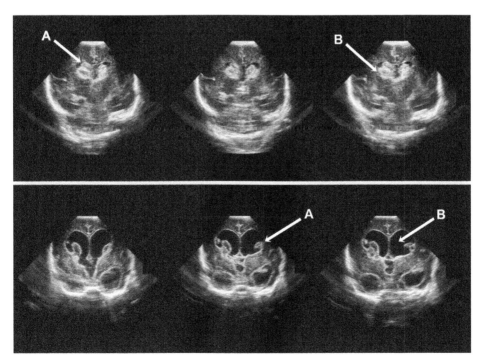

Figure 2   (*Upper panel*) Head ultrasound images (at corrected age of 27 weeks) reveal the presence of bilateral IVH (**A**), right caudate nucleus hemorrhage (**B**), and prominent ventricles. (*Lower panel*) Subsequent head ultrasound images (at corrected age of 29 weeks) of the same patient (shown in upper panel) show evolving IVH (**A**) within both lateral ventricles and interval development of hydrocephalus (**B**).

Although most cases of IVH occur within the first week of life, PHH does not usually develop until the second or third week of life. Therefore, a cranial US is recommended toward the middle to end of the first week of life if PHH is suspected. Although IVH can be detected at earlier time points, scans performed earlier in the week could potentially miss bleeds that develop later in the week. However, if overt clinical signs suggest PHH, earlier USs are recommended. A more detailed discussion of the timing of scans follows in the next section.

MANAGEMENT OF PHH

Most clinicians would concur that the ideal management of PHH would be the prevention of neonatal IVH, and consequently, numerous strategies have been investigated. These include prophylactic administration of indomethacin (13,17,58–67); vitamin E (68–71); antenatal vitamin K (72–74); ethamsylate (13,75–78); phenobarbital, both antenatal (79,80) and postnatal (16,80–82); and expectant neuromuscular paralysis of ventilated newborns (73,83). Unfortunately, none of these approaches has consistently proven to be efficacious in preventing IVH. There are, nonetheless, practical routine precautions that may ameliorate the progression of the hemorrhage. These precautions primarily focus on avoiding abrupt increases in cerebral blood flow and other hemodynamic disturbances as briefly discussed in the section pathogenesis and pathology of PHH of this chapter. For a more inclusive discussion of preventative strategies and practices, please refer to Tortorolo et al. (11), Hansen and Snyder (84), and Duncan and Chiang (16).

Monitoring, Detection, and Initial Intervention

A combination of cranial ultrasonography and clinical assessment is generally used to detect IVH in the preterm infant as well as to monitor for the development of PHH. Perlman and Rollins (85) recommend an ultrasonography protocol based on the infant's birth weight. These protocols are shown below.

For neonates of <1000 g birth weight:

- an initial US on day 3–5 of life (this should identify at least 75% of cases of IVH),
- a second US on day 10–14 (this should identify at least 84% of IVH and also identify early hydrocephalus and early cyst formation),
- a third US on day 28 (this should detect all cases of IVH as well as assess ventricular size in infants previously diagnosed with IVH), and
- a fourth and final US before discharge from the hospital (this should detect ~20% of significant late-onset lesions).

For neonates weighing 1000 to 1250 g at birth:

- an initial US on day 3–5 of life (should detect at least 40% of significant abnormalities),
- a second US on day 28 (should detect at least 70% of significant abnormalities), and
- a third US prior to discharge (should detect all late-onset significant lesions).

For neonates weighing 1251 to 1500 g at birth:

- an initial US on day 3–5 of life and
- a second US before discharge, so long as the clinical course is uncomplicated

Clinical assessment should focus on the signs and symptoms of PHH, as discussed earlier. However, because many of the symptoms do not appear until the hydrocephalus is severe (47), it is important to monitor ICP by serial measurement of the occipitofrontal circumference (36,86).

Unfortunately, there are currently no effective methods for preventing PHH after IVH has occurred. For the majority (65%) of newborns with PHH, the condition resolves spontaneously within a month, either regressing or stabilizing at an acceptable ICP (less than approximately 80–110 mm H_2O), and these patients never require medical or surgical intervention (13,87). Therefore, if the monitored progression continues at a slow rate, surveillance alone is the most appropriate management program. However, if close monitoring reveals rapid progression [increase in serial head circumference measurements of 2 cm/wk with a full fontanel and split sutures (24)] or if the slow progression persists beyond two to four weeks, interventions are indicated (36,84,88).

Medical Interventions

Medical interventions are aimed at maintaining a normal ICP in order to facilitate normal cerebral perfusion pressure and cerebral blood flow as well as to avoid compression of periventricular white matter and cerebral arteries and veins (13). These actions, however, are temporizing measures at best. Although they do not alter the natural course of the disease, they may relieve symptoms while the patient's condition declares itself as either spontaneously resolving or continually progressive. The latter category requires definitive therapy (84).

Medical interventions for PHH fall into two categories: mechanical measures that increase CSF elimination and pharmacotherapeutic measures that decrease CSF production.

Mechanical Approach: Lumbar Punctures

For more than 20 years, lumbar puncture has been a mainstay in efforts to slow the progression of ventricular dilation, the theory being that serial removal of CSF in bulk prevents volume accumulation, thus temporarily reducing ICP and ventricular size by negating the imbalance between CSF production and absorption (22). However, in a 2001 meta-analysis, Whitelaw (89) concluded that although it was a reasonable hypothesis, controlled trials failed to demonstrate any evidence of benefit. Indeed, there is a risk of secondary infection in addition to the discomfort of the procedures. Therefore, on the basis of results of this study, routine use of early lumbar punctures for infants at risk of, or actually developing, PHH cannot be recommended.

Pharmacotherapy

Both acetazolamide and furosemide are carbonic anhydrase inhibitors that act to reduce the production of CSF (88). In two separate studies in 1998, these agents were evaluated for treating PHH. While Hansen and Snyder found a combination of the two drugs to be efficacious (84), the International PHVD (Posthemorrhagic Ventricular Dilation in Infancy) Drug Trial Group reported an increased relative risk of death or shunt placement in neonates randomized to receive this combination diuretic therapy in comparison to those receiving treatment without diuretics (18). In a follow-up study, the Group concluded that the use of such combination diuretic therapy in preterm infants is ineffective in decreasing the rate of shunt placement and is, in fact, associated with increased neurological morbidity (90). In a 2001 Cochrane Report, Whitelaw et al. (91) assessed the results from two controlled trials (18,92), but urged caution on interpretation because of statistical heterogeneity and concerns about the methodological quality of the smaller trial. Given these cautions, his conclusion was that acetazolamide and furosemide combination therapy is neither effective [no reduction in the risk for ventriculoperitoneal (VP) shunt] nor safe (risk for nephrocalcinosis and biochemical anomalies and borderline increased risk for motor developmental anomalies at one year) and cannot be recommended as treatment options.

Several studies have also evaluated the efficacy of intraventricular fibrinolytic therapies, such as streptokinase or tissue plasminogen activator (tPA) (93,94). In a 2001 Cochrane Report (95), Whitelaw examined the results from a small randomized trial of intraventricular fibrinolytic therapy (streptokinase) and found that the number of infants dying or requiring a VP shunt for hydrocephalus was identical in the two groups. He concluded that intraventricular fibrinolytic therapy with streptokinase, starting at a median postnatal age of 12 days in infants developing posthemorrhagic ventricular dilatation, cannot be recommended.

More recently, Whitelaw et al. (96) have piloted a radical new technique they term DRIFT (for drainage, irrigation, and fibrinolytic therapy), the objective of which is to remove as much blood and TGFβ1 as possible while normalizing ICP (see section pathogenesis and pathology of PHH). The procedure involves insertion of two ventricular catheter tubes through which human recombinant tPA and large volumes of artificial cerebrospinal fluid are injected. The combination of fibrinolytic therapy with irrigation and drainage of the fluid removes old blood and debris from the ventricles.

Between May 1998 and October 2002, 25 eligible infants with gestational age varying between 23 and 42 weeks and birth weight between 780 and 3770 g were involved in the DRIFT study. The age at which DRIFT was started varied from 5 to 28 days. Twenty-four infants (96%) survived, two (8%) developed CSF infections, and two developed secondary IVH. Six infants required VP shunt surgery (24%). Although these findings are based on relatively small numbers, it would appear that drainage and irrigation has the potential to reduce ongoing brain injury by normalizing pressure, reducing free radical injury from nonprotein-bound iron, and reducing inflammatory cytokines. Although the figures show a reduction in shunt dependence with trends toward reducing mortality and disability in favor of DRIFT, it is also clear that DRIFT failed to prevent shunt dependence in some cases. This may be because it is impossible to remove enough blood clot from the ventricular system or because the intervention was used too late to prevent TGFβ1-stimulated fibrosis.

Surgical Interventions

Subcutaneous Reservoir and Ventricular Catheter

Placement of a low-profile subcutaneous reservoir connected to an intraventricular catheter remains a viable option for treatment of PHH (25,84,97–102). This device may be indicated in those infants who are below the weight requirement for shunt placement (i.e., not yet 1500 g) or if there is still hope that the patient may recover spontaneously over time (84,101). The reservoir allows easy tapping of CSF as often as needed to normalize CSF pressure and arrest ventricular enlargement. Other advantages, as discussed by Hudgins (25), include ease of insertion and use; low rates of infection, occlusion, and wound complications; and the ability to instill medication into the ventricles. The design of the reservoir also makes it relatively easy to attach an outflow catheter to convert the system into a VP shunt (16). The major drawbacks to the system include problems with erosion of the thin infant skin overlying the reservoir (16) and the fact that ICP is only intermittently controlled (25).

External Ventricular Drainage

External ventricular drainage (EVD) is based on the idea that continuous drainage of CSF will produce a steadier and therefore more physiological ICP profile than intermittent large volume taps (99,103). However, problems of catheter dislodgement (47) and high infection rates (104) may negate any benefits of continuous drainage (16). Although the use of EVD is generally reserved for cases where there is bloody CSF with symptomatic raised ICP that cannot be lowered any other way, it has received favorable reports (105–109). There have been no controlled trials (9).

Serial Ventricular Taps

Multiple percutaneous ventricular taps are not considered an acceptable treatment for PHH (25). There are numerous complications and a high risk of encephalomalacia and porencephaly associated with these taps (25). Hence, most centers tend to avoid them whenever possible.

Third Ventriculostomy

This technique has met with only limited success in premature infants with IVH (110). For third ventriculostomy to be effective, CSF reabsorption pathways must be fully functional.

Ventriculoperitoneal Shunts

Most forms of hydrocephalus are classically treated by the surgical placement of a VP shunt that diverts accumulating CSF from the ventricles to the peritoneal cavity for resorption. However, the decision to shunt preterm infants with PHH must be carefully weighed owing to their relatively high risk for shunt blockage, infection, and skin ulceration (9). Because shunt placement is better tolerated in larger infants who are more physiologically stable (47), shunting is generally delayed until PHH is definitively diagnosed and other treatment options have been explored.

The typical shunt system, consisting of a ventricular catheter, distal tubing, and a one-way anti-siphon valve, is designed to direct CSF from the ventricles to a distal site, such as the peritoneal cavity. The valve controls the rate and directional flow of the fluid and may be classified based either on the pressures at which it inhibits CSF drainage (low, medium, or high) or on flow rate. Although a variety of shunt systems are available, clinical trials designed to assess their relative efficacy in treatment of PHH have yielded no conclusive data to suggest that any one shunt system is superior (111–115).

Despite their role in treatment of PHH in preterm infants, the use of VP shunts is associated with a number of complications that can contribute to the increased rate (20–50%) of shunt revisions in this group (87,103). For example, shunt mechanical malfunction can result in CSF overdrainage or underdrainage, with ventricular collapse and subdural hematoma developing in the former case and a recurrence of hydrocephalus in the latter (25).

Because preterm infants are often below the minimum weight requirement for shunt placement, their risk for recurrent shunt obstruction is increased due to the high viscosity of the CSF and the presence of residual intraventricular blood clots and debris. Shunt erosion, migration, or disconnection can also occur. Inflammatory gliosis secondary to clots in the foramen of Munro or aqueduct of Sylvius may result in the development of isolated ventricles (116) and increasing ICP.

The incidence of postoperative shunt infections, sepsis, and ventriculitis, correlating with poor neurological outcome, is elevated in this group, along with intra-abdominal complications, such as necrotizing enterocolitis (36,117,118). The rate of shunt infections increases with decreasing age, reaching as high as 30% among the most premature infants (119,120), largely due to the immature status of their immune systems.

Long-term or even permanent shunt dependency remains a controversial issue in surgical placement of a VP shunt, with studies showing that shunt placement can result in loss of borderline CSF absorptive capacity such that the patient becomes entirely shunt dependent (16).

In view of the many complications associated with shunting, the procedure should be avoided until all other therapeutic alternatives have been exhausted.

CONCLUSIONS

For preterm infants with PHH, neither medical nor surgical intervention effectively treats the disorder without, at the same time, posing numerous problems. As survival rates for low–birth-weight infants continue to increase, the need for alternative therapies becomes all the more urgent to ensure that these children are given the opportunity to develop to their maximum neurological potential. Clearly, more research is needed in both the prevention and cure of IVH and PHH.

Outcomes appear to be most closely related to the extent of the initial IVH—the severity and duration of elevated ICP with resultant compromise in cerebral perfusion pressure and compression of white matter and cerebral arteries—and not to the PHH per se (84,121,122). Indeed, logistic regression analysis has determined that grade of hemorrhage is the only significant predictor of cognitive and motor outcomes (123). Thus, future research directed at strategies for the prevention of severe IVH will have the greatest impact on prevention of PHH and the requirement for surgical intervention.

In terms of research, one area that may hold promise is the development of therapeutic strategies to remove, block, or prevent release of TGFβ1 and perhaps other cytokines. In addition, as technology advances, tools may become available that will help in better monitoring and managing IVH and subsequent PHH. For example, amplitude-integrated electroencephalogram (aEEG), which allows continuous neurophysiological surveillance, may prove quite useful in defining the optimal timing for intervention in infants with progressive PHH (124). Use of a small, commercially available ICP transducer (e.g., Codman Microsensor) that can directly measure ICP in infants undergoing ventricular reservoir drainage for treatment of PHH may allow the amount and frequency of CSF removal to be customized for each patient (125). Near-infrared spectroscopy, which can measure continuously and noninvasively changes in the cerebral concentration of oxygenated and deoxygenated hemoglobin and oxidized cytochrome oxidase, may also prove useful in detecting impending cerebral ischemia in infants at risk and thereby provide a means to guide the rational management of PHH (126).

REFERENCES

1. Cherian S, Whitelaw A, Thoresen M, et al. The pathogenesis of neonatal post-hemorrhagic hydrocephalus. Brain Pathol 2004; 14:305–311. [Review article].
2. Ghazi-Birry HS, Brown WR, Moody DM, et al. Human germinal matrix: venous origin of hemorrhage and vascular characteristics. Am J Neuroradiol 1997; 18:219–229.

3. Love S. Acute haemorrhagic and hypoxic-ischaemic brain damage in the neonate. Cur Diagn Pathol 2004; 10:106–115.

4. Nakamura Y, Okudera T, Fukuda S, et al. Germinal matrix hemorrhage of venous origin in preterm neonates. Hum Pathol 1990; 21:1059–1062.

5. Volpe JJ. Intraventricular hemorrhage in the premature infant—current concepts. Part I. Ann Neurol 1989; 25:3–11.

6. Papile LA, Burstein J, Burstein R, et al. Incidence and evolution of subependymal and intraventricular haemorrhage: a study of infants with birth weight less than 1500 gm. J Pediatr 1978; 92:529–534.

7. Szymonowicz W, Schafler K, Cussen LJ, et al. Ultrasound and necropsy study of periventricular hemorrhage in preterm infants. Arch Dis Child 1984; 59:637–642.

8. Volpe JJ. Neuronal proliferation, migration, organization and myelination. In: Volpe JJ, ed. Neurology of the Newborn, 4th ed. Philadelphia, PA: WB Saunders, 2001:45–99.

9. Whitelaw A. Intraventricular haemorrhage and posthaemorrhagic hydrocephalus: pathogenesis, prevention and future interventions. Semin Neonatol 2001; 6:135–146. [Review article].

10. Kamei A, Houdou S, Mito T, et al. Developmental change in type VI collagen in human cerebral vessels. Pediatr Neurol 1992; 8:183–186.

11. Tortorolo G, Luciano R, Papacci P, et al. Intraventricular hemorrhage: past, present and future, focusing on classification, pathogenesis and prevention. Childs Nerv Syst 1999; 15:652–661. [Review article].

12. Hambleton G, Wigglesworth JS. Origin of intraventricular haemorrhage in the preterm infant. Arch Dis Child 1976; 51:651–659.

13. Volpe JJ. Intracranial hemorrhage: germinal matrix-intraventricular hemorrhage of the premature infant. In: Volpe JJ, ed. Neurology of the Newborn, 4th ed. Philadelphia, PA: W.B. Saunders, 2001:428–493.

14. Ichord RN. Neurologic complications. In: Witter FR, Keith LG, eds. Textbook of Prematurity. Boston, MA: Little, Brown, and Co, 1993:305–320.

15. de Vries LS, Dubowitz LM, Dubowitz V, et al. Predictive value of cranial ultrasound in the newborn baby: A reappraisal. Lancet 1985; 326:137–140.

16. Duncan CC, Chiang VL. Intraventricular hemorrhage and posthemorrhagic hydrocephalus. In: Albright AL, Pollack IF, Adelson PD, eds. Principles and Practice of Pediatric Neurosurgery, New York: Thieme Medical Publishers, Inc., 1999:107–124.

17. Randomised trial of early tapping in neonatal posthaemorrhagic ventricular dilatation. Ventriculomegaly Trial Group. Arch Dis Child 1990; 65:3–10.

18. International randomised controlled trial of acetazolamide and furosemide in posthaemorrhagic ventricular dilatation in infancy. International PHVD Drug Trial Group. Lancet 1998; 352: 433–440.

19. Korobkin R. The relationship between head circumference and the development of communicating hydrocephalus in infants following intraventricular hemorrhage. Pediatrics 1975; 56:74–77.

20. Volpe JJ. Neonatal intracranial hemorrhage. Pathophysiology, neuropathology, and clinical features. Clin Perinatol 1977; 4:77–102.

21. Ment LR, Duncan CC, Scott DT, et al. Posthemorrhagic hydrocephalus. Low incidence in very low birth weight neonates with intraventricular hemorrhage. J Neurosurg 1984; 60:343–347.

22. Papile LA, Burstein J, Burstein R, et al. Post-hemorrhagic hydrocephalus in low-birth-weight infants: Treatment by serial lumbar punctures. J Pediatr 1980; 97:273–277.

23. Harbaugh RE, Saunders RL, Edwards WH. External ventricular drainage for control of posthemorrhagic hydrocephalus in premature infants. J Neurosurg 1981; 55:766–770.

24. Allan WC, Holt PJ, Sawyer LR, et al. Ventricular dilation after neonatal periventricular-intraventricular hemorrhage. Natural history and therapeutic implications. Am J Dis Child 1982; 136:589–593.

25. Hudgins RJ. Posthemorrhagic hydrocephalus of infancy. Neurosurg Clin N Am 2001; 12:743–751.

26. Murphy BP, Inder TE, Rooks V, et al. Posthaemorrhagic ventricular dilatation in the premature infant: natural history and predictors of outcome. Arch Dis Child Fetal Neonatal Ed 2002; 87:F37–F41.

27. Davis SL, Tooley WH, Hunt JV. Developmental outcome following posthemorrhagic hydrocephalus in preterm infants. Comparison of twins discordant for hydrocephalus. Am J Dis Child 1987; 141:1170–1174.

28. Pierrat V, Bevenot S, Truffert P, et al. Incidence, evolution and prognosis of posthemorrhagic ventriculomegaly in a population of newborns of less than 33 weeks gestational age. Arch Pediatr 1998; 5:974–981.

29. Punt J. Neurosurgical management of hydrocephalus. In: Levene MI, Lilford RJ, eds. Fetal and Neonatal Neurology and Neurosurgery. London, Edinburgh: Churchill Livingstone, 1995:661–666.

30. Guyer B, Hoyert DL, Martin JA, et al. Annual summary of vital statistics—1998. Pediatrics 1999; 104:1229–1246.
31. McIntire DD, Bloom SL, Casey DM, et al. Birth weight in relation to morbidity and mortality among newborn infants. N Engl J Med 1999; 340:1234–1238.
32. Philip AG, Allan WC, Tito AM, et al. Intraventricular hemorrhage in preterm infants: declining incidence in the 1980s. Pediatrics 1989; 84:797–801.
33. Vohr BR, Wright LL, Dusick AM, et al. Neurodevelopmental and functional outcomes of extremely low birth weight infants in the National Institute of Child Health and Human Development Neonatal Research Network. Pediatrics 2000; 105:1216–1226.
34. Sheth RD. Trends in incidence and severity of intraventricular hemorrhage. J Child Neurol 1998; 13:261–264.
35. Whitelaw A, Thoresen M, Pople I. Posthaemorrhagic ventricular dilatation. Arch Dis Child Fetal Neonatal Ed 2002; 86:F72–F74.
36. Roland EH, Hill A. Intraventricular hemorrhage and posthemorrhagic hydrocephalus. Current and potential future interventions. Clin Perinatol 1997; 24:589–605. [Review article].
37. Whitelaw A. We need a new understanding of the reabsorption of cerebrospinal fluid. Acta Paediatr 1997; 86:133–134.
38. Whitelaw A, Christie S, Pople I. Transforming growth factor β-1: a possible signal molecule for post-haemorrhagic hydrocephalus? Pediatr Res 1999; 46:576–580.
39. Galbreath E, Kim SJ, Park K, et al. Overexpression of TGF-beta 1 in the central nervous system of transgenic mice results in hydrocephalus. J Neuropathol Exp Neurol 1995; 54:339–349.
40. Heep A, Stoffel-Wagner B, Soditt V, et al. Procollagen I C-propeptide in the cerebrospinal fluid of neonates with posthaemorrhagic hydrocephalus. Arch Dis Child Fetal Neonatal Ed 2002; 86:F34–F36.
41. Kaiser A, Whitelaw A. Cerebrospinal fluid pressure during post-haemorrhagic ventricular dilatation in newborn infants. Arch Dis Child 1985; 60:920–924.
42. Savman K, Nilsson UA, Blennow M, et al. Non-protein-bound iron is elevated in cerebrospinal fluid from preterm infants with posthemorrhagic ventricular dilatation. Pediatr Res 2001; 49:208–212.
43. Bejar R, Saugstad OD, James H, et al. Increased hypoxanthine concentrations in cerebrospinal fluid of infants with hydrocephalus. J Pediatr 1983; 103:44–48.
44. Leviton A, Paneth N, Reuss ML, et al. Maternal infection, fetal inflammatory response, and brain damage in very low birth weight infants. Developmental Epidemiology Network Investigators. Pediatr Res 1999; 46:566–575.
45. Savman K, Blennow M, Hagberg H, et al. Cytokine response in cerebrospinal fluid from preterm infants with posthaemorrhagic ventricular dilatation. Acta Paediatr 2002; 91:1357–1363.
46. Guzzetta F, Mercuri E, Spano M. Mechanisms and evolution of the brain damage in neonatal post-hemorrhagic hydrocephalus. Childs Nerv Syst 1995; 11:293–296. [Review article].
47. Holt PJ. Posthemorrhagic hydrocephalus. J Child Neurol 1989; 4(suppl):S23–S31. [Review article].
48. Burstein J, Papile L, Burstein R. Subependymal germinal matrix and intraventricular hemorrhage in premature infants: Diagnosis by CT. AJR Am J Roentgenol 1977; 128:971–976.
49. Babcock DS, Han BK. Accuracy of high resolution real-time ultrasonography of the head in infants. Radiology 1981; 139:665–676.
50. Mack LA, Wright K, Hirsch JH, et al. Intracranial hemorrhage in premature infants: accuracy of sonographic evaluation. AJR Am J Roentgenol 1981; 137:245–250.
51. Johnson ML, Rumack CM, Mannes EJ, et al. Detection of neonatal intracranial hemorrhage utilizing real-time and static ultrasound. J Clin Ultrasound 1981; 9:427–433.
52. Sauerbrei EE, Digney M, Harrison PB, et al. Ultrasonic evaluation of neonatal intracranial hemorrhage and its complications. Radiology 1981; 139:677–685.
53. Davies MW, Swaminathan M, Chuang SL, et al. Reference ranges for the linear dimensions of the intracranial ventricles in preterm neonates. Arch Dis Child Fetal Neonatal Ed 2000; 82:F218–F223.
54. Anderson N, Allan R, Darlow B, et al. Diagnosis of intraventricular hemorrhage in the newborn. AJR Am J Roentgenol 1994; 163:893–896.
55. London DA, Carroll BA, Enzmann DR. Sonography of ventricular size and germinal matrix hemorrhage in premature infants. AJR Am J Roentgenol 1980; 135:559–564.
56. Rumack CM, McDonald MM, O'Meara OP, et al. CT detection and course of intracranial hemorrhage in premature infants. AJR Am J Roentgenol 1978; 131:493–497.
57. Levene MI. Measurement of the growth of the lateral ventricles in preterm infants with real-time ultrasound. Arch Dis Child 1981; 56:900–904.
58. Bandstra ES, Montalvo BM, Goldberg RN, et al. Prophylactic indomethacin for prevention of intraventricular hemorrhage in premature infants. Pediatrics 1988; 82:533–542.
59. Volpe JJ. Brain injury caused by intraventricular hemorrhage: Is indomethacin the silver bullet for prevention? Pediatrics 1994; 93:673–677.

60. Fowlie PW. Prophylactic indomethacin: systematic review and meta-analysis. Arch Dis Child Fetal Neonatal Ed 1996; 74:F81–F87.
61. Norton ME, Merrill J, Cooper BA, et al. Neonatal complications after the administration of indomethacin for preterm labor. N Engl J Med 1993; 329:1602–1607.
62. Pryds O, Greisen G, Johansen KH. Indomethacin and cerebral blood flow in premature infants treated for patent ductus arteriosus. Eur J Pediatr 1988; 147:315–316.
63. Pourcyrous M, Leffler CW, Bada HS, et al. Brain superoxide anion generation in asphyxiated piglets and the effect of indomethacin at therapeutic dose. Pediatr Res 1993; 34:366–369.
64. Ment LR, Stewart WB, Ardito TA, et al. Indomethacin promotes germinal matrix microvessel maturation in the newborn beagle pup. Stroke 1992; 23:1132–1137.
65. Fowlie PW. Intravenous indomethacin for preventing mortality and morbidity in very low birth weight infants. Cochrane Database Syst Rev 2000; 2:CD000174.
66. Ment LR, Vohr B, Allan W, et al. Outcome of children in the indomethacin intraventricular hemorrhage prevention trial. Pediatrics 2000; 105:485–491.
67. Schmidt B, Davis P, Moddemann D, et al. Long-term effects of indomethacin prophylaxis in extremely-low-birth-weight infants. N. Engl J Med 2001; 344(26):1966–1972.
68. Sinha S, Davies J, Toner N, et al. Vitamin E supplementation reduces frequency of periventricular haemorrhage in very preterm babies. Lancet 1987; 329:466–471.
69. Poland RL. Vitamin E for prevention of perinatal intracranial hemorrhage. Pediatrics 1990; 85:865–867.
70. Chiswick ML, Johnson M, Woodhall C, et al. Protective effect of vitamin E (DL alpha-tocopherol) against intraventricular haemorrhage in premature babies. Br Med J 1983; 287:81–84.
71. Fish WH, Cohen M, Franzek D, et al. Effect of intramuscular vitamin E in mortality and intracranial haemorrhage in neonates of 1000 grams or less. Pediatrics 1990; 85:578–584.
72. Morales WJ, Angel JL, O'Brien WF, et al. The use of antenatal vitamin K in the prevention of early neonatal intraventricular hemorrhage. Am J Obstet Gynecol 1988; 159:774–779.
73. Pomerance JJ, Teal JG, Gogolok JF, et al. Maternally administered antenatal vitamin K1: effect on neonatal prothrombin activity, partial thromboplastin time, and intraventricular hemorrhage. Obstet Gynecol 1987; 70:235–241.
74. Crowther CA, Henderson-Smart DJ. Vitamin K prior to preterm birth for preventing neonatal periventricular haemorrhage. Cochrane Database Syst Rev 2001; 1:CD000229.
75. Benson JW, Drayton MR, Hayward C, et al. Multicentre trial of ethamsylate for prevention of periventricular haemorrhage in very low birthweight infants. Lancet 1986; 328:1297–1300.
76. Morgan ME, Benson JW, Cooke RW. Ethamsylate reduces the incidence of periventricular haemorrhage in very low birth-weight babies. Lancet 1981; 318:830–831.
77. Chen JY. Ethamsylate in the prevention of periventricular-intraventricular hemorrhage in premature infants. J Formos Med Assoc 1993; 92:889–893.
78. The EC randomised controlled trial of prophylactic ethamsylate in very preterm neonates: early mortality and morbidity. EC Ethamsylate Trial Group. Arch Dis Child Fetal Neonatal Ed 1994; 70:F201–F205.
79. Shankaran S, Papile LA, Wright LL, et al. The effect of antenatal phenobarbital therapy on neonatal intracranial hemorrhage in preterm infants. N Engl J Med 1997; 337:466–471.
80. Crowther CA, Henderson-Smart DJ. Phenobarbital prior to preterm birth for preventing neonatal periventricular haemorrhage. Cochrane Database Syst Rev 2003; 3:CD000166.
81. Kuban KC, Leviton A, Krishnamoorthy KS, et al. Neonatal intracranial hemorrhage and phenobarbital. Pediatrics 1986; 77:443–450.
82. Whitelaw A. Postnatal phenobarbitone for prevention of intraventricular haemorrhage in preterm infants. Cochrane Database Syst Rev 2005; 2:CD0001691.
83. Cools F, Offringa M. Neuromuscular paralysis for newborn infants receiving mechanical ventilation. Cochrane Database Syst Rev 2005; 2:CD0002773.
84. Hansen AR, Snyder EY. Medical management of neonatal posthemorrhagic hydrocephalus. Neurosurg Clin N Am 1998; 9:95–104. [Review article].
85. Perlman JM, Rollins N. Surveillance protocol for the detection of intracranial abnormalities in premature neonates. Arch Pediatr Adolesc Med 2000; 154:822–826.
86. Vannucci RC. Disorders in head size and shape. In: Fanaroff AA, Martin RJ, eds. Neonatal–Perinatal Medicine: Diseases of the Fetus and Infant, Vol. 2, 7th ed. St Louis, MO: Mosby-Year Book, 2001:924–931.
87. Dykes FD, Dunbar B, Lazarra A, et al. Posthemorrhagic hydrocephalus in high-risk preterm infants: natural history, management, and long-term outcome. J Pediatr 1989; 114:611–618.
88. Roland EH, Hill A. Germinal matrix-intraventricular hemorrhage in the premature newborn: management and outcome. Neurol Clin 2003; 21:833–851, vi–vii. [Review article].

89. Whitelaw A. Repeated lumbar or ventricular punctures in newborns with intraventricular hemorrhage. Cochrane Database Syst Rev 2001; Issue 1. Art. No.: CD000216. Review. DOI:10.1002/14651858.CD000216.

90. Kennedy CR, Ayers S, Campbell MJ, et al. Randomized, controlled trial of acetazolamide and furosemide in posthemorrhagic ventricular dilation in infancy: follow-up at 1 year. Pediatrics 2001; 108:597–607.

91. Whitelaw A, Kennedy CR, Brion LP. Diuretic therapy for newborn infants with posthemorrhagic ventricular dilatation. Cochrane Database Syst Rev 2001; Issue 2. Art. No.: CD002270. Review. DOI:10.1002/14651858.CD002270.

92. Libenson MH, Kaye EM, Rosman NP, et al. Acetazolamide and furosemide for posthemorrhagic hydrocephalus of the newborn. Pediatr Neurol 1999; 20:185–191.

93. Whitelaw A, Rivers RP, Creighton L, et al. Low dose intraventricular fibrinolytic treatment to prevent posthaemorrhagic hydrocephalus. Arch Dis Child 1992; 67:12–14.

94. Whitelaw A, Saliba E, Fellman V, et al. Phase I study of intraventricular recombinant tissue plasminogen activator for treatment of posthaemorrhagic hydrocephalus. Arch Dis Child Fetal Neonatal Ed 1996; 75:F20–F26.

95. Whitelaw A. Intraventricular streptokinase after intraventricular hemorrhage in newborn infants. Cochrane Database Syst Rev 2001; Issue 1. Art. No.: CD000498. Review. DOI:10.1002/14651858.CD000498.

96. Whitelaw A, Cherian S, Thoresen M, et al. Posthaemorrhagic ventricular dilatation: new mechanisms and new treatment. Acta Paediatr Suppl 2004; 93:11–14.

97. Brockmeyer DL, Wright LC, Walker ML, et al. Management of posthemorrhagic hydrocephalus in the low-birth-weight preterm neonate. Pediatr Neurosci 1989; 15:302–307, discussion 308.

98. Hudgins RJ, Boydston WR, Gilreath CL. Treatment of posthemorrhagic hydrocephalus in the preterm infant with a ventricular access device. Pediatr Neurosurg 1998; 29:309–313.

99. Marlin AE. Protection of the cortical mantle in premature infants with post-hemorrhagic hydrocephalus. Neurosurgery 1980; 7:464–468.

100. McComb JG, Ramos AD, Platzker AC, et al. Management of hydrocephalus secondary to intraventricular hemorrhage in the preterm infant with a subcutaneous ventricular catheter reservoir. Neurosurgery 1983; 13:295–300.

101. Frim DM, Scott RM, Madsen JR. Surgical management of neonatal hydrocephalus. Neurosurg Clin N Am 1998; 9:105–110. [Review article].

102. de Vries LS, Liem KD, et al.; Dutch Working Group of Neonatal Neurology. Early versus late treatment of posthaemorrhagic ventricular dilatation: results of a retrospective study from five neonatal intensive care units in the Netherlands. Acta Paediatr 2002; 91:212–217.

103. Gurtner P, Bass T, Gudeman SK, et al. Surgical management of posthemorrhagic hydrocephalus in 22 low-birth-weight infants. Childs Nerv Syst 1992; 8:198–202.

104. Mayhall CG, Archer NH, Lamb VA, et al. Ventriculostomy-related infections. A prospective epidemiologic study. N Engl J Med 1984; 310:553–559.

105. Reinprecht A, Dietrich W, Berger A, et al. Posthemorrhagic hydrocephalus in preterm infants: long-term follow-up and shunt-related complications. Childs Nerv Syst 2001; 17:663–669 [Epub October 19, 2001].

106. Berger A, Weninger M, Reinprecht A, et al. Long-term experience with subcutaneously tunneled external ventricular drainage in preterm infants. Childs Nerv Syst 2000; 16:103–109, discussion 110.

107. Weninger M, Salzer HR, Pollak A, et al. External ventricular drainage for treatment of rapidly progressive posthemorrhagic hydrocephalus. Neurosurgery 1992; 31:52–57, discussion 57–58.

108. Allan WC, Sobel DB. Neonatal intensive care neurology. Semin Pediatr Neurol 2004; 11: 119–128.

109. Cornips E, Van Calenbergh F, Plets C, et al. Use of external drainage for posthemorrhagic hydrocephalus in very low birth weight premature infants. Childs Nerv Syst 1997; 13:369–374.

110. Drake JM. Ventriculostomy for treatment of hydrocephalus. Neurosurg Clin N Am 1993; 4:657–666. [Review article].

111. Tuli S, O'Hayon B, Drake JM, et al. Change in ventricular size and effect of ventricular catheter placement in pediatric patients with shunted hydrocephalus. Neurosurgery 1999; 45:1329–1333, discussion 1333–1335.

112. Drake JM, Kestle JR, Milner R, et al. Randomized trial of cerebrospinal fluid shunt valve design in pediatric hydrocephalus. Neurosurgery 1998; 43:294–303.

113. Robinson S, Kaufman BA, Park TS. Outcome analysis of initial neonatal shunts: Does the valve make a difference? Pediatr Neurosurg 2002; 37:287–294.

114. Kestle J, Drake J, Milner R, et al. Long-term follow-up data from the Shunt Design Trial. Pediatr Neurosurg 2000; 33:230–236.

115. Davis SE, Levy ML, McComb JG, et al. The delta valve: How does its clinical performance compare with two other pressure differential valves without antisiphon control? Pediatr Neurosurg 2000; 33:58–63.

116. Eller TW, Pasternak JF. Isolated ventricles following intraventricular hemorrhage. J Neurosurg 1985; 62:357–362.

117. Blount JP, Campbell JA, Haines SJ. Complications in ventricular cerebrospinal fluid shunting. Neurosurg Clin N Am 1993; 4:633–656. [Review article].

118. Hislop JE, Dubowitz LM, Kaiser AM, et al. Outcome of infants shunted for post-haemorrhagic ventricular dilatation. Dev Med Child Neurol 1988; 30:451–456.

119. Ammirati M, Raimondi AJ. Cerebrospinal fluid shunt infections in children. A study on the relationship between the etiology of hydrocephalus, age at the time of shunt placement, and infection rate. Childs Nerv Syst 1987; 3:106–109.

120. Quigley MR, Reigel DH, Kortyna R. Cerebrospinal fluid shunt infections. Report of 41 cases and a critical review of the literature. Pediatr Neurosci 1989; 15:111–120. [Review article].

121. Resch B, Gedermann A, Maurer U, et al. Neurodevelopmental outcome of hydrocephalus following intra-/periventricular hemorrhage in preterm infants: short- and long-term results. Childs Nerv Syst 1996; 12:27–33. [Review article].

122. Ment LR, Vohr B, Allan W, et al. The etiology and outcome of cerebral ventriculomegaly at term in very low birth weight preterm infants. Pediatrics 1999; 104:243–248.

123. Levy ML, Masri LS, McComb JG. Outcome for preterm infants with germinal matrix hemorrhage and progressive hydrocephalus. Neurosurgery 1997; 41:1111–1117, discussion 1117–1118.

124. Olischar M, Klebermass K, Kuhle S, et al. Progressive posthemorrhagic hydrocephalus leads to changes of amplitude-integrated EEG activity in preterm infants. Childs Nerv Syst 2004; 20:41–45.

125. Bass JK, Bass WT, Green GA, et al. Intracranial pressure changes during intermittent CSF drainage. Pediatr Neurol 2003; 28:173–177.

126. Soul JS, Eichenwald E, Walter G, et al. CSF removal in infantile posthemorrhagic hydrocephalus results in significant improvement in cerebral hemodynamics. Pediatr Res 2004; 55:872–876 [Epub January 22, 2004].

8 | Aqueductal Stenosis

Giuseppe Cinalli, Pietro Spennato, Ferdinando Aliberti, and Emilio Cianciulli

Department of Pediatric Neurosurgery, Santobono Children's Hospital, Naples, Italy

INTRODUCTION

The cerebral aqueduct had been recognized as early as Galen's time (AD 130–200); however the eponym "Aqueduct of Sylvius" dates back to the Middle Age. Two medieval anatomists referred to themselves with the name "Sylvius," that is the Latinized version of their surname "de la Boe," equivalent to "Dubois" in French and "Woods" in English (1). The eponym of the aqueduct probably refers to the younger Sylvius: the French physician Jacobus Sylvius (1478–1555), alias Jacques Dubois (2). About one century later, the older Sylvius, Franciscus Sylvius (1614–1672), alias Francois de la Boe, described the "sylvian fissure" and the "sylvian artery."

The sylvian aqueduct is a narrow channel, about 15 mm long, that connects the third and the fourth ventricle. Because of its length and narrowness, it is considered as the most common site of intraventricular blockage of the cerebrospinal fluid (CSF).

Aqueductal stenosis is responsible of 6% to 66% of cases of hydrocephalus in children (more than 50% presenting in the first year of life) and 5% to 49% in adults (3–5). Tisell and coworkers (6) reported an incidence of aqueductal stenosis of 3.7/million/yr in adult Sweden population; Ceddia and coworkers (7) reported an incidence of congenital hydrocephalus of 0.3 to 2.5 per thousand born alive, 20% associated to aqueductal stenosis. There is a mild male prevalence, and there are two peaks of distribution for age: one in the first year of life and the second in the adolescence (3).

NORMAL AQUEDUCT

During embryological life, following closure of the neural tube, the aqueduct is as large as other portions of neural tube. Its adult configuration results from the gradual narrowing that occurs during fetal development due to thickening of surrounding nuclear masses and fiber tracts of the mesencephalon (4,8).

The aqueduct forms a gentle curve with concavity towards the base of the skull. It is situated in the dorsal midbrain, surrounded by the periaqueductal gray matter. The posterior commissure and the superior and inferior colliculi are located behind; oculomotor and trochlear nerves nuclei, medial longitudinal fasciculus, and red nuclei are located in front. The cross section of the aqueduct is highly variable, probably resulting from the influence of different nuclear masses or fiber tracts surrounding it at different levels: it is triangular with the apex directed ventrally at the cranial orifice, under the posterior commissure; it is rounded or oval in the central dilated area under the superior colliculi (ampullae) and assumes the shape of an inverted "U" at the level of the inferior colliculi (4). Two constrictions are regularly present: at the level of superior colliculi and at the level of intercollicular sulcus. The lumen varies considerably—the narrowest part usually being at the level of the superior constriction. Emery and Staschak (9) reported a mean value of 0.5 mm^2 of cross-sectional area in children, and Woollam and Millen (10) reported a mean value of 0.8 mm^2 (range 0.2–1.8 mm^2) in normal adult. A cross-sectional area as narrow as 0.1 mm^2 has been reported in association with normal size ventricles (4,9,11). The internal lumen of the aqueduct is lined by a layer of ependymal cells. This lining often presents variations: it can be absent for some distances (denuded areas) or thicker than one cell layer; it can form small diverticula. In areas lacking in ependyma, glia can overgrow. If this proliferation is excessive, glia can protrude into the lumen and even bridge the canal. At variable short distances from the wall of the main aqueduct, small accessory aqueductules or clusters of ependymal cells can be found (12). The subependymal glial plate also presents numerous variations in position and cell density: it may be situated in only one part or it may surround the entire aqueduct. In some cases it is absent, and the ependymal wall is bordered by the continuance of the brain stem glia (12).

   The CSF, produced mainly in the lateral and third ventricle, flows along the aqueduct to reach the fourth ventricle. Passage of the CSF through the narrow aqueduct is fast [about 10 cm/sec as measured with dynamic MRI techniques (13)] and has a pulsatile nature, with a systolic and diastolic to-and-fro displacement. This pulsatile nature has been well studied by dynamic MRI techniques, which permit to observe a craniocaudal CSF displacement occurring in the aqueduct, basal cisterns, and cervical subarachnoid space during systole (14,15). In fact, during systole an increased amount of blood volume reach the cranial cavity; thereafter the same volume of CSF and venous blood leaves the cranial cavity. This seems to be because of the distensibility of lumbar sac, which acts as a buffer of the changes of intracranial volume, and emptying of veins in spinal and cranial cavities. During diastole the decrease in brain blood volume and recoil of CSF displaced in the lumbar sac reverse the CSF displacement. The net outward movement is equivalent to CSF production (0.0067 mL/sec). The modification of the pulsation nature of the flow through the aqueduct has not been yet proven to have any diagnostic significance in any of the diseases producing abnormal patterns of CSF circulation (16). The presence of a net outward flow of CSF implies that there is a net outward pressure driving it. The pressure drop in the aqueduct is too small to be measured by clinically used pressure transducers. Jacobson et al. developed a computer modeling of the flow dynamics in normal (17) and stenotic (18) aqueducts. Comparing the flow through the aqueduct with flow through a cylinder of comparable dimensions, with inlet area of 1.56 mm^2, they observed that flow increased linearly with pressure at inlet (laminar flow) and calculated that 1 Pa (0.0075 mm Hg) of steady pressure caused a volume flow rate of CSF of 0.0060 mL/sec. Therefore, the pressure drop required to move 0.0067 mL/sec is 1.1 Pa and that required moving the CSF produced above the aqueduct [assuming that this is half of the total (17)] is 0.55 Pa. Comparing these data with the transmantle pressure of 27 Pa (from lateral ventricles to the subarachnoid space) measured by Conner et al. (19), it is evident that the pressure drop across the aqueduct is small, less than 5% of the total. Even applying an unsteady pressure producing a pulsatile flow similar to the physiological CSF pulse, CSF remained laminar at all times and flow continued to follow the wall even when the direction of flow reversed, without recirculation of fluid. Jacobson et al. (17) also discovered that the shape of the aqueduct is important in minimizing the pressure drop for a given flow rate. In fact, it seems to guide a core of fluid centrally away from the wall effect that could slow it down.

PATHOLOGICAL AQUEDUCT

Sylvian aqueduct may become stenotic as a consequence of compression from mass lesions (particularly tectal tumor and vascular malformations) or because of intrinsic pathology (the so-called "nontumoral aqueductal stenosis"). Intrinsic aqueductal stenosis may be congenital or acquired. Even if some morphological appearances of the aqueduct may be suggestive of the nature of the stenosis (acquired or congenital), a complete correlation between pathological findings, age of clinical onset, and etiology has never been demonstrated. The aspect of the aqueduct in cases of aqueductal stenosis is highly variable. Complete obstruction of the aqueduct is referred to as atresia, incomplete obstruction as stenosis. Russell (11) in her histopathological classification in 1949 subdivided nontumoral aqueduct anomalies into four types:

1. *Stenosis*: The aqueduct is narrowed or obliterated and normal ependyma lines the lumen. No gliosis of the surrounding tissue is evident. In more simple cases, an abnormally small aqueduct with normal cells is present. In cases of "congenital atresia" (Fig. 1), the aqueduct may not be discernible on gross inspection. Microscopic examination usually reveals clusters of ependymal nests and channels or aqueductules scattered throughout the midbrain. Real congenital atresia is rare, and it is more probably caused by "developmental" errors in which abnormal infolding of the neural plate results in narrowing of the neural tube with cleaning of the lumen and creating small ependymal rests (4).
2. *Forking*: The aqueduct is split into two or more separate irregular channels (Fig. 2). They can communicate each other, enter the ventricle independently or end blindly. Although a "simple" forking, that is, a smaller channel ventral to the normal aqueduct, can be found also in nonhydrocephalic subjects, this condition usually reduces aqueductal lumen. It results from incomplete fusion of the median fissure.

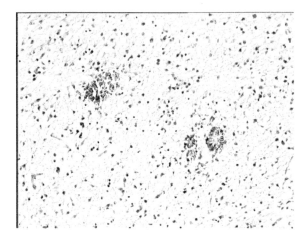

Figure 1 Congenital atresia of aqueduct: instead of lumen there are only minute nests of ependyma.

3. *Septum formation*: The aqueduct is totally or partially obstructed by a thin, translucent membrane. This is usually located at the distal end of the aqueduct and is composed of loose textured fibrillary neuroglia. Small ependymal canaliculi or scattered clumps of ependymal cells can be found on the septum or in the brain adjacent to its attachment. These small openings may provide an incomplete flow of CSF and explain the often very slow onset of symptoms (20). According to Turnbull and Drake (20), septum formation results from the same process that produces other forms of aqueductal stenosis: when the glial overgrowth is restricted to the lower end of the aqueduct, it gradually becomes a tiny sheet from prolonged pressure and dilatation of the canal above. Membranous occlusion, if present at the distal end of the aqueduct, is easily recognized on pre-op MRI because of the funnel dilatation of the proximal part of the aqueduct that is usually well visible, especially in T2 sequences [Fig. 3(A) and 3(B)]. On the contrary, if the membrane is at the very proximal end of the aqueduct, then the deformation of the mesencephalon caused by the long-standing ventricular dilatation can mimic a long-segment aqueductal stenosis, and the membrane can be well visible on the post-ETV studies, after resolution of anatomical deformation [Fig. 4(A) and 4(B)].
4. *Gliosis*: Gliotic stenosis is characterized by proliferation of glial cells and overproduction of glial fibers that are arranged in tangled fasciculi or large bands (12). Gliosis fills completely the area of preexisting aqueduct or leaves a narrow lumen or several little channels that are not outlined by ependyma (Fig. 5). This kind of stenosis may be an expression of developmental disorder due to its association with other developmental alterations, but it can be more often considered an acquired condition. Glial proliferation is a reaction to irritant agents, whether toxic, inflammatory, or traumatic. Gliotic stenosis may be present in

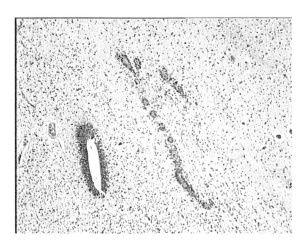

Figure 2 Forking of the aqueduct with two relatively small channels lined by ependymal cells and no surrounding gliosis.

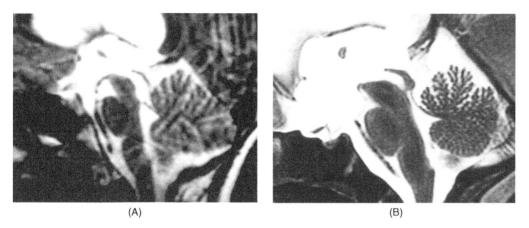

(A)   (B)

Figure 3 (**A** and **B**) Membranous occlusion of the distal end of the aqueduct. Note the dilatation of the proximal part of the aqueduct.

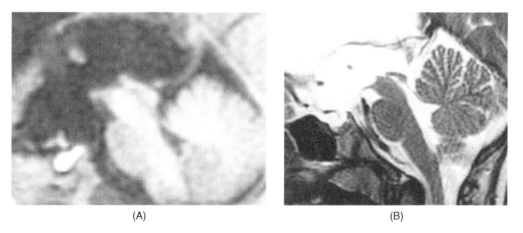

(A)   (B)

Figure 4 Membranous occlusion of the proximal end of the aqueduct (**A**): the tectum is flattened and pushed above the midbrain, and the aqueduct is scarcely visible. After ETV (**B**), with resolution of the pressure gradient, the aqueduct is visible as well as the occluding proximal membrane.

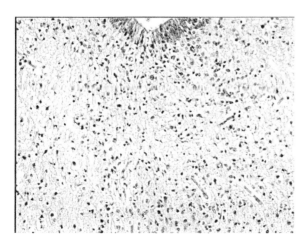

Figure 5 Gliosis surrounding stenotic aqueduct (em.eos. 225×).

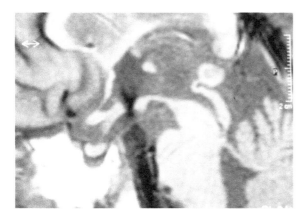

Figure 6 Short segment aqueductal stenosis. The aqueduct is well visible except the tiny segment of stenosis (<5 mm).

only one part of the aqueduct, determining a short-segment stenosis (<5 mm; Fig. 6) or be part of a widespread ependymitis of the ventricles and be extended to a longer part of the aqueduct, therefore determining a long-segment stenosis (>5 mm; Fig. 7). Obstruction of the aqueduct by reactive gliosis has to be distinguished from subependymal astrocytomas, which cause progressive aqueductal stenosis in children and adult (4).

Aqueductal stenosis should not be considered a stable condition. Often, also in the forms of unknown origin (considered secondary to developmental errors), it may be well tolerated for years, but give complications later. Many hypotheses have been advanced to explain this phenomenon. Lapras and coworkers (21) suggested that occlusion can be worsened by head trauma, subarachnoid hemorrhage, or viral infection during life. They also suggested that partial stenosis could be completed by functional mechanisms (21): accumulation of fluid in the supratentorial ventricular system may cause distortion of the brain stem and kinking of the aqueduct, worsening the stenosis in a vicious circle.

Oi et al. (22), studying a group of 20 patients with onset of symptoms in adulthood despite the signs of congenital aqueductal stenosis (such as macrocrania and radiological findings of chronic intracranial hypertension), hypothesized that CSF dynamics could change over time under disturbed conditions: an arrested hydrocephalus could change to progressive hydrocephalus and vice versa. This is possible because of the high compensatory capacity of the brain and skull during neonatal and infantile periods, when progression of the hydrocephalic state can be compensated, due to the activation of some of the three mechanisms described by Johnston et al (23): (*i*) reestablishment of the normal CSF circulation, (*ii*) utilization of an alternative CSF pathway, and (*iii*) changes in CSF production. Oi et al. (22) suggested that further impairment of one of these compensatory mechanisms may revert an arrested hydrocephalus into a progressive hydrocephalus in cases of late onset hydrocephalic state.

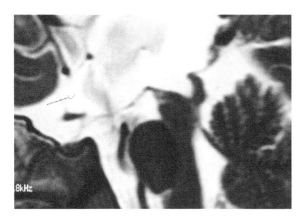

Figure 7 Long-segment aqueductal stenosis. The lower half of the aqueduct is not visible; tectum and tegmentum appear fused together on a long tract (>5 mm).

ETIOLOGY

In about three quarters of patients with aqueductal stenosis, the etiology of the disorder is not known (4). In remaining cases, it can be attributed to different causes.

Genetic Factors

In 1949, Bickers and Adams (24) and in 1961 Edwards (25) described an X-linked syndrome characterized by congenital hydrocephalus, stenosis of the aqueduct, adducted thumbs, and spastic paraparesis. This syndrome has been called "Bickers–Adams–Edwards syndrome" or "X-linked hydrocephalus." It is considered the most common genetic forms of congenital hydrocephalus and occurs in about 1:30,000 births (26). Transmission of the disease is from mother to sons. It has been estimated that 25% of males with aqueductal stenosis have X-linked hydrocephalus (26). Pathological findings in X-linked hydrocephalus are similar to those that occur in sporadic aqueductal stenosis, thus the stenosis was thought to be the primary cause of hydrocephalus. Subsequent observations (27) suggested that the reduction of the aqueduct caliber should be secondary to chronic compression from the lateral and third ventricles. The patency of aqueduct was also demonstrated in some cases by MR images (28). Linkage analysis studies (29) established that a point mutation of the gene for neural cells adhesion molecule L1 may be responsible of X-linked hydrocephalus. L1-CAM, mainly expressed on neurons and Schwann cells, is involved in the mediation of axon and neurite growth, which are necessary for the development of the nervous system. The poor neurological outcome of X-linked hydrocephalus reported in many series (29,30), despite early surgical intervention and good control of hydrocephalus, and the frequent association to other malformations, such as aplasia of the corpus callosum and of the pyramids in the medulla, are expression of cortical malformation and poor differentiation and maturation of cortical neurons (25,26,). Different mutations in the L1-CAM gene at the same locus Xq28 may lead to different clinical manifestations, not always associated with aqueductal stenosis, such as agenesis of the corpus callosum, spastic paraplegia, and MASA syndrome (mental retardation, aphasia, shuffling gait, and adducted thumbs). Prenatal diagnosis is possible: the main ultrasound marker is hydrocephalus, but it does not become apparent until 18 to 20 weeks' gestation. The presence of adducted thumbs in ultrasound examination in the first trimester of pregnancy may be a useful marker for X-linked hydrocephalus, in particular in a male fetus with a family history of X-linked disorders (31). The diagnosis is confirmed by molecular identification of the mutation in the L1-CAM gene by chorionic villus sampling and detection of asymptomatic female carriers.

Hydrocephalus has also been reported to occur as an autosomal recessive trait that affects both sexes and may or may not be associated to aqueductal stenosis (32). The clasped thumbs, characteristic of X-linked hydrocephalus, is not generally observed in this form of hydrocephalus. In fact, adduction–flexion deformity of the thumb in the X-linked hydrocephalus is caused by localized atrophy or agenesis of the abductor and anterior muscles of the thumbs (27), not to spastic flexion of the thumbs that may occur in other forms of hydrocephalus. Electrophysiological findings may help to distinguish these entities. Also, in autosomal recessive hydrocephalus, the role of aqueductal stenosis in inducting hydrocephalus is controversial (32). In both X-linked and autosomal recessive hydrocephalus, the age of onset may vary from child to child even in the same family.

Nontumoral aqueductal stenosis may also be part to some inherited syndromes, such as neurofibromatosis (33; Fig. 8).

Infection

Bacterial meningitis, both intrauterine and infantile, is the most common cause of acquired gliotic obstruction of the aqueduct: the lumen can be filled during the acute or subacute phase by a fibrinopurulent exudate that successively organizes. The stenosis can also develop gradually from proliferation and fusion of glial nodules in diffuse ependymitis (4; Fig. 9). Prenatal infection caused by the protozoan *Toxoplasma gondii* can be typically associated with aqueductal stenosis (Fig. 10), severe hydrocephalus with periventricular calcifications (Fig. 11), microphthalmia (Fig. 12), and other systemic involvements.

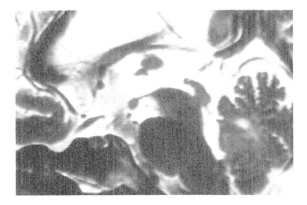

Figure 8 Aqueductal stenosis in a case of neurofibromatosis type I.

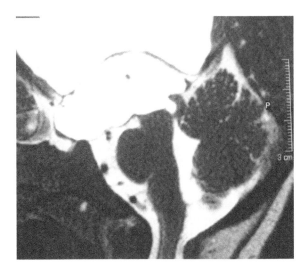

Figure 9 Tiny stenosis with midbrain flattening in an 8-month-old baby who suffered a neonatal bacterial meningitis. The patient was successfully treated by endoscopic third ventriculostomy.

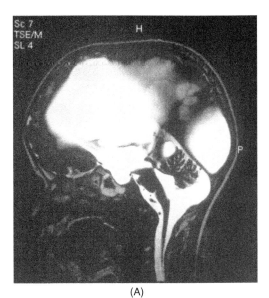
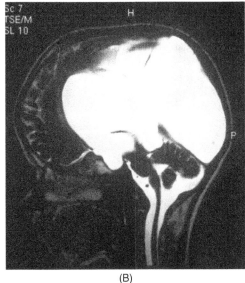

(A)   (B)

Figure 10 Severe hydrocephalus following prenatal toxoplasmosis infection. Note the aqueductal stenosis (**A**) and the pulsion diverticulum (**B**).

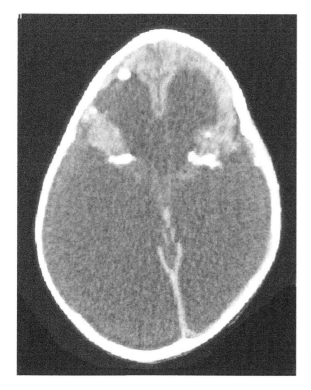

Figure 11 Same case as in Figure 10. Note periventricular calcification.

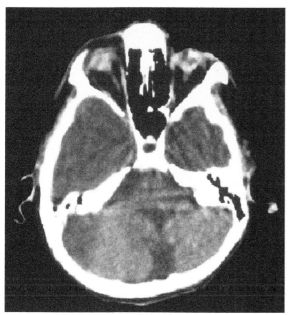

Figure 12 Same case as in Figure 10. Note the microphthalmia.

Aqueductal stenosis may occur as a noninflammatory sequela of a preceding viral infection of ependyma. This phenomenon was first demonstrated for mumps virus (34,35) (Fig. 13); thereafter aqueductal stenosis was observed following cytomegalovirus (CMV), lymphocytic choriomeningitis, influenza A, and parainfluenza II infections (4,36). The pathological findings in virus-induced aqueductal stenosis are usually similar to the "simple stenosis" (without gliosis) described by Russell (11); moreover the viral ependymal infection may be clinically inapparent. Thus, some authors (37) hypothesize a pathogenetic role of viral infection (in

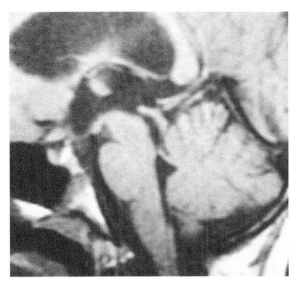

Figure 13 Membranous occlusion of the distal end of the aqueduct diagnosed 9 years after mumps meningoencephalitis.

particular mumps infection) in induction the forms of "unknown etiology" of aqueductal stenosis. Viruses may cause granular ependymitis and ependymal cell loss resulting in desquamation of the ependyma and subsequent aqueduct occlusion (38). Wolinsky et al. (39) suggested an alternative pathogenetic mechanism: viral absorption on the outer surface of the ependymal cell plasmalemma and viral penetration into the cell to determine fusion of the cilia of adjacent cells, thus creating a cross-linking between ependymal cells by viral particles bridges. At the level of the aqueduct, this process is favored by the high concentration of particles that occur in the aqueduct that is continually bathed by CSF into which virions are released.

Hemorrhage
Aqueductal stenosis can be secondary to organization of clots following intraventricular hemorrhage at any age (40; Fig. 14).

Intoxications and Deficiencies
In experimental models, many substances, such as trypan blue, salicylate and cuprizone, administered to the mother in early gestation, were able to induce aqueductal stenosis (4). Similar

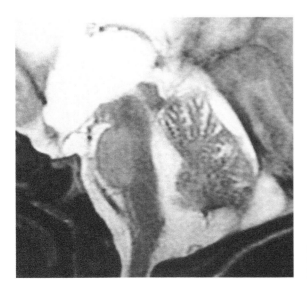

Figure 14 Extensive web occluding the aqueduct and the basal cisterns in a 2-month-old baby affected by neonatal intraventricular hemorrhage.

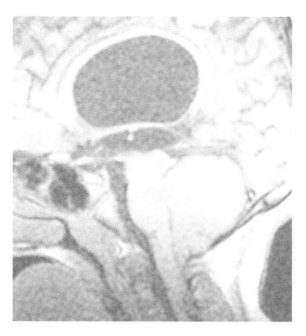

Figure 15 Aqueductal stenosis in a patient affected by Arnold–Chiari malformation and myelomeningocele.

lesions were induced in rabbits by vitamin A deficiency and in rats born from mothers fed with a diet deficient in vitamin B or folic acid (4).

CNS Malformations

Aqueductal stenosis has been reported in association with different CNS malformations, such as Arnold–Chiari in myelomeningoceles (Fig. 15), Dandy–Walker, and retrocerebellar and supracollicular cysts (Fig. 16) (4,41,42). The pathogenesis of the stenosis appears as a result of long-standing hydrocephalus that determines axial herniation and entrapment of the midbrain and secondary compression of the ependymal surfaces of the aqueduct, leading to aqueductal obstruction. In cases of "brain stem cerebellum deformity" or other lesions affecting posterior cranial fossa, the aqueductal stenosis may be related to the transtentorial upward displacement of the cerebellum with compression of the quadrigeminal plate and secondary modifications of the aqueductal ependyma (42). In particular, aqueductal stenosis is found often in case of

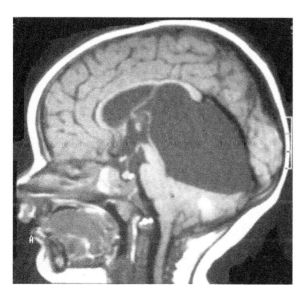

Figure 16 Aqueductal stenosis in a patient affected by a cyst of the quadrigeminal cistern.

Dandy–Walker malformation and its variants (42). It may be secondary to herniation of vermis or cyst through the tentorial hiatus. Upward herniation of contents of the posterior fossa, with subsequent aqueductal obstruction, may follow shunting of the supratentorial ventricular system, or may be secondary to failure of the shunt from the cyst.

Functional Stenosis

Raimondi et al. (43) first observed, in cases of Dandy–Walker cysts, that when there is an increased pressure under the tentorium, the upper vermis may rotate further anteriorly, acting as a valve for the fluid attempted to escape from the fourth ventricle. They called this condition "functional aqueductal stenosis."

Thereafter many authors suggested that a functional mechanism might contribute to the progression of hydrocephalus in patients with initially communicating hydrocephalus: progressive enlargement of the lateral and third ventricles would lead to a distortion of the brainstem and kinking of the aqueduct (44,45).

Aqueductal obstruction may complicate the course of postmeningitic or posthemorrhagic hydrocephalus, leading to isolation of the fourth ventricle (46,47). Pathogenesis is controversial; some cases, according to Oi and Matsumoto (46), are related to overfunctioning supratentorial shunt drainage that determine a pressure gradient between the supratentorial and infratentorial compartments with shifting of the superior cerebellar structures upward and functional occlusion of the aqueduct. Raimondi et al. (43) observed that decreasing the pressure gradient results in reopening of the aqueduct. However, isolated fourth ventricle is not always a reversible condition, but often it may be caused by irreversible changes subsequent to meningitis, hemorrhage, and posterior fossa operation (47).

Acquired Aqueductal Stenosis Following Shunt Malfunction

An acquired aqueductal stenosis may develop following shunting of originally communicating hydrocephalus, explaining the high success rate of surgical procedures of internal diversion of CSF (endoscopic third ventriculostomy, see later in the text) in cases of shunt malfunction (48). These patients generally present initially with communicating hydrocephalus caused by blockage of the subarachnoid spaces and arachnoid granulations with infective/hemorrhagic debris [Fig. 17(A)]. Placement of a VP shunt diverts CSF to the abdominal cavity, allowing the CSF spaces to reexpand. The procedure may also induce an acquired aqueductal stenosis through continuous CSF diversion [Fig. 17(B) and 17(C)], which together with reexpansion of the subarachnoid spaces makes the likelihood of a third ventriculostomy being successfully greater at a later date when a shunt malfunction occurs [Fig. 17(D)].

Tumoral Aqueductal Stenosis

Obstruction of the aqueduct has to be distinguished from small subependymal tectal tumors that can cause progressive aqueductal stenosis in children and adults. Contrarily to the majority of brain stem tumors that are intrinsic, infiltrative, and biologically aggressive, gliomas of the tectal plate have been reported (49,50) to be particularly indolent, often remaining stable in size for several years [Fig. 18(A) to 18(E)]. These tumors characteristically present with late onset aqueductal stenosis, often without associated brain stem signs, and they enlarge slowly, if at all, over time. The management of hydrocephalus usually warrants a favorable long-term prognosis (50).

Aqueductal Stenosis and Vascular Malformations

Obstruction of the aqueduct by vascular malformations is rare at any age (4). Aneurysms of the vein of Galen (11) may compress the quadrigeminal plate, inducing aqueductal stenosis. The stenosis may disappear after shrinking of the vascular malformation following arterial embolization [Fig. 19(A) and 19(B)]. Abnormal draining veins of midbrain arteriovenous malformations may also cross the aqueduct and obstruct the CSF flow (51). Cavernous angiomas of the tectal plate may cause aqueductal stenosis like any other tectal mass [Fig. 20(A) and 20(B)]. In adults, aqueductal stenosis may be caused by large fusiform aneurisms of the basilar artery (4).

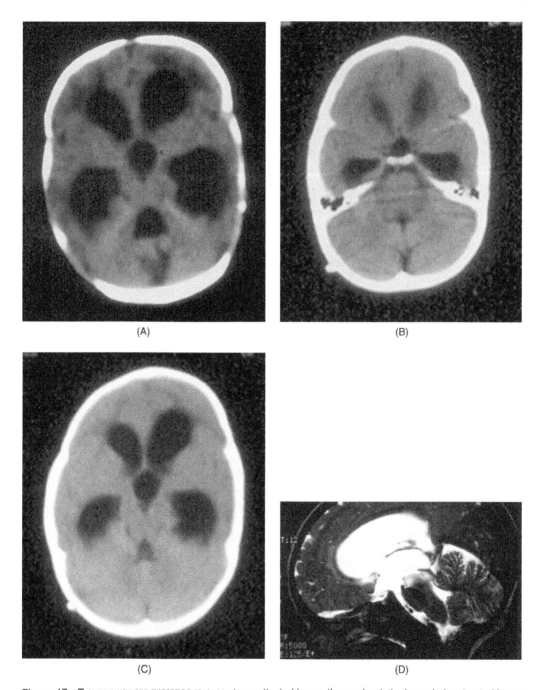

Figure 17 Tetraventricular dilatation in a newborn affected by posthemorrhagic hydrocephalus, treated by ventriculoperitoneal shunt (**A**). Two years later, during a shunt malfunction, the dilatation is triventricular (**B–C**) due to acquired aqueductal stenosis visible on MRI (**D**). The patient was treated by endoscopic third ventriculostomy and the shunt was removed.

CSF DYNAMICS IN AQUEDUCTAL STENOSIS

Aqueductal stenosis is a progressive disease. It is well known, since the ventriculographic era, that many patients presenting with symptoms and signs of intracranial hypertension still present some passage of contrast medium through the aqueduct (Fig. 21). This can also be observed at CT scan with intraventricular injection of contrast medium that also contaminates

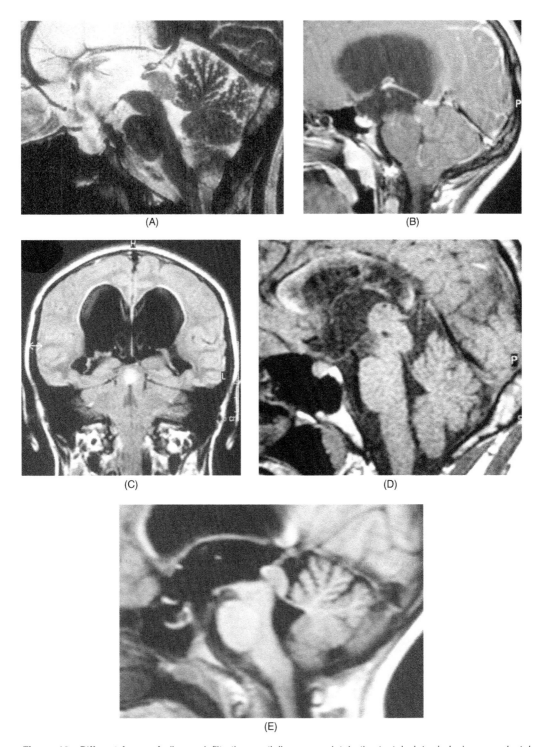

(A)

(B)

(C)

(D)

(E)

Figure 18 Different forms of gliomas infiltrating partially or completely the tectal plate, inducing aqueductal stenosis (**A–E**).

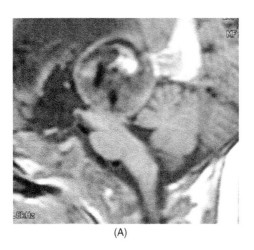
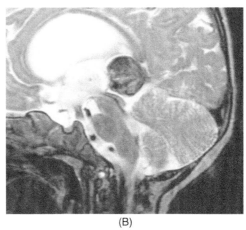

(A)   (B)

Figure 19 Vein of Galen malformation inducing aqueductal stenosis and hydrocephalus (**A**). After embolization of the vascular malformation and endoscopic third ventriculostomy, hydrocephalus resolved and the aqueduct is permeable again with a well-represented flow void inside (**B**).

the fourth ventricle (Fig. 22) or at MRI where residual lumen can be detected in same cases at the level of the stenosis (Fig. 23). The different patterns of progression of the stenosis according to the underlying etiology (gliosis, amartoma, infection, etc.) accounts for the variability of clinical presentation, ranging from rapid onset intracranial hypertension to very long clinical history of endocrine dysfunctions, chronic headaches, and other symptoms that can last for many years. Changes in aqueductal size and shape will alter the volume flow rate and the flow pattern in the aqueduct. As the aqueduct narrows, the flow decreases for a given pressure difference, the velocity increases until a maximum of 10 times the normal velocity, and the wall shear stresses increase (17). This velocity may potentially cause a flow void on MR imaging (see later in the text), falsely leading to the diagnosis of a patent aqueduct. Increasing the wall shear stresses and the pressure inside the aqueduct, gliosis with further narrowing may develop (17), or alternatively the duct may dilate, due to the disruption of the ependymal layer.

Changes in the structural anatomy (for example, forking without stenosis) may also dramatically change the flow pattern: it becomes turbulent and flow stasis occurs just distal to the area of forking.

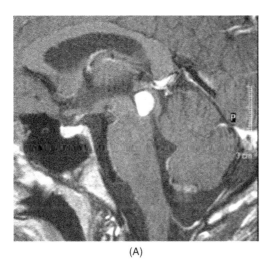
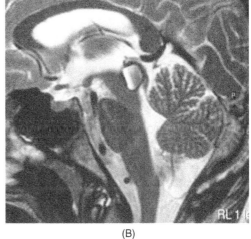

(A)   (B)

Figure 20 Cavernous angioma of the midbrain with recent hemorrhage visible in T1-weighted sequences (**A**) inducing hydrocephalus. Fluid level is visible in T2-weighted sequences (**B**).

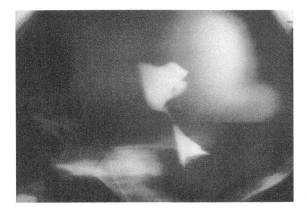

Figure 21 Ventriculography performed in the pre-CT scan era, showing aqueductal stenosis with residual CSF flow through the aqueduct.

In the computer modeling of stenotic aqueduct described by Jacobson et al. (17) to achieve normal physiological CSF flow through two narrow ducts with inlet areas of 0.49 and 0.15 mm², pressure of 10 and 120 Pa are required, respectively. Therefore, significant stenosis may occur without necessarily increasing the ICP to abnormal levels, but the increased wall shear stresses may result in ongoing damage of the aqueduct. The drop pressure required when the cross-sectional area is as little as 0.15 mm², although may not contribute significantly to the total intracranial pressure (120 Pa or 0.9 mm Hg), is significant and measurable in vivo. Any measurable pressure difference between the third and fourth ventricles should be pathological (17). More severe stenosis results in detectable increase in ICP. Kaufmann and Clark (52), in their study on simultaneous supratentorial and infratentorial ICP monitoring in patients with head injury or intracranial space-occupying lesion, observed that when intraventricular CSF pressure exceeds the cervical subarachnoid pressure by more than 10 mm Hg, fatal transtentorial and/or tonsillar herniation occur. Also, in noncommunicating hydrocephalus, the pressure gradient

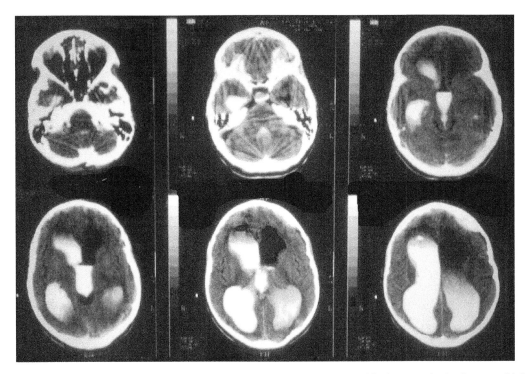

Figure 22 CT scan with intraventricular injection of metrizamide, showing residual communication between third and fourth ventricles. The patient was successfully treated by endoscopic third ventriculostomy.

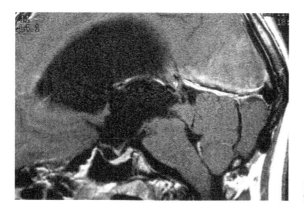

Figure 23 Same case of Figure 22, showing tectal hyperplasia and aqueductal stenosis.

cannot exceed the critical value of 10 mm Hg, because the intraventricular pressure is partially transmitted through the brain parenchyma to the supratentorial subarachnoid spaces that communicate freely with infratentorial compartment, contributing to infratentorial pressure (53,54). The developing of a pressure gradient between the supra and infratentorial compartment may lead to typical anatomical deformations of the third ventricle and to symptoms specific of hydrocephalus secondary to aqueductal stenosis [Fig. 24(A) to 24(C)].

The importance of CSF pulsation in the development of ventricular dilatation has been discussed by many authors (55–58). Mise et al. (58) observed that in experimental aqueductal stenosis, the systolic displacement of CSF is impaired. The CSF pulse during systole may lead to periventricular edema and partial displacement of blood from parenchymal vessels as well as to accumulation of CSF in third and lateral ventricles. This could lead to ischemia, tissue damage, and ventricular dilatation. According to these theories, the cumulative effect of many pulse waves, slowly remolding the brain, should be the cause of the ventricular enlargement in chronic hydrocephalus (57).

Actually, Greitz (57) hypothesizes two different mechanisms in ventricular dilatation differentiating an acute phase from a chronic phase. In case of acute intraventricular block, the CSF is prevented to reach its main absorption site. The ventricles increase in volume because the periventricular capillaries can only absorb part of the CSF produced. The pressure in the ventricles and brain becomes elevated. The ventricular dilatation displaces the brain towards the skull and compresses the cortical veins. This leads to venous congestion with increased blood volume and further increased intracranial pressure. The venous congestion and the brain swelling counteracts the ventricular dilatation, which otherwise would be fatal. At some point a new equilibrium is reached at higher pressure. The arteriolar and capillary regulation of fluid absorption in the periventricular brain capillaries finally balances the production of CSF inside the isolated ventricles. The CSF pressure decreases and a new equilibrium is established at near normal pressure in the chronic phase of obstructive hydrocephalus (57). In this phase, the venous outflow compression and venous congestion disappears; thereafter, there is no force to counteract ventricular dilatation, while the capacitance vessels become compressed. This decreases intracranial compliance, which causes a breakdown of the arterial windkessel mechanism with decreased arterial expansion, increased capillary expansion, increased CSF pulsations, and hyperdynamic CSF flow in the blocked ventricles (57). The increased pulse pressure increases the transmantle pulsatile stress, which continues to dilate the ventricles even if the mean CSF pressure is normal (57).

Compared with other forms of hydrocephalus, obstructive hydrocephalus is characterized by a marked reduction in ventricular compliance (54,57). Compliance (defined as dV/dP ratio) expresses the capacity of the brain to modify its volume, without important increase in intracranial pressure, due to the physical and geometric properties of the brain substance, the presence of interstitial and subarachnoid spaces, such as sulci, fissures and cisterns, and the ready compressibility of the veins. When the aqueduct is obstructed, the ventricles are isolated from the cranial and spinal subarachnoid spaces.

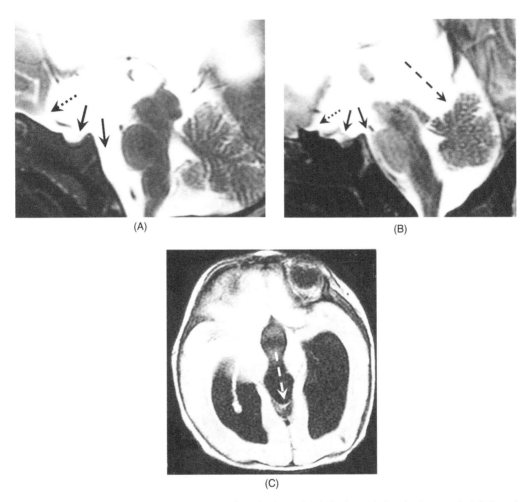

(A)   (B)

(C)

Figure 24 Typical deformations of the outline of the third ventricle in hydrocephalus due to aqueductal stenosis. In part (**A**), the floor of the third ventricle is pushed downward anteriorly and behind the posterior clinoids (*full arrows*), the lamina terminalis is deformed and bulges anteriorly (*dotted arrow*). In part (**B**) same alterations as in part (**A**), with a more significant deformity of the suprapineal recess (*interrupted arrow*). In part (**C**) a very large suprapineal recess is visible (*interrupted arrow*)

TYPICAL ANATOMICAL DEFORMATIONS OF THE VENTRICLES IN AQUEDUCTAL STENOSIS

The presence of a pressure gradient at tentorium (53,59) is specific of hydrocephalus secondary to aqueductal stenosis and determines the application of the most important stress on anatomical structure located at the level of the tentorial hiatus and third ventricle. The floor of the third ventricle is forced to bulge downward into the interpeduncular cistern [Fig. 24(A)]; the suprapineal recess is forced to bulge backward in the quadrigeminal cistern [Fig. 24(B) and 24(C)] and the midbrain is pushed down and flattened (Fig. 25). The more severe deformation is observed at the level of the periaqueductal region, with ballooning and funneling of the aqueduct above the obstruction, depression of its floor, severe compression of the periaqueductal gray matter, and stretching of the posterior commissure (53,59,60).

In case of chronic hydrocephalus, with massive ventricular dilatation, long-standing CSF pulsations against the thinnest segment of the ventricular walls may determine focal enlargement of some portions of the ventricular system, leading to the formation of pulsion diverticula, subependymal dissection and spontaneous ventriculocisternostomies [Fig. 26(A) to 26(C)].

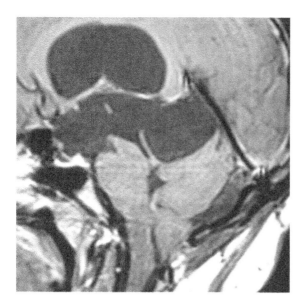

Figure 25 Significant enlargement of the suprapineal recess.

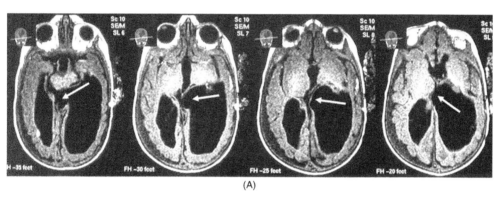

(A)

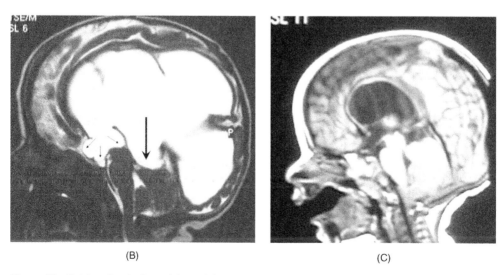

(B)   (C)

Figure 26 Pulsion diverticulum of the atrial wall (**A**); note the herniation of the medial ventricular wall through the tentorial incisura (*arrows*). The pulsion diverticulum is well visible (**B**) on sagittal T2 sequences (*large arrow*) as well as the typical deformations of the third ventricle (*small arrows*). Complete resolution of the diverticulum is observed after VP shunting (**C**).

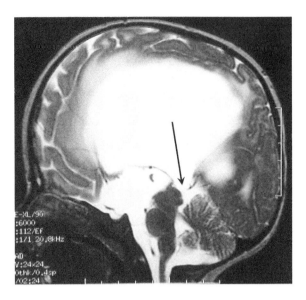

Figure 27   Early stage of formation of a pulsion diverticulum.

Pulsion Diverticula

Diverticula are cystic spaces lined by pia mater that are walled off the subarachnoid spaces and that communicate only with the ventricles (61). The most frequent sites (62) of ventricular rupture and formation of diverticula are the medial wall of the trigone of the lateral ventricles (atrial diverticula) and posterior wall of the third ventricle (expansion of the suprapineal recess). Atrial diverticula (63) occur at the weakest point of the trigone where the wall is formed by splenium of corpus callosum above, crura of fornix inferiorly, and alvei and fimbriae of hippocampus connecting splenium with crura (Fig. 27). With progressive hydrocephalus and progressive expansion of atria, alvei are displaced medially and stretched between the elevated corpus callosum and depressed fornix. With greater atrial dilatation, the alveus and crus became an extremely thinned alvear-crural sheet. This may be denuded by ependyma and may dehisce or shear creating unilateral or bilateral diverticulum ostia of 5 to 20 mm in diameter, boarded by splenium posterolaterally and crura anteromedially (61). Following formation of ostium, CSF pulsations may bulge the pia mater inferomedially to form the pulsion diverticulum. With progressive enlargement, the pial diverticulum and the arachnoid, that surrounds it, may bulge downward through the incisura, driven by the pressure gradient between the supratentorial and infratentorial compartments, forming an incisural and subtentorial "cyst" behind the midbrain within the ambient and superior vermian cisterns (64) [Fig. 28(A) and 28(B)]. The diverticulum typically displaces the quadrigeminal plate, pineal gland, fourth ventricle, and vermis inferiorly; the straight sinus, tentorium, vein of Galen, and occipital lobes superiorly (61). It can be confused (especially on CT scan) with a dilated fourth ventricle, or an arachnoid cyst of the quadrigeminal cistern (61). In this case, the differential diagnosis is important because arachnoid or ependymal cyst should be managed with extirpation, fenestration, or shunting, usually also resolving the associated hydrocephalus. Otherwise, in case of atrial diverticulum, the treatment of hydrocephalus (shunting or third ventriculostomy) is usually sufficient to induce regression of the diverticulum (61) [Fig. 28(C)]. MR imaging, flow-sensitive phase-contrast MR imaging (65) and, in more difficult cases, metrizamide CT ventriculography (61) may be useful to demonstrate direct continuity between lateral ventricle and "quadrigeminal cyst" in case of atrial diverticulum.

The suprapineal, lamina terminalis, and infundibular recesses are the weakest part of the third ventricle. Their walls are not covered by neural or vascular structures, contrary to the lateral and inferior third ventricular walls that are bordered by the two thalami laterally and midbrain inferiorly. The suprapineal recess, in normal subjects, is a diverticulum of ependymal roof (66) and, in cases of aqueductal stenosis, may become markedly dilated to fill the quadrigeminal and superior vermian cisterns, displacing the vermis and cerebellar hemispheres downwards, dislodging and compressing the dorsal midbrain and posterior commissura. In case of massive

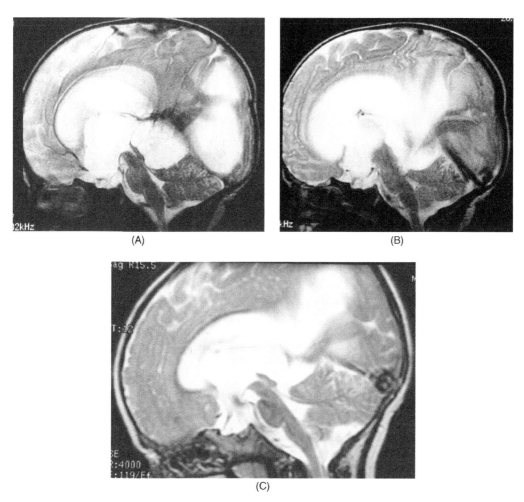

(A)

(B)

(C)

Figure 28 Very large pulsion diverticulum of the lateral ventricle mimicking a quadrigeminal cistern cyst (**A** and **B**). Almost complete resolution is observed following endoscopic third ventriculostomy (**C**).

dilatation of the suprapineal recess, severe cerebellar compression, deformation of the midbrain, and chronic tonsillar herniation may occur (64). An enlarged anterior third ventricle may be responsible for chiasm and hypothalamo–hypophyseal axis compression.

Subependymal Dissection

Subependymal dissection may originate from spontaneous or iatrogenic ruptures of the ependymal layer, with CSF entering the subependymal space and dissecting the ependymal layer from the periventricular white matter. The latter can present severe damage, with formation of enlarge CSF-filled cavities. Intraparenchymal cavities may occur, following ependymal laceration secondary to intracranial pressure monitoring (64). Subependymal dissections connecting the ventricular cavities with the subarachnoid space can act like spontaneous ventriculocisternostomies and account for clinicoradiological stabilization of extreme cases [Fig. 29(A) and 29(B)]

Spontaneous Ventriculocisternostomies

Ventriculocisternostomies may occur when rupture of the ventricular walls, more often at the level of the lamina terminalis and of the posterior wall of third ventricle, leads to free communication between the ventricle and subarachnoid space, allowing in some circumstances to spontaneous compensation of hydrocephalus. Less frequently ventricles may open into the

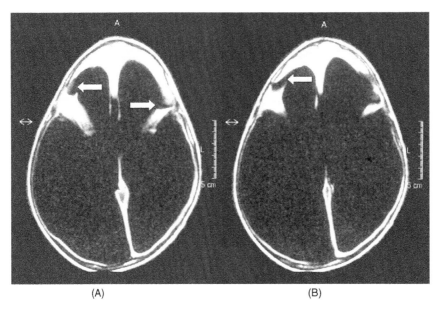

Figure 29 Subependymal dissection. Eight-year-old boy affected by congenital toxoplasmosis and aqueductal stenosis, never operated on due to parents' refusal. Note the interruption of the ependymal layer at the level of both frontal horns, with CSF tracks through the residual white matter that reach the subarachnoid spaces of the convexities, thus creating spontaneous ventriculocisternostomies.

subdural space [Fig. 29(A) and 29(B)] or even into the frontal, sphenoidal sinuses, or ethmoidal cells, whose walls have been thinned progressively by chronic increased intracranial pressure (60,67), with subsequent rhinoliquorrhea. These events are rare and may follow mild head injury.

SYMPTOMS SPECIFIC OF HYDROCEPHALUS SECONDARY TO AQUEDUCTAL STENOSIS

The symptomatology and the course of aqueductal stenosis is highly variable, according to the patient's age and the anatomical deformation of the ventricular system. In first year of life, the clinical presentation usually consists of acute onset and rapid enlargement of the circumference of the head (5,68). In older children, adolescents, and adults, only in a little percentage (15%), the onset is acute with headache, nausea and vomiting, visual disturbances, seizures, changes in mental state, and coma. More often the onset is insidious (68). Some patients with chronic history of symptoms, such as retarded psychomotor development, school difficulties, temporary headache, endocrine disturbances, growth retardation, may show acute progression of symptoms as the result of further decompensation of hydrocephalic state. In some circumstances, the causes of late decompensation may be identifiable in slight cranial trauma, hyperpyretic crises, or subarachnoid hemorrhage (5,68–70,). The clinical presentation of aqueductal stenosis in adults and elderly patients may be correlated with the presence of aqueductal narrowing and hydrocephalus since early life [the so-called "Late onset idiopathic aqueductal stenosis" described by Fukuhara and Luciano (70)]. These patients often report a history of recurrent headache during childhood and adolescence and present cranial enlargement and characteristic radiographic changes, suggestive of intracranial hypertension, such as elongation of anterior wall of the sella turcica (71). When aqueductal stenosis decompensates in the elderly, it usually does so in a normal pressure hydrocephalus fashion (71–73), with the classic triad of gait disturbance, dementia, and incontinence.

In about 15% of cases (72), patients experience seizures during the course of their illness. It appears to be a predilection for development of temporal lobe and generalized seizures (71). Their appearance is related to the distress of the cerebral cortex due to increased intracranial pressure; often seizures do not regress with the treatment of hydrocephalus.

Headache has the characteristics of that associated with raised intracranial pressure, with exacerbation during coughing, sneezing, straining, and stooping. The site is variable and it is usually described as occurring in attacks. These may last for seconds or minutes or may continue for days. During attacks nausea, vomiting, drowsiness, sensation in weakness in the legs, and even falls may occur. Headache and drop attacks are thought to be caused by sudden changes in pressure relationship (71).

Visual Disturbances

Visual disturbances are related to papilledema, with reduction of visual acuity in many cases. The chronic compression of the optic chiasm exerted by enlarged third ventricle warrants the presence of visual field defects. Unilateral or bilateral blurring of vision are frequent and had been variable attributed to compression of chiasma, ischemia of occipital lobes, or paralysis of reflexes of fixing and following due to dorsal midbrain dysfunction (74).

Endocrine Manifestations

Endocrine manifestations have been reported (37,75) occurring in 10% of adolescents and adults with aqueductal stenosis. The chronic compression of the hypothalamo–hypophyseal axis by enlarged anterior third ventricle that, in some cases, bulges into the sella turcica and erodes the clinoids (76) may explain both hypophyseal hypofunction and hyperfunction. Diencephalon–hypophyseal compression can not only reduce secretion of hypophyseal hormones, but also of hypothalamic inhibitor hormones resulting in increase of hypophyseal function. Endocrine findings in order of frequency in the report of Rotilio and coworkers (75) have been in males: obesity, hypogonadism (with impotence and infertility), diabetes insipidus, precocious puberty, and, less frequently, lethargy, gigantism, and acromegaly; in females: amenorrhea, obesity, and, less frequently, diabetes insipidus, hypertrichosis, acromegaly, and dwarfism. Endocrine abnormalities may constitute the only symptoms of the patients and in many cases reverse after treatment of hydrocephalus.

Ocular Disturbances and Sylvian Aqueduct Syndrome

Ocular disorders, ranging from paresis of upward gaze to the complete syndrome of aqueduct of Sylvius are the most characteristic signs of aqueductal stenosis (74). Classically, ocular disorders had been considered the result of compression of tectum and posterior commissure between the dilated suprapineal recess of the third ventricle above and the dilated rostral aqueduct below (77), associated with caudal displacement and distortion of the upper brain stem (78). The identification of the anatomical structures responsible for upward gaze and their location in the periaqueductal gray matter ventral to the aqueduct led to better understanding of the pathogenesis of the ocular disorders, such as upward gaze paralysis (Parinaud's syndrome), abnormality of the pupils (better reaction to accomodative stimulus than to light stimulus), spasm of convergence, nystagmus retractorius on attempted upward gaze, and upper lid retraction (Collier's sign) (74,78). The association of these symptoms has been referred to Koerber—Salus–Elschnig or aqueductal syndrome (53,74,78), and is also known as pretectal (78) and dorsal midbrain syndrome (53,79). Collier's sign associated with upward gaze paralysis corresponds to the "setting sun sign" described in infant patients. The transtentorial pressure gradient, accountable for severe deformation of the periaqueductal region and severe compression of the periaqueductal gray matter ventral to the aqueduct (53,60), is the most likely responsible for aqueductal syndrome. Rostral interstitial nucleus of the medial longitudinal fasciculus (riMLF), a group of cells in the prerubral field of the mesencephalic reticular formation, is considered the location of vertical presaccadic burst neurons (80), while the paramedian pontine reticular formation (PPRF) is the location of both horizontal and vertical gaze controls. The supranuclear control is provided by signals from frontal, parietal, occipital cortex, cerebellum, and superior colliculi. The efferent pathways for upward and downward gaze are segregated: the one for the upward gaze leaves the riMLF dorsolaterally and decussate through the posterior commissure to the contralateral riMLF before projecting bilaterally to the oculomotor nuclei. This long circuit explains the selective damage to this pathway (80). The decussation of the downgaze fibers is probably lower in midbrain (81). Other midbrain structures implicated are interstitial nucleus of Cajal and nucleus of Darkschewitsch (80).

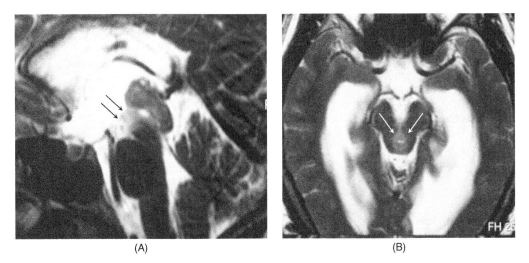

                    (A)   (B)

Figure 30   Shunt malfunction in a patient affected by aqueductal stenosis due to a large mass of the tectal plate, presenting with Parinaud's sign and global dorsal midbrain malfunction. Note the significant deformation of the midbrain in (**A**) due to increased CSF pressure into the third ventricle (*black arrows*) and the typical hyperintensity in the midbrain (**B**) around the aqueduct (*white arrows*).

The anatomical relationship of these structures explains the order of appearance of eye signs during progression of hydrocephalus (74): usually upward gaze paralysis appears before the downward and lateral gaze impairment. The pupillary dilatation and the paralysis of light reflex tend to occur when hydrocephalus is advanced.

Global Rostral Midbrain Dysfunction

With further progression of hydrocephalus in addition to tegmental involvement, signs of ventral midbrain involvement may appear, configuring the "global rostral midbrain dysfunction" (53,79), characterized by (*i*) parkinsonian-like state with tremor, bradykinesia, masked face, and cogwheel rigidity; (*ii*) spastic quadriparesis; and (*iii*) alteration of level of consciousness (79). All these symptoms can be explained by the progressive involvement of substantia nigra, with nigrostriatal and nigrocortical connections, cerebral peduncles, and midbrain reticular formation. The severity of this syndrome is determined by rapidity of onset and severity of hydrocephalus; thus, although it may also occur in patients first presenting with hydrocephalus, it is much more probable following shunt failure and sudden blockage of CSF drainage in patients with aqueductal stenosis (53,78). The functional impairment of the riMLF and of the whole dorsal midbrain during shunt malfunction is explained by the severe and acute deformation of the midbrain [Fig. 30(A) and 30(B)] due to the formation of a pressure gradient between the supra- and infratentorial compartments [Fig. 31(A) and 31(B)]. In this acute phase, sagittal MRI shows marked hyperintensity on T2-weighted sagittal images, probably indicating focal edema. These changes are usually rapidly reversible following third ventriculostomy (53)

Extrapyramidal Signs

Parkinsonian features may be the presenting symptoms of obstructive hydrocephalus or may be manifest during shunt failure (82) as a result of compression of the striatum and midbrain. Curran and Lang (83) suggested that the dysfunction of "ascending" tracts (cortico-striato-pallido-thalamo-cortical motor loop and/or nigro-striatal fibers) would play an important role in pathophysiology of parkinsonism in hydrocephalus. They proposed three potential sites of disconnection: the first is the nigro-striatal dopaminergic system, which explain the levo-dopa responsive parkinsonism, due to torsion or direct compression of the midbrain or its striatal efferents by the expanding third ventricle and rostral aqueduct. The second is at the level of the basal ganglia connections (pallidal efferents to thalamus) and the third at the level of the connection of the thalamus to the supplementary motor cortex in the periventricular matter. These last two sites are less involved in cases of aqueductal stenosis and are responsible for the

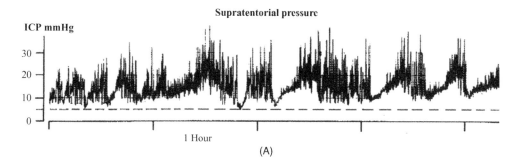

(A)

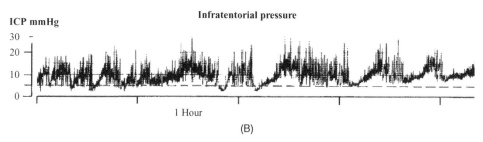

(B)

Figure 31 Evidence of a pressure gradient in a patient affected by global rostral midbrain dysfunction during shunt malfunction. Supratentorial pressure (**A**) is higher than infratentorial pressure (**B**) recorded simultaneously.

levo-dopa resistant parkinsonism typical of normal pressure hydrocephalus. The mechanism of insult of these circuits probably combines varying degrees of direct or indirect mass effect with ischemia (73,83). The degree of reversibility of symptoms in response to shunt should reflect the extent of permanent neuronal damage.

The compromise of nigro-striatal dopaminergic pathway in aqueductal stenosis should explain the presence of other symptoms, such as blepharoclonus (84), inappropriate brief rhythmic contractions of orbicularis oculi resembling clonus in other body segments, and, more important, akinetic mutism. This is a condition characterized by unresponsiveness with the appearance of alertness (85). Typically, the patient may look at the examiner, but remain mute. Commands may be carried out in a feeble, slow, and incomplete manner and painful peripheral stimulation produces slow withdrawal of the limb without manifestation of emotion (86). This rare syndrome may develop after multiple shunt revisions for shunt failure (86,87). Curran and Lang (83) placed akinetic mutism at the extreme end of the hydrocephalus-parkinsonian spectrum, identifying the pathogenetic mechanism in a combination of severe bradykinesia/akinesia plus compromise of ascending reticular activating system. Anderson (88) suggested that the monoaminergic projection fibers from the brain stem in regions adjacent to the third ventricle are exposed to damage when rapid ventricle dilatation occurs in patients with multiple shunt failures in which the repeated bouts of ventricle dilatation and relaxation have induced alterations of the physical characteristics of the brain parenchyma so that expansion at a lower pressure and more rapid dilatation are permitted. Usually, this syndrome responds to dopamine agonists, such as levo-dopa and bromocriptine, with ephedrine added due to the possible damage to noradrenergic fibers (86–88).

NEURORADIOLOGICAL FINDINGS

On CT scan, diagnosis of aqueductal stenosis can be only presumptive: CT criterion for the site of obstruction in hydrocephalus is the point of transition from dilated to nondilated CSF spaces (89)—dilatation of only the lateral and third ventricles suggests obstruction at or near the aqueduct. Actually up to 25% of patients with nonobstructive hydrocephalus shows little or no dilatation of the fourth ventricle (Fig. 32). Moreover, CT may fail to rule out the presence of brain stem tumors, particularly tectal tumors. These tumors are usually small, isodense with

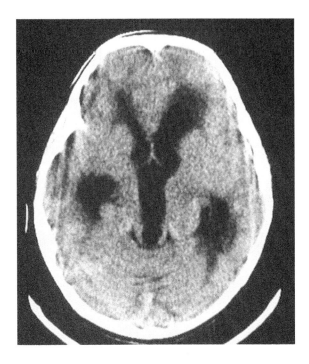

Figure 32 CT scan of a patient with aqueductal stenosis with acute presentation. The shape of the third ventricle with a very large suprapineal recess is highly suggestive for aqueductal stenosis.

the surrounding brain and typically enhance poorly or not at all after administration of contrast material.

An MRI is mandatory for all cases of hydrocephalus; it will easily confirm the status of the aqueduct and, in case of aqueductal stenosis, the primary or secondary nature of the obstruction. Since the advent of MR imaging, it has been possible to visualize, in a noninvasive way, the entire length of the aqueduct.

The optimal view for the evaluation of anatomical details is a midline sagittal section using a T1- and T2-weighted techniques (90,91). On T1-weighted images (WI) sequence the aqueduct has the same signal intensity as CSF, while on T2 WI, as a result of rapid CSF flow pulsations, the signal become hypointense compared to ventricular CSF (92). This "flow-related signal void" is more correctly defined by Kemp and coworkers (91) as "a reduced signal intensity within the center of the aqueduct on both the first and second echoes of the T2 WI, in comparison to the higher signal of the lateral ventricular CSF." "Flow void" often appears extending superiorly into the third ventricle and through the aqueduct into the superior aspect of the fourth ventricle; its presence has been considered as the most important sign for diagnosis of patent aqueduct (93,94). However, the flow-void is not always present: Sherman et al. (95) reported it in about 70% of normal subjects.

In some cases, the aqueduct is poorly visualized on the sagittal plane: these should be explained by distortion or displacement of the aqueduct out of the plane of section. Kemp et al. (91) advises 3-mm-thick contiguous sections for specific evaluations of the aqueduct. If the aqueduct is not seen in either the sagittal plane or the axial plane, a long segment of obstruction is present. In cases of aqueductal stenosis in which the aqueduct remains visible, the obstruction is presumably caused by a membrane (92). Three-dimensional Constructive Interference Steady State (CISS) sequences, by providing greater detail of the ventricular system and basal cistern due to excellent CSF-to-brain contrast and superior spatial resolution, may permit easy identification of aqueductal obstruction by membranes, webs, and hypoplasia or by cysts and tumors (96,97).

Hydrocephalus caused by obstruction at the aqueduct level is not always associated with the loss of flow void (91). In effect narrowing of the aqueduct is likely to cause either pronounced flow, as the same amount of CSF has to pass through a narrow duct, or absence of flow. Only in the latter situation the flow void is absent. Other methods have been introduced to better assess the CSF flow dynamics through the aqueduct, in particular gradient-echo rapid MR imaging

(GRE) and cardiac-gated cine-MRI. On GRE sequences, it is possible to distinguish stationary spins from those that are moving: when appropriate (98) technical variables are used, the flow can be demonstrated as having high signal intensity, the absence of flow as having low signal. Flow-sensitive phase-contrast cine MR imaging is more sensitive than static MRI in detecting the pulsatile motion of CSF (15). A specially designed sequence (flow sensitive gradient echo sequence) can accurately measure the flow perpendicular to the plane of acquisition. It is based on the acquiring of multiple gradient echo images in the same plane (usually the midsagittal) during a cardiac cycle, starting immediately after the R-wave and acquiring successive images at regular intervals. The technical features of the examination are described elsewhere (13). Two different sequences are available: a "cine phase contrast" sequence, in which the flow is coded on gray scale, and a "phase contrast flow" sequence, in which the velocity is coded not only on gray scale, but also on a quantitative scale. Absolute velocity measurement is possible on dedicated software (13). With this technology, aqueductal stenosis is no longer a diagnostic problem as measurement of flow in this structure can readily differentiate between an obstructed and a patent aqueduct (13).

Failure to demonstrate flow in the aqueduct by cine-MRI technique is pathological (15): it has been observed in cases of aqueductal stenosis, midbrain, and aqueduct compression by a mass and in presence of a third ventricular mass lesion, which have resulted in a lack of propagation of the fluid wave. It has been reported (99) that in patients with aqueductal stenosis turbulent flow in the third ventricle may be discernable. Moreover, cine MRI can provide the confirmation that the ventriculomegaly is a consequence of aqueduct kinking or compression in case of mass lesion and can be helpful in determining the level of obstruction in cases of complex hydrocephalus where multiple adhesions or mass may warrant ventriculomegaly. These data are important in assessing whether surgical intervention may be efficacious and whether shunting or third ventriculostomy should be more indicated. Moreover, in cases of long-standing hydrocephalus both MRI and cine MRI may be helpful in detecting and correctly explaining ventricular diverticula, third ventricle bulging in the chiasmatic and interpeduncular cisterns, and cystic expansion of the suprapineal recess.

In some patients with aqueductal stenosis, MRI may reveal focal or diffuse abnormality of morphology (dorsal flattening and thinning) and signal characteristics (hypointensity in T1 and hyperintensity in T2) of the corpus callosum, which may persist after treatment of hydrocephalus despite clinical improvements (100). A combination of factors involving both compression and reexpansion of corpus callosum has been suggested, such as edema, ischemia, and demyelinization, caused by long-standing compression of the corpus callosum against the falx and subsequent ventral collapse after shunt placement with segmental tethering of the dorsal surface at sites where arterial rami of the pericallosal artery perforate the body of the corpus callosum (101). The importance in recognizing these findings is in avoiding misinterpretation of the diagnosis (100).

In the postoperative period, to assess ventricular size after shunting, CT scan alone is sufficient for follow-up (90). However, to assess the permeability of internal shunts, such as endoscopic third ventriculostomy, phase-contrast MRI is needed (90,102). A sagittal scan should be obtained showing a to-and-fro movement of CSF through the stoma between the third ventricle and the prepontine cistern. Quantitative analysis may display a speed of CSF between 2 and 5 cm/sec.

TREATMENT

Treatment of hydrocephalus secondary to aqueductal stenosis can be achieved with both extracranial and intracranial shunting. In the preshunt era (before 1950s), several attempts had been made in order to surgically bypass the aqueductal obstruction. Dandy first in 1922 proposed a subfrontal approach to open the floor of the third ventricle by sacrificing one optic nerve (103), thereafter several authors later attempted to treat obstructive hydrocephalus by creating communications between the third ventricle and chiasmatic or interpeduncular cistern by opening the lamina terminalis or the floor of the third ventricle, using an open craniotomy, via subfrontal or subtemporal approach (104). This intervention failed in one third of cases with a mortality rate as high as 15%. The surgical approach, in fact, destroyed the cisterns where the stomies were performed (104). To increase the successful rate, indirect ventriculostomies, in which the communications between the ventricular cavities and subarachnoid spaces were created via a drain, had been introduced. Among these, the most widely used was the Torkild-sen's ventriculocisternostomy (105), first performed in 1939. Via a posterior fossa craniectomy a catheter going from the lateral ventricle to the cisterna magna was positioned. The introduction of ventriculocervical shunting by Matson in 1949 simplified the procedure by requiring only a second cervical hemilaminectomy to insert the distal catheter anterior to the cervical spinal cord. The cases of Torkildsen procedure were reviewed by Scarff (106) in 1966 who revealed a mortality of 25%, a mechanical dysfunction of 50%, and a failure of 40%, chiefly because of obstruction of the distal stump of the catheter by arachnoidal adhesions. However, this opera-tion had been employed above all in cases of posterior fossa tumors, in which the ambient and the basal cisterns became obstructed by tumor or internal herniations.

Direct cannulation of the aqueduct (interventriculostomy) was first attempted by Dandy in 1920 (107) who forced via a posterior fossa craniectomy a small sound from the fourth ventricle into the aqueduct and inserted a rubber catheter. Variations of this procedure had been performed until 1980s by Lapras and coworkers (21). Only for membranous occlusion a simple perforation of the diaphragm is considered sufficient, while in most cases some types of stents should be positioned into the aqueduct to prevent later occlusion by scarring (108). Although the success rate was satisfactory (59%), the mortality rate of the open direct cannulation of the aqueduct reviewed by Schroeder and Gaab (108) was significant (12%).

In the 1920s, the first attempts of endoscopic approaches were made as well. The first report of an endoscopic third ventriculostomy (ETV) was that of Mixter (109) who in 1923 used a urethroscope to enter the third ventricle through the foramen of Monro. The opening into the interpeduncular cistern was performed by puncturing the floor of the third ventricle with a sound. The presence of contrast dye (previously injected in the lateral ventricle) in the lumbar subarachnoid space demonstrated the success of the first ETV ever realized. In the following years, the efforts were addressed towards the improvement of the endoscopic techniques (110). In fact, although the procedures were correctly carried out and based on a sound theory, the long-term results were not rewarding yet and the morbidity and mortality rate unacceptable. Poor design of the instruments and optical apparatus was the main cause of the disappointing outcomes.

Since the introduction of valvular shunts in the 1950s to carry the CSF from the ventricles to the venous circulation (111), the treatment of hydrocephalus has become more efficient, with very low short-term mortality and morbidity. Therefore, the attempts of internal shunting were virtually abandoned, and ventriculoatrial or ventriculoperitoneal shunting became the treatments of choice for all forms of hydrocephalus, including aqueductal stenosis.

After more than 50 years of widespread use of CSF shunts, the limits of shunt surgery have become evident. Thereafter, since 1980s the interest towards alternatives to shunt, in particular endoscopic and X-ray guided percutaneous techniques, has renewed in cases of noncommunicating hydrocephalus, with the aim to provide a natural route for CSF within the range of physiological intracranial pressure and to avoid all the pathology related to shunt dysfunction, such as subdural effusions, secondary craniosynostosis or slit ventricles, and that related to mechanical dysfunction, such as infections and occlusions, which require reoperations. This became possible because of miniaturization and improvement of surgical tools, in particular concerning endoscopic surgery (112).

Guiot (113) used ventriculographic control to create a communication between the third ventricle and interpeduncular cistern with a leukotome thrust through the floor of the third ventricle. The same technique was used by Hirsch (104) who, reviewing the literature, calcu-lated a mortality rate of 1.2% and a morbidity of 1.7%, including transient oculomotor palsies and infection, and reported, in their series, 80% of success rate in children and 70% in infants (Fig. 33). The selection of the patients was considered by the authors as the most important factor for the success: they performed this procedure only when the third ventricle was large enough and when its floor bulged into the interpeduncular cistern; in these cases, the hypotha-lamic nervous structures are displaced laterally and the floor on the midline consists only of pia mater. In this series, all cases with a history of meningitis or subarachnoid hemorrhage resulted in failure, therefore they advocate to not select these patients due to the incapacity of the sub-arachnoid spaces to absorb CSF normally. Prerequisite for the success of all intracranial shunting

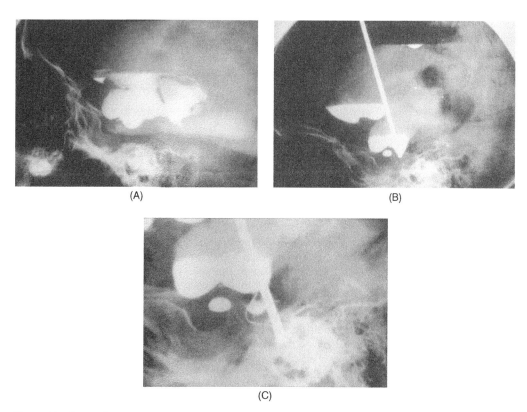

(A)   (B)

(C)

Figure 33   Steps of a ventriculocisternostomy in the pre-CT scan and pre-endoscopy era. Ventriculography shows aqueductal stenosis (**A**). A leukotome is inserted through a bur hole and advanced in the third ventricle under ventriculographic control (**B**). After perforation of the floor, a loop is opened into the cistern and the leukotome is withdrawn to enlarge the hole in the floor (**C**). The risks of this procedure are self-evident.

technique is the patency of the subarachnoid spaces and adequacy of CSF absorptive mechanism. With the evolution of the surgical tools, it became possible to perform third ventriculostomy under stereotactic control. This offers some advantages over ventriculographic guidance (114): it ensures that the leukotome is truly on the midline, reducing the risk of hypothalamic and oculomotor nerves damage; furthermore, stereotactic angiographic target-point cross correlation as reported by Kelly (114) reduces the risk that instrumentation trajectories damage major vascular structures.

Endoscopic third ventriculostomy offers significant advantages over other methods: it combines a minimally invasive approach with brilliant visual control of manipulation, the risk of vascular and neural damage is reduced under direct vision, and the avoidance of radiopaque intraoperative dyes reduces the risk of later closure of the ventriculostomy due to development of arachnoiditis (115). Several factors have contributed to the renaissance of the neuroendoscopy in the last two decades. Among them are the pioneer work of Bosma, who applied an 8-mm film registration in his interventions, and the introduction by Harold Hopkins of a solid-rod lens system during 1960s (102,112). These innovations were the base for the following development of modern instruments, as, for example, the ductile Fukushima ventriculofiberscope introduced in 1973 (116). During the second half of the 1990s, with the publication of results in large clinical series (117–121), neuroendoscopy became widely accepted in the neurosurgical community and is now considered as the first-line treatment of obstructive hydrocephalus (122).

Patients with primitive stenosis of the sylvian aqueduct have been historically considered the ideal candidate for ETV (118,122), whatever the pathologic process responsible for the stenosis and the age of the patient. With strict selection of the patients, the success rate is above 75% (115,119,123). Thereafter, a conspicuous number of patients still require a shunt during their life. As mentioned above, prerequisite of a successful ventriculostomy is the patency of the distal subarachnoid pathways, so a careful examination of preoperative neuroradiological examinations, especially magnetic resonance imaging (MRI), is mandatory to detect further areas of obstruction in order to minimize the number of failures (102).

The indications to perform an endoscopic third ventriculostomy rather than a shunt operation have increased in the last few years. Initially, the ideal candidates had to follow the subsequent criteria: acquired aqueductal stenosis, adequate size of third ventricle (at least 1 cm bicoronal diameter), and extension of the floor of the third ventricle behind and below the dorsum sellae, potentially patency of subarachnoid spaces (115,124). Thus, patients previously shunted and patients who experienced meningitis, subarachnoid hemorrhage or with associated spinal dysraphism were considered poor candidates (104,125,126). Recently, there has been a tendency to include patients with myelomeningocele, Chiari malformation, congenital aqueductal stenosis, previous meningitis, age younger than two years, and prior ventriculoperitoneal shunt (115,127–130). In the presence of history of meningitis, shunt infection, subarachnoid and/or intraventricular hemorrhage, and in hydrocephalus associated with spinal dysraphism, endoscopic third ventriculostomy is effective in approximately two-thirds of patients (112,120,127). Previous shunting could even increase the successful rate after endoscopic third ventriculostomy by decreasing the transmantle pressure, allowing arachnoid granulations to open and mature (112). Controversies are still present in patients younger than one year (112,118,131), because of underdeveloped granulations. Warf (132) suggested to associate endoscopic coagulation of the choroid plexus to ETV in order to increase the success rate in children younger than one-year old. As no clinical tests, even invasive infusion test, can predict outcome, because the opening of the subarachnoid spaces after the operation may take days or even weeks (104), endoscopic third ventriculostomy should be suggested for all cases where an obstructive component of the hydrocephalus is present or strongly suspected, giving the patients the chance to remain or become shunt free, but adequate information regarding mild higher surgical risk and lower success rate (particularly in the first year of life and in case of history of meningitis or hemorrhage) than shunting operation should be addressed in the preoperative informed consent.

Stereotactic guidance of endoscopic third ventriculostomy should help in cases of inferior visual conditions (after infection or intraventricular bleeding), distorted anatomy (malformation, cystic lesions, tumors), or when another procedure, such as biopsy or cyst fenestration, is needed (112). The surgical technique of ETV and shunt implantation is described elsewhere in the book.

As an alternative to ETV, in cases of membranous occlusion or short stenosis of the aqueduct, endoscopic aqueductoplasty could be employed. According with Schroeder and Gaab (108) aqueductoplasty should have some theoretical advantage compared with endoscopic third ventriculostomy: it restores the physiological CSF pathway and does not carry the risks of major vessel injury. Moreover, arachnoid adhesions, which occasionally may be found below the floor of the third ventricle and may interfere with CSF circulation, do not occur around the aqueduct; finally, sometimes the floor of the third ventricle is very tough and considerable force has to be utilized to perform a sufficient fenestration, which can damage hypothalamus, while strictures of the aqueduct are not as tough. On the other hand, aqueductoplasty is generally considered more risky because of the surrounding delicate midbrain structures, with the risk of neurological deficits such as oculomotor and trochlear palsies, Parinaud's or aqueduct syndromes. However, in properly selected cases, aqueductoplasty can be performed effectively and safely. It is the opinion of Schroeder and Gaab (108) that aqueductoplasty of membranous stenosis is less traumatic than third ventriculostomy. In case of membranous occlusion of the aqueduct, they perform simple perforation of the membrane; in case of stenosis of a short segment of the aqueduct, they complete aqueductoplasty with balloon dilatation and often insertion of a stent, to reduce the risk of restenosis (133). In patients with longer stenosis (>5 mm) they advise against aqueductoplasty.

PROGNOSIS AND INTELLECTUAL OUTCOME

Prognosis of patients with aqueductal stenosis is highly dependant on efficacy of surgical treatment. However, even in case of prompt surgical intervention long-term outcome, especially in children, is not always favorable (134,135). The poorest results had been found in X-linked aqueductal stenosis (28,30), where the obstruction of CSF flow is only partly responsible for the very low IQ. Obviously, the presence of associated malformations imply a low survival rate and poor mental developmental.

In most series (3,30,134,135), older patients at the time of clinical presentation have a more favorable neurodevelopmental prognosis. Renier and coworkers (30) in their series of 108 children with congenital hydrocephalus (premature newborn and spina bifida patients excluded) observed a significant difference in outcome between infants with aqueductal stenosis and those with communicating hydrocephalus: the 10-year survival was 80% in aqueductal stenosis and 60% in communicating hydrocephalus; the mean intelligence quotient (IQ) was 67 in aqueductal stenosis, with 46% of children at or above 80; whereas in communicating hydrocephalus, the mean IQ was 52, with only 20% of children at or above 80. They also noted a better outcome in postnatal hydrocephalus (3), with the same difference in intellectual outcome between hydrocephalus due to aqueductal stenosis and communicating hydrocephalus. These data are in disagreement with those of Hanigan et al. (134) and McCullough et al. (136) who found that children with aqueductal stenosis have significant lower IQs than children with communicating hydrocephalus.

In the pediatric series published by Villani et al. (135) 68% of patients with follow-up longer than 15 years were designed as "normal" at the neurodevelopmental evaluation (attending normal school courses or having regular jobs); 24% "moderately disabled" and 8% "severely disabled". However, the 39% of patients designed as "normal" had functional motor skills abnormal for the presence of neurological deficits such as paraplegia, visual disturbances, and mild hemiparesis. The incidence of epilepsy paralleled the degree of mental and motor abnormalities (137), as in hypothalamus–hypophyseal dysfunction.

Many prognostic factors have been studied. Among these, head circumference at birth, the value of the first IQ assessment, and the relevance of postoperative frontal cortical mantle width on MRI or CT scan after surgery had been demonstrated as the most relevant (30,134,135). Failure in reexpansion of the cortical mantle (less than 20 mm) should indicate an irreversible damage and a poor mental neurodevelopment, as well as increase head circumference above 4 standard deviations and low first IQ or development quotient assessment.

In older patients also duration of symptoms affects the prognosis: chronic symptoms and delayed diagnosis usually correlate with partial regression of symptomatology (69). Older children with acute onset of symptoms and prompt surgery have the best prognosis.

Children treated with shunts become shunt dependent: shunt malfunction is often associated with a temporary increase of intracranial pressure, which may be responsible for progressive psychological deterioration (60). It has been observed (128) that shunt malfunction may be more dangerous, with more acute and massive intracranial rises, in hydrocephalus due to aqueductal stenosis, than in communicating hydrocephalus due to reduction in brain compliance (53,54). In some studies, shunt infections are strictly related to poor intellectual development (136). Villani and coworkers (135) reported a global mortality rate of 28.8% for children with aqueductal stenosis treated with shunts followed for a period of 5 to 25 years (mean 15.2 years), and a death rate of 1.2% per year. These data included a mortality rate of 7.7% after shunt revisions.

Compared to the implant of an extrathecal CSF shunt device, the most important difference of endoscopic third ventriculostomy is the effect on the volume of the cerebral ventricles as demonstrated by neuroimaging. The ventricular size usually decreases rapidly and significantly following the shunt implantation, while it decreases much slower and smaller after ETV (138,139). This has been cause of concern regarding neuropsychological outcome following ETV in children affected by aqueductal stenosis. To further complicate this scenario is the lack of multicentric, prospective, randomized studies focused on the long-term outcome of patients treated with ETV or extrathecal shunts. Only few retrospective studies are available (102). Hirsch et al. (3) reviewed 114 children affected by aqueductal stenosis, 70 treated by shunting and 44 by percutaneous third ventriculostomy: the postoperative IQ was not significantly different in the two groups. Sainte-Rose (140) compared two identical series of patients with aqueductal stenosis: 38 were treated by insertion of VP shunt and 30 by third ventriculostomy. From neurological, endocrinologic, social, and behavioral point of view, he found no statistical difference between the two groups. Similar results have been achieved by Tuli et al. (141). A controlled randomized study comparing neuroendoscopic versus nonneuroendoscopic treatment of hydrocephalus in children seems to show that the outcome of the patients treated initially with a neuroendoscopic procedure is significantly better than that of the patients initially treated with a shunt, but this observation requires further investigation in multicenter studies (142).

REFERENCES

1. Van Gijn J. Franciscus Sylvius (1614–1672). J Neurol 2001; 248:915–916.
2. Baker F. The two Sylviuses. An historical study. Bull Johns Hopkins Hosp 1909; 20:329–339.
3. Hirsch JF, Hirsch E, Sainte-Rose C, et al. Stenosis of the aqueduct of Sylvius (etiology and treatment). J Neurosurg Sci 1986; 30:29–39.
4. Jellinger G. Anatomopathology of nontumoral aqueductal stenosis. J Neurosurg Sci 1986; 30:1–16.
5. Robertson JA, Leggate JRS, Miller JD, et al. Aqueductal stenosis-presentation and prognosis. Br J Neurosurg 1990; 4:101–106.
6. Tisell M, Edsbagge M, Stephenson H, et al. Elastance correlates with outcome after endoscopic third ventriculostomy in adults with hydrocephalus caused by primary aqueductal stenosis. Neurosurgery 2002; 50:70–77.
7. Ceddia A, Di Rocco C, Iannelli A, et al. Idrocefalo neonatale ad eziologia non tumorale. Minerva Pediatr 1992; 44:445–450.
8. Catala M. Development of the cerebro-spinal fluid pathways during embryonic and fetal life in humans. In: Cinalli C, Maixner WJ, Sainte-Rose C, eds. Pediatric Hydrocephalus. Milan, Italy: Springer-Verlag, 2004:19–45.
9. Emery JL, Staschak MC. The size and form of cerebral aqueduct in children. Brain 1972; 95:591–598.
10. Woollam DH, Millen JW. Anatomical considerations in the pathology of stenosis of the cerebral aqueduct. Brain 1953; 76:104–112.
11. Russell DS. Observations on the pathology of hydrocephalus. Medical Res Council, spec rep series No. 265. His Majesty's Stationery Office, London, 1949.
12. Beckett RS, Netsky MG, Zimmerman HM. Developmental stenosis of the aqueduct of Sylvius. Am J Path 1950; 26;755–787.
13. Brunelle F. Dynamic MRI of cerebro-spinal fluid in children. In: Cinalli C, Maixner WJ, Sainte-Rose C, eds. Pediatric hydrocephalus. Milan, Italy: Springer-Verlag, 2004:397–403.
14. Enzmann DR, Pelec NJ. Normal flow pattern in intracranial and spinal cerebrospinal fluid defined with phase-contrast cine—MR imaging. Radiol 1991; 178;467–474.
15. Quencer RM, Donovan Post MJ, Hinks RS. Cine MR in the evaluation of normal and abnormal CSF flow: intracranial and intraspinal studies. Neuroradiology 1990; 32:371–391.
16. Czosnyka M, Czosnyka ZH, Whitfield PC, et al. Cerebrospinal fluid dynamics. In: Cinalli C, Maixner WJ, Sainte-Rose C, eds. Pediatric Hydrocephalus. Milan, Italy: Springer-Verlag, 2004:47–63.
17. Jacobson EE, Fletcher DF, Morgan MK, et al. Fluid dynamics of the cerebral aqueduct. Pediatr Neurosurg 1996; 24;229–236.
18. Jacobson EE, Fletcher DF, Morgan MK, et al. Computer modelling of the CSF flow dynamics of aqueductal stenosis. Med Biol Eng Comput 1999; 37(1):59–63.
19. Conner ES, Foley L, Black PM. Experimental normal-pressure hydrocephalus is accompanied by increased transmantle pressure. J Neurosurg 1984; 61:322–327.
20. Turnbull IM, Drake CG. Membranous occlusion of the aqueduct of Sylvius. J Neurosurg 1966; 24; 24–33.
21. Lapras C, Bret P, Patet JD, Huppert J, et al. Hydrocephalus and aqueductal stenosis. Direct surgical treatment by interventriculostomy (Aqueduct cannulation). J Neurosurg Sci 1986; 30:47–53.
22. Oi S, Shimoda M, Shibata M, et al. Pathophysiology of long-standing overt ventriculomegaly in adults. J Neurosurg 2000; 92:933–940.
23. Johnston IH, Kowman-Giles R, Whittle IR. The arrest of treated hydrocephalus in children. A radionuclide study. J Neurosurg 1984; 61:752–756.
24. Bickers DS, Adams RD. Hereditary stenosis of aqueduct of Sylvius as a cause of congenital hydrocephalus. Brain 1949; 72:246–262.
25. Edwards JH. The syndrome of sex-linked hydrocephalus. Arch Dis Child 1961; 36:486–493.
26. Dirks PB. Genetics of hydrocephalus. In: Cinalli C, Maixner WJ, Sainte-Rose C, eds. Pediatric Hydrocephalus. Milan, Italy: Springer-Verlag, 2004:1–17.
27. Landrieu O, Ninane J, Ferriere G, et al. Aqueductal stenosis in X-linked hydrocephalus: a secondary phenomenon? Dev Med Child Neurol 1979; 21:637–652.
28. Yamasaki M, Arita N, Hiraga S, et al. A clinical and neuroradiological study of X-linked hydrocephalus in Japan. J Neurosurg 1995; 83:50–55.
29. Rosenthal A, Jouet M, Kenwrick S. Aberrant splicing of neural cell adhesion molecules L1 mRNA in a family with X-linked hydrocephalus. Nature Genet 1992; 2:107–112.

30. Renier D, Saint-Rose C, Pierre-Kahn A, et al. Prenatal hydrocephalus: outcome and prognosis. Childs Nerv Syst 1988; 4:213–222.

31. Senat MV, Bernard JP, Delezoidë A, et al. Prenatal diagnosis of hydrocephalus-stenosis of the aqueduct of Sylvius by ultrasound in the first trimester of pregnancy. Report of two cases. Prenat Diagn 2001; 21:1129–1132.

32. Castro-Cago M, Alonso A, Eiris-Punal. Autosomal recessive hydrocephalus with aqueductal stenosis. Childs Nerv Syst 1996; 12:188–191.

33. Spadaro A, Ambrosio D, Moraci A, et al. Aqueductal stenosis as isolated localization involving the central nervous system in children affected by von Recklinghausen disease. J Neurosurg Sci 1989; 30:87–93.

34. Johnson RT, Johnson KP, Edmonds CJ. Virus-induced hydrocephalus: development of aqueductal stenosis in hamsters after mumps infection. Science 1967; 157(792):1066–1067.

35. Meyer HM Jr. Central nervous system syndromes of viral etiology. Am J Med 1960; 29:334–347.

36. Cinalli G, Spennato P, Ruggiero C, et al. Aqueductal stenosis 9 years after mumps meningo-encephalitis. Treatment by endoscopic third ventriculostomy. Childs Nerv Syst 2004; 20:61–64.

37. Rotilio A, Salar G, Dollo C, et al. Aqueductal stenosis following mumps infection. Case report. Ital J Neurol Sci 1985; 6(2):237–239.

38. Hower J, Clar HE, Duchting M. Mumps as a cause of hydrocephalus. Pediatrics 1972; 50(2): 346–347.

39. Wolinsky JS. Mumps virus induced hydrocephalus in hamsters. Ultrastructure of the chronic infection. Lab Invest 1977; 37(3):229–236.

40. Boop FA. Posthemorrhagic hydrocephalus of prematurity. In: Cinalli C, Maixner WJ, Sainte-Rose C, eds. Pediatric Hydrocephalus. Milan, Italy: Springer-Verlag, 2004:121–131.

41. McFarlane A, Maloney AFJ. The appearance of aqueduct and its relationship with hydrocephalus in the Arnold–Chiari malformation. Brain 1957; 80:479–491.

42. Cinalli G, Spennato P, Del Basso De Caro ML, et al. Hydrocephalus and Dandy Walker malformation. In: Cinalli C, Maixner WJ, Sainte-Rose C, eds. Pediatric Hydrocephalus. Milan, Italy: Springer-Verlag, 2004:259–277.

43. Raimondi AJ, Samuelson G, Yarzagaray L, et al. Atresia of the foramen of Luschka and Magendie: The Dandy–Walker cyst. J Neursurg 1969; 31:202–216.

44. Raimondi AJ, Clark SJ, McLone DG. Pathogenesis of aqueductal occlusion in congenital murine hydrocephalus. J Neurosurg 1976; 45:66–77.

45. Nugent GR, Al-Mefty O, Chou S. Communicating hydrocephalus as a cause of aqueductal stenosis. J Neurosurg 1979; 51:812–818.

46. Oi S, Matsumoto S. Pathophysiology of aqueductal obstruction in isolated IV ventricle after shunting. Childs Nerv Syst 1986; 2:282–286.

47. Spennato P, Cinalli G, Carannante G, et al. Multiloculated hydrocephalus. In: Cinalli C, Maixner WJ, Sainte-Rose C, eds. Pediatric Hydrocephalus. Milan, Italy: Springer-Verlag, 2004:219–244.

48. O'Brien DF, Javadpour M, Collins DR, et al. Endoscopic third ventriculostomy: an outcome analysis of primary cases and procedures performed after ventriculoperitoneal shunt malfunction. J Neurosurg (5 suppl Pediatrics) 2005; 103:393–400.

49. Chapman PH. Indolent gliomas of the midbrain tectum. Concepts Pediatr Neurosurg 1990; 10;97–107.

50. Pollack IF, Pang D, Albright AL. The long-term outcome in children with late-onset aqueductal stenosis resulting from benign intrinsic tectal tumors. J Neurosurg 1994; 80:681–688.

51. Blackmore CC, Mamourian AC. Aqueduct compression from venous angioma: MR findings. AJNR Am J Neuroradiol 1996; 17;458–460.

52. Kaufmann GE, Clark K. Continuous simultaneous monitoring of intraventricular and cervical subarachnoid cerebrospinal fluid pressure to indicate development of cerebral or tonsillar herniation. J Neurosurg 1970; 33:135–140.

53. Cinalli G, Sainte-Rose C, Simon I, et al. Sylvian aqueduct syndrome and global rostral midbrain dysfunction associated to shunt malfunction. J Neurosurg 1999; 90:227–236.

54. Lim ST, Potts DG, Deonarine V, et al. Ventricular compliance in dogs with and without aqueductal obstruction. J Neurosurg 1973; 39:463–473.

55. Bering EA. Choroid plexus and arterial pulsation of the choroid plexus as a cerebrospinal fluid pump. Arch Neurol Psychiatr 1955; 73:165–172.

56. Di Rocco C, Di Trapani G, Pettorossi VE, et al. On the pathology of experimental hydrocephalus induced by artificial increase in endoventricular CSF pulse pressure. Childs Brain 1979; 5:81–95.

57. Greitz D. Radiological assessment of hydrocephalus: new theories and implications for therapy. Neurosurg Rev 2004; 27:145–165.

58. Mise B, Klarica M, Bulat M, et al. Experimental hydrocephalus and hydromyelia: a new insight in mechanism of their development. Acta Neurochir 1996; 138:862–869.

59. Johnson RT, Yates PO. Clinico-pathological aspects of pressure changes at tentorium. Acta radiol 1956; 46:242–249.
60. Lapras C, Bret P, Tommasi M, et al. Les sténoses de l'aqueduc de Sylvius. Neurochirurgie 1980; 26(suppl 1):1–152.
61. Naidich TP, McLone DG, Hahn YS, et al. Atrial diverticula in severe hydrocephalus. AJNR Am J Neuroradiol 1982; 3:257–266.
62. Wakai S, Narita J, Hashimoto K, et al. Diverticulum of the lateral ventricle causing cerebellar ataxia. Case report. J Neurosurg 1983; 59:895–898.
63. Mott M, Cummins B. Hydrocephalus related to pulsion diverticulum of lateral ventricle. Arch Dis Child 1974; 49:407–410.
64. Cinalli G, Spennato P, Cianciulli E, et al. Hydrocephalus and aqueductal stenosis. In: Cinalli C, Maixner WJ, Sainte-Rose C, eds. Pediatric Hydrocephalus. Milan, Italy: Springer-Verlag, 2004: 280–293.
65. Rovira A, Capellades J, Grive E, et al. Spontaneous ventriculostomy: report of three cases revealed by flow-sensitive phase-contrast Cine MR Imaging. AJNR Am J Neuroradiol 1999; 20:1647–1652.
66. Shallat RF, Pawl RP, Jerva MJ. Significance of upward gaze palsy (Parinaud's syndrome) in hydrocephalus due to shunt malfunction. J Neurosurg 1973; 38:717–721.
67. Cabezudo JM, Vaquero J, Garcia-de-Sola R, et al. Direct communication between the lateral ventricle and the frontal sinus as a cause of CSF rhinorrhea in aqueductal stenosis. Acta Neurochir 1981; 57:95–98.
68. Vindigni G, Del Fabro P, Facchin P, et al. On the neurological complications of internal and external shunt in patients with non-neoplastic stenosis of the aqueduct. J Neurosurg Sci 1986; 30:83–86.
69. Di Rocco C, Iannelli A, Tamburrini G. Idrocefalo da stenosi dell'acquedotto ad insorgenza tardiva. Minerva Pediatr 1995; 47:511–520.
70. Fukuhara T, Luciano M. Clinical features of late-onset idiopathic aqueductal stenosis. Surg Neurol 2001; 55:132–137.
71. Little JR, Houser OW, MacCarty CS. Clinical manifestations of aqueductal stenosis in adults. J Neurosurg 1975; 43:546–552.
72. Harrison MJG, Robert CM, Uttley D. Benign aqueductal stenosis in adults. J Neurol Neurosurg Psychiatry 1974; 37:1322–1328.
73. Vanneste J, Hyman R. Non-tumoral aqueductal stenosis and normal pressure hydrocephalus in the elderly. J Neurol Neurosurg Psychiatry 1986; 49:529–535.
74. Chatta AS, Delong GR. Sylvian aqueduct syndrome as a sign of acute obstructive hydrocephalus in children. J Neurol Neurosurg Psychiatry 1975; 38:288–296.
75. Rotilio A, d'Avella D, de Blasi F, et al. Disendocrine manifestations during non tumoral aqueductal stenosis. J Neurosurg Sci 1986; 30:71–76.
76. Avman N, Gökalp HZ, Arasil E, et al. Symptomatology, evaluation and treatment of aqueductal stenosis. Neurol Res 1984; 6:194–198.
77. Azar-Kia B, Palacios E, Churchil R. Aqueductal stenosis and Parinaud's syndrome. Illinois Med J 1975; 148:532–533.
78. Bleasel AF, Ell JJ, Johnston I. Pretectal syndrome and ventricular shunt dysfunction. Neuro Ophthalmol 1992; 12:193–196.
79. Barrer SJ, Schut L, Bruce DA. Global rostral midbrain dysfunction secondary to shunt malfunction and hydrocephalus. Neurosurgery 1980; 7:322–325.
80. Büttner-Ennever JA, Büttner U, Cohen B, et al. Vertical gaze paralysis and the rostral interstitial nucleus of the medial longitudinal fasciculus. Brain 1982; 105:125–149.
81. Bogousslavsky J, Miklossy J, Regli F, et al. Vertical gaze paralysis and selective unilateral infarction of the rostral interstitial nucleus of the medial longitudinal fasciculus (riMLF). J Neurol Neurosurg Psychiatry 1990; 53:67–71.
82. Jankovic J, Newmark M, Peter P. Parkinsonism and acquired hydrocephalus. Mov Disord 1986; 1:59–64.
83. Curran T, Lang AE. Parkinsonian syndromes associated with hydrocephalus: case reports, a review of the literature and pathophysiological hypotheses. Mov Disord 1994; 9:508–520.
84. Gatto M, Micheli F, Pardal MF. Blepharoclonus and parkinsonism associated with aqueductal stenosis. Mov Disord 1990; 5:310–313.
85. Cairns H, Oldfield RC, Pennybacker JB, et al. Akinetic mutism with an epidermoid cyst of the third ventricle. Brain 1941; 64:273–290.
86. Berger L, Gauthier S, Leblanc R. Akinetic mutism and parkinsonism associated with obstructive hydrocephalus. Can J Neurol Sci 1958; 12:255–258.
87. Messert B, Henke TK, Langheim W. Syndrome of akinetic mutism associated with obstructive hydrocephalus. Neurology 1966; 16:635–649.

88. Anderson B. Relief of akinetic mutism from obstructive hydrocephalus using bromocriptine and ephedrine. J Neurosurg 1992; 76:152–155.
89. Naidich TP, Schott LH, Baron RL. Computed tomography in evaluation of hydrocephalus. Radiol Clin North Am 1982; 20:143–167.
90. Brunelle F. Modern imaging of hydrocephalus. In: Cinalli C, Maixner WJ, Sainte-Rose C, eds. Pediatric Hydrocephalus. Milan, Italy: Springer-Verlag, 2004:79–93.
91. Kemp SS, Zimmerman RA, Bilaniuk LT, et al. Magnetic resonance imaging of the cerebral aqueduct. Neuroradiology 1987; 29:430–436.
92. Lee BCP. Magnetic resonance imaging of peri-aqueductal lesions. Clin Radiol 1987; 38:527–533.
93. Citrin CM, Sherman JL, Gangarosa RE, et al. Physiology of the CSF flow-void sign: modification by cardiac gating. AJNR Am J Neuroradiol 1984; 7:1021–1024.
94. Bradley WG, Cortman KE, Burgoine B. Flowing cerebrospinal fluid in normal and hydrocephalic states: appearance on MR images. Radiology 1986; 159:601–616.
95. Sherman JL, Citrin CM, Gangarosa RE, et al. The MR appearance of CSF flow in patients with ventriculomegaly. AJNR Am J Neuroradiol 1986; 7:1025–1031.
96. McConachie NS. The CISS sequence in the pre-operative assessment of neuroendoscopic third ventriculostomy. In: Cinalli C, Maixner WJ, Sainte-Rose C, eds. Pediatric Hydrocephalus. Milan, Italy: Springer-Verlag, 2004:405–410.
97. Laitt RD, Mallucci CL, McConachie NS, et al. Constructive interference in steady state 3D Fourier transform MRI in the management of hydrocephalus and third ventriculostomy. Neuroradiology 1999; 41:324–327.
98. Fram E, Hedlund L, Dimick R, et al. Parameters determining the signal of flowing fluid in gradient refocused imaging: flow velocity, TR and flip angle. In: Book of Abstracts: Society of Magnetic Resonance in Medicine 1986, Vol. 1. Berkeley, CA: Society of Magnetic Resonance in Medicine, 1986:84–85.
99. Kadowaki C, Hara M, Numoto M, et al. Cine magnetic resonance imaging of aqueductal stenosis. Childs Nerv Syst 1995; 11:107–111.
100. Suh DY, Gaskill-Shipley M, Nemann MW, et al. Corpus callosal changes associated with hydrocephalus: a report of two cases. Neurosurgery 1997; 41:488–494.
101. Lane JI, Luetmer PH, Atkinson JL. Corpus callosal signal changes in patients with obstructive hydrocephalus after ventriculoperitoneal shunting. AJNR Am J Neuroradiol 2001; 22:158–162.
102. Di Rocco C, Cinalli G, Massimi L, et al. Endoscopic third ventriculostomy in the treatment of hydrocephalus in pediatric patients. In: Pickard JD, ed. Adv Tech Stand Neurosurg, 2006; 31:110–220. Rome, Italy: Springer-Verlag/Wien.
103. Dandy WE. An operative approach for hydrocephalus. Bull John Hopkins Hosp 1922; 33:189–190.
104. Hirsch JF. Percutaneous ventriculocisternostomies in non-communicating hydrocephalus. Monogr Neural Sci 1982; 8:170–178.
105. Torkildsen A. New palliative operation in cases of inoperable occlusion of the sylvian aqueduct. Acta Chir Scan 1939; 82:117–123.
106. Scarff JE. Evaluation of treatment of hydrocephalus. Results of third ventriculostomy and endoscopic cauterization of choroid plexus compared with mechanical shunts. Archs Neurol 1966; 14:382–391.
107. Dandy WE. Diagnosis and treatment of hydrocephalus resulting from strictures of the aqueduct of Sylvius. Surg Gynec Obstet 1920; 31:340–358.
108. Schroeder HWS, Gaab MR. Endoscopic aqueductoplasty: technique and results. Neurosurgery 1999; 45:508–518.
109. Mixter WJ. Ventriculoscopy and puncture of the floor of the third ventricle. Preliminary report of a case. Boston Med Surg J 1923; 188:277–278.
110. Putnan TJ. The surgical treatment of infantile hydrocephalus. Surg Gynecol Obst 1943; 76:171–182.
111. Nulsen FE, Spitz EB. Treatment of hydrocephalus by direct shunt from ventricle to jugular vein. Surg Forum 1952; 2:399–402.
112. Cinalli G, Cappabianca P, de Falco R, et al. Current state and future development of intracranial neuroendoscopic surgery. Expert Rev Med Devices 2005; 2(3):351–373.
113. Guiot G. Ventriculo-cisternostomy for stenosis of the aqueduct of Sylvius. Acta Neurochir 1973; 28:274–289.
114. Kelly PJ. Stereotactic third ventriculostomy in patients with nontumoral adolescent/adult onset aqueductal stenosis and symptomatic hydrocephalus. J Neurosurg 1991; 75:865–873.
115. Jones RFC, Stening WA, Brydon M. Endoscopic third ventriculostomy. Neurosurgery 1990; 26:86–92.
116. Fukushima T, Ishijima B, Hirakaw K, et al. Ventriculofiberscope: a new technique for endoscopic diagnosis and operation. J Neurosurg 1973; 38:251–256.
117. Brockmeyer D, Abtin K, Carey L, et al. Endoscopic third ventriculostomy: an outcome analysis. Pediatr Neurosurg 1998; 28:236–240.

118. Cinalli G, Sainte-Rose C, Chumas P, et al. Failure of third ventriculostomy in the treatment of aqueductal stenosis in children. J Neurosurg 1999; 90:448–454.

119. Goumnerova LC, Frim D. Treatment of hydrocephalus with third ventriculostomy: outcome and CSF flow patterns. Pediatr Neurosurg 1997; 27:149–152.

120. Hopf NJ, Grunert P, Fries G, et al. Endoscopic third ventriculostomy: outcome analysis of 100 consecutive procedures. Neurosurgery 1999; 44:795–804.

121. Teo C. Third ventriculostomy in the treatment of hydrocephalus: experience with more than 120 cases. In: Hellwig D, Bauer B, eds. Minimally Invasive Techniques for Neurosurgery. Berlin, Germany: Springer, 1998:73–76.

122. Hellwig D, Grotenhuis JA, Tirakotai W, et al. Endoscopic third ventriculostomy for obstructive hydrocephalus. Neurosurg Rev 2005; 28:1–34.

123. Kim S-K, Wang K-C, Cho B-K. Surgical outcome of pediatric hydrocephalus treated by endoscopic III ventriculostomy: prognostic factors and interpretation of postoperative neuroimaging. Childs Nerv Syst 2000; 16:161–169.

124. Høffman HJ, Harwood-Nash D, Gilday DL. Percutaneous third ventriculostomy in the management of non-communicating hydrocephalus. Neurosurgery 1980; 7:313–321.

125. Oka K, Yamamoto M, Ikeda K, et al. Flexible endoneurosurgical therapy for aqueductal stenosis. Neurosurgery 1993; 33:236–243.

126. Vries JK, Friedmann WA. A quantitative assessment of CSF absorption in infants with meningomyelocele. Surg Neurol 1980; 13:38–40.

127. Siomin V, Cinalli G, Grotenhuis A, et al. Endoscopic third ventriculostomy in patients with cerebrospinal fluid infection and/or hemorrhage. J Neurosurg 2002; 97:519–524.

128. Jones RF, Kwok BC, Stening WA, et al. Third ventriculostomy in patients with spinal dysraphism. Indications and contraindications. Eur J Pediatr Surg 1996; 6(suppl):5–6.

129. Teo C, Jones R. Management of hydrocephalus by endoscopic third ventriculostomy in patients with myelomeningocele. Pediatr Neurosurg 1996; 25:57–63.

130. Cinalli G, Salazar C, Mallucci C, et al. The role of third ventriculostomy in the management of shunt malfunction. Neurosurgery 1998; 43:1323–1329.

131. Fukuhara T, Vorster SJ, Luciano MG. Risk factors for failure of endoscopic third ventriculostomy for obstructive hydrocephalus. Neurosurgery 2000; 46:1100–1111.

132. Warf BC. Comparison of endoscopic third ventriculostomy alone and combined with choroid plexus cauterization in infants younger than 1 year of age: a prospective study in 550 African children. J Neurosurg (6 suppl Pediatrics) 2005; 103:475–481.

133. Fritsch MJ, Kienke S, Manwaring KH, et al. Endoscopic aqueductoplasty and interventriculostomy for the treatment of isolated fourth ventricle in children. Neurosurgery 2004; 55:372–379.

134. Hanigan WC, Morgan A, Shaaban A, et al. Surgical treatment and neurodevelopment outcome for infants with idiopathic aqueductal stenosis. Childs Nerv Syst 1991; 7:386–390.

135. Villani R, Tomei G, Gaini SM, et al. Long-term outcome in aqueductal stenosis. Childs Nerv Syst 1995; 11:180–185.

136. McCullough DC, Balzer-Martin LA. Current prognosis in overt neonatal hydrocephalus. J Neurosurg 1982; 57:378–383.

137. Stellman GR, Bannister CM, Hillier V. The incidence of seizures disorders in children with congenital and acquired hydrocephalus. Z Kinderchir 1986; 41(suppl 1):38–41.

138. Xenos C, Sgouros S, Natarajan K, et al. Influence of shunt type on ventricular volume changes in children with hydrocephalus. J Neurosurg 2003; 98:277–283.

139. St George E, Natarajan K, Sgouros S. Changes in ventricular volume in hydrocephalic children following successful endoscopic third ventriculostomy. Childs Nerv Syst 2004; 20:834–838.

140. Sainte-Rose C. Third ventriculostomy. In: Manwaring KH, Crone KR, eds. Neuroendoscopy. New York: Mary Ann Liebert, 1992:47–62.

141. Tuli S, Alshail E, Drake JM. Third ventriculostomy versus cerebrospinal fluid shunt as a first procedure in pediatric hydrocephalus. Pediatr Neurosurg 1999; 30:11–15.

142. Kamikawa S, Inui A, Kobayashi N, et al. Endoscopic treatment of hydrocephalus in children: a controlled study using newly developed Yamadori-type ventriculoscopes. Minim Invasive Neurosurg 2001; 44:25–30.

9 | Postinfectious Hydrocephalus

Graham Fieggen
Division of Neurosurgery, University of Cape Town, Cape Town, South Africa

Tony Figaji
Paediatric Neurosurgery Unit, Red Cross Children's Hospital and University of Cape Town, Cape Town, South Africa

INTRODUCTION

New technology may bring new insights; there are few better examples of this than the evolution of our understanding of hydrocephalus following the advent of computed tomography (CT) and then magnetic resonance imaging (MRI) (67). The resurgence of interest in neuroendoscopy has likewise stimulated new thinking about hydrocephalus, particularly with respect to the management of the more complex conditions, such as hydrocephalus following either infection or hemorrhage.

Intracranial infection has long been recognized as an important cause of hydrocephalus and the various infectious agents often play their role at a particular age. The term *postinfectious hydrocephalus* (PIH) refers to hydrocephalus following *any* intracranial infection. This encompasses a diverse array of diseases such as antenatal TORCH infections, meningitis, ventriculitis, cerebritis, abscess or empyema, and encephalitis.

Meningitis is the most common serious infection of the CNS and invariably involves the leptomeninges and the subarachnoid space. Meningitis may be classified clinically as either *acute*, which develops within days, or *chronic*, when the symptoms and pleocytosis continue for more than four weeks (54). Most commonly the causative organism is bacterial, encompassing a diverse array of Gram-positive and Gram-negative organisms, actinomycetes (including mycobacteria), and spirochetes, but a wide range of other organisms may be encountered, including fungi and viruses.

In contrast to the term PIH, *postmeningitic hydrocephalus* (PMH) may be used in a more restricted sense to refer to hydrocephalus following acute or chronic inflammation of the meninges, most commonly caused by bacteria. This is an important topic, as PMH is common, particularly in the Developing World, complex in nature, and challenging to treat. Furthermore, the long-term outcome is often disappointing, with an academic outlook less favorable than other etiologies of hydrocephalus (15).

This chapter will consider the incidence of PIH and the possible mechanisms by which infections may lead to hydrocephalus, before reviewing the various infections that cause PIH. An attempt will be made to develop general principles for the management of the condition and the special case of PIH in the setting of the human immunodeficiency virus (HIV) will be examined.

INCIDENCE

Although PMH following acute bacterial meningitis is almost invariably a disease of childhood, tuberculous meningitis (TBM) can be seen at any age and cryptococcal meningitis (CM) is encountered most commonly in adults. Matson noted that the incidence of PMH increased markedly following the introduction of antibiotics for the treatment of meningitis as more children survived the initial infection, only to present later following the gradual occlusion of their subarachnoid CSF pathways (64).

Matson believed that this process occurred more commonly in neonates and this has been borne out by a number of early studies. Lorber and Pickering (57) reported that 31% of neonates who survived meningitis developed PMH. In a report from our institution in 1978, 105 (25%) of 419 hydrocephalic children were diagnosed with PMH and a further 22% had hydrocephalus due to a basal cisternal block, which was most likely meningitic in origin (24). Of the children with proven PMH, 70% presented within the first two years of life and over a quarter of them had suffered neonatal meningitis. In a series from Nigeria, 15% of children who survived nontuberculous bacterial meningitis developed hydrocephalus (1).

Tuberculosis has remained a scourge of Developing Countries despite the availability of effective chemotherapy and has now reemerged as a global health concern on the back of the AIDS pandemic. TBM occurs in 7% to 12% of patients with TB and hydrocephalus is nearly always present at some stage of the disease (103). An audit of children undergoing CSF diversion found that PIH accounted for 35% of cases in Cape Town as compared to 6% in Oxford (76). Warf's series of 300 Ugandan children treated with endoscopic third ventriculostomy (ETV) is notable for a 60% incidence of PIH (116). It is however striking how few recent contributions there have been to the literature on the management of PIH.

CONCEPTS

The authors agree with the assertion that all hydrocephalus (with the exception of those rare cases due to CSF overproduction) are obstructive in origin, with the block being either intra-ventricular or extraventricular (81). The latter manifests as "communicating" hydrocephalus, a term that came into use during the era of ventriculography and referred to the situation when a contrast agent introduced into the lateral ventricles was detected in the lumbar subarachnoid space.

For obvious reasons, meningitis most commonly obstructs the subarachnoid CSF pathways, resulting in communicating hydrocephalus (109). Should there be an accompanying ependymitis or ventriculitis, there may also be accompanying changes such as acquired aqueduct stenosis, which results in typical intraventricular obstructive hydrocephalus (35,118). Indeed, Williams notes that Dandy had considered intrauterine or postnatal infection to be a potential cause of aqueduct stenosis (118).

Obstruction could arise elsewhere in the CSF pathways; of the 105 patients with definite postmeningitic hydrocephalus referred to earlier, 24% had a block at the level of the foramen of Monro, aqueduct, or fourth ventricular outlet foramina on percutaneous ventriculography and air encephalography (24). Of course, more than one mechanism may play a role in an individual patient, particularly in the setting of TBM (103).

CAUSES

Antenatal Infection

TORCH Infections: General
The agents responsible for antenatal fetal brain infections are commonly referred to by the acronym TORCH [Toxoplasmosis, Other (varicella-zoster, HIV, syphilis), Rubella, Cytomegalovirus (CMV), and Herpes simplex]. It is important to emphasize that not all maternal infections affect the fetus but when this does occur, there is a wide range of possible consequences, ranging from fetal death to the birth of an infant who may either be asymptomatic or manifests disease that varies markedly in severity (30).

This section will consider the two most common antenatal infections that adversely affect the CNS, toxoplasmosis and CMV, but it is worth remembering that congenital lymphocytic choriomeningitis virus infections can present in much the same way and hydrocephalus may also occur in this condition (121).

Barkovich and Girard posit that infections in the first two trimesters will result usually in malformations, while those occurring in the third trimester typically manifest as destructive lesions. Fetal imaging using MRI may demonstrate evidence of the acute response, or more commonly features of the chronic response. These include ventricular dilatation, atrophy, parenchymal cystic cavities, ependymal cysts, calcifications and malformations, or delays in cortical development (6).

Toxoplasmosis
Toxoplasmosis is caused by the protozoan parasite *Toxoplasma gondii*; infection is acquired primarily through ingestion of cysts in infected, undercooked meat or oocysts that may contaminate soil, water, or food (66). Although the parasite is found worldwide, seroprevalence is highest

in tropical areas (54% in Southern Europe) and decreases with increasing latitude (77). Fifteen percent of women of childbearing age in the United States have serologic evidence of infection, and it is believed that between 400 and 4000 cases of congenital toxoplasmosis occur each year in that country (49).

Women who become acutely infected during pregnancy, or who have reactivation of disease due to immunosuppression, can transmit the parasite transplacentally. Congenital disease is most severe when contracted in the first trimester, but happily the risk of acquiring the disease is lowest early in pregnancy, at around 10% to 20%, and progressively rises to 60% to 90% in the third trimester (49).

Most pregnant women with acute infection do not manifest specific symptoms or signs, and the diagnosis is typically made when a fetal anomaly is found on ultrasound, or following birth. Some countries, such as France and Austria, perform systematic serological screening of pregnant women, but this is controversial not only on the grounds of cost but also because of uncertainty as to the effectiveness of treatment in preventing fetal disease (66). There various protocols for the interpretation of maternal IgG and IgM and amniocentesis may be indicated (after 18 weeks) to confirm fetal disease by polymerase chain reaction (PCR). If there is evidence of recent infection, one may attempt to prevent vertical transmission by prescribing spiramycin before 18 weeks gestation and the combination of pyrimethamine, sulfadiazine, and folinic acid after 18 weeks gestation (66).

Clinical features

Approximately 85% of infants with congenital toxoplasmosis will be asymptomatic and appear normal at birth, but most will suffer an episode of chorioretinitis and developmental delay is frequent in those who go untreated. This may only manifest years later.

The classic triad found in infants symptomatic at birth consists of chorioretinitis, hydrocephalus, and diffuse intracranial calcifications; the most common extraneural features include hepatosplenomegaly, fever, anemia, and jaundice (30).

The meningoencephalitis caused by toxoplasmosis may culminate in intracerebral calcification and hydrocephalus as mentioned, as well as porencephaly, hydranencephaly, or microcephaly (6). There are various mechanisms for the development of hydrocephalus; the parasite invades the ependyma and the ensuing debris in the CSF may occlude the aqueduct, while an animal model shows severe leptomeningeal inflammation and it has been suggested that aqueduct stenosis may be a secondary phenomenon in this situation (20).

Infants with hydrocephalus may present with features of raised intracranial pressure, seizures, or developmental delay. CT scan shows the typical spotty calcification.

Management

Treatment of affected infants with pyrimethamine, sulfadiazine, and folic acid leads to markedly improved outcomes. In some cases, intracranial calcification diminishes and neurological deficits resolve, but 25% will still have severe handicaps. Progressive hydrocephalus has traditionally required insertion of a shunt. Kaiser reported a series of 10 patients who were shunted; hydrocephalus was present at birth in three and manifested within the first year in most. Nine had aqueduct stenosis and some had narrowing at the foramen of Monro, resulting in asymmetric ventricles. Shunt revision was required 19 times in the cohort of 9 long-term survivors over a period of 9.6 years (50).

Given the preponderance of aqueduct stenosis in this condition, ETV is an attractive alternative (20). Indeed, 23 cases of toxoplasmosis were included in a series of 336 patients with aqueduct stenosis reported from Paris in 1999; the success rate for ETV in this subgroup was a very acceptable (60%), although this was below the overall success rate of 72% (19).

Congenital toxoplasmosis is an avoidable condition, through primary prevention to decrease the incidence of infection, secondary prevention in screening at risk pregnant women, or tertiary prevention in early identification and treatment of affected infants (30).

CMV

Human CMV is a large DNA virus; as a member of the herpes virus family, it has the capacity to establish life-long latency with periodic reactivations in the host. Congenital CMV is the

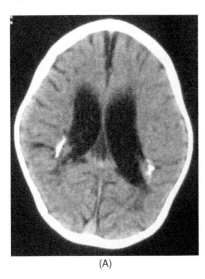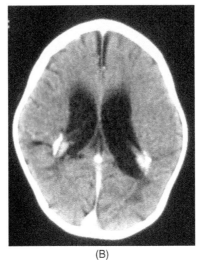

(A)   (B)

Figure 1 Congenital CMV infection in an infant born HIV-positive; CT scans before (**A**) and after (**B**) contrast administration. Note the subependymal calcification and adjacent enhancement.

most common congenital infection worldwide (117) and the leading infectious cause of mental retardation and hearing loss in the developed world (18). CMV infections are endemic and seroprevalence ranges between 35% and 95%, with a prevalence of congenital CMV that varies between 0.15% and 2% (62). The risk of transmission to the fetus is much higher in the setting of primary disease (30–40%) than reactivation (1%) and the consequences more severe when this happens early in pregnancy.

Apart from the occasional mononucleosis-like syndrome, almost all maternal infections are clinically silent. A new infection can be diagnosed serologically; predictors of a bad prognosis for the fetus include structural changes visible on ultrasound and a high viral load on amniocentesis (62).

The typical finding of "owl's eye" intracellular inclusions is the basis of the term CMV inclusion disease (CID). Numerous mechanisms have been implicated in CNS injury and these have been reviewed in detail recently (18). Neuroradiological findings that accompany hydrocephalus in CMV include intracranial calcification in one-third of cases (Fig. 1), cortical atrophy, subdural effusions, porencephaly, and polycystic encephalomalacia (5).

Clinical features

It is estimated that 44,000 CMV-infected infants are born annually in the United States, of whom 10% are symptomatic at birth. The commonest clinical manifestations of CID are a generalized petechial rash, hepatosplenomegaly, and jaundice as well as intrauterine growth retardation. Visual impairment may be caused by chorioretinitis, optic atrophy, and glaucoma, and sensorineural hearing loss occurs in 10% to 15% (62). Intracerebral calcification is present in 50% but, unlike in congenital toxoplasmosis, microcephaly is seen more often than hydrocephalus (117).

Management

A vaccine is not available; hence strategies to reduce the risk of exposure to CMV are important in pregnancy. The antiviral drugs are not recommended during pregnancy due to concerns about potential teratogenicity, but intravenous immunoglobulin is being investigated as an option. Following the isolation of virus from an infected neonate, intravenous ganciclovir has been shown to improve the prognosis for hearing but not the neurodevelopmental outcome (62).

It has been suggested that progressive hydrocephalus in the setting of CMV is best treated with a ventriculoperitoneal (VP) shunt rather than ETV, given the frequent structural abnormalities coupled with involvement of the leptomeninges (20). We have used the endoscope

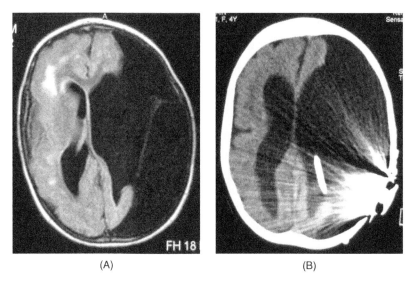

(A)   (B)

Figure 2   Axial CT scan of a 3-year-old child with known congenital CMV (**A**). Initial CT scans showed parenchymal changes with a large left-sided schizencephalic cyst. The child presented two years later with clinical features of acute raised ICP due to expansion of the cyst. This was endoscopically fenestrated into the lateral ventricle but the child's symptoms recurred, necessitating insertion of a shunt (**B**).

on occasion to fenestrate a progressively enlarging cyst into the ventricle, thus simplifying the subsequent treatment of hydrocephalus (Fig. 2).

Viral Meningitis
Viruses have been implicated in the pathogenesis of hydrocephalus through various mechanisms. The role of HIV in setting the stage for other diseases that lead to hydrocephalus is sufficiently important to justify separate consideration (see later). As already discussed, antenatal infection can present with hydrocephalus in the newborn—some viruses selectively infect ependymal cells (mumps, influenza A, parainfluenza 2, CMV, and LCV) and have been shown to cause aqueduct stenosis (20).

CNS infection is the most common extra–salivary gland manifestation of mumps, and CSF pleocytosis is seen in 50% of all cases, often without symptoms or signs; this is, however, almost invariably self-limited and seldom has long-term sequelae (44).

A bewildering array of viruses can afflict the CNS, but the pathological consequences of most viral infections of the brain can be classified into four stereotypic patterns (58):

- Inflammation restricted to the meninges
- Disease restricted to gray matter (polioencephalitis)
- Disease restricted to white matter (leucoencephalitis)
- Disease of both gray and white matter (panencephalitis)

Most viral infections of the CNS cause some degree of meningeal inflammation, but it is rare for this to result in meningitis.

Aseptic Meningitis
This is usually a benign short-lived illness with meningitic features such as headache, photophobia, and neck stiffness predominating. The CSF shows a predominance of lymphocytes, protein may be elevated but glucose is typically normal.

Over 80% of cases are due to non-polio enteroviruses such as echovirus, the coxsackieviruses, and enterovirus 71. Other viruses commonly implicated in aseptic meningitis include Herpes simplex type 2, mumps, arboviruses, measles, parainfluenza, adenovirus, LCV, and HIV (58). One of the clinical challenges in diagnosing aseptic meningitis is to beware of missing another condition, as there is a very wide differential diagnosis (58).

Table 1 Common Bacteria Causing Meningitis at Different Ages

Neonates
   Streptococcus agalactiae (Group B Streptococcus)
   Escherichia coli (*E. coli*)
   Listeria monocytogenes (*L. monocytogenes*)
   Streptococcus pneumoniae
Also:
   Enterobacter species
   Pseudomonas aeruginosa
   Citrobacter species
   Staphylococci (*S. aureus* and *S. epidermidis*)
Infants
   Hemophilus influenzae
   Neisseria meningitides
   Streptococcus pneumoniae
Children and young adults
   Neisseria meningitides
   Streptococcus pneumoniae
Older adults
   Listeria monocytogenes
   Streptococcus pneumoniae

Acute Bacterial Meningitis

General

Acute bacterial meningitis is caused by a variety of infectious agents (Table 1), with age being a major factor in determining which organism is most likely (54). There are few medical conditions where prompt diagnosis and appropriate antibiotic therapy are as essential in diminishing mortality and morbidity.

The incidence of acute bacterial meningitis peaks in the very old and the very young, with neonatal meningitis seen in 2–10 per 10,000 live births (88). A seasonal variation may be seen with meningococcal meningitis, which may occur in epidemics, and meningitis is seen more often in socioeconomically deprived groups (51).

While most cases are spontaneous in origin, in some cases underlying immunological or anatomical factors may play a role. From a neurosurgical point of view, a CSF fistula, which may be spontaneous or due to a congenital defect in the skull base, trauma, surgery, or hydrocephalus, is an important and treatable cause of recurrent meningitis. Meningitis may also complicate craniotomy or CSF diversion procedures such as external ventricular drains or ventriculo-peritoneal shunts (VPS) and all neurosurgeons are aware of the disastrous consequences of infection in the setting of a neonate with open dysraphism (Fig. 3).

Pathogenesis and Pathology

The organisms initially colonize the nasopharynx or other musocal surfaces, invade and spread via the bloodstream to cross the blood–brain barrier at vulnerable sites such as the choroid plexus epithelium or cerebral microvascular endothelium (88). Meningitis can also follow direct implantation due to trauma or at the time of neurological surgery, or can be associated with skull base defects such as a dermal sinus. A local source such as otitis or sinusitis may be present and portend a worse prognosis (112). Host defenses are limited once organisms have entered the CSF, as there are few resident macrophages and low levels of immunoglobulins and complement; however, stimulation of proinflammatory cytokines attracts leucocytes. Increased blood–brain barrier permeability may lead to cerebral edema and the increased protein and number of cells increases the viscosity of the CSF (88).

The hallmark of this condition is a purulent exudate in the subarachnoid space that engulfs vessels and cranial nerves. In the first day or two, this may be visible only as cloudiness in the cisterns or thin creamy lines alongside meningeal veins, but within three to seven days the entire brain may be enveloped in pus (39). Initially, there is virtually no inflammatory change

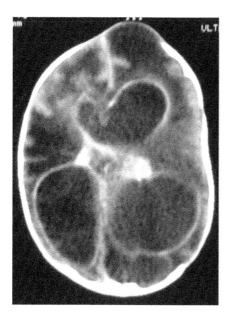

Figure 3 This neonate with a myelomeningocele was referred from a rural area; by the time of presentation the lesion was already infected. CT scan with contrast shows avid enhancement of the ependyma with marked ventriculomegaly; the infant subsequently died.

in the cortex, but fibrinoid necrosis and thrombosis of vessels may later lead to cortical infarcts. If the infection spreads to the ventricles, the ependyma is denuded and ventriculitis may lead to accumulation of thick pus (pyocephalus).

Neuronal injury may be due to direct toxic effects, ischemia, and raised intracranial pressure. In the early phase, an increase in cerebral blood flow is seen, but development of vasculitis leads to ischemia. This can either be focal (because of occlusion of vessels in the subarachnoid space) or global, as a result of raised intracranial pressure. Raised intracranial pressure may be due to cerebral edema (which is vasogenic, cytotoxic, or interstitial in origin), venous sinus thrombosis, extra-axial collections such as effusions and empyema or hydrocephalus.

It is easy to appreciate how thickening of the meninges leads to hydrocephalus, but it is remarkable that hydrocephalus is not a common complication of meningitis in adults, seen in only 3% in one large prospective study (112).

Neonates are particularly vulnerable given their immature immune system and the neurobiology of the developing brain (78). The various pathological features have been documented in a detailed autopsy study; of relevance to this topic is the finding that 56% had hydrocephalus and all those who died more than three days after the onset of their meningitis had hydrocephalus (7). Where the ependyma was denuded, tufts of glial cells herniated through and in some cases formed glial bridges in the aqueduct and fourth ventricle, leading to narrowing or even occlusion. Experimental studies have demonstrated a similar process in the pathogenesis of intraventricular septations (122).

Chronic fibrosis obliterates the subarachnoid space; loss of cerebral cortical tissue and secondary white matter degeneration exacerbate hydrocephalus (7). This leads to the two major neuropathological sequelae of neonatal bacterial meningitis, namely, hydrocephalus and multicystic encephalopathy (52).

Clinical Presentation
It is helpful to consider three broad groups:

(i) Neonates
Two patterns of neonatal meningitis can be discerned (117). Early-onset sepsis (within the first week) is usually caused by infection just before or during labor (such as chorioamnionitis following prolonged rupture of membranes or vaginal infection); later onset is usually caused by neonatal sepsis, which is complicated by meningitis in 25% of cases. Both prematurity and

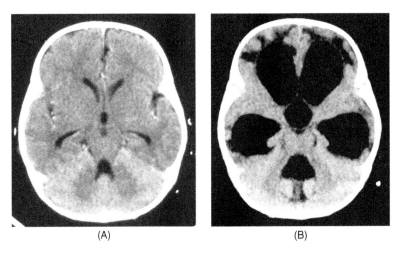

(A)   (B)

Figure 4 Neonate with *Streptococcus agalactiae* (Group B Streptococcus) meningitis. Initial CT with contrast at initial presentation (**A**) and follow-up CT one month later when the infant returned with clinically obvious hydrocephalus despite appropriate antibiotic therapy (**B**).

low birth weight are significant predisposing factors (117). In developed countries, *Streptococcus agalactiae* is the most common pathogen particularly in the first week (Fig. 4), but in developing countries enteric gram-negative bacilli (*Escherichia coli*, *Klebsiella*, *Enterobacter*, and *Salmonella*) are the leading pathogens (88). *Streptococcus pneumoniae*, various staphylococci, and *Listeria monocytogenes* may also be seen. Very low birth weight neonates are particularly vulnerable to nosocomial infections and coagulase-negative staphylococci have been reported to be the most common cause of meningitis in this group (27).

Meningitis may present insidiously in the neonate, with poor sucking, vomiting, recurrent apnea, temperature instability, and seizures.

(ii) Infants and young children

Streptococcus pneumoniae, *Neisseria meningitides*, and *Hemophilus influenzae* are the most common pathogens at this age and their incidence has fallen with routine immunization (88). Typically, the child presents with irritability and a full fontanelle, with fever, vomiting, and seizures.

(iii) Older children and adults

A recent prospective study found that 90% of adults with meningitis have either *S. pneumoniae* or *N. meningitidis* and present with at least two of the symptoms of headache, fever, neck stiffness, and altered mental status (112). Patients presented in coma in 14% of cases, 33% had focal deficits, and 39% had opening pressures above 400 mmH$_2$O on lumbar puncture (LP). Despite this, only 3% had hydrocephalus on CT scan.

In children and adults, the diagnosis is readily confirmed on LP. Neuroimaging usually plays no role in the acute setting, unless there is a contraindication to LP such as a depressed or deteriorating level of consciousness, focal signs or evidence of sinusitis or mastoiditis. In order to avoid delay in commencing treatment in this situation, blood culture should be performed and antibiotics prescribed according to local guidelines.

Meningitis caused by *Listeria* warrants special mention, as this condition is more common at the extremes of age and also in patients who are immunosuppressed, accounting for 8% of cases of bacterial meningitis in the United States (93). The diagnosis may be overlooked, as patients may have no meningeal signs and the CSF cell count may not be raised. Hydrocephalus may occur, but this is not a common complication—in an extensive review analyzing 776 published cases of listerial meningitis, 54 patients underwent a CT scan and 11 had hydrocephalus (68).

Management
Prevention
Universal immunization with conjugated vaccines against *H. influenzae* type B has virtually eradicated this disease in many countries, and the introduction of a polyvalent conjugated vaccine against *S. pneumoniae* is expected to achieve similar results.

Medical
Analgesics and antipyretics are usually indicated and some patients require admission to an intensive care unit. The presence of hyponatremia has sometimes led to fluids being restricted, but cerebral hypoperfusion may ensue and it is now recommended that clinicians aim to maintain euvolemia (60).

Intravenous antibiotics are the mainstay of treatment; there are various regimens, but it is important to choose the correct agent given the most likely organism (this is largely dictated by the patient's age) and use an adequate dose. The choice of antibiotic needs to be reviewed when culture and sensitivities are available; optimum duration of therapy varies from a week for meningococcal meningitis to 10 to 14 days for *S. agalactiae*, *S. pneumoniae*, and *H. influenzae*, and up to 21 days for Gram-negative organisms.

The place of steroids remains controversial. A recent Cochrane review concluded that corticosteroids reduce rates of mortality, severe hearing loss, and neurological sequelae and advised that corticosteroids should be administered together with the first antibiotic dose in adults. In children, data support the use of adjunctive corticosteroids in high-income countries, but evidence for benefit is lacking for children in low-income countries (113).

Neuroimaging is indicated when the patient fails to improve clinically or manifests features of raised intracranial pressure. Usually, CT scan is adequate, but MRI may be more helpful in demonstrating areas of ischemia and vascular studies such as CT or MR venography may be helpful in delineating venous sinus thrombosis. Administration of contrast may demonstrate complications such as ventriculitis or empyema.

Surgical aspects
Although surgery seldom plays a role in the management of acute bacterial meningitis, a number of complications may require surgical intervention. These include the development of hydrocephalus, subdural effusions and empyemas, and brain abscesses.

Hydrocephalus
Ventricular dilatation may occasionally be seen early in the disease, most likely due to blockage of the CSF pathways by inflammatory exudate (64), but hydrocephalus is more commonly seen later as a postmeningitic process. The typical presentation may range from bulging of the fontanelle and altered level of consciousness through to a squint and gradual enlargement of the head.

Management of acute HCP
In the acute setting, an external ventricular drain should be inserted until hydrocephalus has abated; in some cases, the drain can be removed after a short time without need of definitive CSF diversion (80). Hydrocephalus occurs often in newborns during the acute phase of meningitis, but their capacity to accommodate this coupled with the increased risks of an EVD in this group incline us to try to avoid inserting a drain. Hydrocephalus is seldom a clinical problem during the acute phase of nontuberculous bacterial meningitis in older children and adults.

Definitive management
When confronting progressive PMH, the neurosurgeon needs to choose between insertion of a VPS and performing ETV. The following factors are considered for deciding when and how to treat PMH definitively:

• Is the CSF sterile and the infection cured?
• Are there septations or loculations within the ventricles?
• Where is the block?

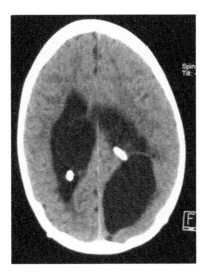

Figure 5 This young child was referred for shunt assessment having been managed at another center for hydrocephalus following *Serratia* meningitis; multiple shunts had been inserted as the child had developed septated ventricles and endoscopy had not been available.

Perhaps the most avoidable complication is reactivating meningitis by inserting a VPS before the infection is cured (24). An important consideration is how well the CSF pleocytosis has responded to treatment; we recommend deferring insertion of a shunt until the polymorphonuclear cell count is below 5 high power field, no organisms are visible on Gram stain and CSF culture is negative. This may be a conservative approach, but it has been our experience that inserting a shunt sooner is not advisable.

The presence of septa within the ventricle has been known since the era of ventriculography; of 105 children with PMH who underwent this investigation in Cape Town between 1971 and 1976, 23% had ventricular septa, ranging from a thin diaphanous membrane to thick bands (42). A number of these patients had previously had elevated CSF protein levels, leading the authors to suggest that this may play a role in the genesis of the septa.

The management of multilocular hydrocephalus will be dealt with elsewhere in this volume, but a few words are apposite as the most common etiology is infection (101); often such patients end up with multiple shunts (Fig. 5). One option is removal of the membranes under the microscope, converting this to a unilocular hydrocephalus (84), but this can now be accomplished in a less-invasive fashion using neuroendoscopy. These patients may well still require a shunt, but the key concept here is the use of the endoscope to simplify complex hydrocephalus and reduce the number of shunts required (101).

The role of ETV. There is remarkably little literature devoted to this topic—it has been pointed out that most children with PIH are reported as a subgroup in larger series (26); in this way, a number of experienced centers have noted that the rate of success of ETV is lower in this group (36,104). The largest series reported to date is a multicenter retrospective study, which comprised patients with a history of CSF infection or hemorrhage undergoing ETV over a seven-year period at seven leading neurosurgical centers on three continents (97). A total of 1294 ETVs were performed, 101 of whom were included in the study. Obstructive hydrocephalus had been triggered by hemorrhage or infection in 87, of whom 73 were children and 28 adults. Of the 42 with a history of infection, 64.3% were successfully managed with ETV; success rates in children and adults were 55.6% and 80%, respectively. The overall success rate in the group with hemorrhage alone was similar at 60.9%, but in those patients with a history of infection *and* hemorrhage, the success rate fell to a paltry 23.1% (97).

A further difficulty in interpreting this data is the fact that 55.4% of the patients had previously had a shunt. This also applies to a study from the United States, which reported an overall success rate of 60% in ETV in the setting of previous CNS infection, but all of the patients who experienced unequivocal success had been previously shunted (100). It has been known for some years that shunt independence may occur in some clinical settings, including PMH (2,24).

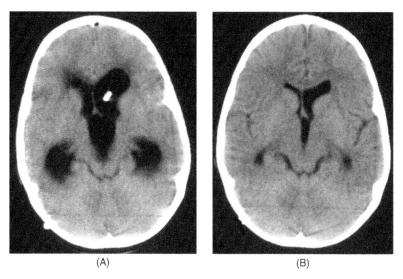

(A)   (B)

Figure 6   This infant presented with acute hydrocephalus (**A**) following *Listeria* meningitis, successfully managed by ETV (**B**).

The largest experience with ETV in the setting of PIH has been that published by Warf, reporting 300 children treated in Uganda in a period of less than two years (116). Infection was considered to be the leading cause of hydrocephalus in this group. As the CSF is usually sterile by the time PIH presents, it is helpful that the criteria for a diagnosis of PIH were clearly specified—there was no history consistent with hydrocephalus at birth, *and* there was either a history of a febrile illness/seizures preceding the onset of progressive enlargement of the head *or* imaging/intraoperative findings indicative of prior ventriculitis. On this basis, the infection was considered to be the cause in 60%, and in three-quarters this occurred in the first month of life. In this setting, the success rate of ETV was 59% for those under one year of age and 81% for those older than one year (116).

In our view, it is certainly worth considering ETV in those cases that have a convincing "triventricular" pattern (Fig. 6).

Empyema/subdural effusions

Subdural effusion was reported as a complication of meningitis in 1950 following the introduction of antibiotics (65). This condition is most commonly seen in *Haemophilus* and *S. pneumoniae* and has now virtually disappeared in countries were routine vaccination occurs. Indications for drainage include a persistently spiking fever or rising septic markers, bulging fontanelle, or increasing head circumference. It may be difficult to rule out a subdural empyema on imaging (although typically there is marked enhancement of the cortical surface), and this may be an indication for drainage (Fig. 7).

Effusions can often be tapped percutaneously (obviously observing strict sterile precautions), but if large or recurrent, may require burr-hole drainage and even occasionally insertion of a subdural-peritoneal shunt.

Abscess

Brain abscesses can occasionally occur as a complication of neonatal meningitis, almost invariably due to the enteric Gram-negative rods *Citrobacter koseri*, *Seratia marcescens*, and *Enterobacter sakazakii* (117) as well as *Proteus mirabilis* (Fig. 8). Brain abscess was reported in 77% of cases of *Citrobacter* meningitis, as compared to a reported incidence of 10% with other types of enteric Gram-negative meningitis (38). *Proteus mirabilis* was the cause of 90% of neonatal brain abscesses reported from Paris; 47% went on to develop hydrocephalus. The authors point out that this condition was seldom reported in clinical series prior to the advent of CT and ultrasound and missing this complication may have contributed to the high morbidity and mortality of neonatal meningitis (83).

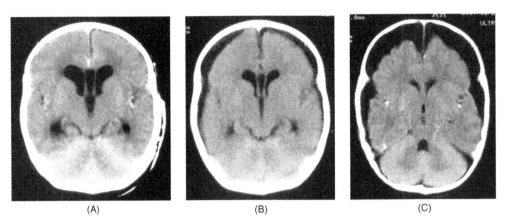

(A)   (B)   (C)

Figure 7   This infant presented with *Haemophilus* meningitis. Initial CT scan showed enhancement of the arachnoid and mild ventriculomegaly (**A**). Follow-up CT two weeks later revealed moderate subdural collections; empyema was considered unlikely due to the absence of pial enhancement (**B**). Despite burr-hole drainage of the subdural effusions, marked progression was evident two weeks later (**C**) and the child eventually required placement of a subdural-peritoneal shunt.

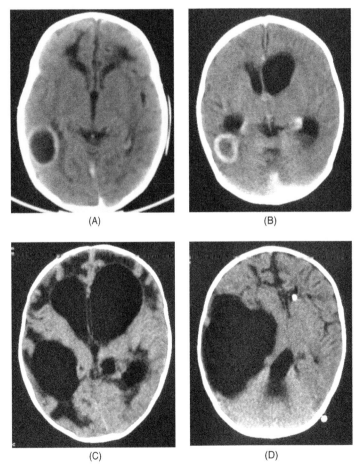

Figure 8   This infant was referred from a peripheral hospital for management of a brain abscess after *Proteus* was isolated on blood culture. As the response to antibiotics was unsatisfactory (**A**), the abscess was tapped via a burr-hole (**B**) and the patient was discharged back to the referring hospital to complete the course of antibiotics. The child returned with severe hydrocephalus (**C**) necessitating insertion of a left VP shunt and subsequently developed an isolated right temporal horn (**D**). A second shunt was required following an unsuccessful attempt to fenestrate this into the cisterns.

Outcome

Neonatal meningitis has a case-fatality rate of 20% to 25% and half of all survivors have significant long-term neurological sequelae such as hearing impairment, mental retardation, cerebral palsy, seizure disorders, and hydrocephalus (117). Although the mortality for PMH has
improved over the years, long-term neurological function is often disappointing. Lorber and
Pickering reported that 5 of their 19 patients with PMH died and only 7 (37%) made a complete
recovery (57). The authors emphasized, however, that predicting outcome was difficult and
advised giving every patient the benefit of the doubt in offering active treatment.

Tuberculous Meningitis

General

Tuberculosis (TB) has afflicted mankind for millennia—the earliest recorded specimen of tuberculous disease in man dates back to 5000 BC. Whytt described the clinical picture and autopsy
findings of 10 cases of hydrocephalus and meningitis in 1768; although some of these patients
would seem to have suffered from tuberculous meningitis (TBM), basal meningitis was only
described as a distinct entity well into the 19th century (103).

Substantial progress in managing TB was made in the 20th century, such that a few decades
ago it was thought that the disease was gradually being vanquished. However, recent years
have seen a major resurgence in TB, particularly in developing countries, to the point that the
WHO recently declared it a global emergency (37). Concerns around the emergence of strains
resistant to two front-line drugs, isoniazid (INH) and rifampicin (RIF) (Multidrug resistant TB
or MDR-TB), have now been compounded by the challenges posed by extended drug-resistant
TB (XDR-TB) (59,82).

TBM is the most lethal form of systemic tuberculosis, particularly when associated with
hydrocephalus, and in some parts of the world, it is now the most common form of bacterial
meningitis; in Sub-Saharan Africa, this has largely happened on the back of the HIV pandemic
(28,59).

Pathogenesis and Pathology

Tuberculosis is caused by infection with *Mycobacterium tuberculosis* (MTB), an aerobic, nonmotile,
rod-shaped bacterium that can be identified on Ziehl–Neelsen stain (acid-fast bacillus). It is
particularly slow growing with a generation time 20 times that of common bacteria and culture
of the organism can take up to eight weeks. Consequently, culture of MTB plays no role in the
initial diagnosis and management of the disease, but this becomes important should one not see
an adequate clinical response, as the specter of multidrug resistance (MDR) or extended drug
resistance (XDR) then looms.

Infection occurs after inhalation of airborne droplet nuclei, which initiate infection in the
lung, resulting in primary pulmonary disease. Phagocytes carry bacilli to regional lymph nodes,
which enlarge and form the co-called "primary complex" with the lung lesion; a cell-mediated,
delayed hypersensitivity immune response is activated in the host.

The patient may remain asymptomatic and never develop clinical disease or may go on
to develop progressive pulmonary disease or experience hematogenous dissemination, which
in its most severe form may present as miliary TB. Reactivated disease may occur later in life.
In general, TBM is typically a disease of young children in countries with a high incidence of
the disease and is seen more often in adults in countries with a low incidence, arising from
reactivation of a dormant focus (23,28).

Involvement of the central nervous system

Conventional understanding of the development of TBM is that the organism spreads via the
blood to the CNS where it develops as a parenchymal or subpial focus as described by Rich
and McCordock (85). Mycobacteria enter the CSF space when this subpial lesion (often referred
to as "Rich's focus") ruptures into the subarachnoid space, giving rise to the typical meningeal
reaction with a thick, yellow, and gelatinous exudate in the basal cisterns (29). The present
authors are not aware of an explanation for this marked predilection for the basal cisterns and
wonder how this relates to the "Rich's focus" model of pathogenesis. Other possible routes into

the CSF include rupture of a focus in the choroid plexus or elsewhere in the ventricle, spread from a contiguous bony structure or delayed rupture of a previously controlled caseous focus.

The two most important consequences of the meningeal reaction are vascular injury and hydrocephalus.

Vascular injury

The basal arteries of the circle of Willis and their perforators are the most commonly involved vessels. They are affected by vasculitis, intraluminal thrombosis, external compression, and vasospasm (22,23). Consequently, cerebral ischemia is common and the development of infarcts portends poor outcome. The distribution of infarcts favors the basal ganglia, thalamus, and internal capsule, but hemispheric infarctions also occur frequently (16,103,108). A major consideration is that infarction may develop even after treatment has been started (108), even when ICP is normalized (34). This is probably the most important reason that patients with tuberculous hydrocephalus (TBH) fail to improve clinically or even deteriorate further despite aggressive medical treatment and early CSF shunting. Future treatment strategies may require modification to address this issue of ongoing ischemia (34).

Hydrocephalus

Hydrocephalus is nearly always present in cases of TBM who survive more than four to six weeks and this is mainly due to blockage of the basal cisterns by tuberculous exudate in the acute stage and adhesive leptomeningitis in the chronic stage.

Although this typically results in communicating hydrocephalus, noncommunicating hydrocephalus is reported to occur in approximately 17% of cases, a figure that is similar in incidence to other forms of infectious hydrocephalus, based on older studies where the level of CSF block was documented (24). Tuberculous exudate may obstruct the outlet foramina of the fourth ventricle (56) or the aqueduct may be narrowed due to circumferential compression by meningeal exudate, mesencephalic edema, or a tuberculoma (103). Of course, more than one of these mechanisms may be relevant in an individual patient.

In treated cases of TBM, the subarachnoid space may be obliterated, as the gelatinous exudate is gradually replaced by connective tissue; areas of caseation may be found within this, as well as granulation tissue that develops from arachnoid trabeculae (103). In the long term, the exudate may resolve or remain in the form of tubercles, encapsulated caseous foci, or scar tissue; the incidence of hydrocephalus is consequently higher in treated than in untreated cases (103). There is a further possibility that venous obstruction may also play a role in the pathogenesis of TBH.

Clinical Presentation and Diagnosis

The diagnosis of TBM in the acute setting is usually made in the context of clinical suspicion with suggestive findings in the CSF and typical features on CT scan (Fig. 9).

Clinical

The prevalence of the disease in the community determines the degree of clinical suspicion. The diagnosis is suggested by a history of a TB contact with a positive tuberculin skin test or Mantoux. The chest X-ray may show findings typical of pulmonary TB and the organism may be identified or cultured from sputum or gastric washings. The greatest challenge is to make the diagnosis early, which is difficult due to the nonspecific early features of TBM; a recent review of 554 pediatric cases seen over a 20-year period found that 91% had poor weight gain or weight loss and this may be an important clue (114).

CSF

The gold standard for the diagnosis of TBM is the demonstration of acid-fast bacilli under the microscope or the culture of the bacillus from a specimen of CSF. There is astonishing variability in the results of direct smear, which has been reported as positive in anywhere between 10% and 90% of cases. Culture rates are generally low, depending on how many specimens and what volumes of CSF are sent; higher rates of culture may be achieved when larger volumes of CSF are processed.

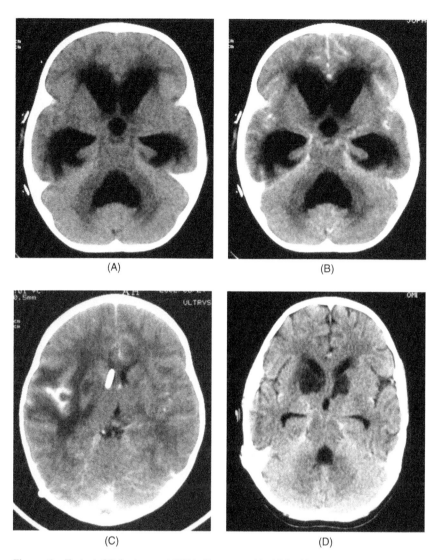

Figure 9 Typical CT features of TBM. Two-year-old child with severe hydrocephalus (**A**), administration of intravenous contrast demonstrates the characteristic basal enhancement (**B**). One month after insertion of a shunt, the hydrocephalus has resolved, but there is residual enhancement in the right Sylvian fissure (**C**). Axial enhanced CT scan of a different patient, demonstrating bilateral caudate infarcts (**D**).

CSF typically shows pleocytosis, with a cell count seldom greater than 500 cells/mm³. Lymphocytes predominate, although polymorphs may be more numerous on occasion, particularly in the early phase of the disease. CSF glucose is typically low. Protein is elevated, usually in the region of 0.8 to 3 g/L, but may be dramatically elevated, especially in lumbar CSF. For all CSF parameters, there is often a discrepancy between ventricular and lumbar specimens. Other specialized tests include the bromide partition test, adenosine deaminase test, and nucleic acid amplification tests, but these are not widely used.

Radiology
Early reports of the value of the CT scan in TBM (13) have stood the test of time; the typical CT appearance of TBM is often described as a triad of contrast enhancement of the basal meninges with hydrocephalus and infarcts (45). Hyperdensity may be noted in the basal cisterns before administering contrast and this represents the cisternal exudate (3). Low densities related to cerebral ischemia are common, particularly in the basal ganglia and occasionally

there may be accompanying tuberculomas or tuberculous abscesses. It is important to note that there is no direct correlation between ventricular size and ICP in TBM (90). Unfortunately, most patients with TBM do not have ready access to MRI—this modality provides additional infor mation about the consequences of the disease and may be useful in evaluating the response to therapy (108).

Staging
In reporting their results in TBM in 1948, the Streptomycin in Tuberculosis Trials Committee of the British Medical Research Council classified patients into three groups, namely, "early," "advanced," and "medium" (10). This has subsequently been modified to

- Stage 1—Normal consciousness, nonspecific symptoms or signs.
- Stage 2—Awake patient with minor focal signs, meningeal irritation, and lethargy.
- Stage 3—Obtunded patient, severe neurological deficits.

Palur and coworkers described a similar classification that included a prognostically significant fourth stage for deeply comatose patients, who experienced a mortality rate of 100% on long-term follow-up if CSF diversion was required (73). More recently, this scale has been modified to include the Glasgow Coma Score (106).

More than half of all patients affected are disabled by or die from the disease (106). Outcome is related to the stage of presentation; however, a decreased level of consciousness in TBM may be due to elevated intracranial pressure, cerebral ischemia, hyponatremia, seizures, and/or tuberculous encephalopathy. Outcome therefore depends also on the cause of the decreased level of consciousness and the speed of intervention. Apart from the presenting level of consciousness, hydrocephalus and infarcts are the most important predictors of outcome (73,91).

Management
Medical management of the infection
As with any chronically ill patient, attention to nutrition, analgesia, and skilled nursing care are fundamental. It is generally accepted that treatment with four drugs should be continued at least for six months, but 9 to 12 months may be better (9,71,106). Antituberculous medication comprises an initial intensive phase with four drugs—isoniazid and rifampicin are pyrazinamide recommended together with streptomycin or ethambutol or ethionamide. This is followed by a continuation phase of 6 to 10 months; pyridoxine should be given with isoniazid (106). Despite early reports as to the efficacy of steroids, controversy surrounded this issue until recently. There is now consensus that they are of benefit in children (92) and adults (105) in reducing mortality and possibly morbidity and this has been substantiated by a recent systematic review (79). Follow-up imaging is helpful in surveillance of hydrocephalus and infarcts (4).

Management of hydrocephalus in TBM
The optimal management of tuberculous hydrocephalus is controversial and has been debated perhaps more than for any other form of hydrocephalus in recent years. It appears that each institution has its own protocol for treatment. The two main areas of contention are the indications for surgery and the choice of operation.

Medical management
Nonsurgical treatment of communicating hydrocephalus is an attractive alternative and will be efficacious in three quarter of all children with proven communicating hydrocephalus (114). This strategy does, however, depend on demonstrating CSF communication convincingly and entails a commitment to monitoring CSF pressures and ventricular dilatation for up to a month before one can be confident that surgery has been avoided. In order to do this safely, air encephalography (32,114) or other dynamic studies are required to demonstrate communication between the ventricular and subarachnoid CSF. An important pitfall in managing patients with TBM is the poor correlation of ventricular size with intracranial pressure (12,90).

Medical treatment for hydrocephalus includes acetazolamide in adequate doses (50 mg/kg) and furosemide (114) and/or repeated lumbar punctures (115). Those who fail medical management, 25% in Schoeman's experience (114), require CSF diversion.

Surgery

Cairns described the various surgical interventions applicable to TBM midway through the 20th century (14), most of which were rendered obsolete by the advent of reliable shunts. Bhagwati was first to report the use of ventriculoatrial shunts in TBM hydrocephalus in 1971, and the following decade saw a number of enthusiastic reports about the results of shunt insertion (8,12,75). Ventriculoperitoneal shunts became the preferred option, as early concerns about the potential for spread of TB to the peritoneal cavity proved unfounded, but two major concerns did, however, arise. Many patients did not do well after shunt insertion, particularly those with a markedly depressed level of consciousness, leading some to propose insertion of an external ventricular drain as a temporary measure and then shunting those who responded (63,73). Furthermore, shunt complications appear to be more common and have been reported in more than half of the patients shunted in some series (53,94). As many of these patients live in Developing Countries, the financial costs of a shunt coupled with difficulty accessing care in the event of complications are real concerns.

Various groups have published their experience with ETV in TBH (Table 2). Most groups advocate performing ETV utilizing the conventional approach through the floor of the third ventricle, but one group described fenestrating the lamina terminalis (70). The indications for ETV in this setting vary from all patients being considered as candidates to stricter selection of patients based on demonstrated noncommunicating hydrocephalus.

ETV has been recommended as the first choice operation for patients with TBH, with shunts reserved for failed ETV cases (43). Outcome of the hydrocephalus in this study was satisfactory in 50% and acceptable in 18%; as medical treatment alone is reported to be successful in 75% (114), the benefit of this approach is debatable. It has been suggested that ETV may be helpful in communicating hydrocephalus (96), perhaps altering pulse pressure, which may play a role in the pathogenesis of chronic hydrocephalus (41).

Various centers use conventional CT imaging in order to distinguish communicating from noncommunicating hydrocephalus. However, conventional imaging is highly inaccurate for this purpose (11,32). In fact, success rates for ETV in TBM for suspected noncommunicating hydrocephalus, or indeed other forms of infectious hydrocephalus, may reflect the fact that up to 40% of patients with communicating hydrocephalus are thought to have noncommunicating hydrocephalus by conventional imaging (32).

Table 2 Reports of Endoscopic Third Ventriculostomy (ETV) in the Management of Hydrocephalus Complicating Tuberculous Meningitis (TBM)

References	Patients	Success	Comments
(31)	2 (Children)	100%	Selection of cases using preoperative modified AEG and postoperative confirmation by column test
(70)	1 (Adult)	100%	EVD placed and contrast ventriculogram performed before and after ETV
(48)	2 (Adults)	100%	Chronic hydrocephalus with VPS dysfunction
(95)	35 (Children and adults)	77% VPS avoidance	Clinical features raised ICP with CT evidence of ventriculomegaly; 16 patients (46%) considered to have communicating hydrocephalus preoperatively
(43)	28 (10 Children and adults)	50% VPS avoidance	Heterogenous group of patients, 9 had additional procedures; ETV if clinical and CT evidence of raised ICP and hydrocephalus
(47)	14 (9 Children and 5 adults)	64.2% VPS avoidance	Patients who required CSF diversion were offered ETV if CT showed triventricular or tetraventricular dilatation
(33)	17 (All children)	41% Confirmed communication postoperatively and VPS avoided	14 acute TBM, selection of cases with noncommunicating hydrocephalus as previously described

Abbreviations: AEG, air encephalogram; CSF, cerebrospinal fluid; VPS, ventriculoperitoneal shunt.

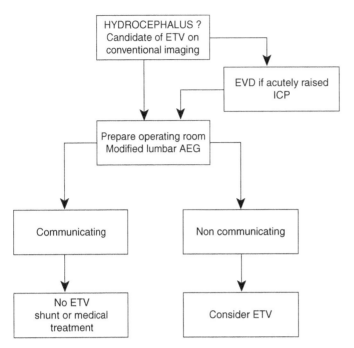

Figure 10   Suggested algorithm for management of tuberculous hydrocephalus. *Source*: From Ref. 32.

As the purpose of ETV is to communicate the ventricular system with the basal cisterns, the present authors are not convinced that there is any value in performing an ETV in the presence of clear communicating hydrocephalus where the block appears to be distal to the prepontine cistern. A case has been described where contrast ventriculography was utilized to demonstrate obstruction prior to endoscopy (70). We have previously published an algorithm (Fig. 10) that was developed in order to try to establish where the block lies in order to rationalize surgical decision making (32). This entails doing a modified air encephalogram as described by Lorber in 1951 (56) to establish whether the patient has communicating or noncommunicating hydrocephalus (Fig. 11). This does entail some risk if noncommunicating hydrocephalus is indeed present, so this is only done in consultation with a neurosurgeon to ensure that there will be no delay in operating, should this be necessary. Some may object that this is invasive, but to our knowledge there is not yet a sufficiently reliable MRI sequence and, even if there

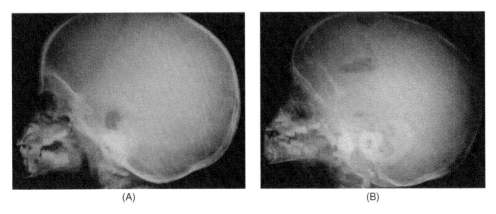

Figure 11   Lateral skull radiograph of an air encephalogram (AEG) demonstrating noncommunicating hydrocephalus with no intraventricular air (**A**). Following successful ETV, air is seen in the lateral ventricle following a repeat AEG (**B**). *Source*: From Ref. 32.

were, most patients with tuberculous hydrocephalus live in places where ready access to MRI is a distant dream.

The technical challenges in performing ETV in the setting of TBM have now been extensively reported (31,33,43,47,95). These include distorted anatomy of the third ventricle, thickened and fibrous third ventricular floor, and extensive exudate in the basal cisterns that makes identification of the cisternal space and the major vessels difficult. These technical challenges increase the difficulty of the procedure, potentially increase the risk of complications (especially in inexperienced hands), and decrease the likelihood of success compared to conventional cases. Therefore, the authors agree with the view that selection of patients is important in order to maximize success and avoid an inappropriate operation in those who would be better off with a shunt ab initio (98).

In view of the challenges encountered in acute TBM, one experienced center reserves ETV for "burnt-out" hydrocephalus when the patient presents with shunt dysfunction (48). Loculation of the ventricular system is common in TBM (33); therefore endoscopic fenestration to simplify the hydrocephalus may also help to avoid multiple shunts. However, it should be remembered that the membranes to be fenestrated may be particularly fibrous. Thorough preoperative planning and adequate endoscopic tools, as in most indications for fenestration, are essential if the procedure is to be successful.

Some patients with predominantly obstructive hydrocephalus may be adequately treated with ETV alone, but it is important to remember that some patients may still have inadequate CSF absorption and will therefore require medical management of their communicating hydrocephalus.

Outcome

Although the majority of children with TBM survive, their long-term neurological, psychometric, and behavioral outcomes are very disappointing—only 16% of children in Schoeman's 20-year experience had a good outcome (114). The presence of hydrocephalus portends a poorer outcome; although this may largely reflect more advanced disease, it presents a challenge to neurosurgeons, as hydrocephalus is a condition we believe we can treat effectively. There is little doubt that much of the damage is a consequence of ischemia and this is an aspect that calls for novel approaches in the years to come (34).

Fungal Meningitis

Fungi are ubiquitous in the environment but seldom pathogenic; the growing number of immunocompromised individuals has, however, seen a rise in the number of fungal opportunistic infections.

Fungal organisms are most commonly seen either in the form of yeasts, up to 20 μm in diameter (Blastomyces, Candida, Coccidioides, Cryptococcus, and Histoplasma) or branching hyphae (Aspergillus). Generally, the smaller forms reach the capillaries and produce meningitis, while the larger hyphae occlude blood vessels, resulting in infarcts (110).

Neurosurgical aspects of fungal infections have been described in detail (89) and specific recommendations regarding antifungal therapy can be sourced elsewhere; attention will be confined to those aspects relevant to hydrocephalus as a complication.

Cryptococcosis

The causative organism, *Cryptococcus neoformans* (formerly known as *Torula histolytica*) is a ubiquitous environmental saprophyte, which is found worldwide. Prior to the AIDS pandemic, fewer than 1000 cases of cryptococcal meningitis (CM) were seen annually in the United States, but the last two decades have seen a dramatic increase in cases worldwide (40). Inhalation of yeasts may lead to an initial pulmonary infection that is either cleared, contained within granulomata, or disseminates, depending on the interplay between the number and virulence of the organisms and the host immune response (46).

Defects in T cell–mediated immunity predispose to dissemination, and the brain is a common target organ. In the setting of HIV, most episodes of CM probably represent reactivation of latent infection in profoundly immunosuppressed patients (CD4 counts <100 cells/μL). The diagnosis is usually straightforward with features of raised intracranial pressure often seen in addition to the typical symptoms and signs of meningitis. India ink staining of CSF is highly likely to be positive and a serological test (CLAT) is also available. It is thought that raised ICP is due to fungal organisms that shed polysaccharide, impairing CSF absorption at the arachnoid villi (46).

Antifungal therapy is usually initiated with intravenous Amphotericin B with or without flucytosine for two weeks, followed by an 8-week consolidation phase with either fluconazole or itraconazole (46). Although this regime is generally well tolerated, Amphotericin B–based regimens are not an option in the resource-poor settings where most of the world's HIV-positive patients live and different treatment approaches are needed (99). High opening pressures and a poor inflammatory response in the CSF are associated with poor outcome, while the most important predictors of death are high organism burden at baseline and abnormal mental status.

Raised ICP

This is a common problem in CM in AIDS, with over half of the patients in a large trial having opening pressures over 25 cm H_2O (40). Despite the high CSF pressure, ventricular size is often normal (Fig. 12). A prospective trial of acetazolamide was terminated prematurely due to adverse effects (72). Most patients are managed with serial lumbar punctures; insertion of a temporary lumbar drain has been recommended as an option in patients whose pressure remains elevated (61). A proportion of patients will develop ventricular dilatation (Fig. 13) and insertion of a VP shunt may be indicated. This has been efficacious in non-HIV CM (74), although patients already in coma may not respond (55). HIV-infected patient may also experience long-term benefit from shunt insertion, even in the absence of ventriculomegaly (120).

Other Fungi

CNS Aspergillosis usually presents as an abscess, and meningitis is not common (87). The most common organism is *Aspergillus fumigatus*; this typically invades vessels, and early surgery together with combination therapy utilizing the newer antifungal drugs improves the outcome (21). Hydrocephalus is occasionally seen as a complication.

Candida spp are normal saprophytes but constitute the most common CNS pathogen in patients dying from AIDS (110). Candida most commonly invades via the gastrointestinal tract but also colonizes central lines, external ventricular drains, and shunts.

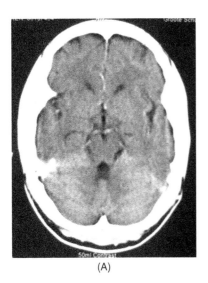
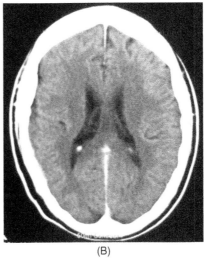

| (A) | (B) |

Figure 12   Adult HIV-positive patient on Amphotericin B for cryptococcal meningitis; (**A**) despite active disease, there is negligible basal enhancement and (**B**) there is minimal ventricular dilatation, although opening pressure on lumbar puncture remained persistently high.

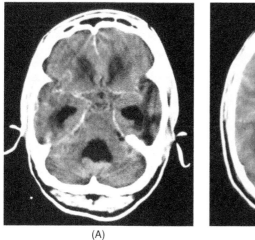
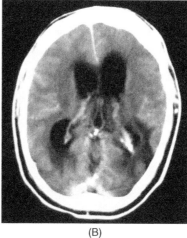

(A) (B)

Figure 13 Adult HIV-positive patient on Amphotericin B for cryptococcal meningitis; **(A)** marked hydrocephalus requiring insertion of a VP shunt. Note the enhancement of the choroid plexus in part **(B)**.

Candida may therefore complicate the treatment of preexisting hydrocephalus, or be the causative organism, particularly in neonates (117).

Coccidioidomycosis is due to infection with *Coccidioides immitis*, a fungus endemic to South and Central America, Mexico, and the southwest United States (102). Although extrapulmonary infection is rare in individuals who are not immunocompromised or diabetic, basal meningitis is the most significant complication. It is important to note that the organism is seldom isolated from the CSF and the diagnosis is usually based on CSF serology (119). The dense arachnoid fibrosis that ensues means that hydrocephalus is a common complication; early shunt placement is recommended and these patients require indefinite antifungal therapy (86).

Hydrocephalus has also been described as a complication of meningitis due to Blastomycosis and Paracoccidioides (89).

Hydrocephalus in HIV–AIDS

UNAIDS estimates that 30 to 36 million people are living with HIV, of whom 67% reside in Sub-Saharan Africa (111). The advent of effective antiretroviral drugs (ARVs) has markedly improved the quality of life and prognosis for those patients who can access such treatment. HIV is a neurotropic virus that has direct effects on the brain, resulting in a wide spectrum of neurocognitive sequelae, opportunistic infections, and neoplasms.

Well thought-out approaches to the diagnostic approach to lesions have been developed (17); with the exception of CM, there is not much literature on the management of hydrocephalus in the setting of HIV.

TBM

Thwaites and coworkers performed a prospective comparison of 528 Vietnamese adults recruited into a trial of dexamethasone treatment in TBM; all received four-drug antituberculous therapy. All were tested for antibodies to HIV; 96 were positive but none received ARVs. Mortality at nine months was significantly higher in the HIV-infected group (64.6% vs. 28.2%). No mention is made of neuroimaging, but it is likely that a number of patients had hydrocephalus, as lumbar opening pressure of up to 41 cm H_2O were recorded (107).

One study has specifically addressed the potential prognostic significance of hydrocephalus in this group of patients. Nadvi et al. reported a series of 30 South African patients who underwent insertion of a VP shunt for presumed tuberculous hydrocephalus and received supervised in-hospital four-drug antituberculous therapy and prednisone; 50% of the patients were HIV+ and again, none received ARVs (69).

Patients were graded on admission as Grade 1 to 4 using the scale described by Palur et al. (73) and at discharge using the Glasgow Outcome Scale of Jennet and Bond. Seventy-four percent of the HIV+ group experienced poor outcomes (GOS 1–3) and no patient experienced a good outcome (GOS 5), while 40% of HIV− patients experienced good recovery (69). The groups were not exactly matched (the HIV− group was predominantly pediatric with a median age of 7 as compared to a median age of 27 in the HIV+ group) but the message was clear. It is possible that increasing availability of ARVs in the Developing World will improve this very dismal picture, but that remains to be investigated.

Immune Reconstitution Inflammatory Syndrome

While commencement of ART usually results in a marked improvement in the patient's clinical condition, a subgroup deteriorates as a direct result of this rapid restoration of antigen-specific immune responses (25). This may be manifest in various ways, most commonly either with a new disease, through the "unmasking" of a previously inapparent infection, or with para-doxical worsening of a condition for which the patient was already being treated. Tuberculous meningitis and cryptococcal meningitis are particularly important conditions in this regard and either may present with worsening hydrocephalus (Fig. 14).

CONCLUDING REMARKS

Public health measures have had a significant impact on the epidemiology of hydrocephalus in the Developed World over the past few decades. Folate supplementation led to a marked reduction in hydrocephalus in the setting of dysraphism, and a similar impact has been seen on the incidence of similar PMH with immunization against *Haemophilus* and *Pneumococcus*. The challenge is to implement these measures in the Developing World where the major-ity of the world's population live. New strategies to curb TBM and HIV are also urgently needed.

New imaging modalities, coupled with the advent of neuroendoscopy, have led to new concepts and a more critical analysis of how the CSF dynamics have been altered in complex conditions such as PIH. This has taken us beyond the point where the discussion centered largely on what type of shunt to insert and it is likely that future advances in imaging CSF flow will take us yet further.

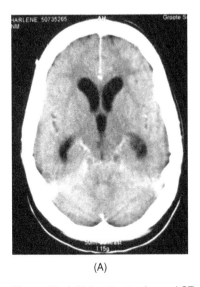 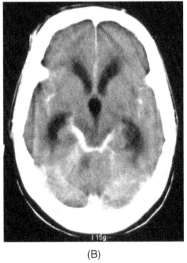

(A)   (B)

Figure 14 Initial contrast-enhanced CT scan in an HIV-positive adult with TBM (**A**). Following commencement of antiretroviral therapy, there is a marked clinical deterioration with evident progression of the basal enhancement and hydrocephalus, compatible with IRIS (**B**).

ACKNOWLEDGMENTS
The authors would like to thank Professor Jonathan C. Peter and Dr. Sally Röthemeyer for their assistance in the preparation of this manuscript.

REFERENCES

1. Adeloye A, Oyedeji GA. Surgical aspects of nontuberculous bacterial meningitis in infancy and childhood. Clin Pediatr 1973; 12(10):589–593.
2. Adeloye A. Cranial and intracranial infections and infestations. In: Neurosurgery in Africa. Ibadan, Nigeria: Ibadan University Press, 1989:161–217.
3. Andronikou S, Smith B, Hatherill M, et al. Definitive neuroradiological diagnostic features of tuberculous meningitis in children. Pediatr Radiol 2004; 34:876–885.
4. Andronikou S, Wieselthaler N, Smith B, et al. Value of early follow-up CT in paediatric tuberculous meningitis. Pediatr Radiol 2005; 35:1092–1099.
5. Bale JF Jr, Bray PF, Bell WE. Neuroradiographic abnormalities in congenital cytomegalovirus infection. Pediatr Neurol 1985; 1(1):42–47.
6. Barkovich AJ, Girard N. Fetal brain infections. Childs Nerv Syst 2003; 19(7–8):501–507.
7. Berman PH, Banker BQ. Neonatal meningitis: a clinical and pathological study of 29 cases. Pediatrics 1966; 38(1):6–24.
8. Bhagwati SN. Ventriculoatrial shunt in tuberculous meningitis with hydrocephalus. J Neurosurg 1971; 35(3):309–313.
9. Blumberg HM, Burman WJ, Chaisson RE, et al. American Thoracic Society/Centres for Disease Control and Prevention/Infectious Diseases Society of America: Treatment of tuberculosis. Am J Respir Crit Care Med 2003; 167(4):603–662.
10. British Medical Research Council Report. Streptomycin treatment of tuberculous meningitis. Lancet 1948; 1:582–596.
11. Bruwer GE, Van der Westhuizen S, Lombard CJ, et al. Can CT predict the level of CSF block in tuberculous hydrocephalus? Child's Nerv Syst 2004; 20(3):183–187.
12. Bullock MRR, van Dellen JR. The role of cerebrospinal fluid shunting in tuberculous meningitis. Surg Neurol 1982; 18:274–277.
13. Bullock MRR, Welchman JM. Diagnostic and prognostic features of tuberculous meningitis on CT scanning. J Neurol Neurosurg Psychiatry 1982; 45:1098–1101.
14. Cairns H. Neurosurgical methods in the treatment of tuberculous meningitis with a note on some unusual manifestations of the disease. Arch Dis Child 1951; 26:373–386.
15. Casey AT, Kimmings EJ, Kleinlugtebeld AD, et al. The long-term outlook for hydrocephalus in childhood: a ten-year cohort study of 155 patients. Pediatr Neurosurg 1997; 27(2):63–70.
16. Chan KH, Cheung RT, Lee R, et al. Cerebral infarcts complicating tuberculous meningitis. Cerebrovasc Dis 2005; 19:391–395.
17. Chappell ET, Guthrie BL, Orenstein J. The role of stereotactic biopsy in the management of HIV-related focal brain lesions. J Neurosurg 1992; 30(6):825–829.
18. Cheeran MC-J, Lokensgard JR, Schleiss MR. Neuropathogenesis of congenital cytomegalovirus infection: disease mechanisms and prospects for intervention. Clin Microbiol Rev 2009; 22(1):99–126.
19. Cinalli G, Sainte-Rose C, Chumas P, et al. Failure of third ventriculostomy in the treatment of aqueductal stenosis in children. J Neurosurg 1999; 90(3):448–454.
20. Ciurea AV, Coman TC, Mircea D. Postinfectious hydrocephalus in children. In: Cinalli G, Maixner WJ, Sainte-Rose C, eds. Pediatric Hydrocephalus. Milan, Italy: Springer Verlag, 2004:201–218.
21. Coleman J, Hogg GG, Rosenfeld JV, et al. Invasive central nervous system aspergillosis: cure with liposomal amphotericin B, itraconazole, and radical surgery—case report and review of the literature. Neurosurgery 1995; 36(4):858–862.
22. Daniel PM. Gross morbid anatomy of the central nervous system of cases of tuberculous meningitis treated with streptomycin. Proc R Soc Med 1949; 42:169–172.
23. Dastur DK, Manghani DK, Udani PM. Pathology and pathogenic mechanisms in neurotuberculosis. Radiol Clin N Am 1995; 33(4):733–751.
24. De Villiers JC, Clüver PF deV, Handler L. Complications following shunt operations for post-meningitic hydrocephalus. In: Wüllenweber R, Wenker H, Brock M, Klinger M, eds. Advances in Neurosurgery, Vol 6: Treatment of Hydrocephalus—Computer Tomography. Berlin, Germany: Springer, 1978:23–27.
25. Dhasmana DT, Dheda K, Wilkinson RJ, et al. Immune reconstitution inflammatory syndrome in HIV-infected patients receiving antiretroviral therapy. Drugs 2008; 68(2):191–208.
26. Di Rocco C, Cinalli G, Massimi L, et al. Endoscopic third ventriculostomy in the treatment of hydrocephalus in pediatric patients. Adv Tech Stand Neurosurg 2006; 31:121–221.

27. Doctor BA, Newman N, Minich NM, et al. Clinical outcomes of neonatal meningitis in very-low-birth-weight infants. Clin Pediatr 2001; 40:473–480.

28. Donald PR, Schoeman JF. Tuberculous meningitis. N Engl J Med 2004; 351:1719–1720.

29. Donald PR, Schaaf HS, Schoeman JF. Tuberculous meningitis and military tuberculosis: the Rich focus revisited. J Infect 2005; 50:193–195.

30. Enright AM, Prober CG. Neurologic sequelae of congenital perinatal infection. In: Stevenson DK, Benitz WE, Sunshine P, eds. Fetal and Neonatal Brain Injury, 3rd ed. Cambridge, MA: Cambridge University Press, 2003:355–376.

31. Figaji AA, Fieggen AG, Peter JC. Endoscopic third ventriculostomy in tuberculous meningitis. Childs Nerv Syst 2003; 19(4):217–225.

32. Figaji AA, Fieggen AG, Peter JC. Air encephalography for hydrocephalus in the era of neuro-endoscopy. Childs Nerv Syst 2005; 21:559–565.

33. Figaji AA, Fieggen AG, Peter JC. Endoscopy for tuberculous hydrocephalus. Childs Nerv Syst 2007; 23:79–84.

34. Figaji AA, Sandler SJI, Fieggen AG, et al. Continuous monitoring and intervention for cerebral ischemia in tuberculous meningitis. Ped Crit Care Med 2008; 9:e25–e30.

35. Foltz EL, Shurtleff DB. Conversion of communicating hydrocephalus to stenosis or occlusion of the aqueduct during ventricular shunt. J Neurosurg 1966; 24(2):520–529.

36. Fukuhara T, Vorster SJ, Luciano MG. Risk factors for endoscopic third ventriculostomy for obstructive hydrocephalus. Neurosurgery 2000; 46(5):1100–1111.

37. Glynn JR. Resurgence of tuberculosis and the impact of HIV infection. Br Med Bull 1998; 54(3): 579–593.

38. Graham DR, Band JD. Citrobacter diversus brain abscesses and meningitis in neonates. JAMA 1981; 245(19):1923–1925.

39. Gray F, Alonso J-M. Bacterial infections of the nervous system. In: Graham DI, Lantos PL, eds. Greenfield's Neuropathology, 7th ed. Oxford: Arnold, 2002:151–194.

40. Graybill JR, Sobel J, Saag M, et al. Diagnosis an management of increased intracranial pressure in patients with AIDS and cryptococcal meningitis. Clin Infect Dis 2000; 30:47–54.

41. Greitz D. Radiological assessment of hydrocephalus: new theories and implications for therapy. Neurosurg Rev 2004; 27:145–165.

42. Handler LC, Wright MGE. Postmeningitic hydrocephalus in infancy. Neuroradiology 1978; 16:31–35.

43. Husain M, Jha DK, Rastogi M, et al. Role of neuroendoscopy in the management of patients with tuberculous meningitis hydrocephalus. Neurosurg Rev 2005; 28:278–283.

44. Hviid A, Rubin S, Mühlemann K. Mumps. New Eng J Med 2007; 371:932–944.

45. Jamieson DH. Imaging intracranial tuberculosis in childhood. Pediatr Radiol 1995; 25:165–170.

46. Jarvis JH, Harrison TS. HIV-associated cryptococcal meningitis. AIDS 2007; 21(16):2119–2129.

47. Jha DK, Mishra V, Choudhary A, et al. Factors affecting the outcome of neuroendoscopy in patients with tuberculous meningitis hydrocephalus: a preliminary study. Surg Neurol 2007; 68:35–42.

48. Jonathan A, Rajshekhar V. Endoscopic third ventriculostomy for chronic hydrocephalus after tuberculous meningitis. Surg Neurol 2005; 63:32–35.

49. Jones J, Lopez A, Wilson M. Congenital Toxoplasmosis. Am Fam Physician 2003; 67(10):2131–2139.

50. Kaiser G. Hydrocephalus following toxoplasmosis. Z Kinderchir 1985; 40(suppl 1):10–11.

51. Katz BZ, Yogev R. Bacterial and viral meningitis and encephalitis. In: McLone DG, ed. Pediatric Neurosurgery, 4th ed. Philadelphia, PA: WB Saunders, 2001:991–1007.

52. Kinney HC, Armstrong DD. Perinatal neuropathology. In: Graham DI, Lantos PL, eds. Greenfield's Neuropathology, 7th ed. Oxford: Arnold, 2002:519–606.

53. Lamprecht D, Schoeman J, Donald P, et al. Ventriculoperitoneal shunting in childhood tuberculous meningitis. Br J Neurosurg 2001; 15(2):119–125.

54. Leib SL, Täuber MG. Acute and chronic meningitis. In: Cohen J, Powderley WG, eds. Infectious Diseases, 2nd ed. Edinburgh, U.K.: Mosby, 2004:251–266.

55. Liliang P-C, Liang C-L, Chang W-N, et al. Shunt surgery for hydrocephalus complicating crypto-coccal meningitis in Human Immunodeficiency Virus-Negative patients. Clin Infect Dis 2003; 37: 673–678.

56. Lorber J. Studies of the cerebrospinal fluid circulation in tuberculous meningitis in children. Part II: a review of 100 pneumoencephalograms. Arch Dis Child 1951; 26:28–44.

57. Lorber J, Pickering D. Incidence and treatment of post-meningitic hydrocephalus in the newborn. Arch Dis Child 1966; 41:44–50.

58. Love S, Wiley CA. Viral diseases. In: Graham DI, Lantos PL, eds. Greenfield's Neuropathology, 7th ed. Oxford: Arnold, 2002:1–106.

59. Maartens G, Wilkinson RJ. Tuberculosis. New Engl J Med 2007; 370:2030–2043.

60. Maconochie IK, Baumer JH, Stewart M. Fluid therapy for acute bacterial meningitis. Cochrane Database Syst Rev 2008; (1):CD004786. DOI:10.1002/14651858.CD004786.pub3.

61. Macsween KF, Bicanic T, Brouwer AE, et al. Lumbar drainage for control of raised cerebrospinal fluid pressure in cryptococcal meningitis: case report and review. J Infect 2005; 51:e221–e224.

62. Malm G, Engman M-L. Congenital cytomegalovirus infection. Semin Fetal Neonatal Med 2007; 12:154–159.

63. Mathew JM, Rajshekar V, Chandy MJ. Shunt surgery in poor grade patients with tuberculous meningitis and hydrocephalus: effects of response to external ventricular drainage and other variables on long-term outcome. J Neurol Neurosurg Psychiatry 1998; 65:115–118.

64. Matson DD. Etiology, classification and diagnosis of hydrocephalus. In: Neurosurgery of Infancy and Childhood, 2nd ed. Springfield: Thomas, 1968:199–221.

65. McKay RJ, Morisette RA, Ingraham FD, et al. Collections of subdural fluid complicating meningitis due to *Haemophilus influenzae* (type B). N Engl J Med 1950; 242:20–21.

66. Montoya JG, Remington JS. Management of *Toxoplasma gondii* infection during pregnancy. Clin Infect Dis 2008; 47:554–566.

67. Mori K. Current concept of hydrocephalus: evolution of new classifications. Childs Nerv Syst 1995; 11(9):523–532.

68. Mylonakis E, Hohmann EL, Calderwood SB. Central nervous system infection with *Listeria monocytogenes*: 33 years' experience at a general hospital and review of 776 episodes from the literature. Medicine 1998; 77(5):313–336.

69. Nadvi SS, Nathoo N, Annamalai K, et al. Role of cerebrospinal fluid shunting for human immunodeficiency virus-positive patients with tuberculous meningitis and hydrocephalus. Neurosurgery 2000; 47(3):644–650.

70. Nakao N, Itakura T. Endoscopic lamina terminalis fenestration for treatment of hydrocephalus due to tuberculous meningitis. J Neurosurg 2003; 99:187.

71. National Collaborating Centre for Chronic Conditions. Tuberculosis: clinical diagnosis and management of tuberculosis and measures for its prevention and control. London, U.K.: Royal College of Physicians, 2006. Available at: www.nice.org.uk/page.aspx?o_297929. Accessed April 30, 2008.

72. Newton PN, Thai LH, Tip NQ, et al. A randomized, double-blind, placebo-controlled trial of acetazolamide for the treatment of elevated intracranial pressure in cryptococcal meningitis. Clin Infect Dis 2002; 35:769–772.

73. Palur R, Rajshekar V, Chandy MJ, et al. Shunt surgery for hydrocephalus in tuberculous meningitis: a long-tem follow-up study. J Neurosurg 1991; 74:64–69.

74. Park MK, Hospenthal DR, Bennett JE. Treatment of hydrocephalus secondary to cryptococcal meningitis by use of shunting. Clin Infect Dis 1999; 28:629–633.

75. Peacock WJ, Deeny JE. Improving the outcome of tuberculous meningitis in childhood. S Afr Med J 1984; 66:597–598.

76. Pereira EAC, Fieggen AG, Kelly D, et al. The etiology of pediatric hydrocephalus: Oxford and Cape Town compared. Childs Nerv Syst 2004; 20(4):266.

77. Petersen E. Toxoplasmosis. Sem Fetal Neonat Med 2007; 12:214–223.

78. Philip AGS. Neonatal bacterial meningitis. In: Stevenson DK, Benitz WE, Sunshine P, eds. Fetal and Neonatal Brain Injury, 3rd ed. Cambridge, MA: Cambridge University Press, 2003:333–354.

79. Prasad K, Singh MB. Corticosteroids for managing tuberculous meningitis. Cochrane Database Syst Rev 2008; (1):CD002244. DOI:10.1002/14651858.CD002244.pub3.

80. Raimondi AJ. Infection. In: Pediatric Neurosurgery. Berlin, Germany: Springer-Verlag, 1987: 401–414.

81. Ransohoff J, Shulman K, Fishman RA. Hydrocephalus: a review of etiology and treatment. J Pediatr 1960; 56:399–411.

82. Raviglione MC. Facing extensively drug-resistant tuberculosis—a hope and challenge. N Engl J Med 2008: 359:636–638.

83. Renier D, Flandin C, Hirsch E. Brain abscesses in neonates. J Neurosurg 1988, 69.877–882.

84. Rhoton AL, Gomez MR. Conversion of multilocular hydrocephalus to unilocular. J Neurosurg 1972; 36(3):348–350.

85. Rich AR, McCordock HA. The pathogenesis of tuberculous meningitis. Bull John Hopkins Hosp 1933; 52:5–37.

86. Romeo JH, Rice LB, McQuarrie IG. Hydrocephalus in coccidioidal meningitis: case report and review of the literature. Neurosurgery 2000; 47(3):773–777.

87. Ruhnke M. CNS Aspergillosis—recognition, diagnosis and management. CNS Drugs 2007; 21(8): 659–676.

88. Sáez-Llorens X, McCracken GH. Bacterial meningitis in children. Lancet 2003; 361:2139–2148.

89. Sharma RR, Lad SD, Pawar SJ, et al. Surgical Infections of the central nervous system. In: Schmidek HH, Roberts DW, eds. Schmidek and Sweet's Operative Neurosurgical Techniques, 5th ed. Philadelphia, PA: Saunders, 2004:1633–1671.

90. Schoeman JF, le Roux D, Bezuidenhout PB, et al. Intracranial pressure monitoring, in tuberculous meningitis: clinical and computerized tomographic correlation. Dev Med Child Neurol 1985; 27: 644–654.

91. Schoeman JF, Van Zyl LE, Laubscher JA, et al. Serial CT scanning in childhood tuberculous meningitis: prognostic features in 198 cases. J Child Neurol 1995; 10:320–329.

92. Schoeman JF, Van Zyl LE, Laubscher JA, et al. Effect of corticosteroids on intracranial pressure, and clinical outcome in young children with tuberculous meningitis. Pediatrics 1997; 99: 226–231.

93. Schuchat A, Robinson K, Wenger JD, et al. Bacterial meningitis in the United States in 1995. Active Surveillance Team. New Engl J Med 1997; 337:970–976.

94. Sil K, Chatterjee S. Shunting in tuberculous meningitis: a neurosurgeon's nightmare. Childs Nerv Syst 2008; 24(9):1029–1032.

95. Singh D, Sachdev V, Singh AK, et al. Endoscopic third ventriculostomy in post-tubercular meningitis: a preliminary report. Minim Invas Neurosurg 2005; 48:47–52.

96. Singh D, Sachdev V, Singh AK, et al. Endoscopic third ventriculostomy in post-tubercular meningitis (response to letter). Minim Invas Neurosurg 2007; 50:251.

97. Siomin V, Cinalli G, Grotenhuis A, et al. Endoscopic third ventriculostomy in patients with cerebrospinal fluid infection and/or hemorrhage. J Neurosurg 2002; 97:519–524.

98. Siomin V, Constantini S. Endoscopic third ventriculostomy in tuberculous meningitis (letter). Childs Nerv Syst 2003; 19:269.

99. Sloan D, Dlamini S, Paul N, et al. Treatment of acute cryptococcal meningitis in HIV-infected adults, with an emphasis on resource-limited settings. Cochran Database Syst Rev 2008; Issue 4. Art. No.: CD005647.DOI:10.1002/14651858.CD005647.pub2.

100. Smyth MD, Tubbs RS, Wellons J, et al. Endoscopic third ventriculostomy for hydrocephalus secondary to central nervous system infection or intraventricular hemorrhage in children. Pediatr Neurosurg 2003; 39:258–263.

101. Spennato P, Cinalli G, Ruggiero C, et al. Neuroendoscopic treatment of multiloculated hydrocephalus in children. J Neurosurg 2007; 106(1 Suppl Pediatrics):29–35.

102. Stevens DA. Coccidioides. New Engl J Med 1995; 332:1077–1082.

103. Tandon PN. Tuberculous meningitis (cranial and spinal). In: Vinken PJ, Bruyn GW, eds. Handbook of Clinical Neurology: Infections of the Nervous System, Vol. 33. Amsterdam, The Netherlands: North Holland, 1978:195–262.

104. Teo C. Third ventriculostomy in the treatment of hydrocephalus: experience with more than 120 cases. In: Hellwig D, Bauer BL, eds. Minimally Invasive Techniques for Neurosurgery. Berlin, Germany: Springer, 1998:73–76.

105. Thwaites GE, Bang ND, Dung NH, et al. Dexamethasone for the treatment of tuberculous meningitis in adolescents and adults. N Eng J Med 2004; 351:1741–1751.

106. Thwaites GE, Hien TT. Tuberculous meningitis: many questions, too few answers. Lancet Neurol 2005; 4:160–170.

107. Thwaites GE, Bang ND, Dung NH, et al. The influence of HIV infection on clinical presentation, response to treatment, and outcome in adults with tuberculous meningitis. J Infect Dis 2005; 192: 2134–2141.

108. Thwaites GE, Macmullen-Price J, Chau TTH, et al. Serial MRI to determine the effect of dexamethasone on the cerebral pathology of tuberculous meningitis: an observational study. Lancet Neurol 2007; 6:230–236.

109. Till K. Paediatric Neurosurgery. Oxford: Blackwell, 1975.

110. Turner G, Scaravilli F. Parasitic and fungal diseases. In: Graham DI, Lantos PL, eds. Greenfield's Neuropathology, 7th ed. Oxford: Arnold, 2002:107–150.

111. UNAIDS—Joint United Nations Programme on HIV/AIDS. Report on the Global AIDS epidemic. 2008. http://www.unaids.org. Accessed April 22, 2009.

112. van de Beek D, de Gans J, Spanjaard L, et al. Clinical features and prognostic factors in adults with bacterial meningitis. New Engl J Med 2004; 351:1849–1859.

113. van de Beek D, de Gans J, McIntyre P, et al. Corticosteroids for acute bacterial meningitis. Cochrane Database Syst Rev 2007; Issue 1. Art. No.: CD004405.DOI: 10.102/14651858 CD004405.pub2.

114. van Well GTJ, Paes BF, Terwee CB, et al. Twenty years of tuberculous meningitis: a retrospective cohort study in the Western Cape of South Africa. Pediatrics 2009; 123(1):e1–e8. DOI:10.1542/peds.2008-1353.

115. Visudhipan P, Chiemchanya S. Hydrocephalus in tuberculous meningitis in children: treatment with acetazolamide and repeated lumbar puncture. J Pediatr 1979; 95:657–660.

116. Warf BC. Hydrocephalus in Uganda: the predominance of infectious origin and primary management with endoscopic third ventriculostomy. J Neurosurg (Pediatrics) 2005; 102:1–15.

117. Weitkamp J-H, Nania JJ. Infectious Diseases. In: Fenichel GM, ed. Neonatal Neurology. Phildelphia, PA: Elsevier, 2007:109–142.
118. Williams B. Is aqueduct stenosis a result of hydrocephalus? Brain 1973; 96:399–412.
119. Williams PL. Coccidioidal meningitis. Ann NY Acad Sci 2007; 1111:377–384.
120. Woodworth GF, McGirt MJ, Williams MA, et al. The use of Ventriculoperitoneal shunts for uncontrollable intracranial hypertension without ventriculomegaly secondary to HIV-associated cryptococcal meningitis. Surg Neurol 2005; 63(6):529–531.
121. Wright R, Johnson DJ, Neumann M, et al. Congenital lymphocytic choriomeningitis virus syndrome: a disease that mimics congenital toxoplasmosis or cytomegalovirus infection. Pediatrics 1997; 100(1):e9.
122. Yamada H, Abe T, Tanabe Y, et al. Experimental and clinical studies on the pathogenesis of intraventricular septations following meningoventriculitis in childhood. Monogr Neural Sci 1982; 8:81–85.

10 | Hydrocephalus in Children with Myelomeningocele

Mark S. Dias and Mark R. Iantosca

Department of Neurosurgery, Section of Pediatric Neurosurgery, Penn State Milton S. Hershey Medical Center, Penn State University College of Medicine, Hershey, Pennsylvania, U.S.A.

INTRODUCTION

Hydrocephalus complicates myelomeningocele in approximately 85% to 90% of patients (1); once the myelomeningocele is closed, the surgical management of hydrocephalus is the cornerstone of ongoing neurosurgical care. Hydrocephalus in the patient with a myelomeningocele presents a number of unusual problems in management that can challenge even the most seasoned clinician. We will review the pathophysiology and presenting features of hydrocephalus in patients with myelomeningocele, and discuss the management of hydrocephalus and shunt complications in this complex disorder.

PATHOPHYSIOLOGY OF HYDROCEPHALUS

Hydrocephalus in patients with myelomeningocele may be caused by any of several pathophysiological mechanisms, alone or in concert (2–4). Aqueductal occlusion, fourth ventricular outlet obstruction, obliteration of the subarachnoid space by the crowded posterior fossa contents, and subarachnoid obstruction at the tentorial hiatus have all been implicated (5). All appear to originate from the Chiari II malformation and its associated hindbrain abnormalities (3,5).

The Chiari II malformation includes a pan-cerebral constellation of malformations (Table 1), the most striking and clinically important of which involve the posterior fossa structures. The inferior vermis and cerebellar tonsils, brainstem, and variably the fourth ventricle are caudally displaced through an enlarged foramen magnum into the cervical spinal canal, while the superior vermis and cerebellar hemispheres are cranially displaced through the tentorial hiatus and lie within the supratentorial compartment. Supratentorial abnormalities include an enlarged massa intermedia of the thalamus, dysgenesis of the corpus callosum, "beaking" of the quadrigeminal plate, "stenogyria" (small, ropy gyri), and cortical heterotopias (Fig. 1).

The Chiari II malformation arises during the first several embryonic weeks and is thought to arise as a result of caudal leakage of cerebrospinal fluid (CSF) through the open myelomeningocele placode during and after the period of spinal neurocele occlusion (1,5). During normal development, the central canal of the spinal cord becomes transiently occluded for two to eight days (6). During this time, the isolated ventricular system enlarges and provides a stimulus to mesenchymal growth of the skull in general, and the posterior fossa in particular (7–11). Experimentally venting CSF through small glass tubes during this embryonic "critical period" results in an inadequate stimulus to skull growth and disorganized brain development (1,6,12–14). In the embryo with a myelomeningocele, venting of the CSF through the placode results in a posterior fossa that is too small to accommodate the rapidly growing hindbrain. The developing rhombencephalon (medulla and cerebellum) is therefore displaced both cranially through the tentorial incisura and caudally through the foramen magnum (1).

The resultant crowding of the posterior fossa impedes the normal flow of CSF from the third to the fourth ventricle, from the fourth ventricle to the posterior fossa subarachnoid space, and from the posterior fossa subarachnoid space to the cerebral convexities (2–5) and leads to hydrocephalus.

The Chiari II malformation also has important practical implications for the management of hydrocephalus in patients with myelomeningoceles. Callosal dysgenesis, cortical heterotopias, and polymicrogyria produce a characteristic shape to the ventricular system with disproportionate enlargement of the ventricular atria and occipital horns (*colpocephaly*) even in the absence of hydrocephalus (Fig. 1). One should not therefore rely exclusively on the size of

Table 1 Chiari II–Associated Central Nervous System Malformations

Disorders of the skull
  "Lückenschädel" of the skull
  Small posterior fossa
  Low-lying tentorium cerebelli with large incisura
  Scalloping of the petrous bone
  Shortening of the clivus
  Enlargement of the foramen magnum
Disorders of the cerebral hemispheres
  Polymicrogyria
  Cortical heterotopias
  Dysgenesis of the corpus callosum
  Large massa intermedia
Disorders of the posterior fossa
  Descent of the cerebellar vermis through foramen magnum
  Caudal displacement of pons and medulla
  Rostral displacement of superior cerebellum through the tentorium
  "Kinking" of the brainstem
  Loss of pontine flexure
  Aqueductal stenosis or forking
  "Beaking" of the tectum

the atria in making an assessment of ventriculomegaly in these patients in the absence of frontal horn enlargement or other signs of progressive ventriculomegaly.

Second, it has been our experience that the standard trajectory for frontal catheter placement—aiming one fingerbreadth anterior to the tragus of the ipsilateral ear—is often too anterior in this population and may result in interhemispheric catheter placement; a slightly more posterior trajectory may be required.

The Chiari II malformation may also interfere with proper shunt function; an enlarged massa intermedia and small third ventricle, an enlarged caudate head, prominent commissural

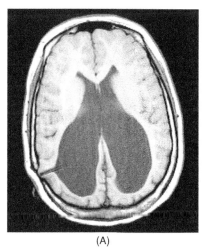 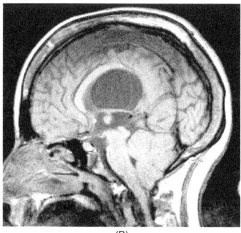

(A)　　　　　　　　　　　　　　(B)

Figure 1 MR scans of a 13-year-old girl who was born with open myelomeningocele that was closed soon after birth and had insertion of ventriculoperitoneal shunt a few days later. (**A**) Axial T1-weighted image, showing the disproportionately dilated atria and occipital horns of the lateral ventricle, a feature called otherwise colpocephaly. In the right lateral ventricle, there is the ventricular catheter of the shunt. (**B**) Sagittal T1-weighted image, showing several of the features of the Chiari II malformation: hindbrain hernia, with the lower edge of the cerebellar tonsils protruding down to the arch of C1, a small crowded posterior fossa, secondary aqueduct stenosis, enlarged massa intermedia, abnormal disposition of the corpus callosum, which is partly absent posteriorly. *Source*: Photo courtesy of Dr. S. Sgouros.

fibers extending across the anterior third ventricle, and anteriorly pointing frontal horns may distort and functionally obstruct the interventricular foramen of Monro and result in isolated lateral ventricles after unilateral shunt placement (15–17). The use of distal slit valves (with strong siphoning effects) may specifically contribute to postshunt isolated ventricles and should be avoided in this population (16).

Finally, hindbrain compression and/or distortion from the Chiari malformation may be exacerbated by hydrocephalus and shunt malfunction, resulting in hindbrain dysfunction, either as an initial manifestation of hydrocephalus in the neonate or as a feature of shunt malfunction in the older child (18–22).

CLINICAL FEATURES AND MANAGEMENT IN CHILDREN WITH MYELOMENINGOCELES AND HYDROCEPHALUS

The clinical features and management of hydrocephalus in the patient with a myelomeningocele can be divided into a neonatal period (lasting up to about five months) during which the decision is made as to whether or not a shunt is required and, for those requiring shunts, a later phase during which the child is surveyed for evidence of shunt malfunction. During both these periods, the myelomeningocele and Chiari II malformation have a profound impact on the evaluation and management of hydrocephalus.

Clinical Features and Management of Hydrocephalus in the Neonate with a Myelomeningocele

Overt hydrocephalus is clinically evident at the time of birth in about 15% of infants with myelomeningocele, usually the result of aqueductal stenosis (23). More frequently, overt hydrocephalus is absent at birth but develops during the days or weeks following myelomeningocele closure and is more frequently the result of obstruction at the incisura or the subarachnoid cisterns (5).

Some of the clinical features of hydrocephalus in the infant with a myelomeningocele are identical to those associated with hydrocephalus from any source and include an enlarging head size, bulging fontanelle, splitting cranial sutures, poor feeding and/or vomiting, sunsetting eyes or limitation of upward gaze, and apnea and/or bradycardia. However, there are two additional features unique to the infant with a myelomeningocele. First, CSF accumulation beneath, or leakage from, the recently closed back wound may occur in the absence of other signs or significant ventricular enlargement. Second, lower brainstem compromise from the Chiari II malformation may cause stridor from vocal cord weakness, a weak high-pitched cry, swallowing difficulties, poor feeding, nasal regurgitation of feeds, aspiration pneumonia, or weakness and hypotonia. Although anatomically related to the Chiari II malformation, these symptoms are exacerbated by the hydrocephalus (21) and will often resolve after shunting.

The decision to treat the hydrocephalus is straightforward in most cases. Infants with obvious macrocephaly and significant ventricular enlargement may be shunted contemporaneously with the back closure without an attendant increase in infectious complications (15). Alternatively, the hydrocephalus can be treated initially with either an external ventricular drain or a ventricular access device at birth, and shunting delayed for several days; this approach requires two procedures and is likely to have increased the infection rate as well.

For the majority of infants who lack signs of overt hydrocephalus at birth, the myelomeningocele is closed and a decision about shunting is deferred. Daily assessments of head circumference, fontanelle fullness, and degree of cranial sutural splitting are supplemented with periodic cranial ultrasounds. Intracranial blood flow measurements, as assessed by pulsed Doppler ultrasound, may provide additional information about evolving hydrocephalus (24) through the Resistive Index (RI) which is calculated by dividing the difference between peak systolic and end diastolic frequencies by the systolic frequency. The averaged values for anterior and middle cerebral and internal carotid arteries should be <0.75, whereas values of >85 suggest evolving hydrocephalus. A *sequential* rise in RI on serial ultrasound examinations in the same infant also suggests worsening hydrocephalus (24).

A small group of infants will have moderate but *nonprogressive* ventricular enlargement, lack signs or symptoms of intracranial hypertension or brainstem compromise, and normal developmental milestones. Under these circumstances, one must carefully weigh the effects of hydrocephalus on subsequent brain development against the well documented and significant lifetime risks of ventricular shunting (25–27). One additional factor that has not been emphasized is the psychological toll that shunting places upon the neurosurgeon, patient, and family. Once a shunt is placed, the child is almost always shunt-dependent for life (25,28) and everyone is committed lifelong to maintain shunt function. The shunt revision rate is 30% to 40% during the first year after insertion, and approximately 5% per year thereafter; 20% require multiple shunt revisions (2,29). Even a functioning shunt wreaks havoc on the patient and the family because every episode of headache, vomiting, or viral syndrome creates angst for the patient and parents and may require a workup to exclude a shunt malfunction.

On the other hand, at what point do the effects of hydrocephalus on neural development and intellectual function outweigh the risks of shunting? Although the effects of experimental hydrocephalus have been well documented in animal models, comparable studies in humans are virtually nonexistent. In one study, postshunt cortical mantle thickness appeared to predict intellectual outcome among shunted hydrocephalic children. In this study, children with a *postshunt* cortical mantle thickness of 2.8 cm or more had essentially normal IQs, whereas those with cortical mantles of less than 2.0 cm had significantly lower IQs. Importantly, *no further* improvement in IQ was observed for those children with cortical mantles thicker than 2.8 cm. Finally, all patients with *preshunt* cortical mantles of less than 2.8 cm achieved this level of mantle thickness when shunted by five months of age (28,30). Therefore, it appears that infants having cortical mantle thickness of at least 2.8 cm may safely be observed if no other clinical abnormalities are evident (25).

Other studies suggest that ventricular size in children with myelomeningoceles is less important than other factors in determining intellectual outcome. In one study, children who did not require shunts had statistically higher IQs (mean IQ of 104) than those who required shunts (mean IQ of 91). However, those who required shunts for the control of hydrocephalus *in the face of complications* (ventriculitis, anoxia, poorly controlled hydrocephalus, or other CNS anomalies) had a worse outcome (mean IQ of 70) than those with uncomplicated shunt placement (mean IQ of 91) (25). Other studies have failed to demonstrate a worsening intellectual outcome among those children with *stable* mild or moderate ventriculomegaly (31,32). In a retrospective comparative study of 285 children with myelomeningoceles, the unshunted group—including both those with normal ventricular size and those with mild or moderate hydrocephalus— had a mean IQ of 98.5, whereas the shunted group had an average IQ of 86. In both groups, the ventricular size did not correlate with IQ *except* those having persistent severe ventricular enlargement *after* shunting. This group also had the highest incidence of severe congenital brain anomalies, meningitis, and/or hypoxia, suggesting that poor outcome is related to underlying conditions and/or complications than to the hydrocephalus per se.

In particular, severe shunt infections *do* adversely affect intelligence (31,32). Among 167 children with myelomeningocele, ventriculitis was the single greatest predictor of poor intel- lectual outcome. Children with ventriculitis had an average IQ of 72, whereas those without ventriculitis had an average IQ of 95 and those who were unshunted had an average IQ of 102 (31). Excluding children with shunt infections, there were no differences in intellectual outcome between the shunted and nonshunted patients.

Although imperfect, these studies nonetheless support nonoperative management for children with mild or moderate nonprogressive ventriculomegaly and cortical mantle thickness of at least 3 cm who are developmentally normal and without signs or symptoms of intracranial hypertension or hindbrain dysfunction. Those who have not required a shunt by five months of age are exceedingly unlikely to need one subsequently (25).

Presenting Features and Management of Shunt Malfunction in the Older Child with a Myelomeningocele

For children with myelomeningocele and shunted hydrocephalus, any clinical change should alert the clinician to the possibility of a shunt malfunction. Nowhere else in pediatric neuro- surgery is clinical judgment so crucial, and misjudgment so treacherous, as in the evaluation of the child with a myelomeningocele and suspected shunt malfunction. Unrecognized/untreated shunt malfunction is the leading cause of death beyond the perinatal period (33). The signs and symptoms of shunt malfunction in these children are both broad and varied and may confuse even the most experienced clinician. Although headache, with or without nausea or emesis, are the most common presenting features of shunt malfunction along with poor feeding, listlessness or lethargy, sunsetting eyes, or extraocular abduction palsies, these "typical" features may be absent in children with myelomeningoceles. Moreover, the presence of the Chiari II malformation, tethering, and syringomyelia all change the way in which a shunt malfunction becomes evident in these patients. Shunt malfunction accordingly can present with any of the following signs and symptoms: (*i*) cognitive changes—declining school performance or worsening behavior; (*ii*) new onset or increased frequency of seizures; (*iii*) lower cranial nerve dysfunction suggesting hindbrain compromise; (*iv*) progressive motor decline (new weakness, loss of previously acquired motor skills, increased spasticity); (*v*) worsening ambulation without another identifiable cause; (*vi*) worsening urinary or bowel function (increasing incontinence or bladder infections, change in catheterization schedule, change in bowel pattern); (*vii*) back or leg pain, particularly pain at the myelomeningocele closure site; and (*viii*) worsening scoliosis or lower extremity orthopedic deformities.

Changes in cognition and/or behavior are among the most frequent manifestations of shunt malfunction in this population (23). Declining school performance, perhaps associated with behavioral changes (declining attention, increased impulsivity, hyperactivity, aggression, or emotional lability) may occur. These cognitive and behavioral changes are often incorrectly attributed to puberty or to changes in the home or school environment but resolve immediately after shunt revision (23). Characteristic "blank spells," during which the child abruptly stops activity and stares blankly with seeming disregard for his surroundings, may occur and may suggest seizures, although the EEG reveals diffuse slowing during these episodes (23).

Seizures occur in approximately 15% to 25% of children with myelomeningoceles (34–37) and are likely related to cerebral malformations such as cortical heterotopias and stenogyria associated with the Chiari II malformation. Prior shunt revisions and ventriculitis may also contribute to seizures (35). However, seizures *as a presenting feature of shunt malfunction* are infrequent, occurring in only 2.6% of children with myelomeningoceles and are usually accompanied by other signs and symptoms of intracranial hypertension (36).

Shunt malfunction may also present as brainstem dysfunction and lower cranial neuropathies from the Chiari II malformation (18–22). Signs and symptoms may include stridor; a weak or high-pitched cry or hoarseness, nasal, or high-pitched voice; frequent choking on foods (particularly liquids); nasal reflux during feeds; repeated bouts of aspiration pneumonia; facial weakness; tongue deviation or fasciculations; or extraocular movement abnormalities. Apnea (19–21) may lead to death if prolonged and untreated. Rarely, motor decline or cerebellar dysfunction may occur.

Shunt malfunction may manifest as progressive motor dysfunction in either arms or legs, presenting as muscle weakness, increased tone, muscle contractures or spasms, and/or worsening gait. These changes are likely mediated through the Chiari II malformation, tethering, or syringomyelia (38), but the underlying problem is shunt malfunction; symptoms may dramatically improve after shunt revision and more complex operations may be avoided.

Changes in urinary function with shunt malfunction are probably mediated through tethering or syringomyelia. Symptoms include increasing incontinence between catheterizations, an increase in the necessity for catheterizations or decrease in bladder volumes, and increasing infections without another cause. Bladder function can be objectively assessed with serial urodynamic tests; abnormalities include reductions in bladder capacity and/or increased bladder pressures, worsening uninhibited bladder contractions, and simultaneous bladder and urethral sphincter contractions ("detrusor-sphincter dyssynergia"). Again, these symptoms and signs may improve after shunt revision.

Progressive orthopedic deformities, including pes cavus or equinovarus deformities, hip subluxation, and "sagging" gait from hamstring flexion contractures are likely mediated by tethering and may occur with shunt malfunction. Progressive scoliosis in the absence of underlying vertebral anomalies may be the only manifestation of shunt malfunction and often will improve following shunt revision (38,39). Shunt malfunction likely causes scoliosis by exacerbating an existing syringomyelia (38), although syringomyelia need not be present in every case and shunt revision may improve or stabilize the scoliosis even when syringomyelia is absent.

Back or leg pain may occur with or without an associated headache. In particular, *pain that occurs at the myelomeningocele closure site*, while often a presenting feature of spinal cord tethering, is also common with shunt malfunction.

Finally, a few children will have few or no symptoms or signs of shunt malfunction, yet have papilledema on physical examination that resolves after shunt revision. A funduscopic examination is therefore recommended at every follow-up encounter with these children.

The diagnostic evaluation of the child with suspected shunt malfunction begins with a CT scan, although the changes in ventricular size may be quite subtle or even nonexistent in some cases, yet symptoms and signs resolve promptly following shunt revision. Several children die each year from unrecognized shunt malfunction, despite a CT scan showing no change in ventricular size. The absence of radiographic change does not necessarily eliminate the possibility of a shunt malfunction in a child having classic signs and symptoms. A shunt tap may be helpful in this setting; poor proximal flow, high pressures with good proximal flow, or prompt resolution of symptoms after removing CSF may all support the diagnosis of shunt malfunction.

In summary, hydrocephalus in patients with a myelomeningocele differs in several respects from other forms of hydrocephalus. The presenting features of shunt malfunction are more diverse and suggest issues related to the Chiari II malformation, syringomyelia, or tethering. When presented with any deterioration, one should always *first* assess shunt function before proceeding with any more complex treatments. This approach has two benefits: (*i*) it obviates the need for a more extensive (and potentially more morbid) surgical procedure, and (*ii*) it may prevent disastrous clinical deterioration from herniation that might otherwise occur after removing CSF caudal to a shunt obstruction. Any child with neurological deterioration should first undergo a CT or other cranial imaging study, and then undergo a shunt revision if an increase in ventricular size is documented. If the clinical circumstances are suspicious for shunt malfunction despite a change in ventricular size, particularly if previous shunt malfunctions have not been associated with ventricular enlargement, the shunt should be tapped or revised empirically. In brief, *"always check the shunt first"* whenever there is any doubt about shunt function.

ENDOSCOPY IN CHILDREN WITH MYELOMENINGOCELES AND HYDROCEPHALUS

As already noted the cause of hydrocephalus in children born with myelomeningocele is usually multifactorial. Traditionally, the use of endoscopic third ventriculostomy (ETV) has been recommended primarily in the treatment of purely obstructive etiologies of hydrocephalus due to higher reported success rates (40–44). Consequently, this treatment for hydrocephalus in the setting of myelomeningocele has not been typically recommended in the past (45). This concept of a link between outcome and hydrocephalus etiology has recently been challenged by several authors (46–48). Most authors also report decreased success rates in infants and young children (42,43,45–48). Unfortunately, the lack of standardized workup, follow-up, and outcome measures across these various case series makes comparison between them difficult. No clear consensus has emerged regarding the indications for endoscopy in patients with myelomeningocele and hydrocephalus. Additionally, there are frequent alterations in the normal ventricular anatomy in these patients, which may complicate standard endoscopic techniques. The authors will generally treat these patients with ventriculoperitoneal shunting at presentation in infancy and reserve ETV procedures for selected difficult, multiple shunt failures or patients with radiographic features suggestive of a predominantly obstructive etiology. Endoscopic techniques for augmenting therapy with shunts, such as fenestration of ventricular loculations, or the septum pelucidum and endoscopic-assisted catheter placement are also employed when necessary.

SHUNT INDEPENDENCE IN CHILDREN WITH MYELOMENINGOCELES AND HYDROCEPHALUS

One final question is whether children with a myelomeningocele and shunted hydrocephalus ever "outgrows" the need for a shunt. Certainly, there are a number of children in every practice in whom the shunt is found to have become disconnected, sometimes with the distal catheter having migrated completely into the peritoneum, on an incidental radiograph obtained for an unrelated reason in an asymptomatic child. One may decide under these circumstances to watch the child expectantly or even to remove the shunt. However, children with myelomeningoceles differ from those with hydrocephalus from other causes in two fundamental ways. First, subtle clinical deterioration in these children may not intuitively be attributed to shunt malfunction and may resolve after shunt revision. In some instances, the deterioration is so insidious that it is only after significant improvement has occurred following shunt revision that the degree of preoperative clinical deterioration becomes apparent. Second, and of greater concern, the Chiari II malformation predisposes these patients to sudden cardiorespiratory arrest, in some cases with few or no premonitory symptoms and with devastating or fatal consequences (23,25,28). Unfortunately, this circumstance may not become apparent until months or years after the shunt has been known to have become disconnected. In one series, sudden death occurred in three patients 24 hours, 9 months, and 5 years following documented shunt nonfunction (28). Whether or not CSF was still capable of draining down a scarred shunt tract for a time in these individuals is unknown. Albright has therefore suggested that a radionuclide study be performed and, if CSF traverses the gap and/or reaches the distal end of the shunt, the shunt should be revised. One should evaluate these children with extreme caution and parents should be warned if observation is chosen under these circumstances. Although there is no absolutely correct answer, the safest approach may be to consider these children "shunt dependent for life."

REFERENCES

1. McLone DG, Knepper PA. The cause of Chiari II malformation: A unified theory. Pediatr Neurosurg 1989; 15:1–12.
2. Caldarelli M, McLone DG, Collins JA, et al. Vitamin A induced neural tube defects in a mouse. Concepts Pediatr Neurosurg 1985; 6:161–171.
3. McLone DG, Mutluer S, Naidich TP. Lipomeningoceles of the conus medullaris. In: Raimondi AJ, ed. Concepts in Pediatric Neurosurgery, Vol. 3. Basel, Switzerland: S. Karger, 1983:170–177.
4. Naidich TP, Maravilla K, McLone DG. The Chiari II malformation. In: McLaurin RL, ed. Spina Bifida: A Multidisciplinary Approach. New York: Praeger Publishing, 1986:164–173.
5. Higbee RG, Nakahara S, Gueye M, et al. Glycoproteins and abnormal neurulation in the delayed splotch mutant. Pediatr Neurosurg 1991.
6. Desmond ME. Description of the occlusion of the spinal cord lumen in early human embryos. Anat Rec 1982; 204:89–93.
7. Desmond ME, Jacobson AG. Embryonic brain enlargement requires cerebrospinal fluid pressure. Dev Biol 1977; 57:188–198.
8. Desmond ME, Schoenwolf GC. Evaluation of the roles of intrinsic and extrinsic factors in occlusion of the spinal neurocele during rapid brain enlargement in the chick embryo. J Embryol Exp Morph 1986; 97:25–46.
9. Kaufman MH. Occlusion of the neural lumen in early mouse embryos analysed by light and electron microscopy. J Embryol Exp Morphol 1983; 78:211–228.
10. Pacheco MA, Marks RW, Schoenwolf GC, et al. Quantification of the initial phases of rapid brain enlargement in the chick embryo. Am J Anat 1986; 175:403–411.
11. Schoenwolf GC. Histological and ultrastructural studies of secondary neurulation in mouse embryos. Am J Anat 1984; 169:361–376.
12. Coulombre AJ, Coulombre JL. The role of mechanical factors in brain morphogenesis. Anat Rec 1958; 130:289–290.
13. Jelínek R, Pexieder T. Pressure of the CSF and the morphogenesis of the CNS I. Chick embryo. Folia Morphol (Praha) 1970; 18:102–110.
14. Pexeider T, Jelínek R. Pressure of the CSF and the morphogenesis of the CNS II. Pressure necessary for normal development of brain vesicles. Folia Morphol (Praha) 1970; 18:181–192.
15. Bell WO, Arbit E, Fraser RAR. One-stage meningomyelocele closure and ventriculoperitoneal shunt placement. Surg Neurol 1987; 27:233–236.
16. Berger MS, Sundsten J, Lemire RJ, et al. Pathophysiology of isolated lateral ventriculomegaly in shunted myelodysplastic children. Pediatr Neurosurg 1990; 16:301–304.
17. Kapron-Brás CM, Trasler DG. Reduction in the frequency of neural tube defects in splotch mice by retinoic acid. Teratol 1985; 32:87–92.
18. Adeloye A, Singh SP, Odeku EL. Stridor, myelomeningocele, and hydrocephalus in a child. Arch Neurol 1970; 23:271–273.
19. Bell WO, Charney EB, Bruce DA, et al. Symptomatic Arnold Chiari malformation: review of experience with 22 cases. J Neurosurg 1987; 66:812–816.

20. Cochrane DD, Adderley R, White CP, et al. Apnea in patients with myelomeningocele. Pediatr Neurosurg 1990–1991; 16:232–239.
21. Holinger PC, Holinger LD, Reichert TJ, et al. Respiratory obstruction and apnea in infants with bilateral abductor vocal cord paralysis, meningomyelocele, hydrocephalus, and Arnold–Chiari malformation. J Pediatr 1978; 92:368–373.
22. Kirsch WM, Duncan BR, Black FO, et al. Laryngeal palsy in association with myelomeningocele, hydrocephalus, and the Arnold–Chiari malformation. J Neurosurg 1969; 28:207–214.
23. Rekate HL. Management of hydrocephalus and the erroneous concept of shunt independence in spina bifida patients. BNI Quart 1988; 4:17–20.
24. Chadduck WM, Seibert JJ, Adametz J, et al. Cranial Doppler ultrasonography correlates with criteria for ventriculoperitoneal shunting. Surg Neurol 1989; 31:122–128.
25. Mapstone TB, Rekate HL, Nulsen FE, et al. Relationship of CSF shunting and IQ in children with myelomeningocele: A retrospective analysis. Childs Brain 1984; 11:112–118.
26. Rekate HL. Shunt revision: Complications and their prevention. Pediatr Neurosurg 1991–1992; 17: 155–162.
27. Scott RM. Preventing and treating shunt complications. In: Scott RM, ed. Concepts in Neurosurgery: Hydrocephalus, Vol. 3. Baltimore, MD: Williams and Wilkins, 1990:115–121.
28. Nulsen FE, Rekate HL. Results of treatment of hydrocephalus as a guide to prognosis and management. In: McLaurin RL, ed. Pediatric Neurosurgery: Surgery of the Developing Nervous System. New York: Grune and Stratton, 1982:229–241.
29. Steinbok P, Irvine B, Cochrane DD, et al. Long-term outcome and complications of children born with meningomyelocele. Childs Nerv Syst 1992; 8:92–96.
30. Young H, Nulsen F, Weiss M. The relationship of intelligence and cerebral mantle in treated infantile hydrocephalus. Pediatrics 1973; 52:38–44.
31. McLone DG, Czyzewski D, Raimondi AJ, et al. Central nervous system infections as a limiting factor in the intelligence of children born with myelomeningocele. Pediatrics 1982; 70:338–342.
32. Storrs BB. Ventricular size and intelligence in myelodysplastic children. Concepts Pediatr Neurosurg 1988; 8:51–56.
33. Bowman RM, McLone DG, Grant JA, et al. Spina bifida outcome: A 25-year prospective. Pediatr Neurosurg 2001; 34:114–120.
34. Bartoshesky LE, Haller J, Scott RM, et al. Seizures in children with myelomeningocele. Am J Dis Child 1985; 139:400–402.
35. Chadduck W, Adametz J. Incidence of seizures in patients with myelomeningocele: A multifactorial analysis. Surg Neurol 1988; 30:281–285.
36. Hack CH, Enrile BG, Donat JF, et al. Seizures in relation to shunt dysfunction in children with myelomeningocele. J Pediatr 1990; 116:57–60.
37. Noetzel MJ, Blake JN. Prognosis for seizure control and remission in children with myelomeningocele. Dev Med Child Neurol 1991; 33:803–810.
38. Hall PV, Campbell RL, Kalsbeck JE. Meningomyelocele and progressive hydromyelia. Progressive paresis in myelodysplasia. J Neurosurg 1975; 43:457–463.
39. Hall P, Lindseth R, Campbell R, et al. Scoliosis and hydrocephalus in myelocele patients. The effects of ventricular shunting. J Neurosurg 1979; 50:174–178.
40. Cinalli G, Sainte-Rose C, Chumas P, et al. Failure of third ventriculostomy in the treatment of aqueductal stenosis in children. Neurosurg Focus 1999; 6:e3.
41. Cinalli G, Salazar C, Mallucci C, et al. The role of endoscopic third ventriculostomy in the management of shunt malfunction. Neurosurgery 1998; 43:1323–1327, discussion 1327–1329.
42. Jones RF, Kwok BC, Stening WA, et al. The current status of endoscopic third ventriculostomy in the management of non-communicating hydrocephalus. Minim Invasive Neurosurg 1994; 37:28–36.
43. Jones RF, Kwok BC, Stening WA, et al. Neuroendoscopic third ventriculostomy. A practical alternative to extracranial shunts in non-communicating hydrocephalus. Acta Neurochir Suppl 1994; 61:79–83.
44. Kelly PJ. Stereotactic third ventriculostomy in patients with nontumoral adolescent/adult onset aqueductal stenosis and symptomatic hydrocephalus. J Neurosurg 1991; 75:865–873.
45. Iantosca MR, Hader WJ, Drake JM. Results of endoscopic third ventriculostomy. Neurosurg Clin N Am 2004; 15:67–75.
46. Drake JM. Endoscopic third ventriculostomy in pediatric patients: The Canadian experience. Neurosurgery 2007; 60:881–886, discussion 881–886.
47. Jones RF, Kwok BC, Stening WA, et al. Third ventriculostomy for hydrocephalus associated with spinal dysraphism: Indications and contraindications. Eur J Pediatr Surg 1996; 6(suppl. 1):5–6.
48. Teo C, Jones R. Management of hydrocephalus by endoscopic third ventriculostomy in patients with myelomeningocele. Pediatr Neurosurg 1996; 25:57–63, discussion 63.

11 | Hydrocephalus in Craniosynostosis

Hartmut Collmann, Jürgen Krauß, and Niels Sörensen

Section of Pediatric Neurosurgery, Neurosurgical Department, University of Würzburg, Würzburg, Germany

INTRODUCTION

Hydrocephalus in primary craniosynostosis, a condition that should not be confused with shunt-induced secondary synostosis (1), is unique in terms of pathogenesis, clinical appearance, and management. First reports about this disorder were published in the very early days of craniofacial surgery (2,3), but knowledge was scarce in former decades, as it was based on incidental findings or on small, highly selected series (4). Only the widespread use of computerized tomography (CT) and magnetic resonance imaging (MRI) permitted systematic studies addressing the questions of incidence, pathogenesis, and clinical significance of dilated ventricles in craniosynostosis (5–8). During the last decade, a number of studies substantially enhanced our knowledge, although many questions still remain (9–16).

From these studies few basic conclusions can be drawn:

1. Ventricular enlargement in craniosynostosis reflects hydrostatic hydrocephalus in some cases, but nonprogressive ventriculomegaly in others (6,8,10,13,17). The term hydrostatic hydrocephalus is meant to imply ventriculomegaly in the presence of raised intracranial pressure.
2. Hydrostatic hydrocephalus predominantly occurs in complex craniosynostosis (6–8,10,13).
3. The diagnosis of hydrostatic hydrocephalus is not always straightforward, inasmuch as raised intracranial pressure may also be caused by craniosynostosis, which in turn interferes with the head expansion usually occurring in infantile hydrocephalus (6,7).

EPIDEMIOLOGY

The reported incidence of progressive hydrocephalus as well as ventriculomegaly in craniosyn-ostosis varies to a great extent (4,10,13). This may be partly due to problems in differentiating hydrocephalus from simple ventriculomegaly, but also to differences of nosologic classifica-tion, which only recently has been improved by molecular genetic testing. The prevalence of active hydrocephalus may only be established by prospective longitudinal studies, which should include repeated imaging studies prior to and after craniosynostosis surgery. No such investigation has been performed, as yet, to the authors' best knowledge.

Irrespective of these difficulties, a low incidence of hydrocephalus comparable to that of the general population has been observed universally in isolated single-suture craniosynos-tosis (7,8,10,13,18). The few reported cases of shunt-dependent hydrocephalus are most often attributable to disorders independent from craniosynostosis (Table 1), such as ventricular hem-orrhage, meningitis, and aqueductal stenosis (4,6–8,10). A remarkable, yet unexplained co-occurrence of coronal synostosis with hydrocephalus related to neural tube defects has also been reported (19). A personal experience of four patients is added to these observations (Table 1). It is conceivable that some of these disorders may also cause a state of compensated shunt-independent ventricular dilatation (13). An important exception from the above-mentioned rule is represented by the rare type of isolated bilateral lambdoid suture synostosis, which is often combined with sagittal suture synostosis to result in the so-called Mercedes-Benz syndrome (20,21). This particular type appears to predispose to hydrocephalus as well as to herniation of the cerebellar tonsils (see below) (Fig. 1).

In contrast, ventricular dilatation is a quite common finding in several craniosynostosis syndromes, the reported incidence ranging from 30% to 70% in patients with Crouzon's and Pfeiffer's syndrome (8,10,22–24) and from 40% to 90% in Apert patients (25–27) (Table 2). Shunting appears necessary predominantly in Crouzon's and Pfeiffer's syndromes, while most cases of Apert syndrome really represent nonprogressive ventriculomegaly (8,26,27). In the

Table 1 Ventricular Size and Prevalence of Hydrostatic Hydrocephalus in Patients with Various Types of Craniosynostosis Examined at the Authors Institution

Type of craniosynostosis	Sample size	Ventricular dilatation (patients)			Shunt-dependent (patients)	Age at shunting min – median – max (mo)
		Mild	Moderate	Severe		
Sagittal	189	13	3	1	2 (a)	1 – N.A. – 8
Frontal	102	9	1	2	1 (b)	2
Unicoronal	64	1	1	2	2 (c)	0.1 – N.A. – 0.2
Bicoronal	29	1	1	2	3 (d)	0.1 – 0.3 – 2
Multiple sutures	16	2	0	0	0	N.A.
Total isolated	400	26	6	7	8	N.A.
Crouzon*	75	17	11	9	13	2 – 22 – 374
Pfeiffer	15	2	4	6	9	3 – 6 – 78
Apert	52	31	8	0	2	18 – N.A. – 42
Saethre-Chotzen	43	3	0	0	0	N.A.
Muenke	28	4	0	0	0	N.A.
Total syndromic	213	57	23	15	24	N.A.

Etiology of shunted hydrocephalus: (a) posthemorrhagic (1 patient), tonsillar herniation (1), (b) cerebral malformation (1), (c) myelomeningocele (2), (d) myelomeningocele (2), amniotic band sequence (1). N.A.: not applicable.
*2 cases of Crouzon syndrome with acanthosis nigricans included.

Saethre-Chotzen or Muenke syndrome, the ventricles are usually found normal, and shunt-dependent hydrocephalus has not been documented so far. This is also true for our own previous study, in which a case of nonprogressive ventriculomegaly had been erroneously classified as Saethre-Chotzen syndrome (6). Progressive hydrocephalus may also occur in other synostosis syndromes including the Crouzon syndrome with acanthosis nigricans: of our two own patients

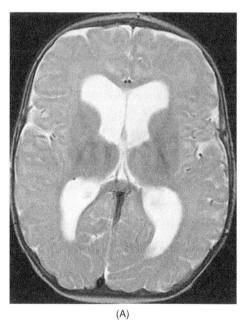
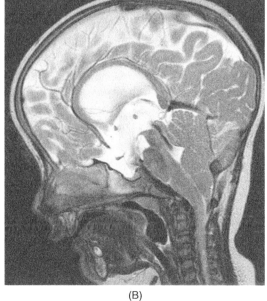

(A)   (B)

Figure 1 (**A**) and (**B**): MRI of a 7-month-old girl with isolated synostosis of the sagittal and lambdoid sutures ("Mercedes-Benz syndrome") and ventriculomegaly. Routine examination revealed papilledema, which resolved after insertion of a ventriculoperitoneal shunt. Note the crowded posterior fossa, ectopic tonsils, and patent aqueduct. *Source*: Courtesy of S. Feuerbach, MD, PhD, Institute of Diagnostic Radiology, and M. Friedrich, MD, Neurosurgical Department, University of Regensburg.

Table 2 Reported Prevalence of Nonprogressive Ventriculomegaly and Progressive
Hydrocephalus in the Most Common Types of Complex Craniosynostosis Syndromes

References	Patients (n)	Normal (%)	Ventriculomegaly (%)	Hydrocephalus (%)
Crouzon				
(8)	12	50	33	17
(24)	35	29	63	9
(10)	86	58	16	26
Würzburg 2006 (unpublished)	75	49	34	17
Pfeiffer				
(8)	5	60	0	40
(23)	11	9	27	64
(10)	18	72	0	28
Würzburg 2006 (unpublished)	15	20	20	60
Apert				
Cohen '92	28	0	93	7
(51)	25	40	48	12
(26)	13	0	92	8
(27)	60	57	35	8
Würzburg 2006 (unpublished)	52	25	71	4

one needed a shunt. In addition, it is described in Carpenter syndrome (8,29), Antley-Bixler syndrome (30), Shprintzen-Goldberg syndrome (31), and some other rare syndromes (32,33) (Table 3). Finally, hydrocephalus is a common feature in thanatophoric dyplasia (34).

PATHOGENESIS
The pathogenesis of hydrocephalus in syndromic craniosynostosis is a matter of ongoing discussion, and reported data are in part conflicting. The former idea of various coincidental disorders is now abandoned as it was based on few exceptional cases (4). The impairment of CSF circulation appears to be related to the site and number of fused sutures and to the time of fusion (9,11,12). No obvious relationship to a specific skull shape has been established except that the Kleeblattschädel deformity in most cases is associated with progressive hydrocephalus (7,10,35). Current authors favor one of the following two pathogenic factors or a combination of both:

- Mechanical obstruction of CSF outflow due to crowding of the posterior fossa (9,11,13–15,36).
- Impaired CSF absorption resulting from venous outlet obstruction (9,10,36,37).

The hypothesis of obstructed CSF pathways was proposed by Rieping (3) as early as 1919 and was later on pursued by David et al. (38) and Venes (39). In fact, with few exceptions,

Table 3 Types of Craniosynostosis in Which Progressive Hydrocephalus or
Nonprogressive Ventriculomegaly are Reported Common Features

Craniosynostosis type	Reference(s)
Mercedes-Benz syndrome	20, 21
Pfeiffer syndrome	7, 10, 13, 23
Crouzon syndrome	6–8, 10, 13, 24, 36
Crouzon syndrome with acanthosis nigricans	28
Beare-Stevenson cutis gyrata syndrome	33
Apert syndrome	4, 8, 10, 13, 17, 26, 27, 51
Carpenter syndrome	8, 10
Shprintzen-Goldberg syndrome	31
Antley-Bixler syndrome	30
Kleeblattschädel deformity	7, 10, 35, 39
Thanatophoric dysplasia	34
Amniotic band sequence	32

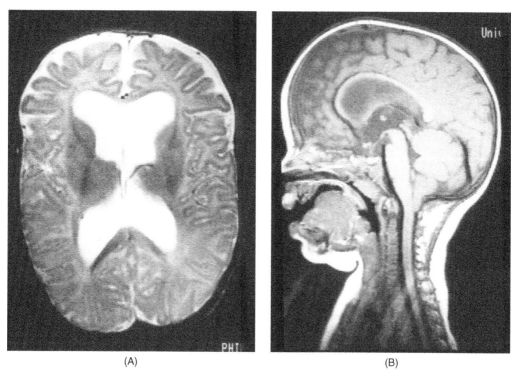

(A)   (B)

Figure 2 (**A**) and (**B**): MRI of a 6-month-old girl with Crouzon syndrome and normal ventricular size at the age of 2 months. Because of progressive ventricular dilatation and papilledema, a VP-shunt was placed. Note herniated cerebellar tonsils and patent aqueduct. *Source*: From Ref. 13.

cases of hydrostatic hydrocephalus exhibit compromised CSF spaces of the posterior fossa, a small fourth ventricle, and herniated cerebellar tonsils (9–12,15,36) (Figs. 1–3). Correspondingly, tonsillar ectopia of varying degree is a common finding in the Crouzon and Pfeiffer syndromes, while it is rarely noted in the Apert syndrome (9,18). Studies of the Paris craniofacial group suggest that crowding of the posterior fossa is an acquired craniocerebral disproportion secondary to deficient occipital cranial expansion, which in turn is related to the time of lambdoid suture fusion (9). This is substantiated by the fact that in the Crouzon and Pfeiffer syndromes, the lambdoid suture closes at an earlier age than in the Apert syndrome (9,12). Additional support comes from experimental findings (40), from estimates of the posterior fossa volume (15,41), and from well-documented postnatal progression of tonsillar ectopia (9,12,16,21). On MR images CSF pathways appear to be compromised at the site of the extracerebral cisterns (11,16,36,42), while the aqueduct is usually shown patent (9,10,15) (Figs. 1 and 2). However, the hypothesis of mechanical CSF pathway obstruction is challenged by some cases of progressive hydrocephalus with absent hindbrain herniation (10). Conversely, many other cases not affected by hydrocephalus do exhibit tonsillar herniation (10,43). Therefore, other causative mechanisms have to be taken into account.

The idea of a defective CSF resorption due to impaired venous outflow was proposed by Hoffman and Hendrick (44), but essentially the same mechanism had been postulated decades before (45,46). The craniofacial group of Paris advanced the concept of venous sinus hypertension as a major factor involved in the evolution of progressive hydrocephalus (10,12,37). Similar to the conditions found in achondroplasia (47,48), these authors documented in some hydrocephalic Crouzon patients a fixed venous sinus hypertension obviously caused by a stenotic jugular foramen (37). Moreover, in one of these patients, they were able to normalize the CSF pressure and the ventricular size by creating a venous bypass between the transverse sinus and the jugular vein. Later on, in a comprehensive study, the group angiographically demonstrated jugular foramen stenosis and an extensive venous collateral

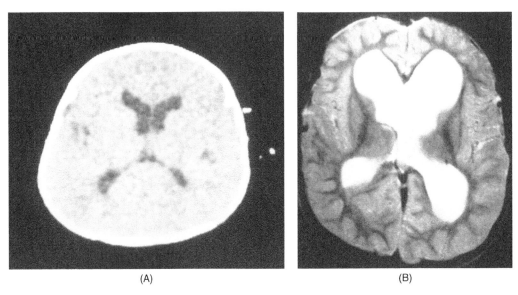

(A)   (B)

Figure 3 (**A**) CT of a 6-month old boy with Pfeiffer syndrome immediately prior to forehead advancement. (**B**) MRI at the age of 30 months showed marked ventricular dilatation in the presence of papilledema, which prompted ventriculoperitoneal shunting. *Source*: From Ref. 13.

network in many Crouzon but few Apert patients (10). Most of these patients actually suffered from shunt-dependent hydrocephalus, whereas only few hydrocephalic patients presented with a normal venous outflow pattern. By applying the vascular theory, the authors provided arguments why progressive hydrocephalus is usually limited to early childhood in that they assumed that venous collateral channels will progressively open with increasing age, thus permitting gradual normalization of the venous sinus pressure. In addition, their findings that the ventricles dilated only in cases in which at least some sutures were still open, comply with the concept of venous hypertension because in a rigid skull the latter should rather induce a pseudotumor-like state (49). Meanwhile, venous hypertension has been accepted as a contributing pathogenic mechanism by other investigators too (15,21,36).

Yet some questions still remain: Given that the same mechanism (i.e., CSF malabsorption) accounts for hydrocephalus in Crouzon syndrome and in achondroplasia, why do patients with achondroplasia only rarely need a shunt, and why do patients with Crouzon syndrome only rarely present with enlarged subarachnoid spaces, which are so common in achondroplasia? In addition, in many cases of severely elevated intracranial pressure and an extensive collateral venous network, actually the ventricles are found normal (43). Finally, although the successful treatment of hydrocephalus by means of a venous bypass provided an argument in favor of an underlying venous problem, unfortunately it could not be substantiated with further patients, since technical problems and the time needed for the small vascular graft to become an efficient shunt prevented further attempts with this kind of treatment (10).

In view of the fact that most patients with progressive hydrocephalus simultaneously exhibit signs of venous outflow obstruction and a crowded posterior fossa, most authors currently favor a combined action of both mechanisms by assuming that venous hypertension causes a CSF absorption deficit as well as brain swelling resulting in tonsillar herniation (36) or that it aggravates the preexistent craniocerebral disproportion by venous engorgement (10,15). The latter appears to be the most accepted theory at present (12).

Nonprogressive, shunt-independent ventriculomegaly is another fairly common phenomenon in complex craniosynostosis. But opinions as to the underlying pathology differ. Early authors postulated brain atrophy (50). This is a conceivable mechanism in a few cases according to our own observations (6). The striking frequency of mild to moderate nonprogressive ventricular dilatation in the Apert syndrome, which so often concurs with other cerebral abnormalities, clearly suggests a primary maldevelopment (8,17,18) (Fig. 4). However, shunt-independent ventriculomegaly is also observed in Crouzon syndrome, which is usually associated with normal

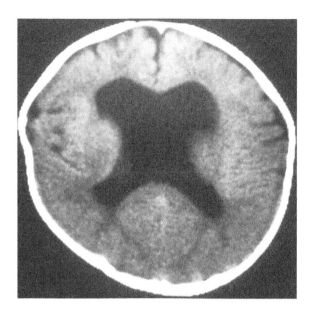

Figure 4 CT of a 12-month-old boy with Apert syndrome showing nonprogressive ventriculomegaly.

cerebral development (Fig. 5). Therefore, Cinalli and coworkers favor the idea of a compensated hydrocephalic state, which they attribute to the same, though less active, mechanisms responsible for progressive hydrocephalus (10). Presently, it may be reasonable to conclude that different mechanisms contribute to nonprogressive ventriculomegaly.

Finally, there is some controversy about the significance of pericerebral CSF collections occasionally noted after cranial surgery, which in some cases prompted treatment with a shunt (10,51). This implied the idea of CSF malabsorption, possibly due to the same mechanism as in progressive hydrocephalus, that is, venous hypertension. Several investigations including intrathecal infusion tests (52,53) and transcranial Doppler sonography (54) seemed to support this idea, although these studies predominantly addressed intracranial pressure and compliance rather than selectively assessing CSF absorption. Consequently, this idea has been doubted (55).

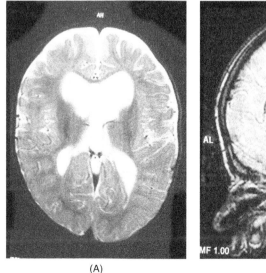 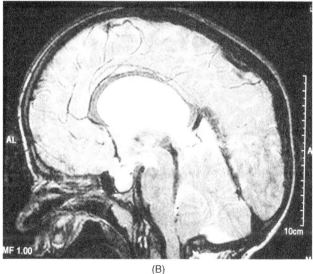

(A)　　　　　　　　　　　　　(B)

Figure 5 (A) A 12-month-old boy with Crouzon syndrome, ventriculomegaly, crowded posterior fossa, and mild tonsillar ectopia. (B) Reexamination at the age of 5 years, 2 months, unchanged. No signs of intracranial hypertension, no surgical treatment, and normal development.

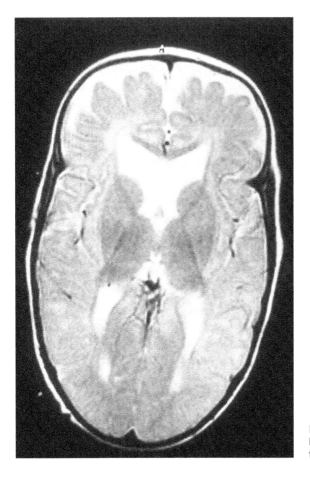

Figure 6 MRI of a 2-month-old boy with iso-lated sagittal synostosis showing extracerebral fluid collections over the frontal lobes.

As a matter of fact, local enlargement of subarachnoid spaces is a quite common phenomenon in craniosynostosis even before surgery (55,56) (Fig. 6). It is mainly confined to regions of compensatory skull expansion and is most pronounced in scaphocephaly (56). Several authors have commented on the possible underlying mechanisms (10,56,57). Modern concepts of calvarial growth in craniosynostosis suggest that the subarachnoid spaces passively dilate to accommodate for the disparate brain shape (58–60). Chadduck et al. suggested that the fluid collections may exert an additional expanding force to the bone by transmitting the brain pulsations without dumping them (55). In addition to this theory, some relationship to the so-called "benign enlargement of subarachnoid spaces" or "external hydrocephalus" has been discussed, since the prominent subarachnoid spaces are usually confined to the first year of age (55,57). In any case, pericerebral fluid collections of major clinical significance, that is, shunt-dependence are rare (10), while transient enlargement of the subarachnoid space is commonly noted after expanding skull surgery at any age (10,13,59–61). In summary, a variety of patients with craniosynostosis, in particular those with Crouzon, Pfeiffer, and Apert syndromes, may present with different patterns of enlarged CSF spaces—progressive hydrocephalus, nonprogressive ventriculomegaly, and dilated subarachnoid spaces. Clinical evaluation will have to focus selecting those patients who require additional shunt treatment.

DIAGNOSTIC EVALUATION

The diagnosis of shunt-dependent hydrocephalus in craniosynostosis is not always straightforward as for instance the accelerated head growth, usually observed in hydrocephalic infants, will be absent if the sutures are fused. In some cases, the ventricles remain small within the synostotic skull only to dilate after decompressive cranial surgery (6,10). In addition, intracranial hypertension is an ambiguous sign attributable to increased CSF outflow resistance, venous hypertension, or the constricting osseous pathology (15). Conversely, even moderate ventricular enlargement in the presence of intracranial hypertension does not necessarily signify shunt-dependent hydrocephalus (13). In difference to other authors (8,10), we do not rely on radio-logical signs of hydrostatic hydrocephalus such as dilated temporal horns, as we hold these signs to be of low significance. In our own series, we were not able to separate nonprogressive ventriculomegaly from true hydrocephalus merely on the basis of ventricular size and shape, except that severe ventricular dilatation usually indicated shunt-dependence.

For practical purposes, some diagnostic guidelines can yet be established. To begin with, ventricular distortion in a towering skull should be clearly separated from true dilatation (45). Also, the enlargement of the intra- and extracerebral CSF spaces following a cranial expansion procedure should not be confused with true hydrocephalus (Fig. 7). It is useful to estimate the individual risk of developing hydrostatic hydrocephalus by looking for the main risk factors: multiple suture craniosynostosis, in particular the Crouzon and Pfeiffer phenotypes, Kleeblattschädel deformity, any progressive synostosis involving the lambdoid suture at an early age, a crowded posterior fossa, and herniated cerebellar tonsils. Routine MR imaging including MR venography should be performed not only in all patients presenting with Crouzon, Pfeiffer, or Apert syndrome (10,18,43), but also in cases of multisutural synostosis or bilateral lambdoid synostosis combined with sagittal synostosis. Gross crowding of the posterior fossa or tonsillar ectopia should prompt careful surveillance of the intracranial pressure and the ventricular size, making use of ophthalmoscopy and ultrasound or computerized tomography as basic diagnostic tools. As in other forms of hydrocephalus, subjective symptoms of intracra-nial hypertension like headaches, nausea, and vomiting may be missed, while, for instance, papilledema is noted frequently.

In 50% (in our series: 33%) of the patients affected by hydrostatic hydrocephalus, the diagnosis is straightforward because of rapidly progressive ventricular dilatation prior to any surgical intervention, and this is mainly confined to early infancy (10,12) (Figs. 1 and 2). In most of the remaining patients, ventricular dilatation of varying degree will only become apparent after skull surgery. In these cases, the indication for shunting is mainly based on gross ventricular expansion and/or persisting intracranial hypertension, which is documented ophthalmoscopi-cally or by invasive pressure monitoring (Fig. 3). It should be kept in mind that cranial expansion can be followed by a distinct dilatation of the intracerebral as well as extracerebral CSF spaces, which subsequently may shrink again (Fig. 7). In such cases, however, the possibility of a com-pensated or even slowly progressive hydrocephalic state should also be taken into consideration. Therefore, it is prudent to keep these patients under careful long-term surveillance.

Finally, a few patients present with mild or moderate, sometimes even slightly progressive ventricular enlargement, and signs of elevated intracranial pressure, who yet may remain shunt-independent after adequate cranial expansion (6,13,62). In these cases, we prefer to first operate on the craniosynostosis and then carefully observe the ventricular size and intracranial pressure afterwards (10).

TREATMENT AND OUTCOME

Although improvement of ventricular dilatation has been anecdotally reported following removal of constricting bony ridges (35), most attempts to relieve progressive hydrocephalus by eliminating its potential causes have failed or could not be established as routine techniques (9,10,11, and comments therein). Nevertheless, some authors recommend suboccipital decom-pression as a first-stage procedure (11,12). To the authors' knowledge, third ventriculostomy has not been evaluated within this context, and a single successful procedure in a personal case of progressive hydrocephalus associated with tonsillar herniation is not conclusive. Hence, shunting appears to be the single feasible mode of treatment. In the presence of hindbrain herniation, there is certainly no place for the lumbar route, as this can result in a fatal course (63). When selecting the valve system, it seems advisable to take particular precautions against overdrainage, because the latter may induce a pseudotumor-like state (49), which in craniosyn-ostosis may add to the preexisting venous problem. We prefer a high-pressure valve with a well-functioning antisiphon device incorporated.

Admittedly, shunting does not cure the venous outlet problem. In fact, the clinical sig-nificance of untreated venous outflow obstruction remains unclear. It is assumed that venous

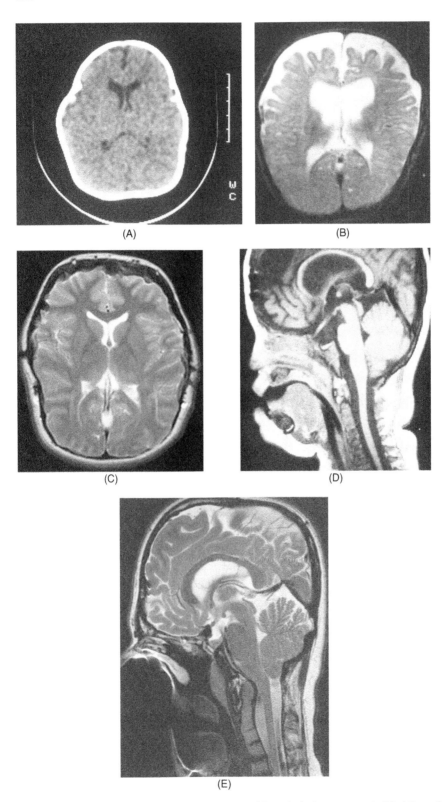

Figure 7   Girl with Pfeiffer syndrome (**A**) at the age of 3 weeks before treatment, (**B**) at 7 months after a two-stage cranial expansion procedure, (**C**) at 16 years. Note progressive tonsillar herniation between the age of 7 months (**D**) and 16 years (**E**).

hypertension persists throughout early childhood until an age of about six years when sufficient collateral channels have opened (16,21,36,62).

It is tempting to treat any kind of ventricular dilatation by shunting with the simple intention of gaining space and avoiding extensive cranial surgery. Without taking in to account the problem of shunt morbidity, this policy at best may be justified occasionally after brain growth has been completed. But it is certainly ill-advised in childhood, because the drained CSF spaces will rapidly be filled up by the growing brain while the skull will be deprived of an important growth stimulus.

Timing of shunt placement in relation to skull surgery is a matter of additional concern because the stability of cranial reconstruction may be endangered if the dura is prevented from rapid expansion due to the depletion of CSF spaces, and the cranial content fails to support the bone plates in due time. One of our patients had to be reoperated because skin tension caused a displacement of some bone segments that had not been firmly secured during the initial procedure. Taking the dynamics of bone healing and brain growth into account, it is reasonable to postpone any reconstructive cranial procedure after primary shunt insertion, until intracranial hypertension recurs. Secondary shunting after cranial remodeling should be deferred for at least two months. If this is not feasible, particular effort should be made to firmly secure the surgical bone plates before impending shunt surgery.

There is little evidence that moderately dilated ventricles per se have an adverse effect on mental outcome (8,27,51), whereas the severe congenital hydrocephalus, as observed in the Kleeblattschädel deformity, obviously carries an increased risk of a subnormal performance level (35,64). As in hydrocephalus of other origin the prognosis mainly depends on concurrent cerebral abnormalities and on the detrimental effect of long-standing elevated CSF pressure.

REFERENCES

1. Kloss JL. Craniosynostosis secondary to ventriculoatrial shunt. Am J Dis Child 1968; 116:315–317.
2. Park EA, Powers GF. Acrocephaly and scaphocephaly with symmetrically distributed malformations of the extremities. Am J Dis Child 1920; 20:235–315.
3. Rieping A. Zur Pathogenese des Turmschädels. Dtsch Z Chir 1919; 148:1–51.
4. Fishman MA, Hogan GR, Dodge PR. The concurrence of hydrocephalus and craniosynostosis. J Neurosurg 1971; 34:621–629.
5. Carmel PW, Luken MG, Ascherl GF. Craniosynostosis: Computed tomographic evaluation of skull base and calvarial deformities and associated intracranial changes. Neurosurgery 1981; 9:366–372.
6. Collmann H, Sörensen N, Krauss J, et al. Hydrocephalus in craniosynostosis. Childs Nerv Syst 1988; 4:279–285.
7. Golabi M, Edwards MSB, Ousterhout DK. Craniosynostosis and hydrocephalus. Neurosurgery 1987; 21:63–67.
8. Noetzel MJ, Marsh JL, Palkes H, et al. Hydrocephalus and mental retardation in craniosynostosis. J Pediatr 1985; 107:885–892.
9. Cinalli G, Renier D, Sebag G, et al. Chronic tonsillar herniation in Crouzon's and Apert's syndromes: The role of premature synostosis of the lambdoid suture. J Neurosurg 1995; 83:575–582.
10. Cinalli G, Sainte-Rose C, Kollar EM, et al. Hydrocephalus and craniosynostosis. J Neurosurg 1998; 88:209–214.
11. Cinalli G, Chumas P, Arnaud E, et al. Occipital remodelling and suboccipital decompression in severe craniosynostosis associated with tonsillar herniation. Neurosurgery 1998; 42:66–73.
12. Cinalli G, Spennato P, Sainte-Rose C, et al. Chiari malformation in craniosynostosis. Childs Nerv Syst 2005, 21:889–901.
13. Collmann H, Krauß J. Sörensen N, Hydrocephalus in craniosynostosis: A review. Childs Nerv Syst 2005; 21:902–912.
14. Hayward R. Venous hypertension and craniosynostosis. Childs Nerv Syst 2005; 21:880–888.
15. Thompson DNP, Harkness W, Jones BM, et al. Aetiology of herniation of the hindbrain in craniosynostosis. Pediatr Neurosurg 1997; 26:288–295.
16. Thompson DNP, Jones BM, Harkness W, et al. Consequences of cranial vault expansion for craniosynostosis. Pediatr Neurosurg 1997; 26:296–303.
17. Cohen MM, Kreiborg S. The central nervous system in the Apert syndrome. Am J Med Genet 1990; 35:36–45.
18. Tokumaru AM, Barkovich AJ, Ciricillo SF, et al. Skull base and calvarial deformities: Association with intracranial changes in craniofacial syndromes. Am J Neuroradiol 1996; 17:619–630.

19. Martinez-Lage JF, Poza M, Lluch T, et al. Craniosynostosis in neural tube defects: A theory on its pathogenesis. Surg Neurol 1996; 46:465–470.

20. Moore MH, Abbott AH, Netherway DJ, et al. Bilambdoid and posterior sagittal synostosis: The Mercedes Benz syndrome. J Craniofac Surg 1998; 9:417–422.

21. Rollins N, Booth T, Shapiro K. MR venography in children with complex craniosynostosis. Pediatr Neurosurg 2000; 32:308–315.

22. Montaut J, Stricker M. Les dysmorphies craniofaciales. Les synostoses prématurées (craniosténoses et faciosténoses). Neurochirurgie 1977; 23(suppl. 2): 1–299.

23. Moore MH, Hanieh A. Hydrocephalus in Pfeiffer syndrome. J Clin Neuroscience 1994; 1:202–204.

24. Proudman TW, Clark BE, Moore MH, et al. Central nervous system imaging in Crouzon's syndrome. J Craniofac Surg 1995; 6:401–405.

25. Cohen MM, Kreiborg S. Unpublished data 1992, cited in Cohen MM. Apert syndrome. In: Cohen MM, McLean RE, eds. Craniosynostosis—Diagnosis, Evaluation, and Management, 2nd ed. New York: Oxford, Oxford University Press, 2000:316–353.

26. Hanieh A, David DJ. Apert's syndrome. Childs Nerv Syst 1993; 9:289–291.

27. Renier D, Arnaud E, Cinalli G, et al. Prognosis for mental function in Apert's syndrome. J Neurosurg 1996; 85:66–72.

28. Meyer GA, Orlow SJ, Munro IR, et al. Fibroblast growth factor receptor 3 (FGFR3) transmembrane mutation in Crouzon syndrome with acanthosis nigricans. Nat Genet 1995; 11:462–464.

29. Taravath S, Tonsgard JH. Cerebral malformations in Carpenter syndrome. Pediatr Neurol 1993; 9:230–234.

30. Lee HJ, Cho DY, Tsai FJ, et al. Antley-Bixler syndrome, description of two new cases and review of the literature. Pediatr Neurosurg 2001; 34:33–39.

31. Greally MT, Carey JC, Milewicz DM, et al. Shprintzen-Goldberg syndrome: A clinical analysis. Am J Med Gen 1998; 76:202–212.

32. Bamforth JS. Amniotic band sequence: Streeter's hypothesis re-examined. Am J Med Genet 1992; 44:280–287.

33. Wang TJ, Hung KS, Chen PK, et al. Beare-Stevenson cutis gyrata syndrome with Chiari malformation. Acta Neurochir 2002; 144:743–745.

34. Cohen MM. Achondroplasia, hypochondroplasia, and thanatophoric dysplasia: Clinically skeletal dysplasias that are also related at the molecular level. Int J Oral Maxillofac Surg 1998; 27: 451–455.

35. Shiroyama Y, Ito H, Yamashita T, et al. The relationship of cloverleaf skull syndrome to hydrocephalus. Childs Nerv Syst 1991; 7:382–385.

36. Francis PM, Beals S, Rekate HL, et al. Chronic tonsillar herniation and Crouzon's syndrome. Pediatr Neurosurg 1992; 18:202–206.

37. Sainte-Rose C, Lacombe J, Pierre-Kahn A, et al. Intracranial venous sinus hypertension: Cause or consequence of hydrocephalus in infants? J Neurosurg 1984; 60:727–736.

38. David DJ, Poswillo D, Simpson D. The Craniosynostoses. Causes, Natural History and Management. Berlin, Germany: Springer, 1982.

39. Venes JL. Arnold-Chiari malformation in an infant with Kleeblattschädel: An acquired malformation? Neurosurgery 1988; 23:360–362.

40. Marin-Padilla M, Marin-Padilla. TM morphogenesis of experimentally induced Arnold-Chiari malformation. J Neurol Sci 1981; 50:29–55.

41. Sgouros S, Natarajan K, Hockley AD, et al. M Skull base growth in craniosynostosis. Pediatr Neurosurg 1999; 31:281–293.

42. Scarfo GB, Tomaccini D, Gambacorta D, et al. Contribution to the study of craniostenosis: Disturbance of the cerebrospinal fluid flow in oxycephaly. Helv Paediatr Acta 1979; 34:235–243.

43. Taylor WJ, Hayward RD, Lasjaunias P, et al. Enigma of raised intracranial pressure in patients with complex craniosynostosis: The role of abnormal intracranial venous drainage. J Neurosurg 2001; 94:377–385.

44. Hoffman HJ, Hendrick EB. Early neurosurgical repair in craniofacial dysmorhism. J Neurosurg 1979; 51:796–803.

45. Gross H. Zur Kenntnis der Beziehungen zwischen Gehirn und Schädelkapsel bei den turricephalen craniostenostischen Dysostosen. Virchows Arch [Pathol Anat] 1957; 330:365–383.

46. Günther H. Der Turmschädel als Konstitutionsanomalie und als klinisches Symptom. Ergeb Inn Med Kinderheilk 1931; 40:40–135.

47. Pierre-Kahn A, Hirsch JF, Renier D, et al. Hydrocephalus and achondroplasia. A study of 25 observations. Childs Brain 1980; 7:205–219.

48. Steinbok P, Hall J, Flodmark O. Hydrocephalus in achondroplasia: The possible role of intracranial venous hypertension. J Neurosurg 1989; 71:42–48.

49. Karahalios DG, Rekate HL, Khayata MH, et al. Elevated intracranial venous pressure as a universal mechanism in pseudotumor cerebri of varying etiologies. Neurology 1996; 46:198–202.

50. Bertelsen TI. The premature synostosis of the cranial sutures. Acta Ophthalmol (Kbh) Suppl 1958; 51:1–176.

51. Murovic JA, Posnick JC, Drake JM, et al. Hydrocephalus in Apert syndrome: A retrospective review. Pediatr Neurosurg 1993; 19:151–155.

52. Di Rocco C, Caldarelli M, Mangiola A, et al. The lumbar subarachnoid infusion test in infants. Childs Nerv Syst 1988; 4:16–21.

53. Lundar T, Nornes H. Steady-state lumbar infusion tests in the management of children with craniosynostosis. Childs Nerv Syst 1991; 7:31–33.

54. Mursch K, Enk T, Christen HJ, et al. Venous intracranial hemodynamics in children undergoing operative treatment for the repair of craniosynostosis—A prospective study using transcranial colour-coded duplex sonography. Childs Nerv Syst 1999; 15:110–118.

55. Chadduck WM, Chadduck JB, Boop FA. The subarachnoid spaces in craniosynostosis. Neurosurgery 1992; 30:867–871.

56. Hassler W, Zentner J. Radical osteoclastic craniectomy in sagittal synostosis. Neurosurgery 1990; 27:539–543.

57. Sawin PD, Muhonen MG, Menezes AH. Quantitative analysis of cerebrospinal fluid spaces in children with occipital plagiocephaly. J Neurosurg 1996; 85:428–434.

58. Delashaw JB, Persing JA, Broaddus WC, et al. Cranial vault growth in craniosynostosis. J Neurosurg 1989; 70:159–165.

59. Moore MH, Abbott AH. Extradural deadspace after infant fronto-orbital advancement in Apert syndrome. Cleft Palate Craniofac J 1996; 33:202–205.

60. Moore MH, Hanieh A. Cerebrospinal fluid spaces before and after fronto-orbital advancement in unilateral coronal craniosynostosis. J Craniofac Surg 1996; 7:102–105.

61. Marchac D, Renier D. Craniofacial Surgery for Craniosynostosis. Boston, MA: Little, Brown and Co., 1982.

62. Gosain AK, McCarthy JG, Wisoff JH. Morbidity associated with increased intracranial pressure in Apert and Pfeiffer syndromes: The need for long-term evaluation. Plast Reconstr Surg 1996; 97:292–301.

63. Chumas PD, Drake JM, Del Bigio MR. Death from chronic tonsillar herniation in a patient with lumboperitoneal shunt and Crouzon's disease. Br J Neurosurg 1992; 6:595–599.

64. Lodge ML, Moore MH, Hanieh A, et al. The cloverleaf skull anomaly: Managing extreme cranio-orbitofaciostenosis. Plast Reconstr Surg 1993; 91:1–9, discussion 10–14.

12 | Uncommon Congenital Malformations and Hydrocephalus

Jerard Ross

Department of Paediatric Neurosurgery, The Royal Hospital for Sick Children, Edinburgh

INTRODUCTION

A number of congenital malformations that are associated with hydrocephalus have been discussed in other chapters, e.g., aqueductal stenosis, Chiari malformations, arachnoid cysts, and craniosynostosis and will not be discussed further here. This chapter will concentrate on the less-common congenital malformations resulting in hydrocephalus, such as the Dandy–Walker malformation, encephalocele, agenesis of the corpus callosum, hydranencephaly, and holoprosencephaly.

DANDY–WALKER MALFORMATION

First described by Dandy in 1914 (1) and further by Taggart (2), the term Dandy–Walker Malformation was later coined to delineate a congenital malformation comprising of cystic dilatation of the fourth ventricle, partial or complete absence of the cerebellar vermis, and hydrocephalus (3). Hydrocephalus is not present in all cases and it has been dropped from the diagnostic criteria.

The classic Dandy–Walker malformation (DWM) is defined by the presence of a large median posterior fossa cyst (more properly a diverticulum) widely communicating with the fourth ventricle, associated with a rotated, elevated, and hypoplastic or aplastic cerebellar vermis contacting an upwardly displaced tentorium and similarly displaced transverse sinuses. There is in addition posterior bossing of the posterior fossa contributing to its enlargement and anterolateral displacement of normal or hypoplastic cerebellar hemispheres (4). The cystic dilatation of the fourth ventricle fills the posterior fossa and extends into the cisterna magna, which is compressed between the dilated fourth ventricle and the posterior fossa dura. The cystic CSF collection in the posterior fossa does not communicate freely with the basal cisterns [Fig. 1(A) and 1(B)].

Dandy Walker: Changing Terminology

However, there is a marked heterogeneity of the conditions grouped under the heading "Dandy Walker" that causes confusion in the literature. Barkovich et al. (5) changed the terminology to that of Dandy–Walker complex (DWC) to denote a spectrum of disorders including classic DWM at one extreme all of which include a cyst communicating with the fourth ventricle. The other members of the DWC are where much of the confusion arises in terminology.

The crucial point according to Barkovich et al. is to assess the axial images at the mid fourth ventricle level; no vermian tissue interposed between the fourth ventricle and the cyst indicates a Type A DWC, which is either a classic DWM or a "Dandy–Walker variant" (DWV). The Dandy–Walker variant being, effectively, the same widely communicating cyst without all of the features of a classic DWM, particularly the enlargement of the posterior fossa (Fig. 2).

If vermis is interposed between the cyst and the fourth ventricle at the level of the mid-fourth ventricle, then this is referred to as a type B DWC lesion, the equivalent, traditional term being mega cisterna magna (MCM). Tortori-Donati et al. (6) introduced the concept of the Blake's Pouch Cyst (BPC) differentiated from the MCM by the presence of hydrocephalus; the difference between these lesions being the lack of communication with the perimedullary basal cisterns in the BPC (7) [Fig. 3(A) and 3(B)].

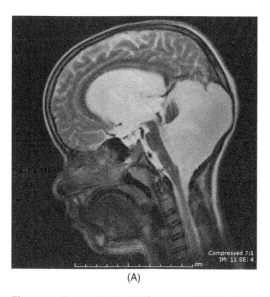
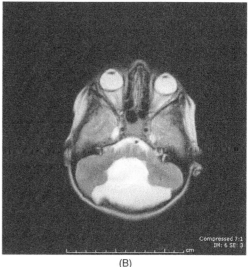

(A)   (B)

Figure 1 Dandy–Walker Malformation (DWM). These MR images in the midsagittal (**A**) and mid-fourth ventricle axial (**B**) plains show the salient features of the classic DWM, namely, the rotated and partially agenetic vermis, the high insertion of the torcular, the enlarged posterior fossa, and the wide communication between the fourth ventricle proper and the "cyst." Note the widely patent aqueduct with flow void.

Other CSF density collections in the posterior fossa include arachnoid cysts (Fig. 4). These generally do not communicate with the fourth ventricle, which they often distort; the vermis and cerebellum are usually normal. CSF flow studies may help differentiate lesions of DWC from arachnoid cysts (8). A prominent cisterna magna may be found in pathology resulting in atrophy of the vermis and cerebellar hemispheres.

Although it appears that much has been made of the classification and the subtleties of diagnosis, there is evidence that the pathoanatomical abnormality may correspond with prognosis (4,9). By the same token, the labeling of posterior fossa CSF collections is fraught with controversy, and MR imaging has confirmed that the displacement of structures, such as the vermis, is of less significance in terms of outcome than the normality or otherwise of those structures (Fig. 5). However, the DWV remains a heterogeneous disorder and is where most of the confusion arises.

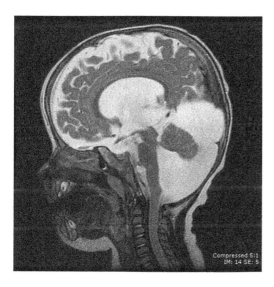

Figure 2 Dandy–Walker variant (DWV).

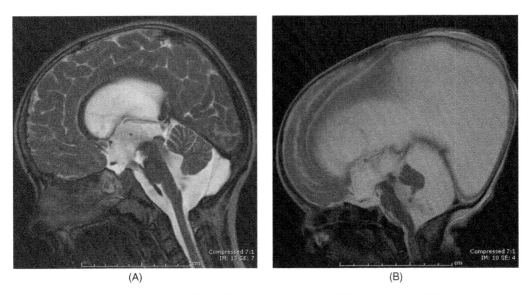

(A)   (B)

Figure 3   These MR images show two different Blakes Pouch Cysts: part (**A**) shows a small BPC with a functioning third ventriculostomy, while part (**B**) shows a giant BPC with a normally formed, fully lobulated vermis.

Etiology of DWC

The Dandy–Walker complex can arise in the context of Mendelian disorders, chromosomal disorders (trisomies, deletions, and duplications), and with teratogen exposure (alcohol, viral infection, drugs). In addition, the DWC may be associated with other brain malformations in 68% of cases (10) including aqueductal stenosis, callosal agenesis, and neural tube defects. In addition, significant extracerebral malformations, particularly of the heart, the kidneys, the palate, the perineum, and the vertebrae, are present in about 45% (11–13). For these reasons, it is imperative that every new case of the DWC is assessed by a clinical geneticist and other abnormalities identified. This in addition allows assessment of the etiology and recurrence risk, of the order of 1% to 10%, out with the context of Mendelian disorders (14) and allows appropriate parental counseling.

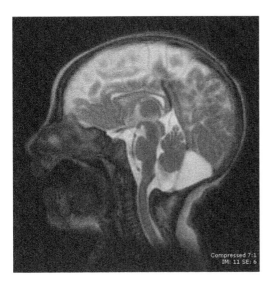

Figure 4   This image shows a posterior fossa arachnoid cyst compressing the normal vermis.

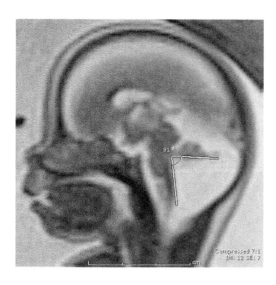

Figure 5 Fetal MRI showing DWM. Note the degree of rotation of the vermis from the tegmentum of the mesencephalon (tegmentovermian angle).

Epidemiology
Incidence of the order of 1:25,000 to 1:30,000 live births (12,13,15) with DWC accounting for around 4% of all cases of hydrocephalus. The majority of fetuses with prenatally diagnosed DWM or DWV will not survive to term (16).

Presenting Features
The majority of children present in the first year of life (11,12,15); the infants tending to present with macrocrania and features of raised intracranial pressure; older children often present with developmental delay and psychomotor retardation. In older children and adults, DWC may present similarly to a posterior fossa tumor.

Treatment Options
The surgical approach to DWC has evolved over the last century, with a move away from the direct surgical approaches to the cyst recommended by the pioneers to management directed toward the hydrocephalus. In recent years, there has been a partial return to surgical therapy of the cyst in limited circumstances.

The advent of CSF shunts changed therapy for DWC, but there are some fundamental questions required before placing a shunt into someone with the DWC.

Does the patient have hydrocephalus? This seems an obvious point but not all cases of DWC have hydrocephalus, so a careful clinical assessment for other features of hydrocephalus and raised pressure should be made. Confirmatory evidence including abnormal cranial growth on the centile charts, bulging fontanelles, or splayed sutures must be sought. Complications from shunting patients with DWC are rife and placement of the shunt should be considered. The figure of 90% of patients with DWC developing hydrocephalus has been used, but given that patients with hydrocephalus are those that present to neurosurgeons, a significant proportion may be asymptomatic (13).

Is the diagnosis of DWC correct? The differential diagnosis of a posterior fossa cystic structure with CSF density on CT includes the prominent cisterna magna, MCM, arachnoid cysts, trapped fourth ventricle, cystic tumors, the DWM, and the DWV. It is imperative that CT is not relied upon solely to make the diagnosis, as placement of a lateral ventricle shunt is unlikely to adequately treat a posterior fossa arachnoid cyst or tumor and is unlikely to be necessary in a prominent cisterna magna.

Is the cerebral aqueduct open? Aqueductal stenosis has been associated with the DWC; however, it is not always present. Shunting of the lateral ventricles alone will not adequately treat a patient with a posterior fossa cyst and aqueductal stenosis.

Where is the transverse sinus? The high position of the transverse sinus in DWM must be considered when placing shunts in the parieto-occipital region.

The major disagreement in the literature is the proximal position of the shunt; whether they should be in lateral ventricle, in the posterior fossa cyst, or in both connected with a "Y" connector. Unsurprisingly, with such a rare condition there have been no comparative trials of neurosurgical strategies. The literature consists primarily of case series from large institutions garnered over many years, as such they consist, largely, of series of different operations done in different periods with the only comparisons being historical controls. If we add the fact that many of the cohorts were accumulated in the pre-MRI era, the value of the literature drops further. However, much pre-MR data is regularly quoted.

Patency of the aqueduct is an absolute requirement for a single shunt in whichever compartment. The incidence of aqueductal stenosis is unclear with and much of the confusion surrounding this topic may be due to the inclusion in the literature of early studies from the pre-MR era. A number of authors have indicated that aqueductal stenosis is uncommon (17–19) on both MRI assessment and ventriculographically. Strict diagnostic categorization is necessary in future studies to answer the question adequately; however, the aqueduct must be assessed radiologically.

Cystoperitoneal shunts, that is, fourth ventricular shunts have found favor over the years, although they are difficult to place and secure as well as being associated with significant complications, for example, posterior fossa hematomas (20), cranial nerve palsies, intraventricular hemorrhage (21), and brainstem tethering with resultant headaches (22). A number of authors have reported favorable results with cyst shunts (12,18); these are, however, mixed series over different epochs. Further complications may accrue depending on the choice of valve employed in the shunt; the use of low-pressure valves can result in significant herniation of the medial aspects of the lateral ventricles through the tentorial hiatus resultant mesencephalic deformation and secondary aqueductal stenosis (23). This may go some way explaining the prevalence of aqueductal stenosis in historical series (24), a finding not borne out in contemporary series.

The perceived risk of aqueductal stenosis resulted in a number of centers placing shunts into both the cyst and the lateral ventricle joined by a Y connector, this allowed pressure equalization across the tent, and a number of groups have reported their experience of this approach as a primary procedure (15,25). Other groups have placed either a VP or a CP shunt as the first procedure and gone on to a second shunt if there developed a failure of communication between the cyst and the ventricles. Bindal et al. (20) were unable to pinpoint any difference in outcome between children with CP and VP shunts, but opted for VP as the first line due to the lesser complication profile. In that study, conversion from single to double shunt secondary to expansion of the unshunted compartment occurred in 42% of CP only and 30% of VP only patients. In the cohort from the Toronto group (18), 35% of those who had a VP shunt went on to develop a noncommunicating cyst. In another mixed cohort (17), 17% of those shunted from the cyst only and none of the VP shunt's required placement of a second shunt. Similarly, a review of the data from the Necker Group in Paris suggests that very few of those infants shunted in one or other compartment require a second shunt, and that supratentorial shunts fail less frequently. They stress in addition that low-pressure valves must be avoided and recommended medium pressure or flow regulating valves (26).

Third Ventriculostomy and Endoscopically Placed Shunts

Given the significant complication rate of shunt surgery in patients with the DWC, third ventriculostomy has been attempted by both radiological techniques and more recently endoscopically. Hirsch et al. (12) and Hoffman et al. (27) reported a 50% success rate with radiologically guided third ventriculostomy albeit with very small numbers in the study. Endoscopic third ventriculostomy (ETV) has superceded this procedure and has been reported by a number of groups. The largest single series is that of Mohanty et al. (17) who as part of a bigger mixed series reported their experiences of ETV either as a stand alone procedure or with additional maneuvers (aqueductal stenting and cyst fenestration) in 21 patients, 5 of the ETV patients required subsequent VP shunt insertion. The report does not indicate why ETV was chosen in some cases and not others, and patient ages are not indicated, although half of the children in the whole cohort were less than one-year old. Cinalli reported the results of his series of four cases in 1999 with successful resolution of the hydrocephalus in three cases (26).

Open fenestration of cysts has been recommended in patients with multiple shunt-related complications and failure of control of hydrocephalus. In a series of six patients, Villavicencio et al. (28) performed small suboccipital craniectomies and cyst fenestration with good outcome in five patients.

Outcome

The mortality of the DWC has dropped in the modern era to around 10%. Children still die of infectious complications, poorly controlled hydrocephalus, and shunt-related complications.

In general, the more normal the brain and the rest of the body, the better the outlook, and in the absence of other major malformations, the early and adequate treatment of hydrocephalus is one of the most important factors in a normal intellectual achievement (15).

Boddaert et al. (9) have suggested that there is a close relationship between the degree of vermian malformation and intellectual outcome. The more complete the lobulation of the vermis, the better the intellectual outcome is likely to be.

Counseling

Perinatal outcome of a prenatally diagnosed case of DWC is related to the fetal karyotype and as indicated associated anomalies (29), and therefore all pregnancies with a prenatal diagnosis of DWC require in-depth ultrasonographic assessment, prenatal MRI, and amniocentesis for karyotype (Fig. 5). Prenatally diagnosed DWC is associated with a poor outcome overall (16,30).

HYDROCEPHALUS AND ENCEPHALOCELE

The term encephalocele is used to describe all congenital cranial herniations. Traditionally, encephaloceles are divisible into posterior and anterior encephaloceles. The more common, at least in western populations, posterior lesions are classified into parietal and occipital lesions with the occipital lesions including supra- and infratorcular subtypes. These are cystic swellings with variable skin coverage. A significant subgroup of these includes the atretic encephalocele, which is usually flat and noncystic. The rarer anterior encephaloceles are herniations through the anterior skull base and they are classified as, sincipital, where the herniation is through the foramen cecum anterior to the cribriform plate, or basal, where the herniation is through the sphenoid bone and sinus.

Posterior encephaloceles are associated with very significant brain abnormalities including hydrocephalus, agenesis of the corpus callosum, DWC, gray matter heterotopias, and venous drainage anomalies (Fig. 6). Parietal lesions are particularly associated with dorsal interhemispheric cysts, which may communicate directly with the ventricular system; in extreme cases, they may be associated with holoprosencephaly. MRI is mandatory before exploring these lesions to delineate other abnormalities, and MRV may help delineate venous anatomy, which is frequently abnormal.

The incidence of hydrocephalus in posterior encephaloceles is variably reported and these series are accrued over long epochs, therefore outcome assessment is difficult as is individual prognostication. Simpson et al. (31) reported a series of 74 encephaloceles and found hydrocephalus in 9, while Docherty et al. (32) noted hydrocephalus requiring treatment in 18 out of 52 patients with ventriculomegaly in a further 11 patients. The frequent combination of parietal encephalocele and hydrocephalus was indicated by Yokota et al. (33). They found that 11 out of 15 cases (mixed cystic and atretic) had hydrocephalus and this was associated with a poor prognosis as regards intellectual outcome. The association between atretic encephaloceles and hydrocephalus has been further confirmed by Martinez-Lage et al. (34) who found 8 from 16 patients with atretic encephaloceles had hydrocephalus, although in his series it was associated with occipital lesions predominantly. Another contemporary series (35) confirms a high incidence of hydrocephalus in posterior encephaloceles; in their series 18 out of 30 required treatment for hydrocephalus.

Hydrocephalus is less common in anterior lesions with an incidence of 13 cases in 103 anterior encephaloceles in a recent study (36). All 13 cases had radiological hydrocephalus, which was treated with a shunt before the surgery for the encephalocele.

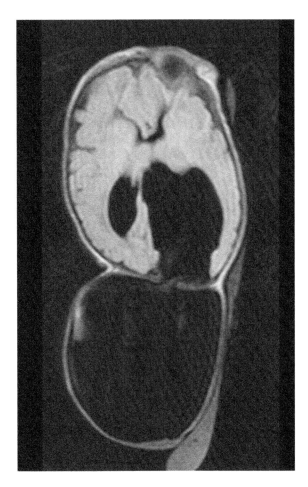

Figure 6 Encephalocele. T1w axial MR scan of a newborn baby with encephalocele and hydrocephalus. There is a large encephalocele sac in direct communication with the ventricular system through the occipital horn of the left lateral ventricle. *Source*: Photograph courtesy of Dr S. Sgouros.

HYDROCEPHALUS AND AGENESIS OF THE CORPUS CALLOSUM

The corpus callosum is the major commissural structure and its complete or partial agenesis is a common brain malformation with a prevalence of 0.5 to 70 per 10,000 in children with developmental delay. It is rarely isolated and is often associated with other serious brain malformations, that is, DWC, Chiari malformations, holoprosencephaly, and interhemispheric cysts (37) [Fig. 7(A) and 7(B)].

A large survey of the etiology of congenital hydrocephalus indicated that agenesis of the corpus callosum was a relatively common cause of fetal and to a lesser extent infantile hydrocephalus (38). In a large literature review encompassing 705 cases of agenesis of the corpus callosum (ACC), hydrocephalus was present in some 23%, often associated with distinct syndromic states (Aicardi, Acrocallosal, Andermann, and Shapiro syndromes) (39). More recently, it has been realized that X-linked hydrocephalus overlaps with X-linked agenesis of the corpus callosum and a number of other conditions, resulting in a spectrum of disorders that include all or some of corpus callosum hypoplasia, mental retardation, adducted thumbs, spastic paraplegia, and hydrocephalus. It has gained the acronym CRASH syndrome and they are related to mutation in the L1 cellular adhesion molecule gene (40).

ACC can be associated with the finding of interhemispheric arachnoid cysts, which again may be related to hydrocephalus. Cinalli et al. (41) treated seven patients with interhemispheric arachnoid cysts of whom six had ACC. They marsupialized the cysts endoscopically into either the ventricles, basal cisterns, or both and five patients required no further intervention. Insertion of a cystoperitoneal shunt has been successfully performed as well (42).

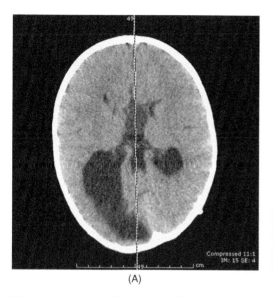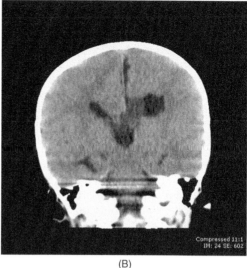

(A)   (B)

Figure 7 Agenesis of the corpus callosum and cyst. These CT images show a partially agenetic corpus callosum and associated cyst in the axial (**A**) and coronal (**B**) plains.

HYDRANENCEPHALY

Hydranencephaly describes a severe brain malformation in which, although remnants of non-functional cortex may be present, there is an extensive reduction in brain parenchyma that has been replaced with CSF. The etiology is variable and infants have a limited lifespan.

Ventriculoperitoneal shunts have been inserted to control head size in infants, and although the literature is sparse, there are reports of relatively prolonged survival (43). However, many of the reports of hydranencephaly predate MR imaging and some may represent cases of maximal hydrocephalus, from which it is important to differentiate this condition (44). Children with hydranencephaly never gain consciousness or awareness regardless of shunt insertion but with aggressive nursing care can have prolonged survival (45), and control of head size reduces the incidence of cranial pressure sores [Fig. 8(A) and 8(B)].

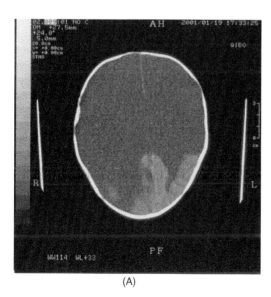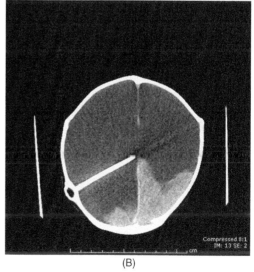

(A)   (B)

Figure 8 Hydranencephaly. This CT shows axial images of hydranencephaly pre and post–VP shunting, note the lack of re-expansion of the hemispheres, which differentiates this from maximal hydrocephalus.

HOLOPROSENCEPHALY

Holoprosencephaly (HPE) is a complex, congenital brain malformation the essence of which is the failure of the forebrain to split into two hemispheres; it is associated with facial anomalies. It occurs in approximately 1:250 pregnancies, but only 3% of fetuses will survive to term, so the live birth prevalence is of the order of 1 in 10,000 (46–48).

HPE is classically divided according to DeMyer's division into three subtypes of decreasing severity, that is, alobar, semilobar, and lobar (49); a more subtle variant termed middle interhemispheric fusion was added by Barkovich and Quint (50). In its most severe form (alobar), there is complete failure of separation of the forebrain and a single midline forebrain ventricle (monoventricle), which communicates with a large dorsal cyst. In the semilobar form, some portions of the posterior hemispheres separate, and in lobar only a small proportion of the most ventral forebrain does not separate.

The incidence of hydrocephalus increases in the more severe forms of the malformation and an important guide is that the majority of children with HPE have microcephaly; when it is not present the child should be investigated for potential hydrocephalus (51). Nearly three quarters of children with alobar HPE and two-fifths of children with dorsal cysts (which also occur in semilobar HPE) develop hydrocephalus. Although the functional status achieved by children with severe forms of HPE is very limited, insertion of a ventriculoperitoneal shunt can make nursing care easier (49).

ACKNOWLEDGMENT

I would like to acknowledge the assistance and advice of Dr. Michelle Fink (Consultant Radiologist, Royal Children's Hospital, Melbourne) in collating the images for this chapter.

REFERENCES

1. Dandy WE, Blackfan KD. Internal Hydrocephalus. An experimental, clinical and pathological study. Am J Dis Child 1914; 8:406–482.
2. Taggart JK, Walker AE. Congenital atresia of the foramen of Luschka and Magendie. Arch Neurol Psychiatry 1942; 48:583–612.
3. Benda CE. The Dandy–Walker syndrome or the so-called atresia of the foramen of Magendie. J Neuropathol Exp Neurol 1954; 13:14–29.
4. Klein O, Pierre-Kahn A, Boddaert N, et al. Dandy-Walker malformation: prenatal diagnosis and prognosis. Childs Nerv Syst 2003; 19:484–489.
5. Barkovich AJ, Kjos BO, Norman D, et al. Revised classification of posterior fossa cysts and cyst-like malformations based on the results of multiplanar MR imaging. Am J Neuroradiol 1989; 153(6):1289–1300.
6. Tortori-Donati P, Fondelli MP, Rossi A, et al. Cystic Malformations of the posterior cranial fossa originating from a defect of the posterior membranous area. Childs Nervous System 1996; 12:303–308.
7. Robinson AJ, Goldstein R. The cisterna magna septa: vestigial remnants of Blake's Pouch Cyst and a potential new marker for normal development of the rhombencephalon. J Ultrasound Med 2007; 26:83–95.
8. Yildiz H, Yazici Z, Hakyemez B, et al. Evaluation of CSF flow patterns of posterior fossa cystic malformations using CSF flow MR imaging. Neuroradiol 2006; 48:595–605.
9. Boddaert N, Klein O, Ferguson, et al. Intellectual prognosis of the Dandy–Walker malformation in children: the importance of vermian lobulation. Neuroradiol 2003; 45:320–324.
10. Hart MN, Malamud N, Ellis WG. The Dandy–Walker syndrome. A clinico-pathological study based on 28 cases. Neurology 1972; 22:771–780.
11. Sawaya R, McLaurin RL. Dandy–Walker syndrome. Clinical analysis of 23 cases. J Neurosurg 1981; 55:89–98.
12. Hirsch JF, Pierre-Kahn A, Renier D, et al. The Dandy–Walker malformation. A review of 40 cases. J Neurosurg 1984; 61:515–522.
13. Pascual-Castroviejo I, Velez A, Pascual-Pascual SI, et al. Dandy Walker Malformation: analysis of 38 cases. Childs Nerv Syst 1991; 7:88–97.
14. Murray JC, Johnson JA, Bird TD. Dandy–Walker malformation: etiologic heterogeneity and empiric recurrence risks. Clin Genet 1985; 28:272–283.
15. Osenbach RK, Menezes AH. Diagnosis and management of the Dandy Walker malformation: 30 years experience. Pediatr Neurosurg 1992; 18:179–189.

16. Has R, Ermis H, Ibrahimoglu L, et al. Dandy–Walker malformation: a review of 78 cases diagnosed by prenatal sonography. Fetal Diagn Ther 2004; 19(4):342–347.
17. Mohanty A, Biwas A, Satish S, et al. Treatment options for Dandy–Walker malformation. J Neurosurg 2006; 105(5 suppl Peds):348–356.
18. Asai A, Hoffman HJ, Hendrick EB, et al. Dandy-Walker syndrome: experience at the Hospital for Sick Children, Toronto. Pediatr Neurosci 1989; 15:66–73.
19. Marinov M, Gabrovski S, Undjian S. The Dandy–Walker syndrome: diagnostic and surgical consideration. Br J Neurosurg 1991; 5:475–483.
20. Bindal AK, Storrs BB, McLone DG. Management of the Dandy–Walker syndrome. Paediatr Neurosurg 1990–1991; 16(3):163–169.
21. Lee M, Leahu D, Weiner HL, et al. Complications of fourth ventricular shunts. Pediatr Neurosurg 1995; 22(6):309–313.
22. Liu JC, Ciacci JD, George TM. Brainstem tethering in Dandy–Walker syndrome: a complication of cystoperitoneal shunting. J Neurosurg 1995; 83:1072–1074.
23. Naidich TP, Radkowski MA, McLone DG, et al. Chronic cerebral herniation in Dandy–Walker malformation. Radiology 1986: 158(2):431–434.
24. Raimondi AJ, Samuelson G, Yarzagaray L, et al. Atresia of the foramina of Luschka and Magendie: the Dandy–Walker cyst. J Neurosurg 1969; 31(2):202–216.
25. James HE, Kaiser G, Schut L, et al. Problems of diagnosis and treatment in Dandy–Walker syndrome. Childs Brain 1979; 5(1):24–30.
26. Cinalli G. Alternatives to shunting. Childs Nerv Syst 1999; 15:718–731.
27. Hoffman HJ, Harwood-Nash D, Gilday DL, et al. Percutaneous ventriculostomy in the management of non-communicating hydrocephalus. Neurosurgery 1980; 7:1330–1337.
28. Villavicencio AT, Wellos JC, George TM. Avoiding complicated shunt systems by open fenestration of symptomatic fourth ventricular cysts associated with hydrocephalus. Pediatr Neurosurg 1998; 29:314–319.
29. Harper T, Fordham LA, Wolfe HM. The fetal dandy-walker complex: associated anomalies, perinatal outcome and postnatal imaging. Fetal Diagn Ther 2007; 22(4):277–281.
30. Forzano F, Mansour S, Ierullo A, et al. Posterior fossa malformation in fetuses: a report of 56 further cases and a review of the literature. Prenat Diagn 2007; 27(6):495–501.
31. Simpson DA, David DJ, White J. Cephaloceles: treatment, outcome and antenatal diagnosis. Neurosurgery 1984; 15(1):14–21.
32. Docherty JG, Daly JC, Carachi R. Encephaloceles: a review 1971–1990. Eur J Pediatr Surg 1991; 1(suppl 1):11–13.
33. Yokota A, Kajiwara H, Kohchi M, et al. Parietal cephalocele: clinical importance of its atretic form and associated malformations. J Neurosurg 1988; 69(4):545–551.
34. Martinez-Lage JF, Sola J, Casas C, et al. Atretic cephalocele: the tip of the iceberg. J Neurosurg 1992; 77(2):230–235.
35. Bui CJ, Tubbs RS, Shannon CN, et al. Institutional experience with cranial vault encephaloceles. J Neurosurg 2007; 107(suppl 1):22–25.
36. Mahapatra AK, Agrawal D. Anterior encephaloceles: a series of 103 cases over 32 years. J Clin Neurosci 2006; 13(5):536–539.
37. Moutard ML, Kieffer V, Feingold J, et al. Agenesis of the corpus callosum: prenatal diagnosis and prognosis. Childs Nerv Syst 2003; 19(7–8):471–476.
38. Moritake K, Nagai H, Miyazaki T, et al. Nationwide survey of the etiology and associated conditions of prenatally and postnatally diagnosed congenital hydrocephalus in Japan. Neurol Med Chir (Tokyo) 2007; 47(10):448–452.
39. Jeret JS, Serur D, Wisniewski KE, et al. Clinicopathological findings associated with agenesis of the corpus callosum. Brain Dev 1987; 9(3):255–264.
40. Fransen E, Van Camp G, Vits L, et al. L1-associated diseases: clinical geneticists divide, molecular geneticists unite. Hum Mol Genet 1997; 6(10):1625–1632.
41. Cinalli G, Peretta P, Spennato P, et al. Neuroendoscopic management of interhemispheric cysts in children. J Neurosurg 2006; 105(suppl 3):194–202.
42. Lena G, van Calenberg F, Genitori L, et al. Supratentorial interhemispheric cysts associated with callosal agenesis; surgical treatment and outcome in 16 children. Childs Nerv Syst 1995; 11(10):568–573.
43. McAbee GN, Chan A, Erde EL. Prolonged survival; with hydranencephaly: report of two patients and literature review. Pediatr Neurol 2000; 23(1):80–84.
44. Sutton LN, Bruce DA, Schut L. Hydranencephaly versus maximal hydrocephalus: an important clinical distinction. Neurosurgery 1980: 6(1):34–38.

45. Dieker T, Bruno RD. Sensory Reinforcement of eye blink rate in decorticate human. Am J Ment Defic 1976; 80(6):665–667.
46. Matsunaga E, Shiota K. Holoprosencephaly in human embryos: epidemioloc studies of 150 cases. Teratology 1977; 16(3):261–272.
47. Cohen MM Jr. Perspectives on holoprosencephaly: Part I. Epidemiology, genetics and syndromology. Teratology 1989; 40(3):211–235.
48. Bullen PJ, Rankin JM, Robson SC. Investigation of the epidemiology and prenatal diagnosis of holo-prosencephaly in the North of England. Am J Obstet Gynecol 2001; 184(6):1256–1262.
49. Hahn JS, Plawner LL. Evaluation of management of children with holoprosencephaly. Pediatr Neurol 2004; 31(2):79–88.
50. Barkovich AJ, Quint DJ. Middle interhemispheric fusion: an unusual variant of holoprosencephaly. Am J Neuroradiol 1993; 14(2):431–440.
51. Plawner LL, Delgado MR, Miller VS, et al. Neuroanatomy of holoprosencephaly as a predictor of function: beyond the face predicting the brain. Neurology 2002; 59(7):1058–1066.

13 | Pericerebral Collections and Subdural Effusions

Matthieu Vinchon and Patrick Dhellemmes
Pediatric Neurosurgery, Lille University Hospital, Lille, France

INTRODUCTION

Pericerebral collections (PCC) are fluid collections located in the subdural and subarachnoid spaces, and the cerebrospinal fluid (CSF) plays a prominent role in most of these. There is still much confusion in the medical literature regarding the classification and nosology of PCC. During the past century, several terms were coined such as subdural effusion (1,2), subdural hydroma, subdural hygroma (3), "meningitis serosa traumatica" (1), and external hydrocephalus (EH) (3); these different names are still often used regardless of the nature of the fluid, of its subdural or subarachnoid location, and of the clinical context. For example, clearly distinct entities like infantile subdural hematoma (SDH) and atrophic SDH in the elderly are both referred to as "chronic SDH"; on the other hand, such terms as SDH, hygroma, hydroma, or effusion, may all refer to a single entity, namely, infantile SDH (iSDH). Similarly, the term "external hydrocephalus" (EH) is often equated to "idiopathic macrocrania," whereas head circumference may stay within normal limits in EH, and macrocrania can persist in a toddler after the excess of subarachnoid fluid has resolved.

In addition to nosological confusion, the anatomical distinction between subarachnoid and subdural collection is often blurred because normal and pathological anatomy are often poorly understood. Historically, the diagnosis of PCC was generally based on data gained from clinical examination, subdural puncture or craniotomy, and neuroradiology, generally limited to angiography and reserved to pseudotumoral cases, showed the PCC indirectly (4). Only recently has imaging afforded noninvasive assessment of the content as well as the limiting structures of PCC. Although the advent of computerized imaging has been decisive in assessing noninvasively PCC, difficulties persist to evaluate the more or less aqueous, albuminous, or hematic nature of the fluid, as well as its precise allocation to the subarachnoid or subdural space, especially in the acute phase. In the absence of an appropriate animal model, advances in the understanding of PCC are still obtained through clinical, radiological, and surgical experience. In this regard, serial imaging of patients with carefully reconstructed history gives useful insight on the temporal alterations of the lesions, the pathogenesis of PCC, and helps dating cases of suspected child abuse (5,6).

This chapter put emphasis on pathophysiology, first collectively for what all of these PCC collections have in common, and what differentiates them, and then more specifically in the systematic study of the main clinicopathological entities. We decided to limit ourselves to the study of PCC related to abnormal CSF circulation; acute traumatic SDH is excluded, as being beyond the scope of this definition; and chronic SDH as well as subdural empyemas is mentioned only for their relation to iSDH and post-meningitis collections, respectively. The main features of these different clinicopathological entities are summarized in Table 1.

ANATOMY AND PHYSIOLOGY

The anatomy, histology, and ontogeny of the meninges are treated in other chapters of this book. In the present paragraph, we shall review briefly the anatomy and physiology of the meninges inasmuch as they are relevant to the pathology and pathophysiology of PCC.

In the normal state, the subdural space is basically a potential or virtual one; the existence of a normal subdural space has been demonstrated in dogs (7). The subarachnoid space is filled with CSF, en route from the ventricular system to its absorption sites. It is limited by the inner and outer arachnoid membranes, which are knit together by spider web–like fibrous bands. The outer arachnoid membrane is considered watertight, on account of desmosomes and tight

Table 1 Main Pathophysiological, Pathological, Diagnostic, and Therapeutic Features of External Hydrocephalus, Infantile SDH, Subdural Hygromas, and Chronic SDH. Note that Macrocrania can be Either a Predisposing Feature, or a Presenting Symptom of Infantile SDH

	External hydrocephalus	Infantile subdural hematoma	Subdural hygroma	Post-meningitis collection	Chronic subdural hematoma
Elective age	3–12 mo	5 mo	After 12 mo	5–8 mo	Elderly
Fluid	CSF	Hemorrhagic CSF	Clear, sometimes xanthochromic	Albuminous CSF/pus	Hemolyzed blood
Membranes	None	Subdural	Thin subdural	Subdural, purulent	Thick subdural, stratified
Favored by	Familial; axial hypotonia	Shaking; macrocrania	Arachnoid cyst	N. meningitidis	Brain atrophy
Presentation	Macrocrania, hypotonia	Raised ICP, macrocrania, seizures	Raised ICP	Fever, inflammation	Raised ICP, deficit
Imaging	Hypodense, large sulci, "vein sign"	Mixed-density, collapsed sulci	Hypodense, collapsed sulci	Hypodense, marginal contrast uptake	Mixed-density, layered, collapsed sulci
Natural history	Stabilization then return to normal values	Rapid progression or chronicization	Severe intracranial hypertension	Spontaneous regression or chronicization or empyema	Slow progression
Treatment	None; acetazolamide	Valveless subduroperitoneal shunt	Subduroperitoneal valve	External drainage	Trephination, external drainage

junctions (8). The arachnoid membranes delimit cisterns, which are crossed by the cerebral vessels and cranial nerves. The presence of bridging veins crossing the subarachnoid space at the periphery of the cerebrum has been considered the cause of subarachnoid and subdural bleeding, caused by both linear and angular traumas (8,9).

The CSF is absorbed by the arachnoid granulations in the adult, arachnoid villi in younger patients, and less well-defined structures in small infants. In the latter, the CSF is considered to be mostly absorbed through accessory sites along the spine and the olfactory nerves, as it is in quadruped species (10,11). The maturation of the arachnoid villi at the vertex is considered by some to be a consequence of the acquisition of the upright position, which causes negative venous pressure in the sagittal sinus (12,13). Detailed anatomical descriptions of the arachnoid granulations show that the arachnoid space extends in the arachnoid granulation (14); the cleavable border cell layer of the external arachnoid membrane extends in the granulation as well, in the vicinity of the venous lumen (15). Cleavage of the subdural space might thus extend in the granulation itself and impair CSF absorption.

PATHOPHYSIOLOGY

Alterations of the Meninges

The arachnoid membrane can be easily cleaved along the weakly knit dural border cell layer, leaving an intact subarachnoid space inside, and opening the subdural space outside (8). Tearing of the border cell layer of the outer arachnoid membrane occurs during surgery and may be caused by trauma, meningitis, or shrinking of the cerebrum due to dehydration or lumbar puncture. The subdural space is contaminated by CSF because the outer arachnoid membrane is initially not absolutely watertight or has been torn (16,17). In addition, subdural bleeding results from tearing of the bridging veins (8), or from cerebral or meningeal trauma, so that the subdural collection has a mixed density from the very beginning (5).

After the initial trauma, secondary phenomena lead to the constitution of subdural membranes. This healing process begins with vascular proliferation, and then accumulation of fibrous material on both the outer and inner membranes (1). In the largest ever published series of SDH in infants treated with craniotomy, Matson reported the presence of thick membranes as early as seven days after the trauma (4). Vascularity is prevalent on the outer membrane and to a lesser extent on the inner membrane (1), and can be evidenced on imaging by contrast enhancement. Angiogenesis is driven by high levels of Platelet-Aggregating Factor, Vascular Endothelial Growth Factor, and other cytokines in the subdural fluid (18,19). The membranes thicken, become watertight, and laden with elastic fibers (7). The membranes are also colonized by fibromyoblasts and smooth muscle cells, which can exert a strangling effect on the underlying brain (1). Unusual colonization of the subdural membranes with eosinophil polymorphonuclears (20) as well as heterotopic erythropoiesis (21) has also been reported. Eventually, the fibrous shell is transformed into a multilayered collagen membrane resembling the dura mater (22), which may ultimately become ossified. Vascular leakage of proteins and blood cells can also alter the subdural fluid, which becomes albuminous and laden with hemosiderin pigment, resulting in the classic appearance of the chronic SDH. Because neovessels bleed easily, this cycle can be repeated, resulting in a multilayered chronic SDH (4). Alternatively, the contamination of the subdural space with CSF can lead to its progressive clearing over one or two weeks (23,24). A third possibility is spontaneous healing of the subdural space, which begins with reexpansion of the arachnoid space (25), after which the subdural space collapses, heals, and returns to its normal virtual status; this evolution is accelerated by surgical drainage.

Very few data are available regarding secondary lesions at the arachnoid villi. In aneurysmal rupture, autopsy shows clogging of the arachnoid villi, and then proliferation of the cap cells, which causes blockage of the absorption of CSF (26). On histopathological specimens, tiny channels stuffed with erythrocytes can also be identified in the dura mater close to the sagittal sinus; these channels represent the likely outlet for CSF, which is obstructed in case of subarachnoid bleeding (15). This finding led Yamashima to consider erythrocytes as a "natural tracer of CSF absorption" in humans.

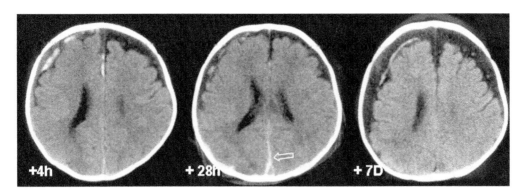

Figure 1   Four-month-old female victim of abuse (shaking and beating). CT scan performed 4 hours after trauma (*left*) showed mixed-density subdural collection over the convexity on the right side and along the anterior part of the falx; CT scan performed 24 hours later (*middle*) shows densification and thickening of the posterior part of the falx and sagittal sinus; 6 days later, a large hypodense SDH has accumulated, which requires drainage (*right*).

Alteration of the Fluids

It is very difficult on initial imaging to allocate the bleeding either to the subdural or to the subarachnoid space because the arachnoid membrane is initially too thin to be identified reliably. In the meninges, extravascular erythrocytes undergo processes of hemolysis, oxidation, dilution, and sedimentation, which alter their physical properties, in particular the way the iron they contain influences magnetic fields (27). Serial imaging also shows temporal modification in the distribution of clots, suggesting not just sedimentation but also migration of the clots toward the sites where the CSF is absorbed (Fig. 1). Blood clots clear rapidly in the subarachnoid space because of the continued flow of CSF, and usually more slowly in the subdural space, although early disappearance of acute SDHs has also been reported; this questions the mechanism underlying such phenomenon (28). In the chronic phase, the SDH is sealed off from the subarachnoid space by watertight membranes; its volume increases not because of the accumulation of CSF but because of rebleeding and oncotic pressure.

In the early phase, clear fluid can accumulate in the subdural space because of inflammation and penetration of CSF. In an electrophoretic study of the subdural fluid in infants, Stroobandt et al. observed that initially the fluid has characteristics of a transudate, produced by extravasation of fluid from leaky vessels with high protein levels; this fluid is gradually replaced by a protein-poor exudate, indistinguishable from CSF (23). Another line of evidence comes from radiological findings: after cisternography, the subdural space is contaminated by radiopaque dye after a variable delay (16,17); on MRI, one can distinguish clearly the blood-like sediment which undergoes oxidation from the CSF-like supernatant, which shows progressive volume increase (6).

The role of impaired CSF absorption in the pathogenesis of iSDH has been suspected long ago; Ford hypothesized that stretching of the cerebral veins due to subdural collections caused impairment of CSF absorption (29). Other authors pushed the same idea a step further by proposing a surgical technique for calvarial reduction aimed at releasing the tension of the corticodural veins (30). More recently, the occurrence of an SDH in a patient with deep cerebral veins thrombosis has been documented (31). Another hypothesis proposed to explain the impairment of CSF absorption after subarachnoid hemorrhage is clogging of the arachnoid villi by erythrocytes. This hypothesis is backed by pathological findings (11,15) and is to be put in perspective with the migration and clearing of the subarachnoid blood seen on serial imaging (Fig. 1). Also, Massicotte and Del Biggio have shown proliferation of the cap cells of the arachnoid granulation of adults after subarachnoid hemorrhage (26). In adults, blockade of CSF absorption causes pseudotumor cerebri rather than an SDH. In infants, however, the presence of open sutures may account for the accumulation of fluid in the subdural space rather than in the cerebral parenchyma. The association of pseudotumor cerebri and subdural collection is a rare occurrence (32), which suggests a common mechanism for these two conditions. The predisposition of infants with EH to develop an SDH also suggests that traumatic bleeding acts by merely decompensating an already borderline CSF circulation.

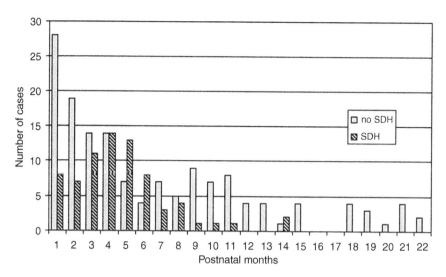

Figure 2 Bar chart showing the age distribution of patients from a prospective series including all infants with head trauma hospitalized in neurosurgery; patients who developed an SDH requiring puncture or drainage (hatched bars) represented more than half of the patients in their fifth month. SDH in newborns required rarely a puncture, and never drainage, and SDH developed exceptionally after 1 year. These data confirm that infants around 5 months are particularly predisposed to developing an SDH.

Age-Related Specificity

In our experience, although SDH are common in neonates after birth trauma, these patients never develop secondary SDH requiring drainage (33). On the contrary, up to 42% of children between 2 and 12 months developed an SDH after head injury, 35% of these requiring subdural drainage (unpublished data). In infants sustaining a head trauma during their fifth month, nearly two-third developed an SDH (Fig. 2). The same age predominance was also observed in posttraumatic, postinfectious, and postoperative PCC (34).

The volume of the subarachnoid space shows variations according to age. Infants have a physiological expansion of CSF spaces, which causes macrocephaly, and usually resolves with time, as discussed below. The production of CSF is low in newborns, especially in preterm infants and is considered to reach adult levels at one year (35), and then diminish in the elderly patients (12). Because maturation of arachnoid villi is considered to take place around the age of 18 months, prompted by the erect position (13), infancy is a period of transition between the neonatal and the adult CSF physiology. The particular vulnerability of infants toward PCC of all causes could thus be explained by a transient inadequacy between the secretion rate of CSF and the absorption capacity.

The role of the open skull in the occurrence of iSDH was suspected by Raimondi and Hirschauer, who considered that the absence of skull closure put the intracranial structures at higher risk of traumatic damage (36). However, neonates, who have the most pliable skull and are submitted to mechanical stress during labor, do not develop progressive SDH, whereas infants tend to develop SDH after several kinds of insult, traumatic or not. We can hypothesize that the open skull, along with the immaturity of CSF circulation, allows expansion of the subdural space in an unspecific response to different causes. Thus, the immaturity of the brain's envelopes is the likely cause of the occurrence of PCC in infants.

CLINICOPATHOLOGICAL ENTITIES

External Hydrocephalus

Nosology and Definition

The old concept of "external hydrocephalus," cited by Dandy and Blackfan in their pioneering work on hydrocephalus published in 1914 (3), has been revised and expanded since the advent of CT scan and ultrasonography. External hydrocephalus (EH), also called benign enlargement of the arachnoid spaces, can be defined as the accumulation of excess CSF in the subarachnoid space and is mostly found in infants. Because EH often causes macrocrania, the terms EH and idiopathic macrocrania are often considered synonymous. However, EH is also found in infants with a normal head circumference (37,38). Conversely, the head circumference of infants having had EH often continues to hover above the 97th percentile even later in life after the subarachnoid spaces have returned to normal. EH should thus be considered a normal, age-specific, developmental variant in relation to the transition between infantile and adult CSF circulation. Because, in the general public, the word "hydrocephalus" is often associated with surgery and/or handicap, the term "benign enlargement of the subarachnoid space" may be preferred.

Pathophysiology

EH is essentially idiopathic, but has often a familial character—one of the child's parents having at least a marginally large skull. It can also be associated with deformation of the skull, and expansion of the frontal subarachnoid space is commonly found in scaphocephaly, which suggests that the brain cannot adapt its shape beyond a certain degree of skull deformity. The progression of EH can be precipitated by several factors, in particular tooth eruption, airway infection, head injury, and iatrogenic factors like steroid treatment (even given percutaneously) or hypervitaminosis A.

The association of SDH with EH is common, as mentioned above. The age distribution and sex ratio of these two conditions are similar, suggesting that EH might facilitate the occurrence of an SDH. The presence of EH is considered to facilitate the occurrence of SDH because the corticodural veins are stretched over the subarachnoid space (39); the physical basis of this phenomenon has been modeled by Papasian and Frim (9). Although connecting EH and SDH appears tempting, clinical studies have failed to confirm that infants with EH are at higher risk of developing an SDH (17). In a previous study, although we did not find a significant correlation between preexisting macrocrania and the occurrence of an SDH, we noted that apparently spontaneous SDH occurred mostly in infants with head circumference above the 97th percentile; these children were often older than the elective age of shaken-baby syndrome and lacked the characteristic retinal hemorrhage (40). A frequently asked question is the risk of SDH due to trivial trauma, in particular at the age of the acquisition of walking. We consider that no special measure is required because at this age, the risk of SDH becomes negligible and the child has already acquired protecting reflexes.

Diagnosis of External Hydrocephalus

The child is generally referred because of enlargement of the head, which can cause positional flattening of the occiput and sometimes delays in the acquisition of the axial tone on account of its weight. The first step is to reconstruct the curve of the head circumference growth, which is typically about the 97th percentile at birth, then shows a regular increase in relative value at about three months, stabilizes around six months, then gradually returns to normal values between two and three years of age (Fig. 3). Because this condition is often familial, measuring the head circumference of the parents may be a good move to reassure the family. Imaging is often unnecessary, however, transfontanel ultrasound, CT scan, and MR are often performed, on demand of anxious parents. Imaging shows PCC of the same density and signal as the CSF, with enlarged cortical sulci and basal cisterns, and often mildly enlarged ventricles (37,41), as shown in Figure 4. The main differential diagnosis is the SDH, which may be associated with EH; this distinction may be difficult on nonenhanced CT scan, but is easily made with ultrasonography, contrast-enhanced CT scan, and MRI. EH should also be differentiated from brain atrophy, which is generally related to serious perinatal incident, and causes progressive microcephaly and not macrocephaly. In a few cases of EH, associated with marked occipital flattening caused by severe axial hypotonia, the advice of a neuropediatrician may be needed to rule out cerebral palsy and other developmental conditions like type 1 glutaric aciduria (Fig. 5).

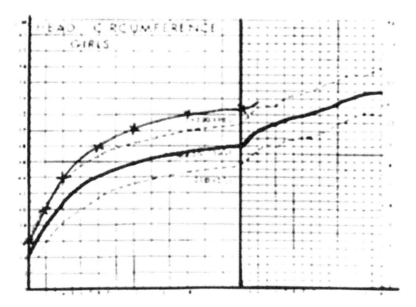

Figure 3 Head circumference curve of a female infant with typical external hydrocephalus. The circumference was at the 97th percentile at birth, began to rise (in relative value) smoothly at four months, stabilized at one year, followed the +4SD curve until the age of three years, then tended to return to the 97th percentile.

Treatment of External Hydrocephalus

In most cases, EH does not require any treatment. In children who have axial hypotonia and mild developmental delay, physiotherapy may be useful to help them acquire control of their head. In severe cases with head circumference beyond +4SD, medical treatment with Acetazolamide® (10 mg/kg daily) may be needed, which has to be continued until the age of 18 months. The efficacy of this treatment is debated; in our experience, in order to show some effect, Acetazolamide® must be administered in three doses, precisely every eight hours (which in an infant requires to wake up for the night dose) and is therefore quite demanding. Poor results

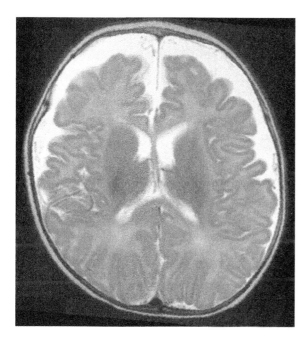

Figure 4 External hydrocephalus: five-month-old male having undergone MRI for seizures. There was no history of trauma; funduscopy was normal. Note the presence of bridging veins in the subarachnoid space. Because head circumference was beyond the 97th percentile and the child had mild axial hypotonia, the child was commenced on Acetazolamide®.

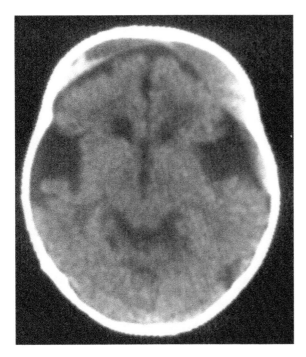

Figure 5 A 14-month-old child with type 1 glutaric aciduria, having a bilateral subdural hematoma diagnosed because of enlarged head circumference. Note the evocative enlargement of the sylvian fissure ("Batman's wing"). The SDH was drained, but had to be reoperated because of recurrence after 4 months. Now aged 23 years, the patient is mentally retarded, epileptic, and has spastic cerebral palsy.

of this treatment can generally be related to lax administration. This treatment also requires supplementation in potassium chloride and monitoring of the blood serum electrolytes.

Outcome
EH does not cause brain dysfunction because intracranial pressure is not elevated (37); however, as mentioned above, the acquisition of the sitting position can be delayed. In rare cases, EH can initiate a vicious cycle, because delay in the acquisition of the erect position can result in delay in the development of adult-type CSF absorption. In the vast majority of cases, however, EH has a benign and self-limiting nature (38). The most common complication of EH is occipital positional plagiocephaly, because the child often reclines on his occiput; this requires only advice on proper positioning.

Traumatic SDH in Infants

Nosology and Definition
Infantile SDH (iSDH) caused by trauma is a common disease, which can be defined anatomically as an accumulation of hemorrhagic CSF in the subdural space. The diagnosis of iSDH is generally made in a patient presenting in emergency: dated observations show that the fluid accumulates in a few days, or even hours after the trauma (5). The term "chronic SDH" is thus inadequate to designate this entity; we think it should be reserved for chronic lesions found mostly in adults, but also in infants with a neglected SDH having undergone the processes of fibrosis and rebleeding, as mentioned above.

Pathophysiology
The issue of iSDH is dominated by the question of child abuse. In our databank on head injuries in infants, we found that iSDH requiring drainage was present in 50% of cases of child abuse, compared with 9.5% of cases of accidental trauma (unpublished data). Infantile SDH are thus not synonymous with child abuse and can develop after any traumatic injury to the infant's head. In road accidents, which are dated and witnessed, and thus not suspect of being concealed child abuse, serial imaging shows the progression of the SDH with mixed density initially, progressively replaced by hypodense fluid (5). Obstetrical trauma represents a counter example, hematomas always disappear within a few weeks (42), and do not give rise to the

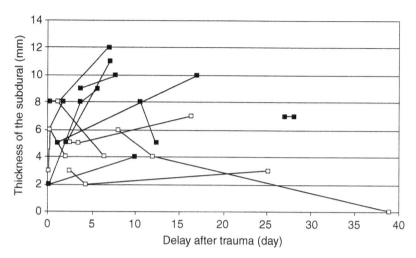

Figure 6 Evolution of the thickness of the subdural hematoma in 14 infants with significant SDH (requiring either puncture or drainage) due to a confirmed trauma and having had at least two CT scans before surgery. Open boxes represent patients who required only subdural puncture; full boxes represent children who required subdural drainage. This figure shows that the natural history of SDH in infants is generally rapid progression requiring drainage. All operated cases were between 2.4 and 9.6 months old. Among the five nonoperated patients, four were less than two months old, and the last was 11 months old.

accumulation of CSF, probably because neonates do not produce enough CSF to develop an infantile-type SDH (33). For unexplained reasons, male infants appear more vulnerable than female, iSDH being much more prevalent in the former (60/103) than in the latter (13/47) (40); the fragility of the male infant may be related to its larger head circumference and wider subarachnoid space.

The spontaneous history of the iSDH is generally one of rapid progression, with signs of raised intracranial pressure appearing within days after trauma (Fig. 6). When iSDH is treated early, in a child without initial brain damage from seizures and hypoxia, anatomical reconstitution with excellent clinical outcome is the rule (43). If left untreated, the iSDH may also stabilize, and then undergo spontaneous healing, with reexpansion of the subarachnoid space (Fig. 7). However, the period of cerebral compression can lead to brain damage, the consequences of which may not be immediately apparent (44); for this reason, we consider that surgical drainage should be performed early. In cases with prolonged brain compression, or with brain atrophy resulting from the initial trauma (especially when complicated by seizures), the iSDH may evolve into a chronic SDH very similar to adult-type SDH, with thickening of the membranes and rebleeding (45). Chronic SDH are thus rare in infants and often represent failure of the treatment of iSDH.

Diagnosis

The diagnostic problem posed by iSDH is twofold: the diagnosis of the lesion and the diagnosis of its cause, with the search for evidence of child abuse. In most legal systems, both tasks, as well as reporting cases of suspected child abuse to the justice, are the treating physician's duty.

The clinical presentation of infants with iSDH is often unspecific, and patients presenting with irritability, drowsiness, floppiness, and vomiting are often misdiagnosed as pyloric stenosis, enteritis, or meningitis. Increased head circumference is found in a minority of cases of iSDH (36% in our experience). In severe cases, the child presents with malaise, convulsion, and apnea and may die rapidly in the absence of immediate and adequate resuscitation. Seizures are especially devastating in infants under three months, because they can initiate status epilepticus and cause extensive brain damage due to excitotoxicity.

Ultrasonography is not well suited to the study of the subdural space, which is in a large measure beyond the reach of the ultrasound cone. The most useful diagnostic tool is the CT scan, because it is readily available in emergency, gives detailed information on the amount

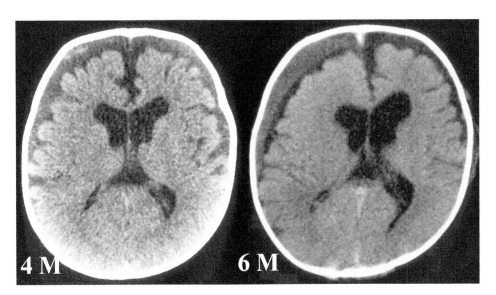

Figure 7 Male infant born on May 1999, seen in outpatient clinic in September 1999 because of increasing head circumference; the child was otherwise asymptomatic, and no history of trauma was reported. The CT scan (*left*) showed enlarged subarachnoid space, but also a subdural hyperdensity suggesting subdural bleeding. The patient was commenced on Acetazolamide®. Two months later, the patient was admitted in emergency for repeated seizures and intracranial hypertension. The new CT scan (*right*) showed an isodense right SDH with mass effect; note the persistence of an open subarachnoid space despite the compression. Funduscopy showed retinal hemorrhages, suggesting shaken baby syndrome, and the case was brought to justice. The SDH was punctured several times before a subdural drainage was put in place, after which the patient recovered completely. Assessed at age 6 years with neuropsychological testing, the patient was clinically normal and followed a normal school curriculum.

and location of meningeal blood, and shows associated lesions of the skull and brain. MRI is performed in selected cases to study the arachnoid membranes, the dura mater (especially in case of growing fracture), lesions of the brain and spinal cord, and in case of suspected repeated trauma. Invasive radiological imaging such as subdurography (16) or cisternography is no longer justified.

Retinal hemorrhage (RH) is of critical importance for the diagnosis of shaken-baby syndrome. Because child abuse is often concealed under alleged household accident, ophthalmologic examination should be systematic in all cases of iSDH without a clear and convincing traumatic history, and more generally in all cases of unwitnessed infantile head injury. Mild RH can be found in accidental trauma, such as car accident or fall from stairs, but severe RH are specific of child abuse (40). The evaluation should be made by a well-trained ophthalmologist, to study the periphery of the retina, and be documented by photographs.

Careful reconstruction of the head perimeter curve can also be of crucial importance in case of possible spontaneous SDH related to macrocephaly. Associated traumatic lesions, like cutaneous stigmata and skeletal lesions, should be searched systematically (46). Study of the child's previous medical history, assay of the child's clotting factors, inquiry about the child's siblings, and information from social workers in contact with the family are also mandatory. Differential diagnoses of child abuse include osteogenesis imperfecta, hemorrhagic diathesis, deep cerebral vein thrombosis, and aneurysmal bleeding (which is exceptional in infants but can be associated with retinal hemorrhage).

Treatment

Subdural tap is necessary to confirm the hemorrhagic nature of the subdural fluid and is both diagnostic and therapeutic. Often, it has to be performed in emergency because of severe intracranial hypertension. Subtraction of 20 mL on each side is often sufficient to alleviate the symptoms; subtracting more may be poorly tolerated.

In the majority of cases (71% in our experience), subdural puncture is not the definitive treatment, and the majority of punctured patients require insertion of a subdural drainage. Our preferred technique is subduroperitoneal valveless shunting, rather than external drainage because the drainage needs to be maintained for at least two weeks, the risk of infection of external drainages is a big concern, and these are difficult to manage in a restless five-month infant on demand for arm care (47). Options left to the judgment of the surgeon include uni- or bilateral drainage and systematic versus optional removal of the drainage after four months (47,48).

When iSDH becomes chronic, the thickness of the membranes and viscosity of the fluid make the drainage ineffective. The only therapeutic option is craniotomy and membranectomy, which is a large operation when performed on a small infant. In our experience, in order to be efficient, it has to be coupled with subduroperitoneal drainage. In "historic" cases with large macrocephalus, reductive craniotomy may be required in order to address massive cranio-cephalic disproportion.

Symptomatic Subdural Hygroma

Definition and Nosology
Subdural hygroma (SDHg), also named subdural hydroma, is probably the most controversial and questionable entity in the spectrum of PCC. These lesions are described in children and young adults, but have many features in common with iSDH. Dorland's medical dictionary (28th edition) defines SDHg as "a collection of fluid in the subdural space resulting from the liquefaction of an SDH," which implies the initial presence of blood. For other authors, the fluid in SDHg is by definition identical to CSF, although some alterations are tolerated, like hemorrhagic (29) or xanthochromic fluid (7). SDHg have been also defined by the lack of subdural membranes, which leaves an ambiguity with expanded subarachnoid spaces (27). The description of SDHg as an "epiphenomenon of head injury... not a mass lesion but a space filling lesion" (49) also suggests that confusion is made between subdural and subarachnoid collections associated with brain atrophy. On CT scan, SDHg have been defined as homogeneous collections with a density less than 20 Hounsfield units and no enhancement after contrast infusion (50). However, more recent studies have described contrast uptake in the external membrane of SDHg (51).

However blurred this issue may be, symptomatic patients do present with subdural hypodense collections, often without trauma, and the fluid is identical to CSF both radiologically and at subdural puncture. In order to avoid confusion, we consider that the term SDHg should be restricted to collections of CSF in the subdural space, limited by thin subdural membranes. These lesions can be present already at the time of diagnosis, represent the evolution of iSDH, or complicate arachnoid cysts, as will be discussed below. SDHg represents thus more a stage in the natural history of PCC than a discrete pathological entity; when SDHg are symptomatic, however, their clinical and radiological findings and the principles of treatment have distinctive features.

Pathophysiology of Subdural Hygromas
Documented cases show progressive volume increase and onset of symptoms of raised intracranial pressure within 10 days after the trauma (50). The supposed mechanism for CSF accumulation is a slit-valve mechanism with influx of CSF in the subdural space (29). The natural history of these collections is to grow progressively and cause intracranial hypertension (50). The severity of clinical presentation is not in relation with the volume of the collection, which may look unimpressive. Observation data indicate that a disturbance of CSF absorption is sometimes associated to the SDHg, as suggested in the case reported by Najjar et al., of a patient who developed pseudotumor cerebri after the subdural collection had disappeared (32). Several authors consider that CSF trapped in the subdural space becomes xanthochromic or hemorrhagic due to secondary phenomena, which include membrane formation and spontaneous bleeding (49,50). Conversely, hygromas can represent the evolution of an SDH under the influence of drainage, the subdural fluid becoming progressively replaced by CSF (23).

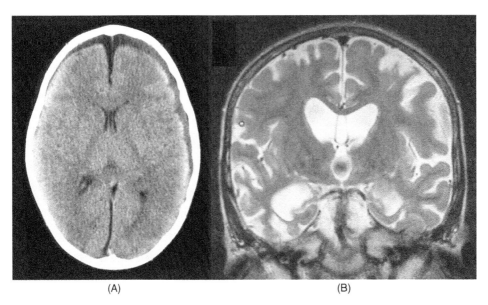

(A)   (B)

Figure 8 Four-year-old boy, victim of child abuse, presenting with severe intracranial hypertension and status epilepticus. (**A**) Initial CT scan shows a thin subdural hypodense collection with severe compression of the cerebral sulci; when surgery performed as an emergency, the pressure of the CSF was extremely high. After seven months, the valveless shunt was removed systematically; the child developed intracranial hypertension due to hydrocephalus, and a ventriculoperitoneal valve was inserted. At last control, the child now aged eight years has developmental delay, spasticity, and loss of vision as sequels of the initial episode. (**B**) Control MRI shows atrophic lesions, especially in the hippocampi.

Diagnosis
Although some SDHg can be asymptomatic and disappear spontaneously, the clinical presentation of symptomatic SDHg is often dramatic, with severe intracranial hypertension and visual loss (32), and can lead to severe sequels due to brain atrophy (Fig. 8).

The main differential diagnosis is between SDHg and subarachnoid collection; the latter is associated with enlargement of the sulci and cisterns, whereas the former is associated with collapse of the subarachnoid space, and mass effect when unilateral (51). CT scan with contrast injection or MRI may be useful, the "vein sign" (corticodural veins crossing the subarachnoid space) indicating a subarachnoid collection (49). As mentioned above, the distinction between SDH and SDHg can be blurred (Table 1). Of note is that hygroma can extend over all the hemisphere convexity and be unilateral, whereas subarachnoid collections are almost always bilateral and in the frontal and temporal regions mostly.

Treatment
The treatment of SDHg is necessary only in case of intracranial hypertension. It is based on subduroperitoneal drainage, using a valve when the fluid is thin, sometimes a valveless shunt when it is hemorrhagic or albuminous. Very often, this cannot be predicted from the imaging, and the choice between valve and valveless shunt can be made only during surgery. When a valveless shunt has been put in place, we opt for systematic removal after four to six months; in a few cases, however, the patient proves shunt dependant of the shunt, and a valve has to be put in place (Fig. 8).

Subdural Collections in Arachnoid Cysts

Nosology
Arachnoid cysts are discussed in another chapter; herein we deal only with subdural collections associated with arachnoid cysts, as these can be the prime presentation of a cyst, or develop after otherwise successful treatment of the cyst. Subdural collections associated with arachnoid

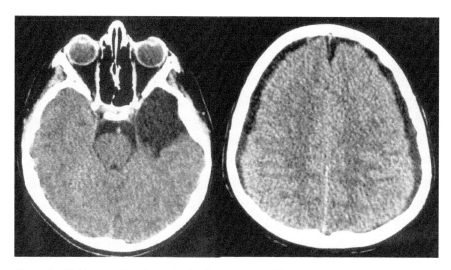

Figure 9 Eight-year-old male presenting in emergency with severe intracranial hypertension of 2-week duration, with papilledema. The CT scan shows a thin bilateral subdural collection and a small arachnoid cyst of the sylvian fissure. We performed shunting in emergency with a left-sided subduroperitoneal valve. At surgery, the liquid was found to be crystal clear and under extremely high pressure. Drainage resulted in immediate relief of the symptoms and complete disappearance of the subdural collection; the cyst remained stable and asymptomatic five years later.

cysts are evenly named acute hematomas, chronic hematomas, or effusion (2); we shall refer to them as SDH.

Pathophysiology

Subdural collections associated with arachnoid cysts are considered to result from a slit-valve mechanism due to rupture of the cyst in the subdural space (52). This pathophysiology suggests the existence of a problem in CSF absorption, which is also suggested by the discrepancy between the unimpressive volume of the collection and the severity of intracranial hypertension (Fig. 9). Mori et al. estimated that SDH complicated the course of 8% to 17% of arachnoid cysts (2). In our experience with 144 arachnoid cysts in children, 33 (23%) were associated with an SDH before surgery and 9 (6.3%) after surgery (unpublished data). SDH associated with arachnoid cysts may be precipitated by trauma, especially angular trauma like shaking or head banging, or occur spontaneously (2). Arachnoid cysts of the sylvian fissure are by far the largest contributors of SDH: among our 42 cases of arachnoid cyst–associated SDH, 36 were due to sylvian cysts (representing 49% of the sylvian cysts), 3 due to interhemispheric cysts, and 3 due to cysts of other locations. Postoperative SDH are more common in younger patients: in our series, the mean age at initial surgery was 10.1 months in the group with SDH versus 68.9 months in the group without SDH ($p = 0.016$), and the oldest patient who developed a postoperative SDH was 25 months old.

Diagnosis and Treatment

Subdural collections causing raised ICP are often the presenting symptom of arachnoid cysts. In other cases, the SDH develops in a patient with a known arachnoid cyst, which has not been considered an indication for surgery (53). After surgery for arachnoid cyst, an SDH may manifest itself early, with symptoms of raised ICP or CSF leakage from the wound (Fig. 10), or later with formation of a chronic SDH (54).

Arachnoid cysts can usually be treated by membranectomy, drainage by shunting or endoscopic fenestration. However, when the arachnoid cyst is revealed by an SDH, drainage of the SDH is often the only option, because the cyst itself is often negligible, or may even disappear spontaneously (53), and because the existence of the SDH often implies a problem of CSF absorption. When the fluid is clear (which is often made evident during surgery only), we put a subduroperitoneal shunt with a valve, and the patient is considered shunt dependent for

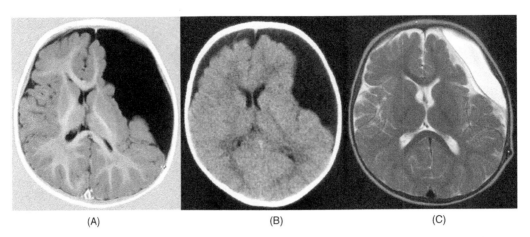

| | | |
| (A) | (B) | (C) |

Figure 10   13-month-old female with a large sylvian arachnoid cyst, causing mass effect (**A**) diagnosed because of enlarged head circumference. After endoscopic fenestration of the cyst in the basal cisterns, symptoms of intracranial hypertension developed, then leakage of CSF from the scalp wound eight days after initial surgery. The CT scan showed bilateral subdural hydroma. The child underwent unilateral external drainage of the subdural collection, followed by a subduroperitoneal valve, with resolution of symptoms. Five months later, a chronic SDH had developed (**B**), and the subdural valve was replaced by a valveless subduroperitoneal shunt, which obtained complete resolution of the lesion and was removed uneventfully 6 months later.

life until proven otherwise; when the fluid is hemorrhagic or albuminous, we insert a valveless subduroperitoneal shunt, which is removed after six months.

Avoidance of postoperative SDH is an important point of the surgical technique for arachnoid cysts; during endoscopic treatment of sylvian arachnoid cysts, suspension of the arachnoid to the dura before entering the cyst aims at reducing the risk of subdural collection, but does not always succeed.

Arachnoid cysts are increasingly diagnosed as incidental findings; although the presence of a small arachnoid cyst represents a small risk of SDH for minor trauma, we do not consider that sports should be avoided in these patients. However, the patient and the family should be aware of the need to consult in emergency in case of persistent headache after minor head injury.

Postoperative Subdural Collections

During opening of the dura, the potential subdural space becomes actual (8); the subdural collection thus created may then evolve autonomously when CSF is trapped in the subdural space. Tanaka et al. hypothesized that SDH were due to opening of the ventricle because of the loss of pulsatility of CSF, and loss of the pressure gradient between the ventricle and brain surface (55). Ventricular opening is a major factor leading to the constitution of an SDH: in our experience with 24 documented cases of SDH after tumor removal, 15 were tumors of the region of the third ventricle, and 12 had been operated through a transcortical route. Patients operated through the transcallosal route might be less prone to develop an SDH. Systemic fluid imbalance may also play a role in tumors of the third ventricle. Young age has a major influence on the risk of postoperative SDH: 16 of our 24 cases of SDH after tumor removal were under 24 months of age; the 8 patients older than 24 months all had a ventricular opening and/or a tumor of the third ventricle. Prevention of postoperative SDH includes choosing the transcallosal rather than the transcortical route when possible and sealing of cortical openings with fibrin glue (56). Transient external drainage of the subdural space may be required in case of severe brain collapse.

SDH may also complicate the postoperative course of neuroendoscopic surgery (56,57). Cartmill and Vloeberghs suggested that during ventriculocisternostomy, the floor of the third ventricle may be fenestrated in the subdural rather than the subarachnoid space (58). The age of the patient also plays a large role, infants being at higher risk of developing an SDH after

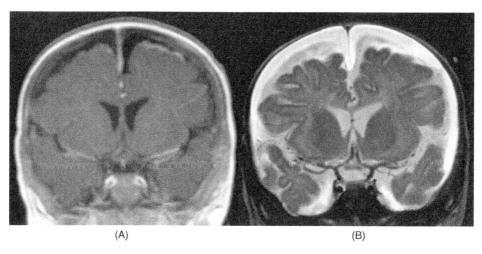

(A)   (B)

Figure 11 Four-month-old female with SDH following meningococcal meningitis. The patient was admitted 28 days after the diagnosis of meningitis because of symptoms of intracranial hypertension and increasing head circumference, and biological signs of inflammation but no fever. MRI showed a subdural collection with partial contrast uptake on the inner membrane; the signal of the fluid was similar to CSF. Subdural puncture showed a xanthochromic fluid with high albumin level, and cultures were sterile. The patient underwent bilateral subduroperitoneal valveless drainage, with total resolution of the SDH, and favorable outcome.

neuroendoscopy (57). The occurrence of this complication should also raise doubts about the existence of communicating hydrocephalus, which requires shunting.

Ex vacuo SDH due to overdrainage and severe dehydration is beyond the scope of the present study.

Postinfectious Subdural Collections
Bacterial meningitis is a common cause of PCC in infants, especially between four and eight months (4). These collections, often named "subdural effusion," may contain purulent, albuminous, or clear CSF-like fluid (59), and the culture may be positive but is more often negative (60). Matson considered that these different types of collections are not different in nature, but represent a continuum from clear-fluid effusion to empyema (4). The more or less aqueous or purulent nature of the fluid depends on the impairment of CSF absorption and the more or less successful immune response by the host (34).

The presentation is typical: after initially favorable evolution of the meningitis under treatment, the patient presents a few days later with secondary elevation of temperature and a tense fontanel, associated with biological stigma of inflammation. Within a few more days, the head circumference may enlarge. On imaging, the subdural collection is hypodense and contrast uptake is generally faint or marginal (Fig. 11). Subdural puncture may be difficult on account of the viscosity of the fluid and of the presence of lumps of purulent material. The majority of post-meningitis collections do not require drainage, because 90% will disappear spontaneously (60). Drainage of the collection may be necessary in order to control infection and to avoid the constitution of an empyema *stricto sensu*. In our experience, *Neisseria meningitidis* was the main organism associated with post-meningitic subdural collections; we estimated that subdural drainage was required in 5% of infantile meningococcal meningitis in our study population (34). The preferred treatment is external drainage, which is replaced by a valveless internal drainage after a few days if the fluid is sterile and clear and does not dry up. Antibiotics should be continued until resolution of fever, inflammation, and contrast uptake on imaging; in situ antibiotics do not appear to be indicated.

CONCLUSION
The issue of PCC is marred by confusion due to the lack of consensus on definitions. The definitions of the different clinicopathological entities often date from historic publications and were

not reappraised with modern neuroimaging and accumulated knowledge of pathophysiology. In the present chapter, we propose a terminology and nosology, being aware that concepts will be challenged and need to be updated. We felt important, however, that clearly separate clinicopathological entities could be identified in a way that helps practical management of the patients.

PCC are another illustration of the fact that physicians have to consider any individual patient the time dimension. In infants, the time course of SDH regularly shows progressive replacement of the initially hematic or albuminous collection by clearer fluid, showing dilution by the influx of CSF. Snapshots of the PCC at different stages of its evolution can identify successively EH, then an SDH, a hygroma, and finally a chronic SDH. Also, if we compare patients of different ages, PCC behave in markedly different fashions, in relation to differences in the physiology of the CSF. Newborns secrete a small amount of CSF and absorb it following archaic pathways; infants are in a process of maturing the absorption pathway and have an open skull; children and young adults have highly reactive cerebral hemodynamics; elderly patients have passive accumulation of CSF due to brain atrophy and cranioencephalic disproportion. Of all groups, infants around five months of age are the most vulnerable and are at particularly high risk of developing an SDH after head injury, meningitis, or surgery. Infantile SDH thus appears as an age-specific, cause-unspecific response to insults to the leptomeninges.

Proper medical and surgical management of these entities requires taking in account the age of the patient, clinical presentation, radiological appearance, and expected spontaneous course of the disease. More dated data on documented patients will be needed to make reliable predictions on the behavior of PCC, and propose adapted treatment of these often difficult patients.

REFERENCES

1. Friede RL. Subdural hematomas, hygromas, and effusions. In: Developmental Neuropathology. Berlin, Germany: Springer Publisher, 1989:198–208.
2. Mori K, Yamamoto T, Horinaka N, et al. Arachnoid cyst is a risk for chronic subdural hematoma in juveniles: Twelve cases of chronic subdural hematoma associated with arachnoid cyst. J Neurotrauma 2002; 19:1017–1027.
3. Dandy WE, Blackfan KD. Internal hydrocephalus: An experimental, clinical and pathological study. Am J Dis Child 1914; 8:406–482.
4. Matson DM. Neurosurgery of Infancy and Childhood. Springfield, IL: Thomas, 1969:328–347.
5. Vinchon M, Noizet O, Defoort-Dhellemmes S, et al. Infantile subdural hematomas due to motor vehicle accidents. Pediatr Neurosurg 2002; 35:245–253.
6. Vinchon M, Noulé N, Tchofo PJ, et al. Imaging of head injuries in infants: Temporal correlates and implications for the diagnosis of child abuse. J Neurosurg (Pediatr) 2004; 101(suppl 2):44–52.
7. Neimann N, Montaut J, Sapelier J. Épanchements sous-duraux chroniques du nourrisson. Paris, France: L'expansion Publisher, 1968.
8. Haines DE, Harkey HL, Al-Mefty O. The "subdural" space: A new look at an outdated concept. Neurosurgery 1993; 32:111–120.
9. Papasian NC, Frim DM. A theoretical model of benign external hydrocephalus that predicts a predisposition toward extra-axial hemorrhage after minor head trauma. Pediatr Neurosurg 2000; 33: 188–193.
10. Davson H, Welch K, Segal MB. The Physiology and Pathophysiology of the Cerebrospinal Fluid. Edinburgh, U.K.: Churchill Livingstone Publisher, 1987:485–521.
11. Papaiconomou C, Zakharov A, Azizi N, et al. Reassessment of the pathways responsible for cerebrospinal fluid absorption in the neonate. Childs Nerv Syst 2004; 20:29–36.
12. Czosnyka M, Czosnyka ZH, Whitfield PC, et al. Cerebrospinal fluid dynamics. In: Cinalli G, Maixner WJ, Sainte-Rose C, eds. Pediatric Hydrocephalus. Milan, Italy: Springer, 2004:47–63.
13. Lasjaunias P. Hydrodynamic disorders. In: Vascular Diseases in Neonates, Infants and Children, 2nd ed. Berlin, Germany: Springer, 1997:31–40.
14. Upton ML, Weller RO. The morphology of cerebrospinal fluid drainage pathways in human arachnoid granulations. J Neurosurg 1985; 63:867–875.
15. Yamashima T. Ultrastructural study of the final cerebrospinal fluid pathway in human arachnoid villi. Brain Res 1986; 384:68–76.
16. Baraton J, Brunelle F, Pierre-Kahn A, et al. Tomodensitométrie couplée à la cisternographie dans les épanchements péri-cérébraux chroniques du jeune enfant. Neurochirurgie 1989; 35:395–400.

17. Hymel KP, Rumack CM, Hay TC, et al. Comparison of intracranial computed tomographic findings in pediatric abusive and accidental trauma. Pediatr Radiol 1997; 27:743–747.

18. Endo S, Hirashima Y, Takaba M, et al. Administration of methylprednisolone acetate into the subdural cavity in an infant with subdural fluid collection. Childs Nerv Syst 1998; 14:354–356.

19. Suzuki K, Takano S, Nose T. Increased concentration of vascular endothelial growth factor (VEGF) in chronic subdural hematoma. J Trauma 1999; 46:532–533.

20. Yamashima T, Tachibana O, Hasegawa M, et al. Liberation of eosinophil granules in the inner capsule of chronic subdural hematomas. Neurochirurgia 1989; 32:168–171.

21. Firsching R, Müller W, Thun F, et al. Clinical correlates of erythropoiesis in chronic subdural hematoma. Surg Neurol 1990; 33:173–177.

22. McLone DG, Guttierez FA, Raimondi AJ, et al. Ultrastructure of subdural membranes of children. Concepts Pediatr Neurosurg 1981; 1:174–187.

23. Stroobandt G, Evrard P, Thauvoy C, et al. Les épanchements péricérébraux du nourrisson à localisation sous-durale ou sous-arachnoïdienne. Neurochirurgie 1981; 27:49–57.

24. Van Calenbergh F, Bleyen J, Lagae L, et al. Long-term external drainage for subdural collections in infants. Childs Nerv Syst 2000; 16:429–432.

25. Haseler LJ, Arcinue E, Danielsen ER, et al. Evidence from proton magnetic resonance spectrography for a metabolic cascade of neuronal damage in shaken baby syndrome. Pediatrics 1997; 99:4–14.

26. Massicotte EM, Del Biggio MR. Human arachnoid villi response to subarachnoid hemorrhage: Possible relationship to chronic hydrocephalus. J Neurosurg 1999; 91:80–84.

27. Fobben ES, Grossman RI, Hackeny DB, et al. MR characteristics of subdural hematomas and hygromas at 1.5T. Am J Neuroradiol 1989; 10:687–693.

28. Tsui EYK, Ma KF, Cheung YK, et al. Rapid spontaneous resolution and redistribution of acute subdural hematoma in a patient with chronic alcoholism: Case report. Eur J Radiol 2000; 36:53–57.

29. Ford FR. Chronic subdural hematoma. In: Diseases of the Nervous System in Infancy, Childhood and Adolescence, 3rd ed. Springfield, IL: Thomas Publisher, 1952:994–999.

30. Guttierez FA, McLone DG, Raimondi AJ. Pathophysiology and a new treatment of chronic subdural hematoma in children. Childs Brain 1979; 5:216–232.

31. Marquardt G, Weidauer S, Lanfermann H, et al. Cerebral venous sinus thrombosis manifesting as bilateral subdural effusion. Acta Neurol Scand 2004; 109:425–428.

32. Najjar MW, Azzam NI, Khalifa MA. Pseudotumor cerebri: Disordered cerebrospinal fluid hydrodynamics with extra-axial collections. Pediatr Neurosurg 2005; 41:212–215.

33. Vinchon M, Pierrat V, Jissendi Tchofo P, et al. Traumatic intracranial hemorrhage in newborns. Childs Nerv Syst 2005; 21:1042–1048.

34. Vinchon M, Joriot S, Jissendi-Tchofo P, et al. Postmeningitis subdural collections in infants: Changing pattern and indications for surgery. J Neurosurg (Pediatr) 2006. In press.

35. Rekate HL. Treatment of hydrocephalus. In: Albright AL, Pollack IF, Adelson PD, eds. Principles and Practice of Pediatric Neurosurgery. New York: Thieme, 1999:47–73.

36. Raimondi AJ, Hirschauer J. Head injury in the infant and toddler. Childs Brain 1984; 11:12–35.

37. Ment LR, Duncan CC, Geehr R. Benign enlargement of the subarachnoid spaces in the infant. J Neurosurg 1981; 54:504–508.

38. Odita JC. The widened frontal subarachnoid space. Childs Nerv Syst 1992; 8:36–39.

39. Kapila A, Trice J, Spiess WG, et al. Enlarged cerebrospinal fluid spaces in infants with subdural hematomas. Radiology 1982; 142:669–672.

40. Vinchon M, Defoort-Dhellemmes S, Desurmont M, et al. Accidental and non-accidental head injuries in infants: A prospective study. J Neurosurg (Pediatr) 2005; 102(suppl 4):380–384.

41. Sgouros S, Tolias C. Benign pericerebral collections in children. In: Cinalli G, Sainte-Rose C, Maixner W, eds. Pediatric Hydrocephalus. Milan, Italy: Springer, 2004:145–153.

42. Whitby EH, Griffiths PD, Rutter S, et al. Frequency and natural history of subdural haemorrhages in babies and relation to obstetric factors. Lancet 2004; 363:846 851.

43. Vinchon M, Defoort-Dhellemmes S, Nzeyimana C, et al. Infantile traumatic subdural hematomas: Outcome after five years. Pediatr Neurosurg 2003; 39:122–128.

44. Marin-Padilla M, Parisi JE, Armstrong DL, et al. Shaken infant syndrome: Developmental neuropathology, progressive cortical dysplasia, and epilepsy. Acta Neuropathol 2002; 103:321–332.

45. Hwang SK, Kim SL. Infantile head injury, with special reference to the development of chronic subdural hematoma. Childs Nerv Syst 2000; 16:590–594.

46. Duhaime AC, Alario AJ, Lewander WJ, et al. Head injury in very young children: Mechanisms, injury types, and ophthalmologic findings in 100 hospitalized patients younger than 2 years of age. Pediatrics 1992; 90:179–185.

47. Vinchon M, Noulé N, Soto-Ares G, et al. Subduroperitoneal drainage for traumatic subdural hematoma in infants: Results with 244 cases. J Neurosurg 2001; 95:248–254.

48. Tolias C, Sgouros S, Walsh AR, et al. Outcome of surgical treatment for subdural fluid collections in infants. Pediatr Neurosurg 2000; 33:194–197.

49. Lee KS. The pathogenesis and clinical significance of traumatic subdural hygroma. Brain Injury 1998; 12:595–603.

50. Park CK, Choi KH, Kim MC, et al. Spontaneous evolution of posttraumatic subdural hygroma into chronic subdural haematoma. Acta Neurochir 1994; 127:41–47.

51. Hasegawa M, Yamashima T, Yamashita J, et al. Traumatic subdural hydroma: Pathology and meningeal enhancement on magnetic resonance imaging. Neurosurgery 1992; 31:580–585.

52. Gelabert-Gonzalez M, Fernandez-Villa J, Cutrin-Prieto J, et al. Arachnoid cyst rupture with subdural hygroma: Report of three cases and literature review. Childs Nerv Syst 2002; 18:609–613.

53. Mori T, Fujimoto M, Sakae K, et al. Disappearance of arachnoid cysts after head injury. Neurosurgery 1995; 36:938–942.

54. Tamburrini G, Caldarelli M, Massimi L, et al. Subdural hygroma: An unwanted result of sylvian arachnoid cyst marsupialization. Childs Nerv Syst 2003; 19:159–165.

55. Tanaka Y, Sugita K, Kobayashi S, et al. Subdural fluid collections following transcortical approach to intra- or paraventricular tumours. Acta Neurochir 1989; 99:20–25.

56. Al-Yamani M, Del Maestro RF: Prevention of subdural fluid collections following transcortical intraventricular and/or paraventricular procedures by using fibrin adhesive. J Neurosurg 2000; 92:406–412.

57. Freudenstein D, Wagner A, Ernemann U, et al. Subdural hygroma as a complication of endoscopic neurosurgery. Neurol Med Chir (Tokyo) 2002; 42:554–559.

58. Cartmill M, Vloeberghs M. The fate of the cerebrospinal fluid after neuroendoscopic third ventriculostomy. Childs Nerv Syst 2000; 16:879–881.

59. Syrogiannopoulos GA, Nelson JD, McCracken GH. Subdural collections in acute bacterial meningitis: A review of 136 cases. Pediatr Infect Dis 1986; 5:343–352.

60. Curless RG. Subdural empyemas in infant meningitis: Diagnosis, therapy, and prognosis. Childs Nerv Syst 1985; 1:211–214.

14 | Shunt-Related Headaches: The Slit Ventricle Syndromes

Harold L. Rekate

Pediatric Neurosciences, Barrow Neurological Institute, St. Joseph's Hospital and Medical Center, Phoenix, Arizona, U.S.A.

Headaches are one of the most common afflictions of mankind. Based on large series of patients, about 4% of the adults in the world suffer headaches every day, with a female-to-male ratio of 2.5:1 (1). A larger but inestimable number of individuals have occasional incapacitating headaches (2). Not surprisingly then, patients with shunts have headache disorders. The presence of the shunt in patients with headaches always leads to the assumption that something is wrong with the shunt. This assumption can lead to large numbers of expensive and possibly dangerous imaging studies, long waits in emergency rooms, and the expenditure of considerable money when the headaches are a chronic condition. There is always the possibility that patients could die or develop severe neurologic dysfunction from high intracranial pressure (ICP) at the time of shunt failure. Medically, therefore, it is reasonable to ascertain that their shunt is working. Doing so, however, is not always straightforward.

Since their development in the 1950s, valve-regulated shunts have probably saved more lives and more cognitive function for more years than anything else neurosurgeons have ever done (3,4). However, shunts have also led to a great many problems that were not easy to predict from the beginning. The most common and most chronic of these newly recognized conditions is the association of chronic headaches with the presence of a shunt. Severe headache disorder in patients with shunts and small ventricles has been called the "slit-ventricle syndrome" (SVS) (5). SVS is not a single condition; rather, several different pathophysiologies can underlie this constellation of findings (6). This chapter defines the various causes of severe headaches in shunted patients, suggests an algorithm for the diagnosis and treatment of this common condition, and suggests a management approach to patients with shunt-related problems.

CLASSIFICATION

As shunting of the ventricles became standard treatment for hydrocephalus, problems related to overdrainage were recognized with increasing frequency (7). Before valve regulation of cerebrospinal fluid (CSF) flow was developed, drainage of the lateral ventricles in children with hydrocephalus was precluded by the routine collapse of the brain with associated lethal subdural hematomas. The development of valve regulation made it possible to treat severe hydrocephalus successfully with much less likelihood of this dreaded complication.

By the mid-1970s problems related to the ventricles becoming too small, leading to intermittent or recurrent obstruction of the ventricular catheter, was recognized as a severe problem. Several strategies, including subtemporal decompression for the management of this condition (8–10), were introduced. In an early report on our experiences with this condition, we defined SVS as a triad involving intermittent headaches lasting 10 to 90 minutes, small ventricles on imaging studies, and slow refilling of the pumping mechanism of the valve (5). In this same article, we demonstrated that it was possible to increase the volume of the lateral ventricles by using valve upgrading and a device that retards siphoning (DRS). We also recommended that the use of low-pressure shunts should be abandoned unless dictated by specific indications.

As experience grew, especially with the ability to track changes in ventricular size using contemporary neuroimaging such as computed tomography (CT) and magnetic resonance imaging (MRI), it became obvious that this view of the SVS was too simplistic and that there were multiple different forms of the problem. Reports dealing with SVS were not describing the same condition (11). In 1993, we published our experiences with ICP monitoring in patients with small ventricles and severe headaches. We identified five distinct pathophysiologies for this condition. There is some overlap, but each condition requires specific treatment paradigms (6). Based on our previous study, it has been our policy to upgrade the valve and include a DRS in all patients. All patients studied had previously undergone the procedure (5).

We intervene surgically only in patients whose headaches significantly interfere with normal life. If children have to leave school or adults need to leave work or discontinue working more than twice a month, we believe that surgical intervention is justified.

There is little consensus about the definition or causes of headaches in shunted patients. Most such patients undergo a valve upgrade and incorporation of a DRS. About one in five of these patients, however, does not improve or improves only temporarily. Before further intervention is pursued, the causes of the patient's headaches and the relationship of the headaches to shunt function and ICP must be understood fully. To understand the causes of the headaches, it is essential to define the relationship of ICP and shunt function to the headaches. Based on chronic monitoring of ICP in these patients with headaches, we have defined five syndromes of shunt-related headaches. Each syndrome leads to specific treatment strategies (6).

Intracranial Hypotension

These patients develop severe headaches that are not present while they are reclined in bed. The headache develops later in the day and gets worse with time as patients maintain an erect position. The headache improves rather rapidly if patients can lie down. Monitoring shows significantly subnormal ICP. We have recorded ICP from −25 to −30 mm Hg. These headaches are analogous to postlumbar puncture headaches and may be associated with enhancement of the meninges on contrast-enhanced imaging studies.

This condition implies that the DRS has failed and that the patient will respond to replacement of the valve mechanism with insertion of an effective DRS and possibly a valve upgrade. Since the publication of the article (6), we now use a programmable valve. We prefer to use the Codman Hakim Programmable Valve with Siphonguard™(Codman Corporation, Raynham, MA), but other adjustable valves with anti-siphon devices exist in the market as well.

Intermittent Proximal Obstruction

This problem is probably the most common of the five conditions and represents patients who were originally described as having SVS. Monitoring shows that patients with this condition have normal to low ICP most of the day, but their ICP increases suddenly with activity. As their ICP increases, the headache worsens until the ventricular catheter reopens and the pressure reverts to normal again. These patients are also managed by placement of a DRS and valve upgrade. In chronically shunted individuals, proximal shunt failure is the most common form of mechanical failure of shunts. For decades my policy has been to assume that this condition is a result of overdrainage of CSF and collapse of the ventricular walls around the ventricular catheter. Therefore, it is a sign that the back pressure or opening pressure of the valve is inadequate to maintain CSF within the ventricular system. I believe that the valve should be upgraded and a DRS should be incorporated into the system any time a proximal obstruction occurs.

Shunt Failure Without Ventricular Enlargement

Engel and colleagues originally described intracranial hypertension with nondistending ventricles, so-called normal volume hydrocephalus (NVH) (12). This enigmatic condition has been studied intensively. It is the most important and difficult to manage of the subtypes of SVS. In the series of Engel and coworkers (12), patients were found to have signs and symptoms of increased ICP with no enlargement of the ventricular system. They recommended exploration of these shunts, which were routinely found to be nonfunctional.

These patients become symptomatic with progressive symptoms of increased ICP with morning headaches progressing to all-day headaches, papilledema, visual loss, and diplopia. If the condition is not treated early, neurologic deterioration is possible and blindness is likely. This problem occurs rarely, if at all, in patients who develop hydrocephalus beyond infancy, but it is a common problem in cases of congenital hydrocephalus (13).

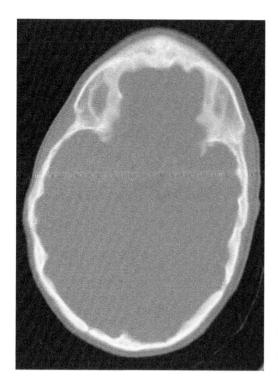

Figure 1   CT scan of a patient with syndromic cranisynostosis and hydrocephalus showing scalloping of the inner table of the bone due to cephalocranial disproportion. With kind permission from Springer Science+Business Media: from Rekate HL: Shunt-related headaches: the slit ventricle syndromes. Childs Nerv Syst 24(4):423–30, 2008.

These patients begin life with hydrocephalus but when older have pseudotumor cerebri. We performed retrograde venographic measurements of sagittal sinus pressure in five such children. All had elevated venous sinus pressure, as have all patients with pseudotumor cerebri that we have tested (14). In general, a shunting strategy that incorporates drainage of the subarachnoid space, such as lumboperitoneal shunts or shunts from the cisterna magna, is needed to manage these patients adequately (15–17).

Increased ICP with a Working Shunt: Cephalocranial Disproportion

Based on shunt flow studies and surgical exploration, these patients have working shunts but show significant signs of increased ICP. In my experience, this problem has been universally associated with hindbrain herniation (Chiari I malformation) and found exclusively in patients with craniofacial disorders such as oxycephaly, Crouzon's syndrome, and Pfeiffer's syndrome (Fig. 1). Other authors have postulated that sutural closure results from decreasing ICP and from insufficient room for the growing brain (18).

With neither a significant abnormality of the shape of the skull and face nor the presence of hindbrain herniation, the problem in these patients is likely NVH and not cephalocranial disproportion. It is best managed with shunts that incorporate the subarachnoid space. Patients with true cephalocranial disproportion need a cranial expansion procedure or large subtemporal decompression. Further manipulation of the shunt is of no benefit. Hindbrain herniation in these patients can be dealt with effectively by enlarging the posterior hemicranium (19).

Shunt-Related Migraine

Patients with shunts can have migraines or other headache disorders that are unrelated to their shunt. Shunt-related migraine usually occurs in the context of a strong family history of migraine and is episodic. As small children these patients usually suffer from seasonal allergies. Their descriptions of their headaches may or may not be typical of migraine.

These patients often improve briefly after shunt manipulation, but the same problems return rather quickly after intervention. Because of the potential medicolegal problems associated with failure to diagnose a shunt malfunction, all these patients have had many visits to the emergency room and a large number of CT scans (because these episodes are usually considered emergencies) and other diagnostic studies. Management of these patients is complicated and frustrating. The patient, family, and neurology staff are often reluctant to believe that the headaches are unrelated to the shunt. Therefore, considerable energy and financial resources are necessary to treat these patients. Documentation by ICP monitoring is often needed to prove that the headaches are unrelated to the shunt before a commitment to medical management can be reached (6).

SHUNT-REMOVAL PROTOCOL
Although most shunted patients have radiographic slit ventricles after years of shunting, only a small number have the symptoms of SVS (20).

Based on my practice, however, I would predict that a third of infants followed for more than five years will have a severe chronic headache disorder that requires intervention. At least 20% will have ventricles that do not expand at the time of shunt failure (NVH). Severe and activity-limiting headaches are common among shunted patients.

As stated, the first step in the management of these patients is to use programmable shunts that incorporate a DRS. In my opinion the prevalence of this problem justifies the routine use of these devices. As Oikonomou et al. noted, avoiding one shunt revision would justify implanting a shunt that cost $50,000 (21).

What are the alternatives for patients with a valve upgrade and incorporation of a DRS who are still incapacitated by headaches? Of the patients described in the discussion of the classification, a specific therapy is available only for those with cephalocranial disproportion—cranial expansion. Before undertaking this procedure, we would always recommend a trial of ICP monitoring to document the problem. MRI often shows a hindbrain herniation in such patients (Fig. 2). These patients require cranial expansion. We agree with Di Rocco and Velardi that occipital expansion is likely to treat both the cephalocranial disproportion and the hindbrain herniation, if the bone around the foramen magnum is removed at the same time (19).

If adequate decompression cannot be achieved from above, occasionally it is necessary to explore the craniovertebral junction directly. Patients with complex craniofacial abnormalities often have an associated set of abnormalities of venous outflow from the intracranial venous sinuses and compression of the jugular foramen. It is essential to obtain either angiographic images or MR venograms to ascertain that this flow is not interrupted (Fig. 3). It is possible that a very large percentage of venous flow is through emissary veins and may need to be saved (22,23). These venous anomalies can lead to a pseudotumor-like picture, and they can coexist with NVH as discussed below.

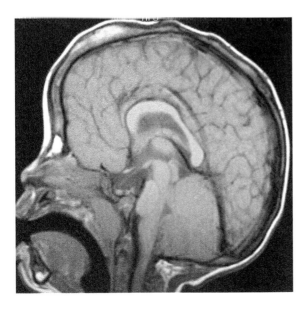

Figure 2 MRI of brain showing hindbrain herniation. With kind permission from Springer Science+Business Media: from Rekate HL: Shunt-related headaches: the slit ventricle syndromes. Childs Nerv Syst 24(4):423–30, 2008.

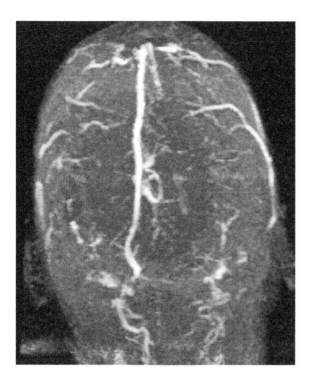

Figure 3 MR venography of patient with normal volume hydrocephalus showing abnormalities of venous drainage leading to late pseudotumor syndrome in NVH. With kind permission from Springer Science+Business Media: from Rekate HL: Shunt-related headaches: the slit ventricle syndromes. Childs Nerv Syst 24(4):423–30, 2008.

We have developed an algorithm for diagnosis and treatment of all other patients with SVS who do *not* improve after a valve change (Fig. 4). This strategy is an attempt to improve understanding of the pathophysiology and treatment of debilitating headaches in individual patients. After prolonged discussions with patients and family, if appropriate, patients are offered the "shunt removal protocol" (24). This procedure has evolved over time. In general, after informed consent is obtained, patients undergo surgery to have their entire shunt system removed and replaced with an external ventricular drain (EVD). After recovering from anesthesia, patients are taken to the intensive care unit where the EVD is used to monitor ICP and to drain CSF if needed. Initially, the drain is left open at 25 cm H_2O above the midposition of the head as long as the setting is tolerated. All participants, the patient, the nurses caring for the patient in the ICU, the family, and the neurosurgical residents are informed of the goals of the procedure and of the parameters for management of the EVD.

The next morning a scan is obtained to determine whether the ventricles have enlarged. If so, this form of treatment is continued for another 24 hours. If not and the patient is only mildly ill from increased ICP, the drain is closed under careful observation in an attempt to increase the size of the lateral ventricles. If the ventricles have enlarged significantly on the third hospital day, the patient returns to the operating room for an endoscopic third ventriculostomy.

We have identified three potential outcomes associated with closure of the drain. In the best scenario, the ventricles enlarge only slightly, ICP normalizes, and the patient is essentially asymptomatic. This hoped-for result has occurred in about 25% of our patients. These patients have usually undergone resection or treatment of a brain tumor or have experienced a subarachnoid or intraventricular hemorrhage. In these cases, ICP is monitored for 48 hours and the drain is removed. The patient remains in close contact with our service and undergoes follow-up scans six weeks and one year after the procedure. These results support findings from our previous study on the possibility of shunt-independent arrest of hydrocephalus (25).

The second possibility is that the ventricles expand and the patient becomes ill. If patients with a coexistent myelomeningocele (Chiari II malformation) are excluded, these patients are excellent candidates for endoscopic third ventriculostomy. The success rate for shunt-independent arrest of the hydrocephalus is 80%.

It is essential to ascertain that patients who have had chronic headaches for a long time are safe and that they have no recurrent increase in ICP. Consequently, over time we have tended to

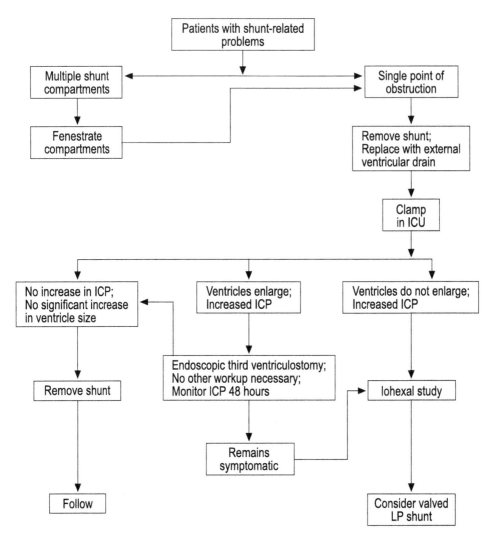

Figure 4 Algorithm for managing shunt-related difficulties with a shunt removal protocol. *Source*: Courtesy of Barrow Neurological Institute.

leave a ventricular access device or tapping reservoir in place after the ETV has been inserted. We affix a butterfly needle into the reservoir for ICP monitoring for 48 hours. If patients return with headaches, the needle remains in place for later assessment of ICP and to inject contrast to ensure that the stoma is open. Using this protocol we have had only one late failure, which occurred one year after the procedure. Reexploration of that patient revealed that the basilar artery had herniated through and sealed the stoma. A second hole was made anterior and lateral to the artery, and the patient's symptoms resolved.

The third possibility is that the ventricles do not expand, ICP increases, and patients seem ill. Such patients have NVH and are not candidates for ETV. There are two reasons why ETV is inappropriate in this condition. The first reason is practical. Even with the use of frameless stereotaxy, it is difficult to manipulate an endoscope within such small ventricles without potential damaging important structures.

The second reason relates to the underlying origin of the hydrocephalus. In our experience, all patients in this series obviously had hydrocephalus during early infancy, when their first shunts were placed. Based on retrograde venous manometry performed in several of these patients, their sagittal sinus pressure is higher than normal. The ventricles have failed to expand in more than 30% of patients undergoing the protocol. It also has occurred in at least 20% of patients with hydrocephalus related to a Chiari II malformation. Consequently, we no longer consider these patients as candidates for the shunt-removal protocol.

Several scenarios frequently result in NVH and respond in this way to attempts at shunt removal. The first group begins life as premature infants and is in the neonatal ICU for prolonged periods. Their hydrocephalus has been attributed to intraventricular hemorrhage, but venous studies reflect abnormal venous drainage either from congenital anomalies or chronic central lines associated with stenosis of the jugular veins or superior vena cava.

The other group is usually diagnosed with congenital aqueductal stenosis. Triventricular hydrocephalus is diagnosed when their heads are discovered to be enlarging and crossing percentile lines. Developmental assessments in these babies are normal, except for some delays in gross motor behavior related to the relatively large head. Later in life at the time of shunt failure, these children develop the signs and symptoms of increased ICP but without ventriculomegaly. At this point, MRI shows open flow through the aqueduct of Sylvius. In such cases, the hydrocephalus has actually caused the closure of the aqueduct (26). In all of these patients and particularly in the two classes of patients discussed here, ETV offers no advantage because communication between the third ventricle and intrapeduncular cistern enables CSF to flow briefly. Intraventricular injection of Iohexol confirms free communication among the ventricles, cortical subarachnoid spaces, and cisterns except in children who experienced severe ventriculitis after their original shunt procedure (17,24). For these patients, it is essential to develop treatment strategies that access the cortical subarachnoid spaces (16).

CONCLUSIONS

Based on reviews of management strategies that treat such headaches, however, narcotic medication must be avoided if possible. Narcotics are widely recognized as leading to the well-defined entity classified as "medication overuse headaches."

The role of neurosurgeons in the management of shunt-related headaches or SVS must be to ensure that ICP dynamics are normalized as much as possible. Doing so requires ascertaining that all CSF compartments communicate without resistance or obstruction. Neuroendoscopic procedures can be used to fenestrate membranes that lead to compartmentalization or by splicing multiple ventricular or subarachnoid space catheters proximal to a single programmable valve containing a DRS. The final step is to monitor ICP over time to ascertain that ICP remains normal during all positions and during sleep.

What should be done if patients return complaining of reexacerbation of their headaches? First, the shunt system must be identified as working as planned. If the ventricles do not expand at the time of shunt failure, which is the likely scenario in these cases, performing CT scans is futile. If it is essential to image the brain, rapid sequence MRIs are preferred. Typically, these patients have undergone many CT scans. At best, patients' risk of cataracts increases. At worst, there is a theoretical possibility that the risk of developing induced malignancies is increased over the ensuing decades.

In NVH patients with worsening symptoms, a reservoir tap is placed. ICP is measured while the patient is recumbent. The patient is asked to sit up to ensure that their ICP falls to a maximum of 5 cm H_2O or lower.

At this point, about 5 mg of Iohexol is injected. The patient is scanned within an hour. The cortical subarachnoid and spinal subarachnoid spaces of the upper cervical spine are analyzed carefully. If there are no obstructions, the system is working as hoped and the headaches are unrelated to the ICP. These patients can then be managed medically with the full understanding that all pressure manipulations that can be done have been done.

REFERENCES

1. Wang SJ, Fuh JL, Lu SR, et al. Chronic daily headache in adolescents: Prevalence, impact, and medication overuse. Neurology 2006; 66(2):193–197.
2. Strine TW, Chapman DP, Balluz LS. Population-based U.S. study of severe headaches in adults: Psychological distress and comorbidities. Headache 2006; 46(2):223–232.
3. Nulsen FE, Becker DP. Control of hydrocephalus by valve-regulated shunt. J Neurosurg 1967; 26(3):362–374.

4. Nulsen FE, Spitz EB. Treatment of hydrocephalus by direct shunt from ventricle to jugular vein. Surg Forum 1951;2:399–403.
5. Hyde-Rowan MD, Rekate HL, Nulsen FE. Reexpansion of previously collapsed ventricles: The slit ventricle syndrome. J Neurosurg 1982; 56(4):536–539.
6. Rekate HL. Classification of slit-ventricle syndromes using intracranial pressure monitoring. Pediatr Neurosurg 1993; 19(1):15–20.
7. Portnoy HD, Schulte RR, Fox JL, et al. Anti-siphon and reversible occlusion valves for shunting in hydrocephalus and preventing post-shunt subdural hematomas. J Neurosurg 1973; 38(6):729–738.
8. Epstein F, Marlin AE, Wald A. Chronic headache in the shunt-dependent adolescent with nearly normal ventricular volume: Diagnosis and treatment. Neurosurgery 1978; 3(3):351–355.
9. Epstein FJ, Fleischer AS, Hochwald GM, et al. Subtemporal craniectomy for recurrent shunt obstruction secondary to small ventricles. J Neurosurg 1974; 41(1):29–31.
10. Holness RO, Hoffman HJ, Hendrick EB. Subtemporal decompression for the slit-ventricle syndrome after shunting in hydrocephalic children. Childs Brain 1979; 5(2):137–144.
11. McLaurin RL, Olivi A. Slit-ventricle syndrome: Review of 15 cases. Pediatr Neurosci 1987; 13(3): 118–124.
12. Engel M, Carmel PW, Chutorian AM. Increased intraventricular pressure without ventriculomegaly in children with shunts: "Normal volume" hydrocephalus. Neurosurgery 1979; 5(5):549–552.
13. Rekate HL. Adults with hydrocephalus treated in infancy and childhood. In: Ellenbogen R, ed. Pediatric Neurosurgery for the General Neurosurgeon. New York: Thieme, 2002:19–28.
14. Karahalios DG, Rekate HL, Khayata MH, et al. Elevated intracranial venous pressure as a universal mechanism in pseudotumor cerebri of varying etiologies. Neurology 1996; 46(1):198–202.
15. Nadkarni TD, Rekate HL. Treatment of refractory intracranial hypertension in a spina bifida patient by a concurrent ventricular and cisterna magna-to-peritoneal shunt. Childs Nerv Syst 2005; 21(7):579–582.
16. Rekate HL, Nadkarni T, Wallace D. Severe intracranial hypertension in slit ventricle syndrome managed using a cisterna magna-ventricle-peritoneum shunt. J Neurosurg 2006; 104(suppl. 4):240–244.
17. Rekate HL, Wallace D. Lumboperitoneal shunts in children. Pediatr Neurosurg 2003; 38(1):41–46.
18. Albright AL, Tyler-Kabara E. Slit-ventricle syndrome secondary to shunt-induced suture ossification. Neurosurgery 2001; 48(4):764–769.
19. Di Rocco C, Velardi F. Acquired Chiari type I malformation managed by supratentorial cranial enlargement. Childs Nerv Syst 2003; 19(12):800–807.
20. Walker ML, Fried A, Petronio J. Diagnosis and treatment of the slit ventricle syndrome. Neurosurg Clin N Am 1993; 4(4):707–714.
21. Oikonomou J, Aschoff A, Hashemi B, et al. New valves—New dangers? 22 valves (38 probes) designed in the "nineties in ultralong-term tests (365 days)". Eur J Pediatr Surg 1999; 9(suppl 1):23–26.
22. Chumas PD, Drake JM, Del Bigio MR. Death from chronic tonsillar herniation in a patient with lumboperitoneal shunt and Crouzon's disease. Br J Neurosurg 1992; 6(6):595–599.
23. Thompson DN, Harkness W, Jones BM, et al. Aetiology of herniation of the hindbrain in craniosynostosis. An investigation incorporating intracranial pressure monitoring and magnetic resonance imaging. Pediatr Neurosurg 1997; 26(6):288–295.
24. Baskin JJ, Manwaring KH, Rekate HL. Ventricular shunt removal: The ultimate treatment of the slit ventricle syndrome. J Neurosurg 1998; 88(3):478–484.
25. Rekate HL. Establishing the diagnosis of shunt independence. Monogr Neural Sci 1982; 8:223–226.
26. Borti A. Communicating hydrocephalus causing aqueductal stenosis. Neuropadiatrie 1976; 7(4): 416–422.
27. Rekate HL, Williams FC Jr, Brodkey JA, et al. Resistance of the foramen of Monro. Pediatr Neurosci 1988; 14(2):85–89.

15 | Acquired Hydrocephalus in Adults

Jörg Baldauf and Henry W. S. Schroeder

Department of Neurosurgery, Ernst-Moritz-Arndt University, Greifswald, Germany

INTRODUCTION

Acquired hydrocephalus in adults is a frequent complication after subarachnoid hemorrhage or head trauma. Additonally, it is seen in patients with intracranial tumors. These clinical entities require different diagnostic and therapeutic strategies. This chapter will discuss the pathophysiological background, the diagnostic criteria, and the surgical management according to the published scientific work and our own experience.

HYDROCEPHALUS AFTER SUBARACHNOID HEMORRHAGE

Incidence and Pathophysiological Considerations

Hydrocephalus is a well-recognized complication following aneurysmal subarachnoid hemorrhage (SAH). The incidence of hydrocephalus after SAH varies between 6% and 67% (1–4). However, different stages must be separated in this setting, such as acute (0–3 days after SAH), subacute (4–13 days after SAH), and chronic (≥14 days after SAH) (1,5). The pathogenesis of the development of hydrocephalus related to SAH is based on the disturbance of cerebrospinal fluid (CSF) hydrodynamics and altered CSF absorption resulting from blood in the subarachnoid space. Several theories exist to explain the background of these problems. Acute hydrocephalus can develop whenever CSF pathways are suddenly obstructed by blood clots, especially within the ventricular system at the aqueduct of Sylvius or at the outlet foramina of Luschka and Magendie (5–9). This fact is frequently seen after rupture of posterior circulation aneurysms or associated intraventricular hemorrhage, whereas bleeding from anterior circulation aneurysms might cause obstruction of arachnoid granulations over the cerebral convexities (7,10).

Experimental studies have shown the resistance to CSF absorption to be increased after SAH and remain elevated for weeks (11). Additionally, there is an indication that an increase of ICP after SAH is associated with an increase in outflow resistance to CSF pathways (9,12). As reported by Fuhrmeister et al., the CSF outflow resistance can be elevated threefold in patients with SAH (13). Although CSF hydrodynamics become normalized in the majority of patients, physiological CSF outflow resistance may not occur until 40 to 50 days after SAH. In cases of arachnoid scarring and blockade of arachnoid granulations, CSF outflow resistance can remain elevated and a state of chronic hydrocephalus may develop (11,14). This fact may be supported by clinical data. In different series, permanent shunting after SAH for chronic hydrocephalus was required after a mean interval of 36 to 44.3 days (2,15). Additionally, we agree with others that the pathogenesis of the chronic phase involves arachnoid adhesions that form as a result of meningeal reaction to blood products, impairing CSF absorption at the arachnoid villi (5,11,16).

Risk Factors Related to Subarachnoid Hydrocephalus

Different factors have been described contributing to the development of shunt-dependent hydrocephalus after SAH, including ventricular enlargement or acute hydrocephalus at the time on admission, amount of diffuse subarachnoid blood, intraventricular hemorrhage, bleeding from posterior circulation aneurysms, increased aneurysm size, severe neurological grade at admission [low-grade Glasgow Coma Scale (GCS); Hunt & Hess grades III–IV], aneurysmal rebleeding, symptomatic vasospasm, focal ischemic deficits, use of antifibrinolytic drugs, hyponatremia, hypertension, alcoholism, pneumonia, meningitis, increasing age, female sex (1,3–6,17–20).

In general, some degree of asymptomatic ventricular enlargement is common after SAH and seems to occur within the first three days after SAH in most patients (4,21). Some patients deteriorate from hydrocephalus after admission. These patients more often demonstrate a lower

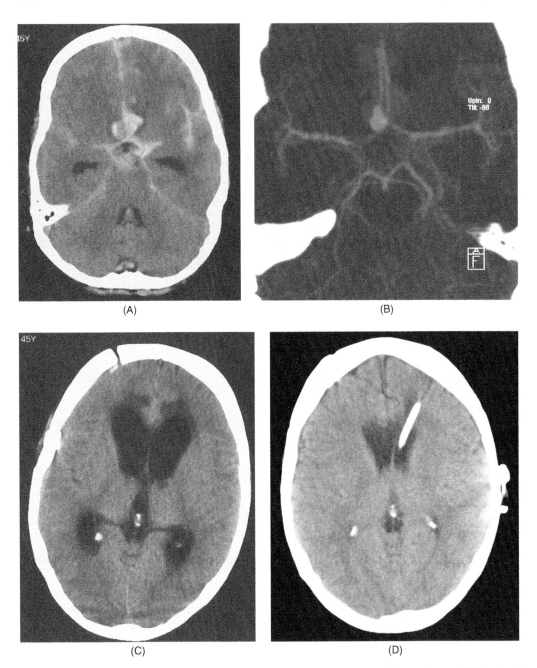

(A)   (B)

(C)   (D)

Figure 1 This 45-year-old female patient presented with a severe subarachnoid hemorrhage (H&H grade IV). (A) The initial CT scan shows already enlarged temporal horns of the lateral ventricles as a sign of an acute hydrocephalus because of SAH. (B) The bleeding originated from an aneurysm of the AComA. (C) An insertion of an external ventricular drainage was performed in the early stage. Two months after SAH a chronic hydrocephalus developed. (D) Ventriculoperitoneal shunting was done with resolution of hydrocephalus.

GCS on admission, a higher amount of cisternal blood on the initial CT, or associated intraventricular bleeding (18). However, the presence of acute hydrocephalus does not always lead to the development of shunt dependency but is a strong predictor of the latter (3,5,6,18).

An example of a severe SAH and an associated hydrocephalus in a patient is presented in Figure 1(A) to 1(D).

Treatment

Dorai et al. reported the need of permanent CSF shunts in 31.1% of patients who demonstrated hydrocephalus at the time of admission (5). The common procedure to treat acute hydrocephalus after SAH is the temporarily placement of an external ventricular drainage (EVD). Some patients improve rapidly in the level of consciousness. During the following period of time, continuous drainage of CSF is necessary and a weaning phase from the device mandatory. Nevertheless, there seems to be no advantage to avoid permanent shunt dependency when compared to rapid, gradual, or multistep EVD weaning (22). The placement of a lumbar drainage is an alternative treatment option in patients with a communicating hydrocephalus. Lumbar drainage is routinely done before surgery by many surgeons for different reasons. The ventricular system may decrease in size and the ICP decreases with the effect that it makes the brain slack for easy surgical access. Secondly, blood can be removed from the basal subarachnoid spaces more effectively than with an external ventricular drain and may therefore prevent vasospasm by removing spasmogens from the subarachnoid space. Although, the influence of this procedure related to later development of a chronic hydrocephalus after SAH has not been sufficiently analyzed yet, we prefer lumbar drainage whenever possible. One might speculate that continuous lumbar cisternal drainage or repeat lumbar puncture could promote the normalization of the CSF dynamics with the result of avoidance of chronic hydrocephalus.

The intraoperative point of view offers another possibility during aneurysm surgery to prevent persistent hydrocephalus requiring shunt placement. The microsurgical fenestration of the lamina terminalis creates an anterior ventriculostomy that may facilitate CSF dynamics and reduce leptomeningeal inflammation and subarachnoid fibrosis (23). The study by Komotar et al. identified a significantly lower rate of shunting in patients who underwent fenestration of the lamina terminalis. The procedure reduced both the overall shunt rate and the rate of conversion from acute hydrocephalus on admission to shunt-dependent hydrocephalus by more than 80% compared to a control group (7).

Bleeding from posterior circulation aneurysms appears to induce a considerably higher rate of chronic hydrocephalus (5,17,19,20). Although, other reports found a positive correlation of ruptured AComA aneurysms and shunt dependency (24). An example of a SAH due to rupture of an AComA aneurysm and a hydrocephalus with shunt dependency in a patient is presented in Figure 1(A) to 1(D). In summary, diffuse and thick layering of subarachnoid blood or blood located strategically in the CSF pathway, such as in the ventricle or near the fourth-ventricular outlet, is more likely to result in hydrocephalus (17).

The surgical approach to ruptured cerebral aneurysms offers the possibility to evacuate blood from the subarachnoid space. One could therefore argue that patients who receive early endovascular treatment for ruptured aneurysms are at greater risk for suffering from chronic hydrocephalus than are those who undergo early aneurysm surgery (24). However, different studies found no evidence for a higher incidence of shunt-dependent hydrocephalus after endovascular treatment of ruptured aneurysms compared to surgery (2,24,25).

The occurrence of chronic hydrocephalus is variable in time. However, definitive ventriculoperitoneal (VP) shunt insertion is performed at a mean interval after SAH of 40 days (2,15,24). Other authors stated that the time span of chronic hydrocephalus seems to be within a six-month period after SAH (1). The gold standard of the treatment of persistent hydrocephalus after SAH is VP shunting. The efficacy of lumboperitoneal shunts after SAH has been proven less successful (26).

POSTTRAUMATIC HYDROCEPHLUS

Incidence

Posttraumatic hydrocephalus is a frequent complication after severe head injury. Still, there are difficulties to differentiate between posttraumatic ventricular dilation, in which the underlying process is brain atrophy, and true hydrocephalus with a cerebrospinal fluid absorptive deficit (27). The incidence of hydrocephalus and ventricular enlargement after head injury varies from 0.7% to 72% (28,29). This high variation may be a result of the definition of diagnostic criteria in head injury.

Diagnostic Criteria

Delayed ventricular enlargement is well recognized after head injury. Kishore et al. performed computerized tomography in 100 consecutive patients after traumatic head injury (30). Ventricular enlargement was present in 29 patients. Clinical outcome was significantly worse in these patients. Only four patients met their CT criteria for hydrocephalus. These included the presence of "distended" appearance of the anterior horns of the lateral ventricles, enlargement of the temporal horns and third ventricle, and abnormal or absent sulci. Additionally, they mentioned the enlargement of the basal cisterns and fourth ventricle. In accordance to Mori et al., periventricular decreased density was confirmed as communicating hydrocephalus (31). Gudeman et al. reported a total of 61 of 200 patients with posttraumatic ventricular dilation (32). Nearly 90% of them showed this by 90 days postinjury. Eleven of them were evaluated for hydrocephalus criteria. These patients underwent radionuclide cisternography. Evidence of communicating hydrocephalus was confirmed when ventricular filling with the radionuclide was delayed or absent. Three patients had abnormal studies and underwent shunting. In comparison to a group of 79 patients without dilation of the ventricles on admission, the patients with ventricular enlargement demonstrated a significantly worse outcome.

The issue whether posttraumatic ventriculomegaly means hydrocephalus or atrophy was discussed by Marmarou and coworkers (27). They analyzed cerebrospinal fluid dynamics in comparison to the changes in ventricular size and Glasgow Outcome Scale (GOS) score at 3, 6, and 12 months posttrauma in patients with severe head injury (GCS $\leq$ 8 on admission). CSF dynamics were studied by using the bolus injection technique measuring the baseline intracranial pressure (ICP), pressure volume index, and resistance for CSF absorption (R0) (33,34). The study demonstrated that approximately 45% of patients with posttraumatic ventriculomegaly have CSF dynamic changes characteristic of hydrocephalus, and these patients have the worst outcome among survivors of head injury. The authors suggested a scheme for the diagnosis of posttraumatic hydrocephalus presented in Table 1. They recommended the testing after one month posttrauma or earlier if deterioration of neurological symptoms occurs. A posttraumatic hydrocephalus after a severe head injury (GCS 5) in a patient is demonstrated in Figure 2(A) to 2(C).

Another method introduced by Yoshihara et al. to differentiate ventricular dilation secondary to brain atrophy and NPH involves the measurement of intracranial and ventricular CSF volume with 3D FASE (Fast Asymmetric Spine-Echo) MR imaging sequence with region growing method (35). The researchers included 21 patients with enlarged ventricles in the study. Eleven of them presented clinically as normal-pressure hydrocephalus (NPH) (shunted group), and the remaining 10 patients were considered to have cerebral atrophy (nonshunted group). Ventricular/intracranial CSF volume ratio was also calculated. Ten out of 11 patients improved in clinical symptoms and/or dementia scale after shunting. Their results indicated that the ventricular volume in the shunted group was enlarged and the ventricular/intracranial CSF ratio was significantly higher. The authors concluded that enlarged ventricles with high ventricular/intracranial CSF volume ratio strongly suggested NPH.

Table 1 Scheme for the Diagnosis of Posttraumatic Hydrocephalus According to Marmarou et al. (27)

Measurements	Proposal
Frontal horn index on CT scan, index >0.3	CSF dynamic studies required via lumbar puncture
Lumbar pressure $\geq$15 mm Hg, independent of R0	High-pressure hydrocephalus, shunt placement is recommended
Lumbar pressure <15 mm Hg, R0 $\geq$ 6.0 mm Hg/mL/min	Normal-pressure hydrocephalus, shunt placement is recommended
Normal pressure and R0	Posttraumatic ventriculomegaly secondary to an atrophic process, benefit from shunt placement unlikely

Abbreviation: R0, resistance for CSF absorption.

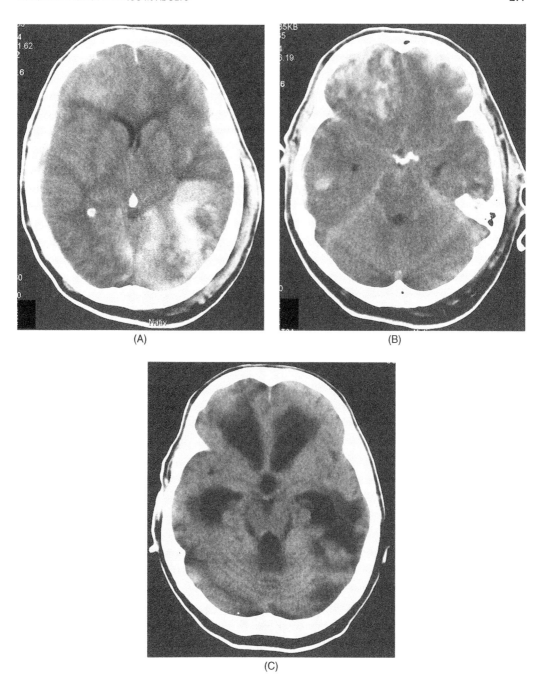

(A)

(B)

(C)

Figure 2 (A) and (B): CT scan of a 09-year-old male demonstrating a severe head injury with multiple contusions and traumatic subarachnoid hemorrhage. At the time of admission, the patient was comatose with a Glasgow coma scale of 5. The patient was treated conservatively under ICP monitoring. The patient was discharged for rehabilitation in a vegetative state. (C) The follow-up CT scan one month after head injury revealed a marked posttraumatic hydrocephalus.

Treatment

The treatment of choice in patients with posttraumatic hydrocephalus is shunting. Tribl and Oder reported the incidence of posttraumatic hydrocephalus requiring shunt implantation from 1% to 8% (36). In their own retrospective series of 3426 patients with severe head injury, 48 (1.4%) patients underwent ventricular shunting because of posttraumatic hydrocephalus. The best predictive parameter for outcome after shunt placement was a preoperative GOS score of 3. Within the first three months after shunt placement, six patients improved from GOS 3 to 2, six patients improved from GOS 4 to 3, and further 13 patients of GOS 3 clearly improved, but did not enter GOS 2. Patient's age at injury did not seem to influence the outcome.

True posttraumatic hydrocephalus is frequently seen after severe head injury. Besides the previously discussed features, a higher risk of developing posttraumatic hydrocephalus is additionally related to subarachnoid or intraventricular hemorrhage on the admission CT scan (27,28,37).

TUMOR-RELATED HYDROCEPHALUS

Tumors obstructing the CSF pathways are a common cause of hydrocephalus. Management strategies are discussed controversially depending on tumor location and clinical presentation. One should distinguish tumors that arise within the ventricles or have tumor extension into the ventricles from tumors that compress the ventricles (extraventricular tumors).

Hydrocephalus Related to Intra- and Paraventricular Tumors

Incidence

Intraventricular tumors are rare. Approximately one-third of tumors arise in the third ventricle or are predominantly parenchymal with extension into it. In adults, colloid cysts, central neurocytomas, subependymomas, astrocytomas, tumors of the pineal region, and metastatic carcinomas are frequently seen (38). Suprasellar lesions such as pituitary macroadenomas, craniopharyngiomas, or arachnoid cysts may extend into the third ventricle.

Whereas tumors of the anterior part of the third ventricle frequently become symptomatic because of an occlusion of the foramen of Monro with a resulting uni- or bilateral hydrocephalus, posterior third ventricular lesion might occlude the aqueduct and a triventricular hydrocephalus develops. Colloid cysts represent the most common lesions of the third ventricle and will be discussed extensively in chapter 14.

Clinical Presentation

Clinical presentation of patients with an acquired tumor-related hydrocephalus of intraventricular origin regularly demonstrates a history of headache followed by intermittent nausea and vomiting. There might be a periodic occlusion of the CSF pathways when symptomatic intervals occur. In most of the cases, microsurgical or neuroendoscopic tumor removal relieves hydrocephalic symptoms (39). However, the surgical approach depends on different clinical and diagnostic features. An immediate management is necessary in cases of acute hydrocephalus.

Hydrocephalus related to intraventricular lesions rarely becomes acutely symptomatic. Planning of surgical management is dependent on tumor size and location. Once the decision to treat the hydrocephalus is made, options include EVD; placement of permanent shunts; internal CSF diversion by ETV, aqueductal stenting, or ventriculocisternal shunting (Torkildsen's procedure); and urgent tumor resection in which CSF is not diverted (40).

Neuroendoscopic Treatment

Neuroendoscopy offers the opportunity to combine techniques to treat hydrocephalus, get a tumor biopsy, or make a complete tumor removal if possible. If a biopsy has to be taken, we prefer to perform neuroendoscopic exploration to obtain biopsy samples under direct view of the field, especially for pineal tumors as presented in Figure 3(A) to 3(C). Any obstruction of CSF pathways that accompanies a lesion can easily be resolved by third ventriculostomy or by stenting the aqueduct using the same approach (41). Limiting factors concerning tumor removal are size and consistency. In general, a solid tumor exceeding 2 cm in diameter might unnecessary prolong the time of endoscopic tumor removal and microsurgery should be preferred. However,

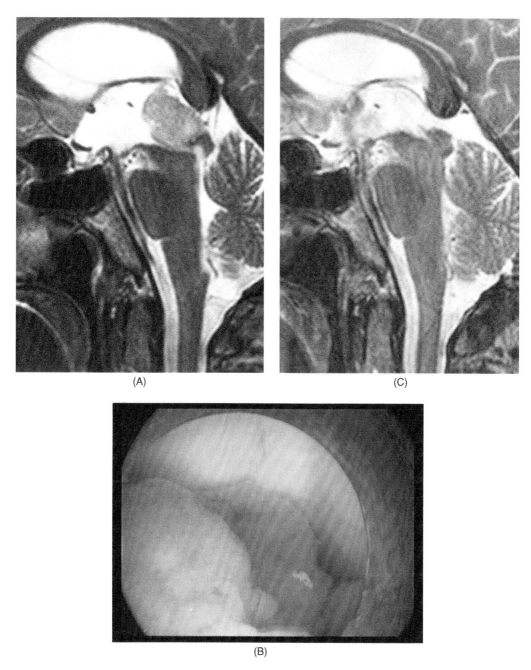

(A)

(C)

(B)

Figure 3 (**A**) A 49-year-old male patient with a tumor of the pineal region and associated hydrocephalus (T2 weighted MR image). The patient became symptomatic with nausea and vomiting. The first step of therapy included ETV and tumor biopsy. (**B**) Endoscopic view on the tumor is presented. Histopathological examination revealed a neurocytoma WHO Grade I. After a short interval, microsurgical tumor removal was performed via a supracerebellar infratentorial approach. (**C**) T2-weighted MR imaging three months after surgery demonstrated complete tumor removal, a patent stoma at the floor of the third ventricle with CSF flow through, and relief of the hydrocephalus.

soft and cystic tumors can be approached endoscopically even if they are larger. In surgery for small intraventricular tumors, we usually start with an endoscopic procedure and switch to microsurgery when necessary. Although, the endoscopic technique is safe and effective in experienced hands, one has to be aware of intraoperative complications that might occur. A huge tumor reduces ventricular size and makes the approach more difficult. Surrounding anatomical structures must be carefully visualized to avoid traumatic injuries to the thalamus or fornix.

Another point worth stressing is precise guidance of neuroendoscopic maneuvres. Especially, lesions that are not approached via a standard precoronal burr hole such as colloid cyst or tumors of the septum pellucidum are candidates for neuronavigation. Additionally, neuronavigation is very useful in approaching intraventricular lesions located in narrow ventricles.

The success rate of endoscopic procedures for obstructive hydrocephalus because of intraventricular tumors as reported by many authors is promising. Gaab and Schroeder reported a series of 30 patients with intraventricular lesions in whom 22 patients revealed an associated hydrocephalus (41). The procedures performed, included septostomies, stent implantations, ETVs, and tumor/cyst removal or resection. The symptoms related to increased pressure resolved in all patients, and all implanted stents remained in place. All third ventriculostomies were patent. In conclusion, no shunt implantation was required.

As reported by MacArthur et al., neuroendoscopic third ventriculostomy in managing brain tumor–associated hydrocephalus is a reliable tool for both short-term and long-term success (42). In their series, ETV was successful in relieving hydrocephalus in the short term in 63/66 (95%) cases and in the longer term in 55/66 (83%) cases.

Hydrocephalus Related to Infratentorial Tumors

Management Strategies
Patients with infratentorial brain tumors often develop hydrocephalus. There is still much controversy on how to manage obstructive hydrocephalus under these circumstances. In several patients, removal of the obstructing tumor restores CSF pathway without further treatment. Difficulties exist in some cases to differentiate between symptoms related to the tumor or hydrocephalus. Moreover, life-threatening complications may result from obstruction of CSF circulation. Therefore, in the past, some authors preferred a preoperative placement of a CSF shunt as most advantageous prior to surgical tumor removal (43,44). However, only a small number of patients suffer from a persistent hydrocephalus after tumor removal. Therefore, we do not advocate preoperative shunting. Shunts are prone to overdrainage with a potential risk of tentorial herniation, when pressure rises within the posterior fossa. Furthermore, shunts frequently become infected or malfunction. The risk of metastasis from shunting in adults is very rare and more common in children (45–47). Other neurosurgeons recommend pre-, peri-, or postoperative EVD to control hydrocephalus after tumor resection (48–51). The procedure is easily done via a frontal or occipital burr hole. The drain can be removed shortly after tumor removal. Prolonged external CSF diversion should be avoided due to the risk of either further shunt dependency or CNS infection. The implantation of an EVD is a reliable technique but has its disadvantages.

Endoscopic Third Ventriculostomy
A third alternative approach is endoscopic third ventriculostomy (ETV). This technique has become a widely accepted treatment option for obstructive hydrocephalus secondary to posterior fossa lesions with less complications (52–58). In most cases, the technique can be performed in the standard fashion. The perforation of the floor of the third ventricle has to be made just behind the clivus, halfway between the infundibular recess, and the mammillary bodies in the midline. Sometimes the interpeduncular cistern may be distorted or narrowed because of the elevation of the brainstem and compression of the brainstem in clival direction. Therefore, planning of ETV with MR images is preferred. However, in emergency situations, a CT scan is sufficient to localize the basilar artery and brainstem.

Our therapeutic strategy depends on the clinical presentation of the patient. If the hydrocephalus is symptomatic, we recommend to perform ETV first with further tumor removal. In our experience, ETV resolves hydrocephalus reliably prior to tumor surgery with often dramatic clinical improvement. In patients without clinical symptoms or mild hydrocephalus, only tumor removal is indicated. If hydrocephalus persists after tumor removal, ETV is promising when CSF outflow is compromised. ETV can be also performed as a palliative procedure in patients with inoperable intracranial lesions and associated hydrocephalus. If possible a tumor biopsy is taken simultaneously. After getting the histological diagnosis, radiotherapy and/or chemotherapy is initiated if considered to be indicated.

In our opinion, the neuroendoscopic techniques are advantageous compared to shunt implantation or external drainage. The risk of ventriculitis or meningitis can be minimized by ETV compared to the higher rate of infections caused by prolonged ventricular drainage or shunting (52,54,59–62).

CONCLUSION

Hydrocephalus after subarachnoid hemorrhage and posttraumatic hydrocephalus are indications for ventriculoperitoneal shunting. A real posttraumatic hydrocephalus has to be differentiated from ventricular dilation after head injury. This is sometimes difficult and requires ICP measurement as well as diagnostic testing of the CSF absorptive capacity. In tumor-related hydrocephalus, tumor removal is the best option to treat the hydrocephalus. If a tumor removal is not possible, neuroendoscopic techniques can restore the CSF circulation.

REFERENCES

1. Vale FL, Bradley EL, Fisher WS III. The relationship of subarachnoid hemorrhage and the need for postoperative shunting. J Neurosurg 1997; 86:462–466.
2. Dehdashti AR, Rilliet B, Rufenacht DA, et al. Shunt-dependent hydrocephalus after rupture of intracranial aneurysms: A prospective study of the influence of treatment modality. J Neurosurg 2004; 101:402–407.
3. Sheehan JP, Polin RS, Sheehan JM, et al. Factors associated with hydrocephalus after aneurysmal subarachnoid hemorrhage. Neurosurgery 1999; 45:1120–1127.
4. Black PM. Hydrocephalus and vasospasm after subarachnoid hemorrhage from ruptured intracranial aneurysms. Neurosurgery 1986; 18:12–16.
5. Dorai Z, Hynan LS, Kopitnik TA, et al. Factors related to hydrocephalus after aneurysmal subarachnoid hemorrhage. Neurosurgery 2003; 52:763–769.
6. Yoshioka H, Inagawa T, Tokuda Y, et al. Chronic hydrocephalus in elderly patients following subarachnoid hemorrhage. Surg Neurol 2000; 53:119–124.
7. Komotar RJ, Olivi A, Rigamonti D, et al. Microsurgical fenestration of the lamina terminalis reduces the incidence of shunt-dependent hydrocephalus after aneurysmal subarachnoid hemorrhage. Neurosurgery 2002; 51:1403–1412.
8. Milhorat TH. Acute hydrocephalus after aneurysmal subarachnoid hemorrhage. Neurosurgery 1987; 20:15–20.
9. Black PM, Tzouras A, Foley L. Cerebrospinal fluid dynamics and hydrocephalus after experimental subarachnoid hemorrhage. Neurosurgery 1985; 17:57–62.
10. Gjerris F, Borgesen SE, Sorensen PS, et al. Resistance to cerebrospinal fluid outflow and intracranial pressure in patients with hydrocephalus after subarachnoid haemorrhage. Acta Neurochir (Wien) 1987; 88:79–86.
11. Blasberg R, Johnson D, Fenstermacher J. Absorption resistance of cerebrospinal fluid after subarachnoid hemorrhage in the monkey; effects of heparin. Neurosurgery 1981; 9:686–691.
12. Kosteljanetz M. CSF dynamics in patients with subarachnoid and/or intraventricular hemorrhage. J Neurosurg 1984; 60:940–946.
13. Fuhrmeister U, Ruether P, Dommatsch D. Alterations of CSF Hydrodynamics Following Meningitis and Subarachnoid Hemorrhage. Intracranial Pressure IV. Berlin, Germany: Springer Verlag, 1980:241–244.
14. Marmarou A, Maset AL, Ward JD, et al. Contribution of CSF and vascular factors to elevation of ICP in severely head-injured patients. J Neurosurg 1987; 66:883–890.
15. Hirashima Y, Hamada H, Hayashi N, et al. Independent predictors of late hydrocephalus in patients with aneurysmal subarachnoid hemorrhage—Analysis by multivariate logistic regression model. Cerebrovasc Dis 2003; 16:205–210.
16. Ellington E, Margolis G. Block of arachnoid villus by subarachnoid hemorrhage. J Neurosurg 1969; 30:651–657.
17. Graff-Radford NR, Torner J, Adams HP Jr, et al. Factors associated with hydrocephalus after subarachnoid hemorrhage. A Report of the Cooperative Aneurysm Study. Arch Neurol 1989; 46:744–752.

18. Vermeij FH, Hasan D, Vermeulen M, et al. Predictive factors for deterioration from hydrocephalus after subarachnoid hemorrhage. Neurology 1994; 44:1851–1855.

19. Tapaninaho A, Hernesniemi J, Vapalahti M, et al. Shunt-dependent hydrocephalus after subarachnoid haemorrhage and aneurysm surgery: Timing of surgery is not a risk factor. Acta Neurochir (Wien) 1993; 123:118–124.

20. Pietila TA, Heimberger KC, Palleske H, et al. Influence of aneurysm location on the development of chronic hydrocephalus following SAH. Acta Neurochir (Wien) 1995; 137:70–73.

21. Wenig C, Huber G, Emde H. Hydrocephalus after subarachnoid bleeding. A correlation of clinical findings, the results of radioisotope Cisternography and computer-assisted tomography. Eur Neurol 1979; 18:1–7.

22. Klopfenstein JD, Kim LJ, Feiz-Erfan I, et al. Comparison of rapid and gradual weaning from external ventricular drainage in patients with aneurysmal subarachnoid hemorrhage: A prospective randomized trial. J Neurosurg 2004; 100:225–229.

23. Tomasello F, d'Avella D, de Divitiis O. Does lamina terminalis fenestration reduce the incidence of chronic hydrocephalus after subarachnoid hemorrhage? Neurosurgery 1999; 45: 827–831.

24. Gruber A, Reinprecht A, Bavinzski G, et al. Chronic shunt-dependent hydrocephalus after early surgical and early endovascular treatment of ruptured intracranial aneurysms. Neurosurgery 1999; 44:503–509.

25. Sethi H, Moore A, Dervin J, et al. Hydrocephalus: Comparison of clipping and embolization in aneurysm treatment. J Neurosurg 2000; 92:991–994.

26. Kang S. Efficacy of lumbo-peritoneal versus ventriculo-peritoneal shunting for management of chronic hydrocephalus following aneurysmal subarachnoid haemorrhage. Acta Neurochir (Wien) 2000; 142:45–49.

27. Marmarou A, Foda MA, Bandoh K, et al. Posttraumatic ventriculomegaly: Hydrocephalus or atrophy? A new approach for diagnosis using CSF dynamics. J Neurosurg 1996; 85:1026–1035.

28. Cardoso ER, Galbraith S. Posttraumatic hydrocephalus—A retrospective review. Surg Neurol 1985; 23:261–264.

29. Levin HS, Meyers CA, Grossman RG, et al. Ventricular enlargement after closed head injury. Arch Neurol 1981; 38:623–629.

30. Kishore PR, Lipper MH, Miller JD, et al. Post-traumatic hydrocephalus in patients with severe head injury. Neuroradiology 1978; 16:261–265.

31. Mori K, Murata T, Nakano Y, et al. Periventricular lucency in hydrocephalus on computerized tomography. Surg Neurol 1977; 8:337–340.

32. Gudeman SK, Kishore PR, Becker DP, et al. Computed tomography in the evaluation of incidence and significance of post-traumatic hydrocephalus. Radiology 1981; 141:397–402.

33. Marmarou A, Shulman K, LaMorgese J. Compartmental analysis of compliance and outflow resistance of the cerebrospinal fluid system. J Neurosurg 1975; 43:523–534.

34. Marmarou A, Shulman K, Rosende RM. A nonlinear analysis of the cerebrospinal fluid system and intracranial pressure dynamics. J Neurosurg 1978; 48:332–344.

35. Yoshihara M, Tsunoda A, Sato K, et al. Differential diagnosis of NPH and brain atrophy assessed by measurement of intracranial and ventricular CSF volume with 3D FASE MRI. Acta Neurochir Suppl 1998; 71:371–374.

36. Tribl G, Oder W. Outcome after shunt implantation in severe head injury with post-traumatic hydrocephalus. Brain Inj 2000; 14:345–354.

37. Beyerl B, Black PM. Posttraumatic hydrocephalus. Neurosurgery 1984; 15:257–261.

38. Pietila TA, Berweiler U, Brock M. Tumors of the third ventricle and pineal region. In: Moskopp D, Wassmann H, eds. Neurochirurgie. Stuttgart, New York: Schattauer, 2005:454–460.

39. Bruce JN. Posterior third ventricular tumors. In: Kaye AH, Black PM, eds. Operative Neurosurgery. London, Edinburgh, New York, Philadelphia, St. Louis, Sidney, Toronto: Churchill Livingstone, 2000:669–775.

40. Teo C, Young R. Endoscopic management of hydrocephalus secondary to tumors of the posterior third ventricle. Neurosurg Focus 1999; 7:e2.

41. Gaab MR, Schroeder HW. Neuroendoscopic approach to intraventricular lesions. J Neurosurg 1998; 88:496–505.

42. MacArthur DC, Buxton N, Punt J, et al. The role of neuroendoscopy in the management of brain tumours. Br J Neurosurg 2002; 16:465–470.

43. Albright L, Reigel DH. Management of hydrocephalus secondary to posterior fossa tumors. J Neurosurg 1977; 46:52–55.

44. Jamjoom AB, Jamjoom ZA, Ur RN. Low rate of shunt revision in tumoural obstructive hydrocephalus. Acta Neurochir (Wien) 1998; 140:595–597.

45. Jamjoom ZA, Jamjoom AB, Sulaiman AH, et al. Systemic metastasis of medulloblastoma through ventriculoperitoneal shunt: Report of a case and critical analysis of the literature. Surg Neurol 1993; 40:403–410.

46. Berger MS, Baumeister B, Geyer JR, et al. The risks of metastases from shunting in children with primary central nervous system tumors. J Neurosurg 1991; 74:872–877.

47. Kessler LA, Dugan P, Concannon JP. Systemic metastases of medulloblastoma promoted by shunting. Surg Neurol 1975; 3:147–152.

48. Papo I, Caruselli G, Luongo A. External ventricular drainage in the management of posterior fossa tumors in children and adolescents. Neurosurgery 1982; 10:13–15.

49. Rappaport ZH, Shalit MN. Perioperative external ventricular drainage in obstructive hydrocephalus secondary to infratentorial brain tumours. Acta Neurochir (Wien) 1989; 96:118–121.

50. Taylor WA, Todd NV, Leighton SE. CSF drainage in patients with posterior fossa tumours. Acta Neurochir (Wien) 1992; 117:1–6.

51. Schmid UD, Seiler RW. Management of obstructive hydrocephalus secondary to posterior fossa tumors by steroids and subcutaneous ventricular catheter reservoir. J Neurosurg 1986; 65:649–653.

52. Schroeder HW, Niendorf WR, Gaab MR. Complications of endoscopic third ventriculostomy. J Neurosurg 2002; 96:1032–1040.

53. Hopf NJ, Grunert P, Fries G, et al. Endoscopic third ventriculostomy: Outcome analysis of 100 consecutive procedures. Neurosurgery 1999; 44:795–804.

54. Hellwig D, Grotenhuis JA, Tirakotai W, et al. Endoscopic third ventriculostomy for obstructive hydrocephalus. Neurosurg Rev 2005; 28:1–34.

55. Ruggiero C, Cinalli G, Spennato P, et al. Endoscopic third ventriculostomy in the treatment of hydrocephalus in posterior fossa tumors in children. Childs Nerv Syst 2004; 20:828–833.

56. Sainte-Rose C, Cinalli G, Roux FE, et al. Management of hydrocephalus in pediatric patients with posterior fossa tumors: The role of endoscopic third ventriculostomy. J Neurosurg 2001; 95:791–797.

57. Roux FE, Boetto S, Tremoulet M. Third ventriculocisternostomy in cerebellar haematomas. Acta Neurochir (Wien) 2002; 144:337–342.

58. Baldauf J, Oertel J, Gaab MR, et al. Endoscopic third ventriculostomy for occlusive hydrocephalus caused by cerebellar infarction. Neurosurgery 2006; 59:539–544.

59. Beems T, Grotenhuis JA. Long-term complications and definition of failure of neuroendoscopic procedures. Childs Nerv Syst 2004; 20:868–877.

60. Choi JU, Kim DS, Kim SH. Endoscopic surgery for obstructive hydrocephalus. Yonsei Med J 1999; 40:600–607.

61. Holloway KL, Barnes T, Choi S, et al. Ventriculostomy infections: The effect of monitoring duration and catheter exchange in 584 patients. J Neurosurg 1996; 85:419–424.

62. Park P, Garton HJ, Kocan MJ, et al. Risk of infection with prolonged ventricular catheterization. Neurosurgery 2004; 55:594–599.

16 | Idiopathic Normal Pressure Hydrocephalus

Rachid Bech-Azeddine and Flemming Gjerris

University Clinic of Neurosurgery, Neuroscience Centre, Rigshospitalet, Capital Region, Copenhagen, Denmark

HISTORY AND EPONYMS

Normal pressure hydrocephalus (NPH) was introduced as a treatable clinical entity by Hakim and Adams in 1965 (1). They described a syndrome consisting of gait disturbance, urinary incontinence, dementia, normal intracranial pressure (ICP), and ventriculomegaly on radiological examination. The symptoms improved after shunt operation, and notably the recognition of a "reversible" form of dementia brought great attention to NPH. Subsequently, patients fulfilling the description were enthusiastically shunted. However, less-encouraging shunt results ensued, and research into the selection of shunt responsive patients and understanding the underlying pathophysiology has been ongoing since.

To underline the apparent lack of an inciting event causing the hydrocephalus, the term *idiopathic* NPH (INPH) has become widely accepted, as opposed to secondary NPH, which is precipitated by disorders known to compromise the CSF absorption, such as subarachnoid hemorrhage, meningitis, head injury, and intracranial surgery. However, no final consensus on the name exists, and several eponyms are used: adult hydrocephalus syndrome, chronic adult hydrocephalus, hydrocephalic dementia, communicating hydrocephalus, low-pressure hydrocephalus, and occult hydrocephalus. We have preferred to stick to INPH in the present chapter, although we acknowledge, that the name is misleading, as the intracranial pressure conditions are not truly normal.

Some authors advocate using the term INPH only for the patients improving after shunting—and applying the term INPH *syndrome* for the patients not improving by shunt surgery despite fulfilling the diagnostic criteria (2).

Only recently have standardized guidelines of the clinical management of INPH been elaborated and published by an international independent study group, based on an extensive evidence-based literature review and expert opinion. The guidelines address the diagnosis of INPH (3), the value of supplemental tests (4), the surgical management (5), and the postoperative outcome assessment (6). It is striking that despite 40 years of ongoing research after the initial description of INPH, the recommendations presented only amount to "options" or "guidelines" but not "standards" (7), due to the lack of class I and class II evidence.

DEFINITION

INPH is classically described as a clinical triad of progressing gait disturbance, cognitive deficit, and urinary disturbance. Hydrocephalus is evidenced by computed tomography (CT) or magnetic resonance imaging (MRI). A state of cerebrospinal fluid (CSF) dynamic disequilibrium is presumed and the ventriculomegaly is demonstrated by an Evans index ≥ 0.3 (8).

The ICP is considered normal; however, INPH possibly begins with a transient increased pressure with subsequent ventricular enlargement. With further enlargement of the ventricles, CSF pressure decreases, but averages slightly higher than normal (9). Consequently, an ICP no higher than 18 mm Hg is usually recommended for the diagnosis of INPH (3).

The clinical picture may vary considerably, partly due to the increased age of the patients and the consequently high frequency of comorbidity. The cardinal symptom is the gait impairment, which may present alone. As the onset is insidious, the symptoms should be presented for at least three months at the time of diagnosis. It is imperative for the definition of INPH, that there is no known triggering event of the hydrocephalus, including any structural abnormalities such as aqueductal stenosis.

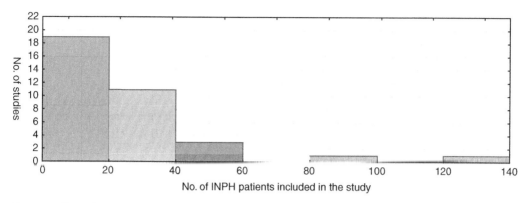

Figure 1 Thirty-five clinical studies of shunted INPH patients subgrouped according to the included patient number. Calculation based on data from review by Hebb and Cusimano (2001).

EPIDEMIOLOGY

INPH is a disease of the elderly people, and usually presents in the sixth or seventh decade (10). The exact incidence is not known, but recent estimations are around 1.0 to 5.5/100,000 (11–13). In a population of residents of assisted-living and extended-care facilities, an estimated incidence of INPH ranging from 9% to 14%, depending on the diagnostic criteria, has been reported (14). Because of increased longevity and the greater awareness of INPH, the incidence is presumed to increase in the following years.

Obtaining a patient material sufficiently extensive to ascertain significant relations has posed a substantial problem in the ongoing clinical INPH research. A meta-analysis from 2001 was restricted, according to well-defined predetermined criteria, to 35 independent studies of shunted INPH patients out of 535 hits on Medline. A low mean value of 25 patients per study was revealed (Fig. 1) (15). Only recently have larger series of 101 to 151 shunted patients been published (16–18).

PATHOGENESIS AND PATHOPHYSIOLOGY

INPH is generally perceived as caused by a complex heterogeneous etiology, and with no obvious and constant underlying pathology.

The perception of the pathophysiology of INPH has over the years gradually shifted from a pure mechanical view of a CSF malabsorption being the main cause, as in secondary NPH, to a more sophisticated view encompassing several factors involved in the pathophysiology (19). However, evidence is still elusive of the exact pathophysiological mechanisms in INPH.

Complete or incomplete obstruction in any place of the CSF pathways causes at least a temporary increase in ICP followed by ventricular enlargement. The CSF production in INPH may be reduced (20), but results are contradictory (9). A compromised CSF absorption surely plays a role, although it is no longer thought to be the only hallmark of INPH. Meningeal fibrosis as a cause of defect CSF absorption over the convexities has not been proven by biopsy studies (19). CSF vasopressin probably regulates some absorptive mechanism of intracranial water, and a linear correlation between ICP and concentration of CSF vasopressin has been found (21).

Cerebrovascular disease (CVD) is often implicated: it is speculated that ischemia in the deep white matter reduces the tensile strength and elasticity, facilitating the enlargement of the ventricles, especially in the case of a concomitant presence of a decreased CSF absorption. The involvement of CVD in INPH is favored by clinical (22) autopsy (23), biopsy (24), and MRI findings (25) of CVD in patients with INPH, including those improving after surgery. However, it is unclear, whether the periventricular degenerative findings are to be perceived as primary or secondary to the progression of INPH, and to which degree a CSF malabsorption is a prerequisite for the progression of INPH.

A marked coexistence of Alzheimer's disease (AD) has likewise been reported in INPH patients, based on cerebral biopsy findings (24,26,27) and clinical findings (28).

Thus, INPH may very well share pathophysiological elements with both CVD and AD. With CVD, more specifically subcortical arteriosclerotic encephalopathy, the pathophysiological overlap could be increasing white matter microangiopathy (29). With AD, it could be CSF stasis resulting in reduced clearance of potentially neurotoxic macromolecules (30). Supporting this view, studies have also indicated that vascular dementia and AD share common risk factors, possibly also reflecting common pathogenic pathways (31).

In recognition of the possible multifaceted etiology, it has even been proposed to perform shunt surgery on patient diagnosed with only subcortical arteriosclerotic encephalopathy (29), and shunt insertion in AD patients not suspected of INPH has been reported to show a trend towards improvement of the cognitive deficits (32). This aspect, obviously, only renders the selection of shunt responsive INPH patients even more difficult.

Other suggested factors implicated in the pathophysiology of INPH are impaired cerebral autoregulation (33), decreased cerebral blood flow (34), and increased superficial venous pressure (35).

CSF Dynamics

As INPH basically has been perceived as caused by an impairment of the CSF absorption, the initial research focused on demonstrating disturbed CSF dynamics assessing the CSF absorption and CSF pressure–volume relations by measuring the so-called resistance to the CSF outflow (R_{out}), intracranial compliance, and B-waves (36).

Whether impairment of these parameters is a prerequisite for the development of INPH is still unclear. In general, however, a decreased intracranial compliance, an increased R_{out} and a high percentage of B-waves are believed to be typical findings of disturbed CSF dynamics in INPH.

Resistance to CSF Outflow, R_{out}

Although the sites of CSF absorption in man and their relative contribution are not fully elucidated, measuring R_{out}, that is, the converse of conductance, gives an estimation of the total CSF absorptive capacity of the system.

R_{out} can be measured by bolus, infusion, or perfusion techniques, based on analogous principles of injecting, infusing, or perfusing artificial CSF into the ventricles or the lumbar subarachnoid space, at either a constant rate or a constant pressure (10). Common to the methods is the attainment of a correlation line, the slope of which is an expression of the conductance to CSF outflow, and the reciprocal value the resistance to CSF outflow, R_{out}.

Importantly, when comparing R_{out} from different studies, values obtained by the bolus injection technique are lower compared to R_{out} values obtained by the infusion technique.

Normal values of R_{out}

At which cut-off value R_{out} is to be considered pathological in a hydrocephalic patient is debated.

R_{out} values below 12 mm Hg/mL/min are generally considered to be normal (Table 1) based on studies of patients initially suspected of CSF disturbances (37–39), young healthy volunteers (40), and patients with spinal diseases (41).

Furthermore, R_{out} increases with age, approximating 0.075 mm Hg/mL/min per year, in patients with no known CSF disorders (Fig. 2) (41). In hydrocephalic patients aged $\geq$ 56 years and presenting R_{out} values above 12 mm Hg/mL/min, an even stronger correlation between

Table 1   Normal R_{out} Values (mm Hg/mL/min)

References	Materials	R_{out}
(38)	Patients	<8.33
(39)	Patients	<10.00
(37)	Patients	<12.00
(40)	Normal individuals	<9.10
(41)	Patients (spinal diseases)	<10.00

Source: From Ref. 10.

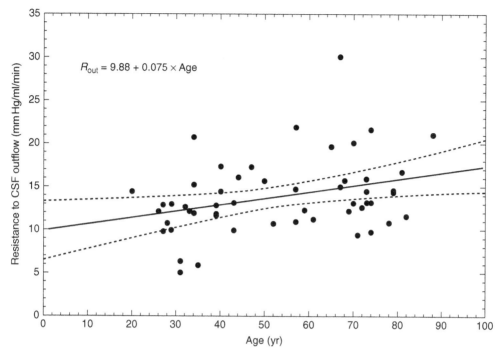

Figure 2 Resistance to CSF outflow, R_{out}, versus age in a cohort of non-hydrocephalic adults with spinal disorders. R_{out} increases with increasing age. *Source*: From Ref. 41.

R_{out} and age, 0.19 mm Hg/mL/min per year, has been demonstrated (42). Accordingly, R_{out} values can be expected to be at least 5 mm Hg/mL/min higher in a patient in the eighth decade compared to a younger patient.

B-waves
B-waves are slow rhythmic oscillations in the ICP. They were originally described by Lundberg in 1960 and are defined as periods of 0.5 to 2 minutes with amplitudes ranging from discernible levels to 50 mm Hg (43).

It is commonly agreed that B-waves are associated to oscillations of the cerebral blood volume (44), probably secondary to cerebral vasomotor waves and representing the autoregulatory response to fluctuations of the cerebral perfusion pressure (45).

In patients evaluated for INPH, a high time percentage of B-waves are generally perceived as a sign of disturbed CSF dynamics, although no consensus exists concerning to which degree the B-wave activity should be increased. Accordingly, various cut-off levels of the time percentage of B-waves, ranging from $\geq 50\%$ (37) to $\geq 10\%$ (46) and $\geq 5\%$, have been advocated as predictors of shunt improvement.

Some studies strongly suggest that the morphology of the B-waves or increased mean intracranial pulse pressure amplitudes are predictive for the outcome of shunt operation (47,48).

SYMPTOMS AND SIGNS
The insidious onset of gait disturbances, cognitive impairment, and/or urinary incontinence should prompt for a suspicion of INPH. The predominant part of the symptoms should be unexplained by other disorders, as a variety of diseases of the elderly people may mimic one or several of the INPH triad symptoms (Table 2). Headache, nausea, seizures, and speech impairment are uncommonly seen. Often, coexisting disorders with symptoms superimposed on the INPH symptoms are the case (49).

Most centers so far agree upon that gait disturbance should be present with or without cognitive deficits. The incontinence, if present, often may be attributed to other common disorders (3). The reported frequency of the triad symptoms is influenced by the inclusion criteria

Table 2 Primary Diagnoses After Evaluation of 71 Patients Initially Referred with a
Clinical and Radiological Suspicion of Idiopathic Normal-Pressure Hydrocephalus

Primary diagnosis	Number of patients
Idiopathic normal pressure hydrocephalus	14
Sequelae from stroke	12
Vascular dementia (probable)	4
Congenital stenosis of the mesencephalic aqueduct	3
Epilepsy	3
Vascular dementia (possible)	2
Dementia without specification	2
Depression	2
Alzheimer's disease (possible)	2
Alcoholic brain damage	2
Organic amnestic syndrome (exclusive alcohol)	2
Diffuse traumatic brain injury	2
Spinal stenosis	2
No disorder identified	2
Atypical Alzheimer's disease	1
Arnold-Chiari type 1 malformation	1
Communicating ("arrested") hydrocephalus	1
Transitory cerebral ischemia	1
Occlusion of the vertebral artery	1
Cerebral anoxia	1
Focal traumatic brain injury	1
Posttraumatic brain syndrome	1
Wernicke's encephalopathy	1
Sequelae of viral encephalitis	1
Age related degeneration of the nervous system	1
Lumbar disc prolapse	1
Ataxia	1
Disseminated cancer of the urinary bladder	1
Porphyria	1
Hodgkin's lymphoma	1
Multiple system atrophy	1

Source: From Ref. 49.

of the studies. Accordingly, the frequency of the full clinical triad in shunted series of INPH
patients varies from 50% to 86% (16).

Gait Disturbances and Other Motor Problems
Several descriptive terms are used to characterize the typical gait of INPH patients: shuffling,
magnetic, apraxic, dyspraxic, glue-footed, and bradykinetic. The gait is short stepped, with
increased outward angle and width of the feet (broad based), and reduced step height and
counter rotation of the shoulders (50).

A subcortical motor control impairment is suggested, resulting in a dysfunction of the
executive motor function with increased activity in the antigravity muscles of the legs (51).
The postural function and balance are impaired with a tendency to fall backwards (52), and
difficulties with fine finger movements, tremor, and impairment of handwriting are common.
However, drop attacks or sudden falls without loss of consciousness are uncommon.

Cognitive Symptoms
The mental changes in INPH represent a spectrum from none to severe. A neuropsychological evaluation is important, especially to assess subclinical deficits and improvement of the
cognitive deficits after shunt surgery.

The cognitive impairment is subcortical with disturbed executive functions of the frontal
lobes. Accordingly, the patient may present with inattentiveness, apathy, slowness of thought,
reduced psychomotor speed, and visuospatial and visuoconstructional deficits (53,54). With

progression, the deficits can extend to a more severe and global pattern including both subcortical and cortical deficits.

Psychiatric manifestations such as depression, mania, and psychosis are uncommon but have been reported (3).

Urinary Disturbances

The micturition disturbance consists of a hyperreactive bladder caused by impairment of the supraspinal bladder control (55). The clinical result is an urge incontinence, which can progress into frank incontinence (56). Possibly, a frontal subcortical pathway from cortex to the brainstem, involved in the micturition control, is affected. A "frontal lobe incontinence" where the patient becomes indifferent to the incontinence may develop in the late stages of the disease, suggesting additional impairment of the executive functions. Rarely fecal incontinence is present.

IMAGING INVESTIGATIONS

CT and MRI

CT and MR imaging illustrate the dilated ventricular system, and in some cases an "edematous" periventricular white matter, typically observed at the tip of the frontal and occipital horns (Fig. 3). It is not clearly elucidated, whether these periventricular hypodensities result from a transependymal exudation, a stagnation of the extracellular fluid in the periventricular region, a combination or possibly periventricular gliosis representing the "endstage" (57). In either case, metabolic disturbances due to a defective turnover of the interstitial fluid might be an underlying cause of the clinical symptoms.

Findings further suggestive of INPH are marked enlargement of third ventricle and temporal horns and flattened cortical sulci (58). Importantly, increased size of the cerebral sulci, normally suggesting cerebral atrophy, does not preclude improvement after shunt operation. Focally widened hemispheric sulci, so-called "transport sulci", may normalize following surgery. It has even been suggested that their presence favors the diagnosis of INPH (59).

Advantages of MRI are the possibility of assessing findings further supportive of shunt improvement:

(a) Limited periventricular and deep white matter changes, although the presence does not exclude clinical effect of shunt surgery (25).

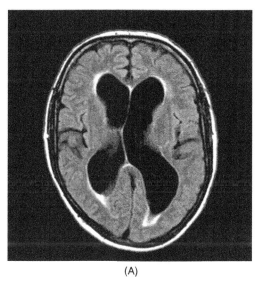 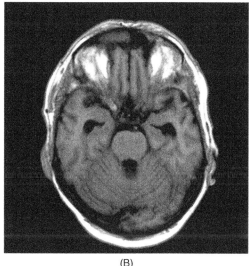

(A)   (B)

Figure 3 MRI demonstrating hydrocephalus in a 65-year-old man, who presented a full INPH clinical triad and improved after shunt operation. Part (**A**) is with flair sequences, showing discrete transudation of CSF at the frontal and occipital horns, and part (**B**) shows dilation of the temporal horns, both factors favoring shunt improvement in INPH.

(b) Thinning of the corpus callosum (18).
(c) No dilatation of perihippocampal fissures, which suggest atrophy from other dementing diseases (60).

Whether increased CSF flow volume in the cerebral aqueduct predicts shunt outcome (61,62) or not (63), remains to be further elucidated.

Functional Brain Imaging Techniques

Radionuclide cisternography, single-photon emission tomography (SPECT), and position emission tomography (PET) are not routinely used in the preoperative evaluation of suspected INPH patients, as none of them are strong predictors of clinical improvement after shunt surgery.

In cisternography, ventricular filling and absence of the radionuclide over the cerebral convexities 24 to 48 hours after application are suggestive of INPH (64); however, correlation with shunt outcome is poor (65).

Findings in SPECT and PET studies suggest a decreased global cerebral blood flow (CBF) compared to normal controls and a decreased regional CBF flow in the periventricular and frontal regions (66–68). Whether an impaired reactivity of the cerebral circulation, as assessed by an acetazolamide test, predicts shunt outcome is still unclear (69).

SUPPLEMENTAL TESTS

No single ancillary test, or combination of clinical and paraclinical findings, can with certainty predict shunt outcome in a patient suspected of INPH. However, increasing the shunt success rate is achievable by employing various supplemental tests. The limitation is mainly the risk of false-negative results, which can deprive a shunt responder from a shunt operation.

Testing of the CSF Dynamics

To which degree the presence of abnormal CSF dynamic parameters prognosticates the outcome of shunt operation is still strongly debated.

Measurement of R_{out} by infusion tests is well established in the preoperative evaluation of patients with INPH (10). An elevated R_{out} seems so far to be one of the most potent single predictors of clinical improvement following shunt surgery (17,37,44).

However, shunt improvement may also be obtained in several cases despite low R_{out} values (16,17), and not all studies have demonstrated a correlation between R_{out} and clinical improvement (2,70).

R_{out} values below 12 mm Hg/mL/min are generally considered normal, whereas R_{out} values above 18 mm Hg/mL/min carry a high positive predictive value (PPV) of 92% of shunt improvement, although the negative predictive value is as low as 34% (17,53). Consequently, R_{out} values between 12 and up to 18 mm Hg/mL/min can be perceived as constituting a gray zone. The decision upon shunt surgery should in such cases be carefully contemplated and primarily judged from the clinical and radiological findings.

Protagonists of the intraventricular assessment and long-term ICP monitoring stress the possibility of estimating B-wave activity and pulse pressure amplitude. We believe it is questionable, whether any significant additional prognostic value is gained by a supplemental intracranial ICP monitoring, if a lumbar infusion test has been performed (71).

CSF Drainage Testing

CSF drainage tests basically mimic the effect of a potentially forthcoming shunt.

CSF Tap Test

With the CSF tap test, 40 to 50 mL of CSF is removed by a single lumbar puncture, and clinical improvement, primarily of the gait impairment, is judged during the next 24 hours (64).

An advantage is the possibility of performing the test in the settings of an outpatient clinic, and the test can be performed right after a lumbar infusion test, during the same lumbar puncture. The PPV is high, up to 100% (72), but the drawback is a low sensitivity, ranging from 26% to 61% (4).

External Lumbar Drainage

With external lumbar drainage (ELD) a continuous drainage of approximately 240 mL of CSF daily is performed via a lumbar catheter for three to five days, and clinical improvement is evaluated. Disadvantages are the necessity of several days of hospitalization and a slight risk of infection (1.3% in the study by Marmarou et al.) (16). The important advantage of ELD is an increased negative predictive value up to 80% (16), thus not depriving to many potentially shunt responders from shunt surgery, if positive outcome of the test is used as a shunt criterion.

Cerebral Biopsy Sampling

Brain biopsies of patients shunted for INPH have shown a high frequency of vascular changes or degenerative disorders in up to 50% of the cases, most often Alzheimer's disease (26). However, cerebral biopsies are of no prognostic value concerning shunt outcome, as patients may improve despite pathological cerebral parenchymal findings (24). Consequently, routine biopsy sampling is not warranted, if at all considered ethically acceptable. However, cerebral biopsies demonstrating a coexistence of a progressive cerebral disorder, most often AD or CVD, may in some cases explain absence of or only short-term cognitive improvement after shunt surgery.

In the future, it is very likely that plain CSF sampling with analysis of CSF biomarkers will play a more important role in the diagnosis and distinction of INPH from CVD and AD (73).

DIAGNOSTIC WORK UP

No combination of clinical and radiological findings and supplementary tests can yet with certainty predict who will benefit from shunt operation. Thus, the main aim of a proficient diagnostic work up is to select the patients with the highest probability of shunt improvement without applying too rigorous criteria depriving shunt responders from shunt operation.

The suspicion of INPH is frequently raised based on initially clinical and/or radiological findings. However, a multiplicity of disorders from the fields of neurology, neurosurgery, psychiatry, and internal medicine may confound, mimic, or overlap with the triad symptoms of INPH (49). The diagnosis of INPH can in most cases not be upheld after a thorough and systematic assessment by an experienced and multidisciplinary team (Fig. 4). In our own series, outpatient evaluation involving a neurologist, a neurosurgeon, a neuropsychologist, and in most cases also a psychiatrist, disproved a shunt responsive symptomatology in over half of the patients referred under the suspicion of INPH. The remaining underwent ICP monitoring and CSF infusion test. Eventually, only 20% of the referred patients were finally diagnosed with INPH and shunted (Fig. 5).

The main question for the clinician contemplating shunt operation is very often not whether the patient suffers from INPH *or* a concurrent irreversible disorder, but whether the hydrocephalus or the presence of a nonshunt responsive comorbidity—most often CVD or AD—is the major contributor to the symptomatology.

For the selection of patients for shunt surgery, we propose the algorithm presented in Figure 6, incorporating clinicoradiological and CSF dynamic findings and results of CSF withdrawal tests.

Clinicoradiological Findings

First, the evaluation consists of estimating, whether the patient presents a clinical and radiological convergence of symptoms and findings suggestive of INPH. We require the presence of at least gait disturbances in the context of hydrocephalus (74). Some centers require one more symptom beside the gait impairment (16).

Based on the clinical and radiological findings, it is very useful, as originally applied by Vanneste et al. (75) and proposed in the published guidelines of INPH (3), to distinguish between probable, possible, and unlikely INPH.

Probable INPH fulfils some or all of the typical INPH clinicoradiological findings, with no coexistence of another disorder, which might explain the symptomatology. Possible INPH covers the cases with an atypical presentation and/or if symptoms may be explained by a concurrent disorder. Unlikely, INPH are cases in which symptoms are fully explained by a disorder other than INPH.

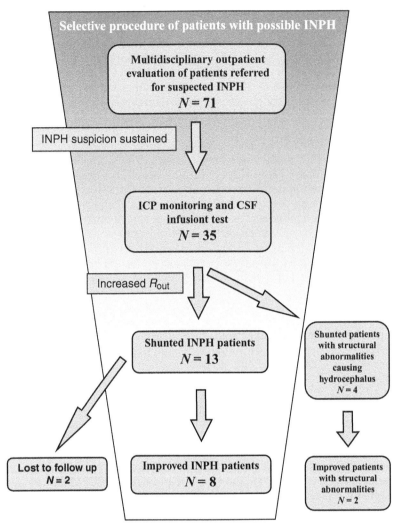

Figure 4 Flowchart representing the selection of patients with a sustained suspicion of INPH during the proceedings of the evaluation program. *Source*: From Ref. 49.

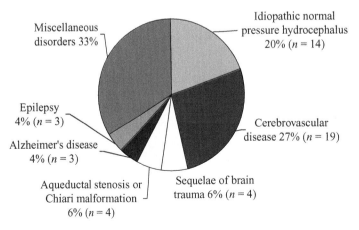

Figure 5 Distribution of the most frequently applied final primary diagnoses in a cohort of patients referred to our tertiary center for evaluation of suspected INPH. *Source*: From Ref. 49.

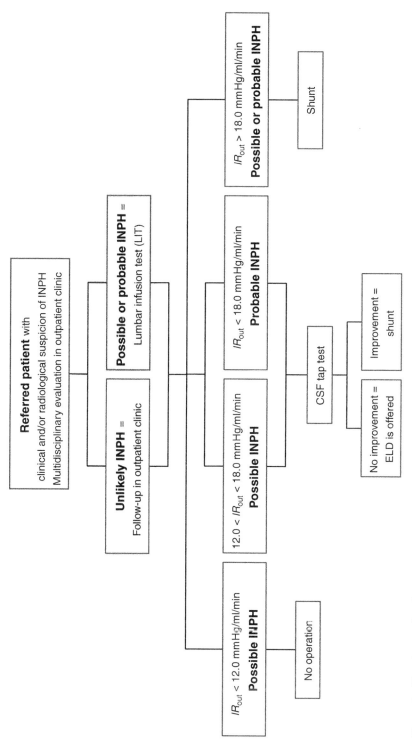

Figure 6 Flowchart of the diagnostic workup and shunt criteria in patients evaluated for INPH.

CSF Dynamic Evaluation

In patients with probable or possible INPH, we proceed with a lumbar steady state infusion test measuring ICP and R_{out} (44), immediately followed by a CSF tap test. All patients with R_{out} equal to or above 18 mm Hg/mL/min, or a positive tap test are shunted. In the gray zone of values between 18 and 12 mm Hg/mL/min and no improvement after CSF tap test, only probable INPH patients are shunted. So far, the evaluation is performed in an outpatient setting.

In cases of probable INPH presenting a R_{out} below 12 mm Hg/mL/min and a negative CSF tap test, we offer an ELD during hospitalization. Shunt operation is then offered, if clinical improvement is obtained during the ELD.

Some centers adhere to one to two days of ICP monitoring by either a lumbar drain (18) or intracranially estimating ICP and the presence of A- and B-waves (74) before deciding upon shunt surgery.

SURGICAL TREATMENT

If shunting is needed, a ventriculoperitoneal shunt is the treatment of choice. Most neurosurgical clinics routinely use prophylactic antibiotics preoperatively.

Some authors recommend low-pressure shunts as opposed to medium-pressure shunts, although the risk of subdural effusions may be higher (76).

Other centers argue that a programmable variable pressure shunt is the treatment of choice (77). With a programmable shunt, the opening pressure, when placing the shunt, can be adjusted according to the measured preoperative ICP. If needed, the opening pressure can successively be lowered stepwise until a satisfactory clinical improvement is obtained. In this setting, the risk of overdrainage may be reduced. In the presence of subdural effusions or hematomas, some cases may resolve by successively increasing the opening pressure of the shunt, thus avoiding surgery.

The most frequent complications of shunt surgery in INPH are infections (3–6%), subdural hematomas (2–17%), and seizures (3–11%) (5). Shunt revision due to shunt malfunction should be expected in 20% to 40% of the patients during a 5-year follow-up (78,79).

Alternative Treatments

A singly study reports a 72% success rate with a 3-year follow-up after endoscopic third ventriculostomy (ETV) in 25 INPH patients (80). The ETV is thought to either modify the CSF pulse pressure wave or relieve a CSF block at the tentorial incisura. The authors suggest ETV for INPH patients with prevalence of gait disturbances and with symptom duration below one year. The intriguing results await further confirmation.

No medical treatment has until now shown any effect in INPH. Although both acetazolamide and furosemide lower ICP, especially in animal research, these drugs are clinically not effective in controlling an uncompensated hydrocephalic state.

PROGNOSIS

INPH is a progressive condition, which means that the symptoms gradually worsen if not treated.

A clinical improvement rate approximating 90%, with no relation to age up to the ninth decade, can be obtained in expert centers by careful patient selection and employing CSF dynamic and drainage tests (4,16). However, in general, published shunt success rates vary widely from 25% to 100% with an overall 59% improvement rate (15).

Some patients improve dramatically after surgery, although most often the symptoms only partially improve. Analysis of recent larger series of shunted INPH patients suggests that the presence of the full clinical triad is not related to a higher shunt success rate, contrary to earlier belief (16,18).

In all patients not improving or in patients deteriorating after an initial improvement, an evaluation of shunt dysfunction should be performed (81).

When evaluating the outcome of shunt surgery, it is important to apply scales for each of the triad symptoms as well as functional scales (6). The gait disturbances are most likely to improve (18). However, it is our experience that with pre- and postoperative psychometric

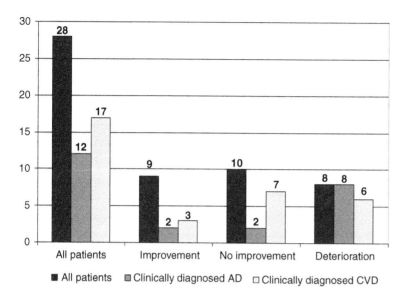

Figure 7 Prevalence among 28 shunted INPH patients with concomitant clinically diagnosed cerebrovascular disease (CVD) or Alzheimer's disease (AD) according to the NINCDS-ADRDA criteria. Eight patients fulfilled criteria for both CVD and AD. The patients are subgrouped according to improvement after shunt operation ($n = 9$), no clinical change ($n = 10$), and clinical deterioration ($n = 8$). One patient was lost to follow-up. *Source*: From Ref. 28.

testings, a slight cognitive recovery can often be demonstrated, despite no subjective improvement by the patient or the relatives.

The postoperative follow-up should always include a one-year post shunt evaluation, as shorter follow-up is more prone to be influenced by shunt-associated complications. The shunt success rate tend to decrease when following the patients above one year, which primarily is explained by the impact of comorbidity (82).

Comorbidities such as CVD and AD is an indicator of poorer prognosis, but does not exclude shunt improvement (Fig. 7) (22,28), likewise with long duration of symptoms (18).

In **summary**, the ideal INPH candidate for shunting is a patient with

- Gait impairment as the initial presenting symptom.
- Gait impairment as the predominant symptom, with or without slight cognitive subcortical deficits.
- Symptom duration below two years and the absence of comorbidity, especially CVD.
- Periventricular lucency, increased temporal horns, and no cortical atrophy on CT or MRI.
- A $R_{out} \geq 18$ mm Hg/mL/min on CSF dynamic investigation.
- Clinical improvement after CSF withdrawal (CSF tap test or prolonged lumbar drainage).
- Decreased global CBF and regional CBF flow in the periventricular and frontal regions on SPECT or PET investigations.

REFERENCES

1. Hakim S, Adams RD. The special clinical problem of symptomatic hydrocephalus with normal cerebrospinal fluid pressure. Observations on cerebrospinal fluid hydrodynamics. J Neurol Sci 1965; 2(4):307–327.
2. Delwel EJ, de Jong DA, Avezaat CJ. The prognostic value of clinical characteristics and parameters of cerebrospinal fluid hydrodynamics in shunting for idiopathic normal pressure hydrocephalus. Acta Neurochir (Wien) 2005; 147(10):1037–1043.
3. Relkin N, Marmarou A, Klinge P, et al. Diagnosing idiopathic normal-pressure hydrocephalus. Neurosurgery 2005; 57(suppl. 3):S4–S16.
4. Marmarou A, Bergsneider M, Klinge P, et al. The value of supplemental prognostic tests for the preoperative assessment of idiopathic normal-pressure hydrocephalus. Neurosurgery 2005; 57(suppl. 3):S17–S28.

5. Bergsneider M, Black PM, Klinge P, et al. Surgical management of idiopathic normal-pressure hydro-cephalus. Neurosurgery 2005; 57(suppl. 3):S29–S39.

6. Klinge P, Marmarou A, Bergsneider M, et al. Outcome of shunting in idiopathic normal-pressure hydrocephalus and the value of outcome assessment in shunted patients. Neurosurgery 2005; 57(suppl. 3):S40–S52.

7. Marmarou A, Bergsneider M, Relkin N, et al. Development of guidelines for idiopathic normal-pressure hydrocephalus: Introduction. Neurosurgery 2005; 57(suppl. 3):S1–S3.

8. Evans WA. An encephalographic ratio for estimating ventricular enlargement and cerebral atrophy. Arch Neurol 1974; 47:931–937.

9. Malm J, Kristensen B, Karlsson T, et al. The predictive value of cerebrospinal fluid dynamic tests in patients with the idiopathic adult hydrocephalus syndrome. Arch Neurol 1995; 52(8):783–789.

10. Gjerris F, Børgesen SE. Pathophysiology of the CSF Circulation. In: Crockard A, Hayward RD, Hoff JT, eds. Neurosurgery—The Scientific Basis of Clinical Practice, 3rd ed. Boston, MA: Blackwell Science, 2000:147–168.

11. Hoglund M, Tisell M, Wikkelso C. Incidence of surgery for hydrocephalus in adults surveyed: Same number afflicted by hydrocephalus as by multiple sclerosis. Lakartidningen 2001; 98(14):1681–1685.

12. Krauss JK, Halve B. Normal pressure hydrocephalus: Survey on contemporary diagnostic algorithms and therapeutic decision-making in clinical practice. Acta Neurochir (Wien) 2004; 146(4):379–388.

13. Brean A, Eide PK. Prevalence of probable idiopathic normal pressure hydrocephalus in a Norwegian population. Acta Neurol Scand 2008; 118(1):48–53.

14. Marmarou A, Young HF, Aygok GA. Estimated incidence of normal pressure hydrocephalus and shunt outcome in patients residing in assisted-living and extended-care facilities. Neurosurg Focus 2007; 22(4):E1.

15. Hebb AO, Cusimano MD. Idiopathic normal pressure hydrocephalus: A systematic review of diagnosis and outcome. Neurosurgery 2001; 49(5):1166–1184.

16. Marmarou A, Young HF, Aygok GA, et al. Diagnosis and management of idiopathic normal-pressure hydrocephalus: A prospective study in 151 patients. J Neurosurg 2005; 102(6):987–997.

17. Boon AJ, Tans JT, Delwel EJ, et al. Dutch normal-pressure hydrocephalus study: Prediction of outcome after shunting by resistance to outflow of cerebrospinal fluid. J Neurosurg 1997; 87(5):687–693.

18. McGirt MJ, Woodworth G, Coon AL, et al. Diagnosis, treatment, and analysis of long-term outcomes in idiopathic normal-pressure hydrocephalus. Neurosurgery 2005; 57(4):699–705.

19. Bech RA, Juhler M, Waldemar G, et al. Frontal brain and leptomeningeal biopsy specimens correlated with cerebrospinal fluid outflow resistance and B-wave activity in patients suspected of normal-pressure hydrocephalus. Neurosurgery 1997; 40(3):497–502.

20. Silverberg GD, Huhn S, Jaffe RA, et al. Downregulation of cerebrospinal fluid production in patients with chronic hydrocephalus. J Neurosurg 2002; 97(6):1271–1275.

21. Sorensen PS, Gjerris F, Hammer M. Cerebrospinal fluid vasopressin and increased intracranial pressure. Ann Neurol 1984; 15(5):435–440.

22. Boon AJ, Tans JT, Delwel EJ, et al. Dutch Normal-Pressure Hydrocephalus Study: The role of cere-brovascular disease. J Neurosurg 1999; 90(2):221–226.

23. Akai K, Uchigasaki S, Tanaka U, et al. Normal pressure hydrocephalus neuropathological study. Acta Pathol Jpn 1987; 37:97–110.

24. Bech RA, Waldemar G, Gjerris F, et al. Shunting effects in patients with idiopathic normal pressure hydrocephalus; correlation with cerebral and leptomeningeal biopsy findings. Acta Neurochir (Wien) 1999; 141(6):633–639.

25. Tullberg M, Jensen C, Ekholm S, et al. Normal pressure hydrocephalus: Vascular white matter changes on MR images must not exclude patients from shunt surgery. AJNR Am J Neuroradiol 2001; 22(9):1665–1673.

26. Golomb J, Wisoff J, Miller DC, et al. Alzheimer's disease comorbidity in normal pressure hydrocephalus: Prevalence and shunt response. J Neurol Neurosurg Psychiatry 2000; 68(6):778–781.

27. Savolainen S, Paljarvi L, Vapalahti M. Prevalence of Alzheimer's disease in patients investigated for presumed normal pressure hydrocephalus: A clinical and neuropathological study. Acta Neurochir (Wien) 1999; 141(8):849–853.

28. Bech-Azeddine R, Hogh P, Juhler M, et al. Idiopathic normal-pressure hydrocephalus: Clinical comor-bidity correlated with cerebral biopsy findings and outcome of cerebrospinal fluid shunting. J Neurol Neurosurg Psychiatry 2007; 78(2):157–161.

29. Tullberg M, Hultin L, Ekholm S, et al. White matter changes in normal pressure hydrocephalus and Binswanger disease: Specificity, predictive value and correlations to axonal degeneration and demyeli-nation. Acta Neurol Scand 2002; 105(6):417–426.

30. Silverberg GD. Normal pressure hydrocephalus (NPH): Ischaemia, CSF stagnation or both. Brain 2004; 127(5):947–948.

31. Skoog I. The interaction between vascular disorders and Alzheimer's disease. In: Ikbal K, Swaab DF, Winblad B, Wisniewski HM, eds. Alzheimer's Disease and Related Disorders: Etiology, Pathogenesis and Therapeutics. Chichester: J. Wiley, 1999:219–229.

32. Silverberg GD, Levinthal E, Sullivan EV, et al. Assessment of low-flow CSF drainage as a treatment for AD: Results of a randomized pilot study. Neurology 2002; 59(8):1139–1145.

33. Czosnyka ZH, Czosnyka M, Whitfield PC, et al. Cerebral autoregulation among patients with symptoms of hydrocephalus. Neurosurgery 2002; 50(3):526–532.

34. Owler BK, Momjian S, Czosnyka Z, et al. Normal pressure hydrocephalus and cerebral blood flow: A PET study of baseline values. J Cereb Blood Flow Metab 2004; 24(1):17–23.

35. Bateman GA. The pathophysiology of idiopathic normal pressure hydrocephalus: Cerebral ischemia or altered venous hemodynamics? AJNR Am J Neuroradiol 2008; 29(1):198–203.

36. Gjerris F, Børgesen SE. Current concepts of measurement of cerebrospinal fluid absorption and biomechanics of hydrocephalus. Adv Tech Stand Neurosurg 1992; 19:147–177.

37. Børgesen SE, Gjerris F. The predictive value of conductance to outflow of CSF in normal pressure hydrocephalus. Brain 1982; 105:65–86.

38. Ekstedt J. CSF hydrodynamic studies in man. 2. Normal hydrodynamic variables related to CSF pressure and flow. J Neurol Neurosurg Psychiatry 1978; 41(4):345–353.

39. Sklar FH. Non-steady-state measurements of cerebrospinal fluid dynamics. Laboratory and clinical applications. In: Wood JH, ed. Neurobiology of Cerebrospinal Fluid. New York: Plenum, 1980:365–379.

40. Albeck MJ, Børgesen SE, Gjerris F, et al. The intracranial pressure and conductance to cerebrospinal outflow in healthy subjects. J Neurosurg 1991; 74:597–600.

41. Albeck MJ, Skak C, Nielsen PR, et al. Age dependency of resistance to cerebrospinal fluid outflow. J Neurosurg 1998; 89(2):275–278.

42. Czosnyka M, Czosnyka ZH, Whitfield PC, et al. Age dependence of cerebrospinal pressure–volume compensation in patients with hydrocephalus. J Neurosurg 2001; 94(3):482–486.

43. Lundberg NG. Continuous recording and control of ventricular fluid pressure in neurosurgical patients. Acta Psychiatr Scand Suppl 1960; 149:1–193.

44. Czosnyka M, Whitehouse H, Smielewski P, et al. Testing of cerebrospinal compensatory reserve in shunted and non- shunted patients: A guide to interpretation based on an observational study. J Neurol Neurosurg Psychiatry 1996; 60(5):549–558.

45. Newell DW, Aaslid R, Stooss R, et al. The relationship of blood flow velocity fluctuations to intracranial pressure B waves. J Neurosurg 1992; 76(3):415–421.

46. Crockard HA, Hanlon K, Duda EE, et al. Hydrocephalus as a cause of dementia: Evaluation by computerized tomography and intracranial pressure monitoring. J Neurol Neurosurg Psychiatry 1977; 40(8):736–740.

47. Raftopoulos C, Chaskis C, Delecluse F, et al. Morphological quantitative analysis of intracranial pressure waves in normal pressure hydrocephalus. Neurol Res 1992; 14(5):389–396.

48. Eide PK, Brean A. Intracranial pulse pressure amplitude levels determined during preoperative assessment of subjects with possible idiopathic normal pressure hydrocephalus. Acta Neurochir (Wien) 2006; 148(11):1151–1156.

49. Bech-Azeddine R, Waldemar G, Knudsen GM, et al. Idiopathic normal-pressure hydrocephalus: Evaluation and findings in a multidisciplinary memory clinic. Eur J Neurol 2001; 8(6):601–611.

50. Stolze H, Kuhtz-Buschbeck JP, Drucke H, et al. Comparative analysis of the gait disorder of normal pressure hydrocephalus and Parkinson's disease. J Neurol Neurosurg Psychiatry 2001; 70(3): 289–297.

51. Knutsson E, Lying-Tunell U. Gait apraxia in normal-pressure hydrocephalus: Patterns of movement and muscle activation. Neurology 1985; 35(2):155–160.

52. Blomsterwall E, Svantesson U, Carlsson U, et al. Postural disturbance in patients with normal pressure hydrocephalus. Acta Neurol Scand 2000; 102(5):284–291.

53. Thomsen AM, Børgesen SE, Bruhn P, et al. Prognosis of dementia in normal-pressure hydrocephalus after a shunt operation. Ann Neurol 1986; 20(3):304–310.

54. Devito EE, Pickard JD, Salmond CH, et al. The neuropsychology of normal pressure hydrocephalus (NPH). Br J Neurosurg 2005; 19(3):217–224.

55. Stolze H, Kuhtz-Buschbeck JP, Drucke H, et al. Gait analysis in idiopathic normal pressure hydrocephalus—Which parameters respond to the CSF tap test? Clin Neurophysiol 2000; 111(9): 1678–1686.

56. Gjerris F, Børgesen SE, Schmidt JF, et al. Resistance to cerebrospinal outflow in patients with normal pressure hydrocephalus. In: Gjerris F, Børgesen SE, Schmidt JF, et al., eds. Outflow of cerebrospinal fluid. Copenhagen, Denmark: Munksgaard, 1989:329–338.

57. Gjerris F. Hydrocephalus and other disorders of cerebrospinal fluid circulation. In: Bogousslavsky J, Fisher M, eds. Textbook of Neurology. Boston, MA: Butterworth & Heinemann, 1998:655–674.

58. Wikkelsø C, Andersson H, Blomstrand C, et al. Computed tomography of the brain in the diagnosis of and prognosis in normal pressure hydrocephalus. Neuroradiology 1989; 31(2):160–165.
59. Holodny AI, George AE, de Leon MJ, et al. Focal dilation and paradoxical collapse of cortical fissures and sulci in patients with normal-pressure hydrocephalus. J Neurosurg 1998; 89(5):742–747.
60. Holodny AI, Waxman R, George AE, et al. MR differential diagnosis of normal-pressure hydrocephalus and Alzheimer disease: Significance of perihippocampal features. AJNR Am J Neuroradiol 1998; 19(5):813–819.
61. Luetmer PH, Huston J, Friedman JA, et al. Measurement of cerebrospinal fluid flow at the cerebral aqueduct by use of phase-contrast magnetic resonance imaging: Technique validation and utility in diagnosing idiopathic normal pressure hydrocephalus. Neurosurgery 2002; 50(3):534–543.
62. Bradley WG, Scalzo D, Queralt J, et al. Normal-pressure hydrocephalus: Evaluation with cerebrospinal fluid flow measurements at MR imaging. Radiology 1996; 198(2):523–529.
63. Kahlon B, Annertz M, Stahlberg F, et al. Is aqueductal stroke volume, measured with cine phase-contrast magnetic resonance imaging scans useful in predicting outcome of shunt surgery in suspected normal pressure hydrocephalus? Neurosurgery 2007; 60(1):124–129.
64. Wikkelsø C, Andersson H, Blomstrand C, et al. Predictive value of the cerebrospinal fluid tap-test. Acta Neurol Scand 1986; 73:566–573.
65. Vanneste J, Augustijn P, Davies GA, et al. Normal-pressure hydrocephalus. Is cisternography still useful in selecting patients for a shunt? Arch Neurol 1992; 49(4):366–370.
66. Owler BK, Pickard JD. Normal pressure hydrocephalus and cerebral blood flow: A review. Acta Neurol Scand 2001; 104(6):325–342.
67. Momjian S, Owler BK, Czosnyka Z, et al. Pattern of white matter regional cerebral blood flow and autoregulation in normal pressure hydrocephalus. Brain 2004; 127(5):965–972.
68. Waldemar G, Schmidt JF, Delecluse F, et al. High resolution SPECT with (99m-tc)-d,1-HMPAO in normal pressure hydrocephalus before and after shunt operation. J Neurol Neurosurg Psychiatry 1993; 56:655–664.
69. Klinge P, Berding G, Brinker T, et al. The role of cerebral blood flow and cerebrovascular reserve capacity in the diagnosis of chronic hydrocephalus—A PET-study on 60 patients. Acta Neurochir Suppl 2002; 81:39–41.
70. Malm J, Kristensen B, Fagerlund M, et al. Cerebrospinal fluid shunt dynamics in patients with idiopathic adult hydrocephalus syndrome. J Neurol Neurosurg Psychiatry 1995; 58:715–723.
71. Bech-Azeddine R, Gjerris F, Waldemar G, et al. Intraventricular or lumbar infusion test in adult communicating hydrocephalus? Practical consequences and clinical outcome of shunt operation. Acta Neurochir (Wien) 2005; 147(10):1027–1036.
72. Walchenbach R, Geiger E, Thomeer RT, et al. The value of temporary external lumbar CSF drainage in predicting the outcome of shunting on normal pressure hydrocephalus. J Neurol Neurosurg Psychiatry 2002; 72(4):503–506.
73. Agren-Wilsson A, Lekman A, Sjoberg W, et al. CSF biomarkers in the evaluation of idiopathic normal pressure hydrocephalus. Acta Neurol Scand 2007; 116(5):333–339.
74. Poca MA, Mataro M, del Mar MM, et al. Is the placement of shunts in patients with idiopathic normal-pressure hydrocephalus worth the risk? Results of a study based on continuous monitoring of intracranial pressure. J Neurosurg 2004; 100(5):855–866.
75. Vanneste J, Augustijn P, Tan WF, et al. Shunting normal pressure hydrocephalus: The predictive value of combined clinical and CT data. J Neurol Neurosurg Psychiatry 1993; 56:251–256.
76. Boon AJ, Tans JT, Delwel EJ, et al. Dutch Normal-Pressure Hydrocephalus Study: Randomized comparison of low- and medium-pressure shunts. J Neurosurg 1998; 88(3):490–495.
77. Zemack G, Romner B. Adjustable valves in normal-pressure hydrocephalus: A retrospective study of 218 patients. Neurosurgery 2002; 51(6):1392–1400.
78. Hanlo PW, Cinalli G, Vandertop WP, et al. Treatment of hydrocephalus determined by the European Orbis Sigma Valve II survey: A multicenter prospective 5-year shunt survival study in children and adults in whom a flow-regulating shunt was used. J Neurosurg 2003; 99(1):52–57.
79. Raftopoulos C, Massager N, Baleriaux D, et al. Prospective analysis by computed tomography and long-term outcome of 23 adult patients with chronic idiopathic hydrocephalus. Neurosurgery 1996; 38(1):51–59.
80. Gangemi M, Maiuri F, Buonamassa S, et al. Endoscopic third ventriculostomy in idiopathic normal pressure hydrocephalus. Neurosurgery 2004; 55(1):129–134.
81. Gjerris F. Hydrocephalus in adults. In: Kay AH, Black PM, eds. Operative Neurosurgery. London, U.K.: Churchill Livingstone, 2000:1236–1247.
82. Malm J, Kristensen B, Stegmayr B, et al. Three-year survival and functional outcome of patients with idiopathic adult hydrocephalus syndrome. Neurology 2000; 55(4):576–578.

NPH and ETV

J. André Grotenhuis

Department of Neurosurgery, Radboud University Nijmegen Medical Center, Nijmegen, The Netherlands

In the literature, there are conflicting reports about the usefulness of ETV in patients with NPH. Personally, concerning NPH and ETV, I am still ambiguous. I have had some very good and often unexpected good results but also a number of patients with none or only short-term result.

The problem is simply NPH itself; it is a receptacle of many different types of hydrocephalus in adults and elderly people. But knowing that, why did I try ETV in NPH patients in the first place, because NPH has always been considered to be a form of communicating hydrocephalus, and ETV is considered to be only effective in obstructive hydrocephalus.

The answer is that adult people with hydrocephalus present mostly with the triad of memory deficit, gait disturbance, and urine incontinence regardless of the cause of hydrocephalus, and furthermore, MRI scan in older patients with hydrocephalus and low-to-normal lumbar CSF pressure sometimes clearly showed a triventricular hydrocephalus, enlarged lateral ventricles and third ventricle and normal-sized fourth ventricle. The only feature not congruent with obstructive hydrocephalus was an anatomically open aqueduct and no bulging of the floor of the third ventricle. But even without this, in the early and mid-1990s, I performed ETV as a first choice for hydrocephalus anyway (which I do not do now!).

But when I looked further into this category of NPH patients, I found that on T2-sagittal image, there was a turbulent flow void sign in front of the open aqueduct but not within it or within the fourth ventricle and I started to consider this as a sign of functional CSF obstruction at the entrance of the aqueduct. In 16 years, I have performed ETV in NPH in 44 cases. Patients that (retrospectively) met the aforementioned criteria of triventricular hydrocephalus and turbulent flow in front of an open aqueduct (26 of the whole group of 44) actually had long-term relieve of symptoms after ETV in 54% (14 out of 26), and improvement, especially in gait and memory problems, in another 15% (4 out of 26). Patients that did not meet these criteria either never improved or showed only a very short period of slight improvement. So, as a total, there was only 41% of improvement in the whole group of 44 patients. But in the group that failed after ETV, there were many who received a shunt and none of them responded to that too in the long term. What we need urgently are better clinicoradiological criteria that can identify the adult hydrocephalus patients that will benefit from ETV. I hope that we can find out more about it and come up with a protocol of preoperative work-up and postoperative follow-up (neurological assessment, imaging) for this group of patients.

17 | Hydrocephalus in Chiari Malformation and Other Craniovertebral Junction Abnormalities

Daniel J. Guillaume

Department of Neurosurgery, Oregon Health & Science University, Portland, Oregon, U.S.A.

Arnold H. Menezes

Department of Neurosurgery, University of Iowa Hospitals and Clinics, Iowa City, Iowa, U.S.A.

INTRODUCTION

Chiari malformations are a group of conditions with different etiologies. They are all similar; however, in that they involve abnormalities in the posterior fossa and craniovertebral junction. These abnormalities often are associated with the presence of hydrocephalus due to changes they cause in cerebrospinal fluid (CSF) flow at the level of the craniovertebral junction. Any posterior fossa/craniovertebral junction abnormality has the potential to affect CSF flow by fourth ventricular outlet atresia or obstruction, venous flow abnormalities or, rarely, other mechanisms. This chapter reviews the most common Chiari malformations associated with hydrocephalus and other similar conditions and discusses development and pathology, presentation, imaging, and management options.

CHIARI I MALFORMATION

Development and Pathology

The Chiari I malformation (CM I), or hindbrain herniation syndrome, consists of downward herniation of the cerebellar tonsils through the foramen magnum into the cervical spinal canal (1,2). The degree of displacement is typically greater than 5 mm below the plane of the foramen magnum on sagittal magnetic resonance image (MRI) (3–7). The vermis, fourth ventricle and brainstem are relatively normal. It is usually associated with osseous abnormalities of the craniovertebral junction and overcrowding of the hindbrain within a relatively small posterior fossa (6,8–12). Syringomyelia occurs in 45% to 68% of cases (6,7,9). It is associated with scoliosis in 42% cases, abnormal retroflexed odontoid process in 26% cases, and basilar invagination in 12% cases (3,6,13–15). The average age of onset is in the mid-30s, but it can occur in those as young as three months (13).

Chronic tonsillar herniation in CM I is most likely secondary to underdevelopment of the occipital bone and overcrowding of the cerebellum in a small posterior fossa. The fundamental defect is thought to involve underdevelopment of the occipital somites originating from the paraxial mesoderm (6,16). Reduction of the height of the occipital bone, accentuation of the slope of the tentorium cerebelli, and underdevelopment of the clivus associated with herniation of the cerebellar tonsils argues in favor of the mesodermal origin of this malformation (6,17). Volume measurements demonstrate a reduction in the volume of the posterior fossa and the amount of CSF that it contains, whereas the volume of nervous tissue is normal (6,18,19). Compression of fluid spaces by cerebellar tissue in the small posterior fossa interferes with CSF circulation and this accounts for many of the symptoms observed (6,20).

Presentation

Presentation in CM I is most often attributed to syringohydromyelia, brainstem compression, or cerebellar compression (Table 1). The presence of hydrocephalus exacerbates these symptoms. The mean age of presentation in the mid 30s, (6), with a female preponderance. The presence of syringomyelia lowered the age of presentation to the mid 20s in the series by Milhorat and colleagues (6). More than a third of presenting patients report lifelong complaints of headaches or clumsiness (6).

Table 1 Pathology, Clinical Presentation, MRI Findings, and Association with Hydrocephalus in Chiari I and Chiari II Malformations

	Pathology	Presentation	MRI	Hydrocephalus
CM I	(1) Overcrowding of cerebellum in relatively small posterior fossa	(1) Average onset in mid-30s	(1) Overcrowded posterior fossa, tonsillar herniation of >5 mm	(1) Seen in 6–11% (most with syrinx)
	(2) Downward herniation of cerebellar tonsils into cervical canal	(2) Most present with headache that is worse with Valsalva	(2) Abnormal CSF circulation with cine	(2) Likely multifactorial: 4th ventricular outlet obstruction common
	(3) Syringomyelia in more than 50% of cases	(3) Other symptoms from brainstem compression, syrinx, or cerebellar dysfunction		(3) Treat hydrocephalus before Chiari
	(4) Other brain anomalies are uncommon			(4) Treat with shunt or ETV
CM II	(1) Associated with MMC	(1) Present in neonate or child	(1) Vermis, 4th ventricle and medulla displaced into cervical canal	(1) Seen in 90%
	(2) Descent of vermis, 4th ventricle, and brainstem through widened foramen magnum	(2) <2 yr present with respiratory and GI problems from cranial nerve and brainstem abnormalities	(2) Many other brain anomalies typically seen	(2) Can be related to aqueductal stenosis, anomalous venous drainage, 4th ventricular outlet obstruction
	(3) Cerebellar inversion, low-lying tentorium, absent cisterna magna	(3) >2 yr present with symptoms from spinal cord dysfunction		(3) Treat hydrocephalus before Chiari
	(4) Other brain anomalies are common			(4) Treated with shunt (ETV with low success in neonates)

The most common symptom, occurring in up to 81% of patients, is suboccipital headache that is worsened with head dependency and Valsalva-type maneuvers such as coughing, straining, and exertion (6,13,21–23). Over 70% of patients present with either ocular disturbances such as diplopia, blurred vision, or retro-orbital pain; or otoneurological disturbances such as dizziness, disequilibrium, tinnitus, or ear pressure (24). Lower cranial nerve, brainstem, and cerebellar findings include dysphagia, sleep apnea, dysarthria, tremors, impaired gag reflex, and poor coordination. Permanent nocturnal central hypoventilation requiring ventilation has been reported (25). Sensory and motor findings due to spinal cord dysfunction are common, especially when associated with syringomyelia. Over 90% of patients with syringomyelia present with spinal cord disturbances such as paresthesias, pain, burning dysesthesias or anesthesia, weakness, spasticity, atrophy, incontinence, trophic phenomena, impaired position sense, or hyperreflexia (6). Scoliosis, which can occur in children with Chiari I–related syringomyelia, has been shown to improve following craniovertebral decompression (26).

Imaging
Prior to the advent of MRI, diagnosis was based on clinical suspicion supported by plain radiography, myelography, computed tomography (CT), and sometimes vertebral angiography. Plain

radiographs are abnormal in 89% of cases (3). Abnormalities including shallow posterior fossa, scoliosis, widened spinal canal, shortened clivus, retroflexion of the odontoid process, basilar invagination, Klippel–Feil syndrome, and atlanto-occipital assimilation (failure of segmentation between the fourth occipital sclerotome and the first spinal sclerotome) can be demonstrated by plain radiographs (3).

MRI has revolutionized the diagnosis of all Chiari malformations. MRI abnormalities include crowding of the CSF spaces within the region of the craniocervical junction, tonsillar herniation below the foramen magnum of at least 5 mm, reduced height of the supraocciput, and increased slope of the tentorium (6). MRI can also demonstrate abnormalities of CSF circulation including compression of the fourth ventricle, empty sella, hydrocephalus, syringobulbia, and syringomyelia. Patients who undergo phase-contrast cine-MRI show evidence of abnormal CSF velocity/flow in the cisterna magna and subarachnoid space posterior to the cerebellum and in the premedullary and prepontine spaces anterior to the brainstem (6).

It is important to note that the clinical significance of radiological studies depends on the patient's presentation. A subgroup of patients exists with Chiari malformation who do not have frank tonsillar ectopia but have syringes that respond to posterior fossa decompression (27). Likewise, there is known to be a great variance in tonsillar position in asymptomatic individuals (4,5).

Hydrocephalus in Chiari I

Chiari's original description included an autopsy case in which the patient died of hydrocephalus (17). In reported case series, hydrocephalus is rare in CM I, occurring in only 6% to 11% of cases (6,23). The majority (84%) of CM I patients with hydrocephalus also present with syringomyelia. The mechanism of hydrocephalus formation in patients with Chiari malformation is likely multifactorial and may differ between patients. At least part of the etiology of hydrocephalus formation is explained by fourth ventricular outlet stenosis (19,28–33), resulting in increased compression of the cisterna magna by the herniated cerebellar tonsils. This relationship is further complicated by the observations that hindbrain herniation can both be the result of hydrocephalus and result in hydrocephalus.

In Chiari malformations, the foramen of Magendie is often encased in scarred arachnoid, with the brainstem descended into the area of the foramen magnum occluding the lateral exiting foramina of the fourth ventricle. This scarring effect is a well-recognized cause of obstruction of the outlet foramina of the fourth ventricle. At surgery this adhesive arachnoiditis is often opened as part of the procedure. A history of a traumatic birth and dense adhesive arachnoiditis is especially prominent in cases of CM I associated with syringomyelia (34).

Most evidence suggests that compression of the cisterna magna by herniated cerebellar tonsils is responsible for the formation of syringomyelia (6,20). However, this interference with CSF flow only rarely results in hydrocephalus. One explanation is that the foramen of Luschka often remains open, allowing CSF to exit the fourth ventricle.

Treatment Options for Hydrocephalus in CM I

When hydrocephalus is observed in a patient with hindbrain herniation, it is often difficult to ascertain which came first. As described above, herniation of cerebellar tonsils can lead to hydrocephalus, and the presence of hydrocephalus can lead to hindbrain herniation. Moreover, each problem may worsen the other. The consensus of management involves first addressing the hydrocephalus (3,13,35).

In 25 patients presenting with hydrocephalus and CM I with syringomyelia at the University of Iowa, all underwent ventriculoperitoneal shunting, with complete resolution of symptoms in eight (Fig. 1). The other 17 required posterior fossa decompression (13).

The standard treatment of obstructive hydrocephalus has been CSF diversion with placement of shunt. Endoscopic third ventriculostomy (ETV), an effective treatment for obstructive hydrocephalus (36–44), has been used to treat cases of obstruction of the foramen of Magendie with aqueductal patency (33,36,45,46). More recently, ETV has been shown to be effective treatment for obstructive hydrocephalus associated with CM I and communicating syringomyelia (38,47,48).

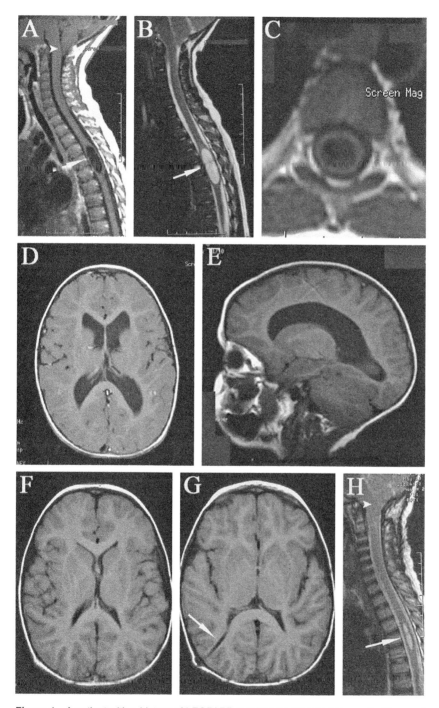

Figure 1 A patient with a history of LEOPARD syndrome presented at age 2 with symptoms of syringomyelia. Sagittal T1-weighted (**A**) and T2-weighted (**B**) cervical and cervicomedullary junction MRI demonstrated evidence of Chiari I malformation (*arrowhead*) and syringomyelia extending from T4 to T6 (*arrows*). Axial T1-weighted MRI (**C**) further detailed the large cervical cord syrinx. Axial (**D**) and sagittal (**E**) T1-weighted MRI demonstrated moderate hydrocephalus. The patient underwent placement of right posterior ventriculoperitoneal shunt with resolution of symptoms. Repeat MRI (**F**) and (**G**) three months later showed interval decompression of the ventricular system and the presence of ventricular catheter entering the occipital horn of the right lateral ventricle (*arrow in G*). Sagittal T2-weighted cervical spine MRI one year later (**H**) demonstrated a significant decrease in the size of the syrinx (*arrow*) and mild improvement in tonsillar descent (*arrowhead*). When last seen in clinic at age 4, the patient continued to do well.

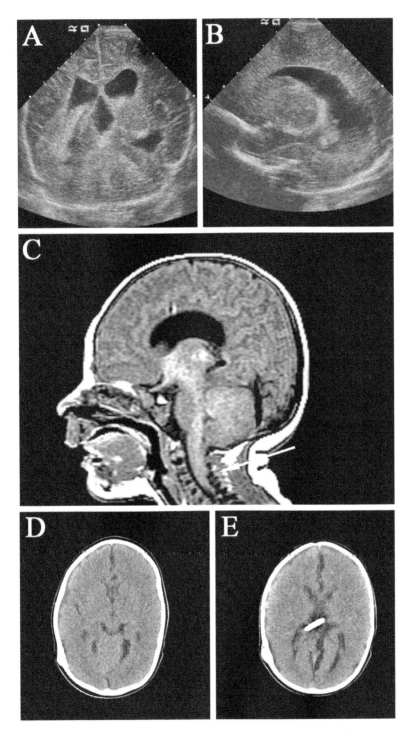

Figure 2 A patient, born at term by caesarian section, was noted to have a lumbosacral myelomeningocele (MMC) by prenatal ultrasound. Coronal (**A**) and sagittal (**B**) head ultrasound on day-of-life 1 showed marked hydrocephalus and evidence of Chiari malformation. Sagittal T1-weighted MRI (**C**) revealed hydrocephalus and a Chiari II Malformation with tonsillar herniation to the level of C4, low-lying tentorium, torcular herophili near foramen magnum, tectal beaking, low-lying inion, small aqueduct, and low-lying fourth ventricle. The patient underwent closure of the MMC on day-of-life 1 with placement of ventricular catheter/reservoir. Ten days later, the patient underwent placement of ventriculoperitoneal shunt. Head CT (**D**) and (**E**) performed two weeks later reveals good ventricular decompression.

Decq and colleagues (38) studied five patients with hydrocephalus and CM I, with a mean third ventricular transverse diameter of 12.79 mm and a mean herniation of cerebellar tonsils of 13.75 mm below the basion-opisthion line. All patients presented with noncommunicating hydrocephalus related to obstruction of the fourth ventricular outlet, demonstrated by the absence of visible CSF flow on cine-MRI. All patients underwent ETV, with resolution of symptoms, reduction in ventricular size, and significant decrease in cerebellar tonsillar herniation (from 13.75 to 7.76 mm). Along these same lines, a case of noncommunicating syringomyelia (syrinx that does not communicate with the fourth ventricle) associated with hydrocephalus was successfully treated with ETV (49).

CHIARI II MALFORMATION

Development and Pathology

The Chiari II malformation (CM II) is intimately associated with myelomeningocele (MMC) and involves vermian herniation with descent of the brainstem and fourth ventricle through a widened foramen magnum. The vermian "peg" may descend as low as the upper thoracic level (35,50,51). Other findings include cerebellar inversion with absent cisterna magna ("banana sign" on ultrasonography), hypoplastic tentorium that inserts very low placing the torcular herophili just above the foramen magnum, and a medullary "kink" in two-thirds of patients due to posterior displacement of a relatively mobile medulla along with a fixed spinal cord (35,50,51).

As opposed to CM I, where associated brain anomalies are rare, CM II is associated with many brain anomalies. Skull findings include enlarged foramen magnum, craniolacunia, scalloping of the petrous bones, jugular tubercles and frontal bone (known as the lemon sign on ultrasound), increased concavity of the basioccipital clivus, low inion, and sometimes basilar impression and assimilation of the atlas (35,52,53). Cerebral findings include enlarged massa intermedia (50), polygyria (54), and agenesis of the corpus callosum. Below-average intelligence occurs in over half of patients (55). Other findings include prominent anterior commissure, absence of the falx with interdigitation of the occipital and parietal lobes, agenesis of the olfactory tract, absence of the cingulate gyrus, heterotopic gray matter, fusion of the colliculi (tectal beaking), cranial nerve nuclei malformation, and decreased cerebellar volume with dysplastic or absent folia. In CM II, cranial and upper cervical nerves display an upward course (35).

CSF flow abnormalities are abundant in CM II. Hydrocephalus requiring treatment is seen in approximately 90% (35,56). Other common ventricular abnormalities include a small, elongated low-lying fourth ventricle that can be displaced into the cervical canal, with outwardly projecting choroid plexus (embryological location), small aqueduct, "shark tooth deformity" of the third ventricle (anterior diverticulum) (50), colpocephalic lateral ventricles, "beaking" of the frontal horns, occasionally absent inferior medullary velum, and occasionally absent foramen of Magendie (35).

Meningeal abnormalities include low-lying and hypoplastic tentorium cerebelli, resulting in a vertical straight sinus and torcular herophili near the foramen magnum as well as fenestrated falx cerebri. Syringohydromyelia occurrence ranges from 20% to 95% in CM II (35,57).

Development of the CM II is likely associated with the open neural tube defect and drainage of CSF through the central canal during development (58). Without ventricular distention, the posterior fossa does not develop normally. This theory also explains the development of hydrocephalus, because of blocked CSF outflow at the foramina of Lushka and Magendie (58,59).

Presentation

Nearly every patient with CM II presents initially with an open neural tube defect. Frequently, the diagnosis is made in utero. Symptoms attributable to CM II vary with age. In all age groups, symptoms are worsened with the presence of hydrocephalus.

Patients younger than two years of age most commonly present with respiratory and gastrointestinal problems related to cranial nerve and brainstem abnormalities (60,61). Signs and symptoms include inspiratory stridor, vocal cord paresis or paralysis, apnea, dysphagia, aspiration, nasal regurgitation, absent gag reflex, and emaciation (35,62). Respiratory symptoms can be life threatening, and often require emergent treatment.

In patients greater than two years of age, symptoms are typically not life threatening. Signs and symptoms are more commonly related to spinal cord dysfunction such as spasticity, weakness, atrophy, dissociated sensory abnormalities and scoliosis, and cerebellar dysfunction such as ataxia and nystagmus (59,62). In adults, ophthalmic problems are common (35).

Imaging
In utero, ultrasonography is typically the first modality, showing the characteristic banana sign (cerebellar hemispheres that are curved anteriorly with a small or absent cisterna magna) and lemon sign (scalloping of the frontal bones) as well as associated anomalies including myelomeningocele and hydrocephalus.

In the neonate, plain radiographs and CT can reveal the small, shallow posterior fossa, scalloping lacunar skull, large foramen magnum, and concave clivus and petrous pyramids.

MRI is the imaging modality that best defines the abnormality and associated CNS findings already discussed. In contrast to CM I in which syringes occur in the upper cervical cord, CM II malformations tend to develop syringes in the lower cervical and upper thoracic cord. The tentorium arises laterally from low-lying transverse sinuses and can be deficient, with an enlarged incisura that is heart-shaped. The interhemispheric fissure is serrated and apposing gyri cross the midline and interdigitate through the fenestrated falx. Postcontrast MRI can show enhancing choroid plexus at the caudal pole of the displaced vermis (62).

Hydrocephalus in Chiari II
Hydrocephalus requiring diversion is seen in approximately 90% of patients with CM II (35,56). In his initial theory, Chiari attributed the hindbrain herniation to the presence of hydrocephalus (17). Although hydrocephalus can lead to worsening of signs and symptoms associated with CM II, there is significant evidence against hydrocephalus as the cause of the CM II. In CM II, the posterior fossa is abnormally small, with a low-lying tentorium insertion (sometimes just above the foramen magnum). Oftentimes upward herniation is seen, arguing against hydrocephalus as a cause of CM II. Further arguing against hydrocephalus as a cause of CM II, CM II has been demonstrated prior to hydrocephalus on prenatal imaging (51), and over 10% of those born with myelomeningocele and CM II do not develop hydrocephalus or require CSF diversion (63).

There is evidence that many factors contribute to the hydrocephalus associated with CM II (64). Some associations include the CM II itself, aqueductal stenosis, anomalous venous drainage, closure of the myelomeningocele, and other CNS malformations (64).

In CM II, the posterior fossa is small, the fourth ventricle is caudally displaced and there is tonsillar herniation. The caudal displacement of the brainstem can cause increased resistance of CSF flow through the tentorial hiatus. There can also be occlusion of the outlets of the fourth ventricle, as in CM I (64).

The cerebral aqueduct can be stenotic, stretched, kinked, laterally compressed, or forked (35). This may add to the other abnormalities within the posterior fossa, creating functional obstruction.

Additionally, problems with venous drainage due to a small posterior fossa have been implicated as contributing to hydrocephalus (63,64). The small posterior fossa volume and crowding at the foramen magnum can lead to compression of the sigmoid sinuses, leading to venous hypertension. Also, compression of the deep venous drainage system due to deformation of the midbrain can further contribute (53,64).

Closure of the MMC often contributes to hydrocephalus formation. This is intuitive, and the presence of hydrocephalus can cause a cyclic phenomena in which the hydrocephalus worsens the cerebellar herniation, worsening the aqueductal stenosis, worsening the hydrocephalus, and so on.

It has been reported that patients who have undergone intrauterine MMC repair had a 59% incidence of hydrocephalus compared to 91% in historical controls (65,66). It was postulated that the lower incidence of hydrocephalus was due to the absence of the obstructing effect of the hindbrain herniation (64). Long-term follow-up data are not yet available.

Treatment Options for Hydrocephalus in CM II

As stated above, the majority of patients with MMC and CM II will have hydrocephalus. This is in stark contrast to those with CM I, which develop hydrocephalus much less frequently. Approximately 90% of those with CM II and MMC will develop hydrocephalus requiring a shunt (35,50,51) compared to less than 10% with CM I. Asymptomatic children with CM II, MMC, and mild or moderate ventriculomegaly and normal head circumference often need no treatment and can be observed. Rekate has developed criteria in deciding which children with dysraphism should not have shunts placed. Shunts may be avoided in those with cerebral mantle thickness of more than 3.5 cm and, at five months, normal development and no lower cranial nerve problems (63).

As with CM I, all algorithms for treatment of CM II involve first addressing and appropriately treating hydrocephalus (see Figure 2). This means thoroughly evaluating the shunt in a shunted patient and evaluating the need for a shunt in an unshunted patient. Compared to CM I, patients with CM II and MMC present with hydrocephalus requiring treatment at a much younger age, and this influences the type of CSF diversion as well as complication rate. The most frequent means of CSF diversion in those with CM II and hydrocephalus remains ventriculoperitoneal shunting. As with other forms of hydrocephalus, alternative distal sites such as atrium, gall bladder, pleural space, or ureter are possible.

Shunts require careful monitoring. At 10 years, up to 80% of shunts placed in this setting require revision (67). There is a higher infection rate during the first few months, possibly related to the open MMC (64) and this can be decreased if the defect is closed as soon as possible after birth.

Endoscopic third ventriculostomy has been used to treat hydrocephalus in patients with CM II and MMC, with a lower rate of success (68,69). The success rate is approximately 30% when used as a primary mode of therapy (68). When used in shunted children returning with shunt malfunction, the success rate range increases from 50% to 80% (45,64,69). The increased success rate in patients with CM II and shunt malfunction can be explained by at least two reasons. First, many of these children have obstruction due to aqueductal stenosis, which may be more treatable by ETV. Secondly, ETV has a higher success rate in older children, and those presenting with shunt failure tended to be older (69).

When contemplating ETV, it is important to study the CSF flow with dynamic sequence MRI, paying particular attention to flow through the aqueduct (64). It is also important to understand the abnormal anatomy of the patient with CM II and MMC. Often the floor of the third ventricle is thicker, the third ventricle is smaller and the septum pellucidum is absent (60).

There is a higher incidence of scoliosis in those with MMC and hydrocephalus, and the scoliosis worsens in the presence of untreated hydrocephalus and improves with proper function of shunt (70,71).

OTHER CRANIOVERTEBRAL JUNCTION ANOMALIES CAUSING HYDROCEPHALUS

In addition to Chiari malformation, hydrocephalus can result from virtually any anatomic abnormality of the posterior fossa or craniovertebral junction that impairs flow of CSF from the fourth ventricle and/or venous drainage. Examples include achondroplasia, craniofacial syndromes such as Crouzon or Pfeiffer syndromes, and arachnoid scarring caused by infection or hemorrhage.

Marked stenosis of the jugular foramen with subsequent pressure differential has been demonstrated in achondroplastic patients (72,73). This has been successfully treated with a venous bypass from the transverse sinus to jugular vein (74).

An analysis of intracranial venous drainage was studied angiographically in patients with craniosynostosis-related syndrome or nonsyndromic multisutural synostosis. Fifty-one to ninety-nine percent stenosis or no flow at all was observed in the sigmoid-jugular sinus complex bilaterally in 11 patients or unilaterally in 7 patients. The authors, however, found no obvious correlation between ICP and degree of abnormality in venous anatomy. In many patients, a florid collateral circulation through the stylomastoid emissary venous plexus was noted (75).

Venous hypertension is thought to inhibit the absorption of CSF because, in order for CSF to be absorbed by the arachnoid granulations, the ICP must exceed the sagittal sinus pressure by 5 to 7 mm Hg (76–78). Venous hypertension is thought to be the cause of hydrocephalus in several syndromes including achondroplasia and craniofacial syndromes such as Crouzon and Pfeiffer syndromes. It may also develop as a consequence of congenital heart disease, diaphragmatic hernia, superior vena cava syndrome and, as mentioned above, can occur with myelomeningocele and CM II (34). When it occurs prior to fontanelle and suture closure, ventriculomegaly develops because the skull is able to enlarge. If it occurs after closure of sutures, pseudotumor cerebri develops (34).

Hydrocephalus often resolves in achondroplastic patients with continued growth of the skull base (73,79). Papilledema is rare. For this reason, a period of observation and monitoring is recommended. Some suggest that imaging studies be reserved for patients whose head circumference crosses percentiles on the achondroplastic chart or those with unexplained neurological deficits (73). When patients exhibit signs and symptoms of hydrocephalus severe enough to warrant CSF diversion, ventriculoperitoneal shunting is generally recommended, as opposed to jugular foramen decompression in both achondroplastic patients (73) and those with syndromic craniosynostosis (80).

CONCLUSIONS

Chiari I and Chiari II malformations are two conditions associated with abnormal posterior fossa and craniovertebral junction anatomy that have different etiologies, presentations, and imaging findings. CM I and CM II are associated with hydrocephalus in approximately 10% and 90%, respectively, related to changes they cause in CSF flow at the level of the craniovertebral junction. Any posterior fossa/craniovertebral junction abnormality has the potential to affect CSF flow, most commonly by fourth ventricular outlet atresia or obstruction or by abnormalities in venous flow. In nearly all symptomatic cases presenting with both hydrocephalus and Chiari malformation, the hydrocephalus must first be addressed. Hydrocephalus in the presence of CM I has been successfully treated with CSF diversion by shunting or ETV. Hydrocephalus occurring with CM II is most commonly treated with shunting alone, with limited success of ETV reported.

REFERENCES

1. Chiari H. Uber Veranderungen des Kleinhiens, des pons und der medulla oblongate. Folge von congenitaler hydrocephalie des grossherns. Deskschr Akad Wiss Wien 1895; 63:71–116.
2. Cleland J. Contribution to the study of spina bifida, encephalocele and anencephalys. J Anat Physiol 1883; 17:257–291.
3. Dyste GN, Menezes AH, VanGilder JC. Symptomatic Chiari malformations: An analysis of presentation, management and long-term outcome. J Neurosurg 1989; 71:159–168.
4. Elster AD, Chen MY. Chiari I malformations: Clinical and radiologic reappraisal. Radiology 1992; 183:347–353.
5. Mikulis DJ, Diaz O, Egglin TK, et al. Variance of the position of the cerebellar tonsils with age: Preliminary report. Radiology 1992; 183:725–728.
6. Milhorat TH, Chou MW, Trinidad EM, et al. Chiari I malformation redefined: Clinical and radiographic findings for 364 symptomatic patients. Neurosurgery 1999; 44:1005–1017.
7. Park JK, Gleason PL, Madsen JR, et al. Presentation and management of Chiari malformation in children. Pediatr Neurosurg 1997; 26:190–196.
8. Elisevich K, Fontaine S, Bertrand G. Syringomyelia as a complication of Paget's disease. J Neurosurg 1987; 67:611–613.
9. Greenlee JDW, Donovan KA, Hasan DM, et al. Chiari I malformation in the very young child: The spectrum of presentations and experience in 31 children under age 6 years of age. Pediatrics 2002; 110:1212–1219.
10. McRai DL. The significance of abnormalities of the cervical spine. Caldwell Lecture 1959. AJR Am J Roentgenol 1960; 84:3–25.
11. Menezes AH. Craniovertebral anomalies and syringomyelia. In: Cho M, Di Rocco C, Hockley A, Walker M, eds. Pediatric Neurosurgery. London, U.K.: Churchill Livingstone, 1999:151–184.
12. Schady W, Metcalfe RA, Butler P. The incidence of craniocervical bony anomalies in the adult Chiari malformation. J Neurol Sci 1987; 82:193–203.
13. Menezes AH, Greenlee JDW, Donovan KA. Honored Guest presentation: Lifetime experiences and where are we going: Chiari I with syringohydromyelia—Controversies and development of decision trees. Clin Neurosurg 2005; 52:297–305.
14. Dyste GN, Menezes AH. Presentation and management of pediatric Chiari malformations without myelodysplasia. Neurosurgery 1988; 23:589.

15. Menezes AH. Comments: Incidentally identified syringomyelia associated with Chiari I malformations: Is early interventional surgery necessary. Neurosurgery 2001; 49:641.
16. Nishikawa M, Sakamoto H, Hakuba A, et al. Pathogenesis of Chiari malformation: A morphometric study of the posterior fossa. J Neurosurg 1997; 86:40–47.
17. Chiari H. Uber Veranderungen des Kleinhirs infolge von Hydrocephalie des Grosshirns. Dtsch Med Wschr 1891; 17:1172–1175.
18. Badie B, Mendoza D, Batzdorf U. Posterior fossa volume and response to suboccipital decompression in patients with Chiari I malformation. Neurosurg 1995; 37:214–218.
19. Sgouros S, Kountouri M, Natarajan K. Posterior fossa volume in children with Chiari malformation Type I. J Neurosurg 2006; 105(suppl 2):101–106.
20. Oldfield EH, Muraszko K, Shawker TH, et al. Pathophysiology of syringomyelia associated with Chiari I malformation of the cerebellar tonsils. Implications for diagnosis and treatment. J Neurosurg 1994; 80:3–15.
21. Alzate JC, Kothbauer KF, Jallo GI, et al. Treatment of Chiari type I malformation in patients with and without syringomyelia: A consecutive series of 66 cases. Neurosurg Focus 2001; 11:1–9.
22. Menezes AH. Chiari I malformations and hydromyelia—Complications. Pediatr Neurosurg 1991–1992; 17:146–154.
23. Tubbs RS, McGirt MJ, Oaks WJ. Surgical experience in 130 pediatric patients with Chiari malformations. J Neurosurg 2003; 99:291–296.
24. Rowlands A, Sgouros S, Williams B. Ocular manifestations of hindbrain-related syringomyelia and outcome following craniovertebral decompression. Eye 2000; 14:884–888.
25. Bhangoo R, Sgouros S, Walsh AR, et al. Hindbrain-hernia-related syringomyelia without syringobulbia, complicated by permanent nocturnal central hypoventilation requiring non-invasive ventilation. Childs Nerv Syst 2006; 22:113–116.
26. Bhangoo R, Sgouros S. Scoliosis in children with Chiari I-related syringomyelia. Childs Nerv Syst 2006; 22:1154–1157.
27. Williams B. Pathogenesis of syringomyelia. In: Batzdorf U, ed. Syringomyelia: Current concepts in diagnosis and treatment. Baltimore, MD: Williams & Wilkins, 1991:59–90.
28. Aesch B, Goldenberg N, Maheut-Lourmiere J, et al. Hydrocephalie par obstruction des foramens de Luschka et Magendie chez l'adult. Rapport d'un cas. Neurochirurgie 1991; 37:269–271.
29. Amacher AL, Page LK. Hydrocephalus due to membranous obstruction of the fourth ventricle. J Neurosur 1971; 35:672–676.
30. Barr ML. Observations on the foramen of Magendie in a series of human brains. Brain 1948; 71:281–289.
31. Dandy WE. The diagnosis and treatment of hydrocephalous due to occlusions of the foramen of Magendie and Luschka. Surg Gynecol Obstet 1921; 32:112–124.
32. David M, Djahanchahiha A, Aboulker J. Obstruction of the foramina of Luschka and Magendie. Neurochirurgie 1961; 7:210–227.
33. Suehiro T, Inamura T, Natori Y, et al. Successful neuroendoscopic third ventriculostomy for hydrocephalus an syringomyelia associated with fourth ventricle outlet obstruction. Case Report. J Neurosurg 2000; 93:326–329.
34. Rekate HL. Hydrocephalus in children. In: HR Winn, eds. Youman's Neurological Surgery, 5th ed. Philadelphia, PA: WB Saunders Co., 2005:3387–3404.
35. Oakes WJ, Tubbs RS. Chiari Malformations. In: HR Winn, eds. Youman's Neurological Surgery, 5th ed. Philadelphia, PA: WB Saunders Co., 2005:3347–3361.
36. Cinalli G, Saint-Rose C, Chumas P, et al. Failure of third ventriculostomy in the treatment of aqueductal stenosis in children. J Neurosurg 1999; 90:448–454.
37. Cohen AR. Endoscopic ventricular surgery. Pediatr Neurosurg 1993; 19:127–134.
38. Decq P, LeGuerinel C, Sol JC, et al. Chiari I malformation: A rare cause of noncommunicating hydrocephalus treated by third ventriculostomy. J Neurosurg 2001; 95:783–790.
39. Goodman RR. Magnetic resonance imaging-directed stereotactic endoscopic third ventriculostomy. Neurosurgery 1993; 32:1043–1047.
40. Grant JA, McLone DG. Third ventriculostomy: A review. Surg Neurol 1997; 47:210–212.
41. Hellwig D, Heinemann A, Riegel T. Endoscopic third ventriculostomy in treatment of obstructive hydrocephalus caused by primary aqueductal stensosis. In: Hellwig D, Bauer BL, eds. Minimally Invasive Techniques for Neurosurgery. Berlin, Germany: Springer-Verlag, 1998:65–72.
42. Hoffman HJ, Harwood-nash D, Gilday DL. Percutaneous third ventriculostomy in the management of noncommunicating hydrocephalus. Neurosurgery 1980; 7:313–321.
43. Hopf NJ, Grunert P, Fries G, et al. Endoscopic third ventriculostomy: Outcome analysis of 100 consecutive procedures. Neurosurgery 1999; 44:795–806.
44. Teo C. Third ventriculostomy in the treatment of hydrocephalus: Experience with more than 120 cases. In: Hellwig D, Bauer BL, eds. Minimally Invasive Techniques for Neurosurgery. Berlin, Germany: Springer-Verlag, 1998:73–76.

45. Jones RF, Stening WA, Brydon M. Endoscopic third ventriculostomy. Neurosurgery 1990; 26: 86–92.
46. Mohanty A, Anandh B, Kolluri VR, et al. Neuroendoscopic third ventriculostomy in the management of fourth ventricular outlet obstruction. Minim Invasive Neurosurg 1999; 42:18–21.
47. Nishihara T, Hara T, Suzuki I, et al. Third ventriculostomy for symptomatic syringomyelia using flexible endoscope: A case report. Minim Invasive Neurosurg 1996; 39:130–132.
48. Zerah M. Syringomyelia in children. Neurochirurgie Suppl 1999; 1:37–57 [French].
49. Metellus P, Dufour H, Levrier O, et al. Endoscopic third ventriculostomy for treatment of noncommunicating syringomyelia associated with a Chiari I malformation and hydrocephalus: Case report and pathophysiological considerations. Neurosurgery 2002; 51:500–504.
50. el Gammal T, Mark EK, Brooks BS. MR imaging of Chiari II malformation. Am J Roentgenol 1988; 150:163–170.
51. McLone DG, Nakahara S, Knepper PA. Chiari II malformation: Pathogenesis and dynamics. Concepts Pediatr Neurosurg 1991; 11:1–17.
52. Nicolaides KH, Campbell S, Gabbe SG, et al. Ultrasound screening for spina bifida: Cranial and cerebellar signs. Lancet 1986; 2:72–74.
53. Naidich TP, Pudlowski RM, Naidich JB. Computed tomographic signs of Chiari KK malformation II: Midbrain and cerebellum. Radiology 1980; 134:391–398.
54. McLendon RE, Crain BJ, Oakes WJ, et al. Cerebral polygyria in the Chiari Type II (Arnold–Chiari) malformation. Clin Neuropathol 1985; 4:200–205.
55. Venes JL, Black KL, Latack JT. Preoperative evaluation and surgical management of the Arnold–Chiari II malformation. J Neurosurg 1986; 64:363–370.
56. Rauzzino M, Oakes WJ. Chiari II malformation and syringomyelia. Neurosurg Clin N Am 1995; 6:293–309.
57. Iskandar B, Oakes W. Chiari malformation and syringomyelia. In: Albright L, Pollack I, Adelson P, eds. Principles and Practice of Pediatric Neurosurgery. New York: Thieme, 1999:165–187.
58. McLone DG, Knepper PA. The cause of Chiari II malformation: A unified theory. Pediatr Neurosci 1989; 15:1–12.
59. Stevenson KL. Chiari type II malformation: Past, present and future. Neurosurg Focus 2004; 16:E5.
60. McLone DG, Naidich TP. Developmental morphology of the subarachnoid space, brain vasculature, and contiguous structures, and the cause of the Chiari II malformation. Am J Neuroradiol 1992; 13:463–482.
61. McLone DG. Continuing concepts in the management of spina bifida. Pediatr Neurosurg 1992; 18: 254–256.
62. Weprin BE, Oakes WJ. The Chiari malformations and associated syringohydromyelia. In: McLone DG, ed. Pediatric Neurosurgery: Surgery of the Developing Nervous System, 4th ed. Philadelphia, PA: W.B. Saunders Co., 2001:214–235.
63. Rekate HL. To shunt or not to shunt: Hydrocephalus and dysraphism. Clin Neurosurg 1985; 32: 593–607.
64. Sgouros S. Hydrocephalus with myelomeningocele. In: Cinalli G, Maixner WJ, Sainte-Rose C, eds. Pediatric Hydrocephalus. Milan, Italy: Springer, 2004:133–144.
65. Bruner JP, Tulipan N, Paschall RL, et al. Fetal surgery for myelomeningocele and the incidence of shunt-dependent hydrocephalus. JAMA 1999; 282:1819–1825.
66. Tulipan N, Bruner JP, Hernanz-Schulman M, et al. Effect of intrauterine myelomeningocele repair on central nervous system structure and function. Pediatr Neurosurg 1999; 31:183–188.
67. Saint-Rose C, Piatt JH, Renier D, et al. Mechanical complications of shunts. Pediatr Neurosurg 1991; 17:2–9.
68. Jones RF, Kwok BC, Stening WA, et al. Third ventriculostomy for hydrocephalus associated with spinal dysraphism: indications and contraindications. Eur J Pediatr Surg 1996; 6(suppl 1):5–6.
69. Teo C, Jones R. Management of hydrocephalus by endoscopic third ventriculostomy in patients with myelomeningocele. Pediatr Neurosurg 1996; 25:57–63.
70. Geiger F, Parsch D, Carstens C. Complications of scoliosis surgery in children with myelomeningocele. Eur Spine J 1999; 8:22–26.
71. Hall P, Lindseth R, Campbell R, et al. Scoliosis and hydrocephalus in myelocele patients. The effect of ventricular shunting. J Neurosurg 1979; 50:174–178.
72. Steinbok P, Hall J, Flodmark O. Hydrocephalus in achondroplasia: The possible role of intracranial venous hypertension. J Neurosurg 1989; 71:42–48.
73. Carson BS, Rigamonti D, Haroun RR. Achondroplasia and other dwarfism. In: Winn HR, eds. Youman's Neurological Surgery, 5th ed. Maryland Heights, MO: Elsevier Inc., 2005:3362–3373.
74. Saint-Rose C, LaCombe J, Pierre-Kahn A, et al. Intracranial venous sinus hypertension: Cause or consequence of hydrocephalus in infants? J Neurosurg 1984; 60:727–736.

75. Taylor WJ, Hayward RD, Lasjuanias P, et al. Enigma of raised intracranial pressure in patients with complex craniosynostosis: The role of abnormal intracranial venous drainage. J Neurosurg 2001; 94:377–385.
76. Olivero WC, Rekate HL, Chizeck HJ, et al. Relationship between intracranial and sagittal sinus pressure in normal and hydrocephalic dogs. Pediatr Neurosci 1988; 14:196–201.
77. Rekate HL, Brodkey JA, Chizeck HJ, et al. Ventricular volume regulation: A mathematical model and computer simulation. Pediatr Neurosci 1988; 14:77–84.
78. Schulman K, Ranshohoff J. Sagittal sinus venous pressure in hydrocephalus. J Neurosurg 1965; 23: 169–173.
79. Erdincler P, Dashti R, Kaynar MY, et al. Hydrocephalus and chronically increased intracranial pressure in achondroplasia. Childs Nerv Syst 1997; 13:345–348.
80. Collmann H, Sorenson N, Krauss J. Hydrocephalus in craniosynostosis: A review. Childs Nerv Syst 2005; 21:902–912.

Management of Chiari I Malformation Associated with Intracranial Hypertension

Caroline Hayhurst and Conor Mallucci

Department of Neurosurgery, The Walton Centre for Neurology and Neurosurgery, Liverpool, U.K.

Chiari I malformation is associated with symptomatic hydrocephalus in 7% to 10% of cases (1). Most authors advocate treatment of any associated hydrocephalus first as this may alleviate symptoms and prevent the need for subsequent hindbrain decompression, even in the presence of syringomyelia (2).

In our institution, we routinely manage symptomatic ventriculomegaly associated with Chiari I malformation using endoscopic third ventriculostomy (ETV). This technique was first reported in 1996 by Nishihara et al. (3). There were early concerns that the prepontine cistern is effaced in this patient group, potentially increasing operative risks. However, several subsequent case reports have demonstrated the efficacy of ETV for treatment of hydrocephalus in Chiari I malformation and in addition for resolution of symptoms and radiographic improvement of syringomyelia (4–7). Between 1996 and 2006 we managed 16 patients with hydrocephalus and Chiari I malformation with initial ETV. In our series, the mean age at presentation was 31.9 years and the mean duration of follow-up was 42 months. Fifteen patients underwent primary ETV and one patient underwent ETV at the time of shunt malfunction. Six patients in the series had a spinal syrinx on preoperative spinal imaging and this was asymptomatic in one patient. All patients had symptoms and signs of raised intracranial pressure. Three patients had symptoms of raised ICP only and five had syringomyelia, the remaining eight patients had classical Chiari related symptoms, such as strain-induced headache, facial numbness, ataxia, upper limb weakness, and dysesthesia.

Fifteen patients remain shunt free following ETV (94%). The single case of ETV failure is a 54-year-old female who had previously had a ventriculoperitoneal shunt for hydrocephalus associated with Chiari I malformation. The patient presented with headaches and right facial numbness secondary to shunt obstruction, with ventriculomegaly and aqueduct stenosis with Chiari I malformation on MR imaging. Following ETV and removal of the shunt the patient continued to experience cough-induced headaches and facial numbness and underwent foramen magnum decompression two months after ETV. The patient's symptoms resolved for two years then recurred at which time re-do ETV showed a patent stoma and a ventriculoperitoneal shunt was inserted.

The ventricular size reduced in only five patients following ETV, and the mean level of tonsillar descent form the basion-opisthion line changed from 15 mm prior to ETV and 13.3 mm after ETV.

All patients had improvement of raised ICP-related symptoms. Table 1 shows the impact of ETV according to symptom category. Of the 16 patients, 6 (37.5%) required foramen magnum decompression following initial management with ETV. The mean time to decompression surgery was six months after the initial ETV (range 0.5–12 months). All six patients demonstrated minimal improvement in symptoms (other than symptoms of raised ICP) following initial ETV, including strain-related headache. All six patients had resolution of strain-related headache following hindbrain decompression and no patients suffered complications at the time of decompression related to hydrocephalus. All patients had improvement of their facial and upper limb symptoms; however, four patients continue to have intermittent upper limb sensory disturbance.

In the six patients with a spinal syrinx, the syrinx reduced in length and caliber or disappeared following ETV alone in five patients. One patient had an asymptomatic syrinx. Two patients (33%) with syringomyelia had persistent marked symptoms following ETV, despite radiological improvement of the appearance of the syrinx cavity

Table 1 Outcome Following ETV by Symptom Category

Symptom category	Symptoms resolved with ETV alone			Syrinx reduction	FMD
	ICP	Chiari	Syrinx		
Raised ICP only (8)	3/3 (100%)	–	–	0/1	–
Chiari (3)	7/8 (88%)	4/8 (50%)	–	–	4/8 (50%)
Syringomyelia (2)	5/5 (100%)	3/3 (100%)	3/5 (60%)	5/5	2/5(40%)

and progressed to hindbrain decompression following which the symptoms improved leaving upper limb sensory changes in one patient and upper limb dysesthesia in the other.

There were no complications at the time of ETV related to raised ICP. One patient had a small extradural hematoma found on postoperative imaging after ETV. This was asymptomatic and was managed conservatively. In patients who progressed to hindbrain decompression, there were no complications as a result of raised intracranial pressure, such as CSF leak, which one would expect if the hydrocephalus is inadequately treated.

We would advocate that ETV replaces the ventricular shunt in the management of Chiari I malformation associated with overt hydrocephalus. In up to 60% of cases, ETV may provide definitive management avoiding unnecessary hindbrain decompression, using a single technique with a very low complication rate.

Decq et al. (5) suggest there is a subset of patients whose symptoms are solely attributable to a disturbance of CSF flow and that treatment of the Chiari malformation in such cases is not mandatory. However, identifying this subset of patients prior to any intervention is difficult, as it does not appear to be solely those who have ventricular dilatation. It is clear that a proportion of patients with Chiari malformation may have acquired tonsillar ectopia due to primary aqueduct stenosis or idiopathic intracranial hypertension (IIH) (8). Conversely, Chiari malformation has been noted in up to 6% of patients diagnosed with IIH (9). In patients with small ventricles who demonstrate any symptoms or signs of raised ICP, we routinely perform ICP monitoring and place a VP shunt if monitoring confirms high pressure (Fig. 1).

The pathophysiology of Chiari I malformation remains poorly understood. However, a proportion manifests either overt hydrocephalus or idiopathic intracranial hypertension, and addressing this can provide definitive long-term resolution.

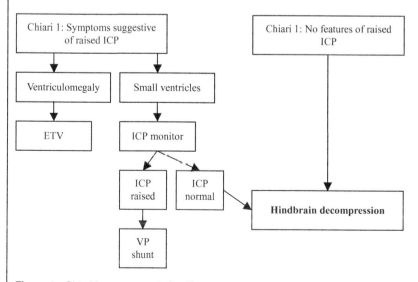

Figure 1 Chiari I management algorithm.

REFERENCES

1. Tubbs RS, McGirt MJ, Oakes WJ. Surgical experience in 130 pediatric patients with Chiari I malformations. J Neurosurg 2003; 99:291–296.
2. Krayenbuhl H. Evaluation of the different surgical approaches in the treatment of syringomyelia. Clin Neurol Neurosurg 1975; 77:111–128.
3. Nishihara T, Hara T, Suzuki I, et al. Third ventriculostomy for symptomatic syringomyelia using flexible endoscope: Case report. Minim Invasive Neurosurg 1996; 39:130–132.
4. Buxton N, Jaspan T, Punt J. Treatment of Chiari malformation, syringomyelia and hydrocephalus by neuroendoscopic third ventriculostomy. Minim Invasive Neurosurg 2002; 45:231–234.
5. Decq P, Le Guerinel C, Sol JC, et al. Chiari I malformation: A rare cause of noncommunicating hydrocephalus treated by third ventriculostomy. J Neurosurg 2001; 95:783–790.
6. Metellus P, Dufour H, Levrier O, et al. Endoscopic third ventriculostomy for treatment of noncommunicating syringomyelia associated with a Chiari I malformation and hydrocephalus: Case report and pathophysiological considerations. Neurosurgery 2002; 51:500–503, discussion 503–504.
7. Mohanty A, Suman R, Shankar SR, et al. Endoscopic third ventriculostomy in the management of Chiari I malformation and syringomyelia associated with hydrocephalus. Clin Neurol Neurosurg 2005; 108:87–92.
8. Fagan LH, Ferguson S, Yassari R, et al. The Chiari pseudotumor cerebri syndrome: Symptom recurrence after decompressive surgery for Chiari malformation type I. Pediatr Neurosurg 2006; 42:14–19.
9. Johnston I, Jacobson E, Besser M. The acquired Chiari malformation and syringomyelia following spinal CSF drainage: A study of incidence and management. Acta Neurochir (Wien) 1998; 140:417–427, discussion 427–418.

The Treatment of Hydrocephalus in Children with Achondroplasia

Triantafyllos Bouras and Spyros Sgouros

Department of Neurosurgery, "Attikon" University Hospital, University of Athens, Athens, Greece

Achondroplasia is often accompanied by neurological complications attributed commonly to compression of neural structures by osseous and ligamentary abnormalities. Neural disorders per se (i.e., cortical atrophy, aqueductal stenosis) exist as well but are less frequent (1). A variety of neurological findings, which can be present in an achondroplastic child (Table 1), may trigger further imaging and neurophysiologic evaluation. Hydrocephalus, which is often present in imaging studies performed as a part of the diagnostic process, raises a challenging neurosurgical problem, as the mechanism, clinical significance, and ideal treatment in these cases remain ambiguous. The rate of ventricular dilatation among achondroplastic patients has been cited to be between 15% and 50% (2,3). However, the percentage of cases where operative treatment is necessary is estimated to be much lower.

The possible mechanism for the pathogenesis of ventricular dilatation in an achondroplastic patient is in dispute. Occasionally, an aqueductal stenosis is the evident cause of an obstructive hydrocephalus (1); besides, another mechanism described as leading to noncommunicating hydrocephalus is the obstruction of the foramina of Magendie and Luschka caused by foramen magnum stenosis (4). Nevertheless, in the majority of cases the hydrocephalus is communicating (1,5–7). Although various pathogenic mechanisms have been proposed, brain venous outflow impairment caused by jugular foramen stenosis is currently considered the most valid (2,5,7–10). This hypothesis is supported by findings of both digital subtraction angiography (8) and, more recently, magnetic resonance venography (MRV) (2,9), while intracranial venous hypertension has been substantiated by direct venous sinus pressure measurement (8). Another important finding is that, at least in some cases, high intraventricular pressure coexists with high pressure in the subdural spaces (5), which may be correspondingly dilated.

The clinical course of ventricular dilatation in achondroplastic patients varies. Usually, there are no signs of intracranial hypertension, while, even in initially symptomatic cases the size of the ventricles often stabilizes and the patient compensates and remains asymptomatic (1). On the other hand, a wide spectrum of symptoms attributable to hydrocephalus and the concomitant intracranial hypertension may persist, necessitating its prompt treatment. Notwithstanding this, it is difficult to document a certain etiologic relation, as various symptoms may result from other pathologies (1,11). Macrocephaly, which could be attributed to hydrocephalus, has been advocated to be a primary disorder of the syndrome (12,13). The majority of the most frequent symptoms (myelopathy, sleep disorders, and in infants hypotonia, feeding problems, apnea, poor head control) are convincingly attributed to medullary compression, characteristically complicating the course of many of these patients (1,3,11). The sudden infant death syndrome, whose prevalence among achondroplastic infants is three-times the one of general population, is also a consequence of cervicomedullary compression (1,11). Finally, psychomotor delay is often attributed to chronic hypoxemia due to pneumonopathy, recurrent pulmonary infections, and apnea (11).

INDICATIONS FOR TREATMENT

Given the above-mentioned ambiguities, it is evident that the first question to be answered when facing an achondroplastic child with ventricular dilatation is whether to treat or not. In general, a conservative strategy is proposed at first in most cases (3). Observation of head circumference is of vital importance, along with careful watch for possible signs of raised intracranial pressure (bulging fontanels, prominent scalp veins, Parinaud's sign),

Table 1 Neurological Symptoms and Signs in
39 Pediatric Patients with Achondroplasia (14)

Sign/symptom	Percentage
Hypotonia	58.9
Weakness	30.7
Hyporeflexia	30.7
Macrocephaly	28.2
Quadriparesis	15.4
Hyperreflexia	12.9
Sensory deficit	10.2

which, when present, should precipitate surgical intervention. However, the course of slight macrocephaly and ventricular dilatation, even when accompanied by mild delay in achieving normal developmental milestones, is often benign as they both stabilize and the affected children return within normal (or borderline) limits concerning growth indices.

In any case, when neurological symptoms are present, a possibly coexistent cervicomedullary compression should be carefully sought, as it is more likely as their probable cause and more urgent to be treated. In the absence of neurological symptoms and signs, in general, it is avoided to perform decompression of the foramen magnum before the age of two years, as despite the dramatic radiological appearance often after the age of two, it improves and never requires surgical treatment (Fig. 1).

A probable role for detailed imaging may rise in doubtful cases. Indeed, the demonstration of ventricular dilatation alone may not be enough as an indication for treatment, and this may be the case even in symptomatic patients. Venous narrowing in the jugular foramina presented in MRV has been shown to correlate with hydrocephalus, but it is not discussed whether this finding is correlated with outcome after certain treatment methods (2). Moreover, another study implies that venous outflow obstruction does not always result in hydrocephalus and suggests that MRV should be performed only when cervicomedullary decompression is scheduled (9).

The study of cerebrospinal fluid (CSF) dynamics may also provide information (9); performance of phase-contrast flow studies could be justified in cases where hydrocephalus

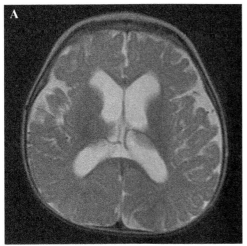 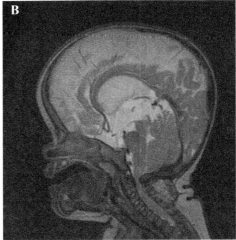

Figure 1 MR scans of a 12-month-old girl with achondroplasia and macrocephaly. Left: Axial T2-weight. Right: Sagittal T2-weight image. There is mild ventricular dilatation and compression at the cranio-cervical junction. The child was observed as she did not develop symptoms and signs of intracranial hypertension or medullary compression. She did not require neither shunting, nor.

coexists with severe medullary compression programmed to be operated upon. A possible deterioration of CSF dynamics and/or the presence of increased intraventricular pressure could jeopardize the result of foramen magnum decompression (7).

Finally, invasive intracranial pressure measurement has been used in order to document the need for shunting (14), although this would be regarded too invasive for most patients.

TREATMENT OPTIONS

In the vast majority of cases, standard ventriculoperitoneal shunting is the indicated method for the treatment of hydrocephalus in achondroplastic children (7,8,14). The usual communicating underlying mechanism renders the realization of third ventriculostomy inappropriate. However, it is described as a viable option in cases of triventricular hydrocephalus. In these cases, the operation can prove demanding as malformation of the floor of the third ventricle can be present (15).

The decompression of foramen magnum only rarely leads to recession of hydrocephalus, even in cases with obstruction of the foramina of the fourth ventricle caused by stenosis of the foramen magnum, and a shunting procedure is almost always needed. Nevertheless, the effectiveness of decompression considering the treatment of hydrocephalus is not negligible according to other authors (7) and it has been cited as being more effective in cases with poor collateral venous outflow (5).

Finally, at least one patient has been reported as treated by venous decompression in the jugular foramen (5), based on the fact that increased intracranial venous pressure and the concomitant deterioration of CSF absorption are the possible underlying mechanisms of hydrocephalus in achondroplasia.

REFERENCES

1. Gordon N. The neurological complications of achondroplasia. Brain Dev 2000; 22(1):3–7.
2. Moritani T, Aihara T, Oguma E, et al. Magnetic resonance venography of achondroplasia: Correlation of venous narrowing at the jugular foramen with hydrocephalus. Clin Imaging 2006; 30(3):195–200.
3. Ryken TC, Menezes AH. Cervicomedullary compression in achondroplasia. J Neurosurg 1994; 81:43–48.
4. Yamada H, Nakayama S, Tajima M, et al. Neurological manifestations of pediatric achondroplasia. J Neurosurg 1981; 54:49–57.
5. Lundar T, Bakke SJ, Nornes H. Hydrocephalus in an achondroplastic child treated by venous decompression at the jugular foramen. Case report. J Neurosurg 1990; 73(1):138–140.
6. Steinbok P, Hall J, Flodmark O. Hydrocephalus in achondroplasia: The possible role of intracranial venous hypertension. J Neurosurg 1989; 71:42–48.
7. Yamada Y, Ito H, Otsubo Y, et al. Surgical management of cervicomedullary compression in achondroplasia. Childs Nerv Syst 1996; 12(12):737–741.
8. Friedman WA, Mickle JP. Hydrocephalus in achondroplasia: A possible mechanism. Neurosurgery 1980; 7(2):150–153.
9. Rollins N, Booth T, Shapiro K. The use of gated cine phase contrast and MR venography in achondroplasia. Childs Nerv Syst 2000; 16(9):569–575, discussion 575–577.
10. Sainte Rose C, LaCombe J, Pierre A, et al. Intracranial venous sinus hypertension: Cause or consequence of hydrocephalus in infants? J Neurosurg 1984; 60(4):727–736.
11. Ruiz-Garcia M, Tovar-Baudin A, Del Castillo-Ruiz V, et al. Early detection of neurological manifestations in achondroplasia. Childs Nerv Syst 1997, 13(4):208–213.
12. Hecht JT, Butler IJ. Neurologic morbidity associated with achondroplasia. J Child Neurol 1990; 5:84–97.
13. Horton WA, Rotter JI, Rimoin DL, et al. Standard growth curves for achondroplasia. J Pediatrics 1978; 93:435–438.
14. Erdinçler P, Dashti R, Kaynar MY, et al. Hydrocephalus and chronically increased intracranial pressure in achondroplasia. Childs Nerv Syst 1997; 13(6):345–348.
15. Etus V, Ceylan S. The role of endoscopic third ventriculostomy in the treatment of triventricular hydrocephalus seen in children with achondroplasia. J Neurosurg 2005; 103(suppl 3):260–265.

18 | Syringomyelia

Spyros Sgouros

Department of Neurosurgery, "Attikon" University Hospital, University of Athens, Athens, Greece

INTRODUCTION

Syringomyelia is defined as the condition of cystic cavitation of the spinal cord extending over a distance more than two spinal segments. The term is derived from the word "syrinx," an ancient Greek word meaning "tube," also describing an ancient Greek reed musical organ similar to a flute, in direct reference to the ancient Greek legend of Pan, who was chasing a nymph by a river, when she preferred to turn to a nest of reeds rather than be molested by Pan. The syringomyelia cavity contains fluid with consistency similar to cerebrospinal fluid (CSF). It was described first in 1892 (1). The advent of magnetic resonance imaging (MRI) in the last 15 years has contributed greatly to the understanding of syringomyelia, and its wide use has resulted in an apparent increase in the incidence of diagnosis both in adults and in children, but the pathophysiology surrounding the formation of the syrinx and its propagation is still unclear. Syringomyelia can cause major neurological dysfunction in arms and legs and bulbar dysfunction. If untreated or if treatment fails to control its progress, it can lead to paraplegia, quadriplegia, bulbar palsy, and death.

EPIDEMIOLOGY

Syringomyelia has a prevalence of 8.4 cases per 100,000 population (2). It is estimated that in the United States only 21,000 individuals suffer from syringomyelia. Chiari I malformation has an estimated incidence of 7% in the general population (2). The incidence of posttraumatic syringomyelia is around 1% to 3% of all paraplegics (3–10). There is a male predominance and with relatively young age. The time between spinal injury and symptomatic presentation may vary from a few months to 30 years with an average interval of seven years.

PATHOPHYSIOLOGY

In the majority of patients, the presence of syringomyelia is associated with impaired cranio-caudal flow of CSF in the spinal subarachnoid space (2,11–14). Significant laboratory research has been done to simulate the creation of syringomyelia (15–18). The commonest association is with hindbrain herniation in the context of Chiari I malformation, which is the prolapse of the cerebellar tonsils for 5 mm or more beyond the foramen magnum. In large clinical series, 50% to 80% of patients with symptomatic Chiari I malformation may have syringomyelia (19–32). Chiari II malformation is less frequently associated with syringomyelia. Less often the block in CSF flow is due to tethered cord secondary to a variety of dysraphic malformations (diastematomyelia, spinal lipoma), as well as spinal cord tumors, spinal arachnoid cysts, posttraumatic or postinfective arachnoiditis, or rare congenital abnormalities around the region of the foramen magnum such as achondroplasia (14,33–35). On very rare occasions no other pathology can be found to coexist or cause syringomyelia, which is thus regarded as idiopathic. Syringomyelia commonly affects the cervical and upper thoracic spinal cord, although it can extend throughout the entire spinal cord, holocord syringomyelia. It can expand cranially to occupy the medulla, syringobulbia.

Although the presence of abnormal fluid dynamics can explain in part the propagation of syringomyelia, it is still unclear how the syrinx cavity is formed on the first place. Several theories have been proposed on the formation and propagation of syringomyelia. The most notable ones in chronological order are Gardner's theory of "water hammer" effect of CSF pulsations, Williams' theory of "suck" and "slosh," and Heiss' and Oldfield's theory of increased subarachnoid CSF pressure. Potential spaces along the vessels of the cord have been described by Virchow and Robin. In experimental studies, dye injected in the spinal subarachnoid space has been found in the central canal (36) and is believed to have arrived there traveling along the

Virchow–Robin spaces. There have been reports of a presyringomyelia state seen in MR scans of patients with Chiari I malformation, as judged by the presence of upper cervical spinal cord swelling, which subsequently developed syringomyelia cavity (37–39).

Gardner observed that the foramen of Magendie was occluded by a membrane, and as the fourth ventricle was partially obstructed, he believed that fluid entered the central canal in the region of the obex at the floor of the fourth ventricle due to the "water hammer" effect of the arterial pulsations on CSF flow. Subsequently, fluid accumulated inside the central canal and created syringomyelia cavity—the so-called communicating syringomyelia (40,41). This view was reinforced by contrast studies that showed that after injection in the cerebral ventricles, contrast reached the syringomyelia cavity. This led to the operative concept of obex plugging, where a piece of muscle or cotton wool was used to plug or obliterate the obex, hoping to disrupt the influx of CSF in the syringomyelia cavity (41). With the advent of MR scan, it became evident that this theory was not entirely accurate, as in the majority of patients there was no communication seen between the obex and the syringomyelia cavity—noncommunicating syringomyelia (42). Another classification stemming from that era was that of canalicular (within the central canal) and extracanalicular (beside the central canal) syringomyelia (42), which is less relevant today, after MR observations.

Williams described in the pre-MR era a mechanism of expansion of the syringomyelia cavity. He described the concept of pressure dissociation between the head and the spine secondary to the block of the hindbrain hernia. Every time a Valsalva maneuver takes place (e.g., coughing, straining), the pressure from the cavities of the chest and abdomen is transmitted to the inside of the spinal canal through the valveless venous plexus around the vertebral bodies. In the presence of a partial subarachnoid block, fluid is forced upwards past the block more efficiently than it can run down again. This leads to a collapsed theca below the block, which exerts a suction effect on the spinal cord. This is the "suck" mechanism. In response to pressure changes, the movement of the syrinx fluid can be violent enough to extend the excavation of the cavity both cranially and caudally. This is the "slosh" mechanism (14,43–45). Williams believed that in cases where no communication with the obex was present, CSF was forced in to the cord along the Virchow–Robin spaces, but could not explain adequately the formation of syringomyelia cavity. Williams' theories were partly verified by MRI scan observations. Using phase-contrast (PC) MR it has been shown that in the presence of hindbrain hernia, CSF movement in the region of the foramen magnum differs between systole and diastole. Nevertheless, Williams' observations of pressure differential were not confirmed by other studies of intraoperative CSF pressure measurements and is believed that the sitting position that he used to obtain his measurements contributed to exaggerated pressure readings due to CSF leakage from the site of the spinal measuring needle (2).

From studies based on phase-contrast MR scanning, Oldfield's group observed that during systole the syrinx cavity contracts, whereas if Gardner's theory was correct it should expand under the force of influxing CSF. CSF velocity was increased at the region of the foramen magnum but CSF flow was decreased, cervical subarachnoid CSF pressure was increased, spinal CSF compliance was decreased, and syrinx CSF flowed caudally during systole and cranially during diastole. The cerebellar tonsils act like a piston partially occluding the subarachnoid space. This creates increased CSF pressure wave along the length of the syringomyelic cord, which has been measured intraoperatively (2,13,46). It is believed that raised subarachnoid CSF pressure in the site of syrinx formation leads to CSF been forced within the spinal cord. While these observations have given new insights in the movement of CSF in and around the spinal cord, they do not adequately explain as yet the mechanism of creation of the syringomyelia cavity.

In patients who suffer spinal cord trauma, cord contusion leads to edema, blood effusion, and subsequent liquefaction leading in a proportion of cases, up to 50%, to cavity formation opposite the fracture site, the so-called a "primary cyst" (47). There may be more than one primary cyst. Syringomyelia cavities are much bigger and longer above and/or below the primary cysts and are separated from them by a septum (9,10). The syrinx may go flat above and below the injury site following treatment, while the primary cysts may remain unchanged. As the acute injury settles, the inflammation is followed by adhesions in the subarachnoid space and gliosis in the cord (47). Narrowing of the bony spinal canal from the spinal fracture can compound further the obstruction of the CSF pathways at the fracture site, where fluid may enter the cord (10).

In patients with spinal cord tumors, it is believed that the presence of tumor causes dilatation of the spinal cord and contributes to subarachnoid obstruction of CSF circulation. In most cases, removal of the tumor leads to disappearance of syringomyelia (48). For forms of syringomyelia associated with other pathologies (dysraphic states, spinal cord tumors, spinal arachnoid cysts), there has been no satisfactory explanation of how CSF enters the spinal cord, and an analogy to the hindbrain hernia–related syringomyelia is currently considered as valid. Of interest is that in contrast to diastematomyelia or spinal lipoma, patients with tethered cord due to thickened filum terminale almost never develop syringomyelia, which further strengthens the view that the presence of arachnoid adhesions contributes to the development of subarachnoid CSF circulation block.

In principle, it is believed that the presence of an obstruction in the subarachnoid space is important in the propagation of syringomyelia, and for this reason surgical treatments are designed to remove such a subarachnoid obstruction.

Posterior Fossa Volume in Chiari I Malformation

Early two-dimensional studies on lateral skull radiographs demonstrated that the height or the area of the posterior fossa is small in patients with Chiari I malformation (49). Recent studies used advanced image analysis techniques to calculate posterior fossa volume in CT or MR scans. All these studies conclude that the posterior fossa is smaller than normal in patients with Chiari I malformation due to presumed maldevelopment of the occipital endochondrium (21,50–52). In a study of children with symptomatic Chiari I malformation requiring surgical treatment, it was demonstrated that patients with Chiari I alone have posterior fossa of normal volume, whereas patients with Chiari I and syringomyelia have posterior fossa volume significantly smaller than normal. This difference was more pronounced in children who presented before the age of 10 years (53,54). After the age of 10 years, there is no significant change in the growth of the cranium overall and little change in the growth of the skull base. The presence of a small posterior fossa underpins to a large extent the philosophy of surgical treatment of hindbrain hernia with craniovertebral decompression that has evolved in the last two decades. Recently, growth hormone deficiency has been identified in children with Chiari I malformation (52).

Although in most patients the Chiari I malformation is considered congenital, acquired Chiari I malformation is well described (e.g., following lumbar or ventricular shunting, in the presence of a posterior fossa tumor) (55), which may imply that the new development of Chiari I malformation may be related more to altered CSF dynamics than posterior fossa dimensions.

In addition to the size of the posterior fossa, it has been postulated that localized venous hypertension and possible altered geometry of the posterior fossa could initiate the downward migration of the cerebellum, which subsequently is perpetuated by CSF movement and impaction. Thus, it appears that foramen magnum decompression probably works by allowing disimpaction of the tonsils from the craniovertebral junction, rather than by "enlarging" the posterior fossa, as the tonsils never move to occupy the newly enlarged cisterna magna, but ascend to a normal location (56). In that line, there is a universal tendency for reduction of the size of the craniectomy in the foramen magnum.

Recently, it has been postulated that patients with normal posterior fossa and Chiari I malformation may suffer in fact from an occult tethered cord syndrome, whereby the spinal cord is "pulled" by a filum terminale under tension, even though the spinal cord ends at the normal level. Some of these patients have responded to division of the filum (57).

CLINICAL FEATURES

Presenting Symptoms

The symptoms can be grouped into those of pain, sensory and motor deficits, and disordered autonomic functions. Severity of symptoms can vary and there are patients who remain completely symptom free for long time periods. A significant proportion (up to 14%) of patients with radiologically identified Chiari I malformation do not experience any symptoms and their malformation is identified incidentally during investigations for other reasons (58).

Patients with hindbrain hernia–related syringomyelia often present with symptoms from the Chiari I malformation, and the syringomyelia is discovered when an MR scan is performed on suspicion of hindbrain hernia. Symptoms associated with Chiari I malformation include headaches usually occipital but often poorly localized, worse on physical exertion and straining, occasionally clumsiness and poor coordination with hands, and ocular symptoms such as blurred vision, diplopia, or oscillopsia. Other rare symptoms are dizziness, unsteadiness (disequilibrium), tinnitus, vertigo, hyperacusis, nystagmus, dysphagia, sleep apnea, dysarthria, tremor, facial pain or numbness, shortness of breath, and syncopal (drop) attacks.

Symptoms relevant to the presence of syringomyelia include weakness or clumsiness of arms and/or legs, which may not be following a myotomal distribution, paraesthesia, dysesthesiae, and pain, which may not be following a dermatomal distribution, unsteady gait, muscle atrophy, and spasticity. Pain is commonly a prominent feature. Urinary and fecal incontinence and impotence in male patients are seen infrequently. The location of symptoms may not be correlated with radiology and can be even unilateral. Syringobulbia can be life threatening. The commonest symptom of syringobulbia is spreading facial numbness. Swallowing and voice may also be affected, as well as vision, hearing, and respiratory function.

Clinical Examination Findings

In patients with Chiari I malformation or syringobulbia, clinical examination findings include lower cranial nerves and cerebellar sings. In patients with syringomyelia, long tract signs are common. Neuro-ophthalmological findings include impaired visual acuity, extraocular muscle palsy, nystagmus, and papilledema in a small minority. Other signs from lower cranial nerves include facial sensory loss, sensorineural hearing loss, impaired vestibular function, vocal cord palsy, and impaired gag reflex. Cerebellar sings such as dysmetria or truncal ataxia are not uncommon.

Clinical examination findings associated with syringomyelia include weakness of arms and/or legs, not always following a myotomal distribution and sensory deficits over arms and/or legs, not always following dermatomal distribution. Unilateral weakness of one upper limb, not infrequently associated with a sudden strain and associated pain, is commonly seen. The small muscles of the hand are often affected first and wasted as well as the triceps or the shoulder musculature. In advanced cases, claw deformity in the hand with wasting of all the forearm and arm musculature can occur. Sensory loss can be of spinothalamic and/or dorsal column type, occasionally in patchy distribution. It is usually unilateral and tends to involve the upper limb early. The traditionally described pain/temperature dissociation, which is loss of pain and temperature sensation with preserved light touch and joint position sense, is uncommon. Dystrophic (Charcot) joints can develop. Hyper- or hyporeflexia can be present depending on the level of syringomyelia. Asymmetry is not uncommon and certain reflexes may be unexpectedly spared. Spasticity can affect upper and/or lower limbs. Scoliosis is a common symptom/sign of syringomyelia in young children or in previously undiagnosed young adults. Short neck and low hair line is seen in patients with basilar invagination. Horner's syndrome is seen infrequently. Dry skin or hyperhidrosis can be observed.

In patients with spinal cord injury, incomplete paraplegia, which deteriorates, or the development of new autonomic features may be associated with syringomyelia. The most important features are those that ascend. Descending syrinx is rarely diagnosed. In complete paraplegia, improvement of leg spasms, alteration of sweating patterns, and impairment of other autonomic functions such as bladder and bowel control and sexual function could imply downward extension of the syrinx. Pain is common in posttraumatic syringomyelia, a paraplegic complaining of severe pain has syringomyelia until proven otherwise. It is frequently associated with straining and progression of neurological deficit. Although it is commonly experienced at the level of the deficit, it can affect sites above or below that level and can be misleading. It can be confused with chest or abdominal pathology. Often it is soon replaced by dysesthetic sensory loss.

RADIOLOGY

Once a patient is suspected to harbor syringomyelia, MRI scan is the investigation of choice, which confirms the diagnosis in most cases. In the pre-MR era, CT scan with intrathecal

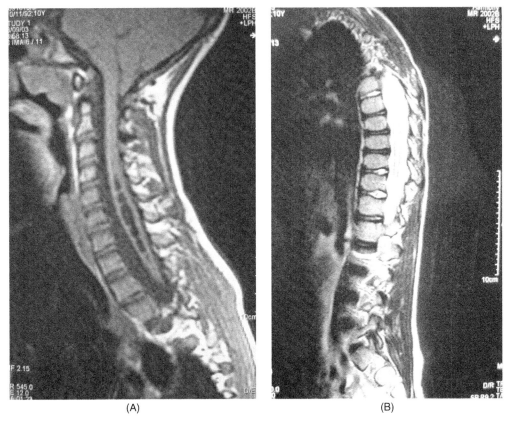

(A)   (B)

Figure 1   MR scans of a 10-year-old boy who presented with progressive scoliosis and persistent headaches, mostly at the back of the head. (**A**) T1W sagittal MR scan of the posterior fossa and the upper cervical spine. There is a Chiari I malformation with tonsillar herniation down to C1. There is a significant syringomyelia cavity starting from C5, with septations. Because of scoliosis, the thoracic part of the spine is not seen well. (**B**) T2W sagittal MR of the lower thoracic and lumbar spine. The syringomyelia cavity is extending down to the lower thoracic spine. Because of the scoliosis, the spine is not seen in all its length in a single image, and hence it is difficult to count the spinal level of the inferior border of the syringomyelia cavity.

metrizamide was employed, acquiring late views to see contrast in the syringomyelia cavity. Post-myelography CT scan remains still useful in patients with severe claustrophobia or magnetic implants. Plain radiographs of the spine are useful in patients with scoliosis and when a bony malformation of the craniocervical junction is suspected. Whenever the issue of possible instability arises, flexion-extension views can provide more information on spinal stability. In patients with posttraumatic syringomyelia, plain radiographs often show posttraumatic kyphosis and associated narrowing of the spinal canal.

MRI scanning shows the presence of Chiari malformation and the extent of the syringomyelia cavity and septa (Fig. 1). T2-weighted sequences are particularly useful in visualizing the fluid filled syringomyelia cavity. In a small percentage of patients (around 15%) hydrocephalus exists at presentation in association to the Chiari I malformation and syringomyelia. Information relating to the CSF circulation around the cord can be obtained with phase-contrast cardiac-gated MR, but its practical usefulness in the surgical management is currently limited, as it cannot differentiate symptomatic from asymptomatic patients (59–62). Sequential MR imaging is useful in assessing the results of treatment or in observing patients who have not been treated over periods of time (63).

Diastematomyelia and spinal lipomas are clearly seen, and commonly the syringomyelia cavity is not as dilated as when Chiari-related (Fig. 2). Posttraumatic syringomyelia shows well in MR scans, although in some patients with extensive spinal fractures, it may be difficult to identify the extent of the bony injury (Fig. 3). This is not a problem usually from the management

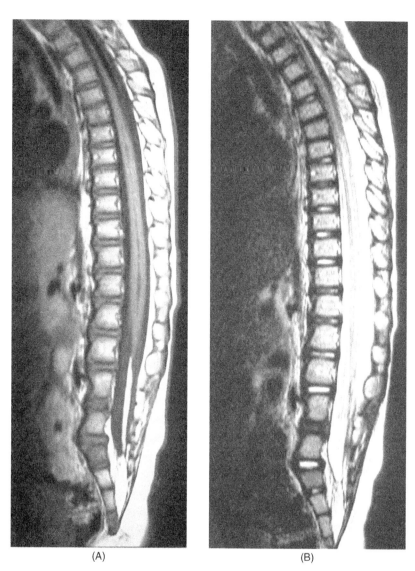

(A) (B)

Figure 2 MR scans of a 13-month-old girl who was born with a red discoloration of the skin in the midline of the lumbar region. (**A**) Spinal sagittal T1W scan. A lipoma of the filum is seen causing spinal cord tethering. A syringomyelia cavity is seen extending from T7 to L1. (**B**) Spinal sagittal T2W scan. The extent of the syringomyelia cavity is shown better.

point of view, because posttraumatic syringomyelia presents well after the injury and spinal stability is not an issue. The relation of the syringomyelia cavity with any primary cysts is usually shown well. Children with profound scoliosis can be difficult to visualize in MR scanning due to the curvature of the spine, making impossible to have the entire spinal cord in a single sagittal view (Fig. 1). Children with significant scoliosis can have syringomyelia in the absence of Chiari I malformation. Spinal cord tumors are clearly identified in contrast-enhanced MR sequences (Fig. 4). Whenever a patient is found to have syringomyelia in the absence of a clearly identifiable associated lesion, contrast-enhanced sequences should be obtained to exclude the presence of spinal cord tumors. There is a small minority of patients in whom no associated lesion is identified, hence they have idiopathic syringomyelia. In some of these patients, arachnoid webs are present in the spinal subarachnoid space, which may be difficult to visualize with any radiological examination.

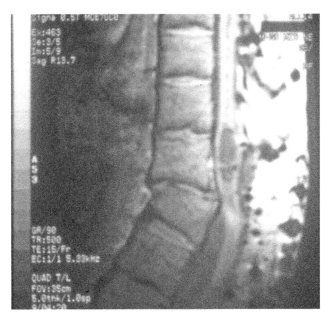

Figure 3 T1W sagittal MR scan of the thoracic spine of a 35-year-old man who was victim of a motor vehicle accident, during which he sustained a spinal fracture and remained paraplegic ever since. For the last few months prior to this scan, the patient had started experience increasing pain down the legs. A wedge fracture of the body of T8 vertebra is seen, the spinal cord is damaged at the fracture site, and a small primary cyst is shown. Just above the fracture site there is a significant syringomyelia cavity, significantly large for one spinal level, but extending much thinner for several levels higher.

Neurophysiological Tests

Nerve conduction studies, brain stem evoked potentials (BSEP), and somatosensory evoked potentials (SSEP) have been used in the study of patients with syringomyelia. It has not been easy to use such tests to tailor the indication for surgery, as normal neurophysiological tests do not imply the absence of threat of neurological deterioration (64,65). Usually, they are abnormal when clinical symptoms or signs have been established. Nevertheless, they may prove useful in the follow up of patients treated surgically. BSEP and SSEP can be useful intraoperatively in selected patients, for example, with spinal cord tumors.

Natural History of Chiari I Malformation and Syringomyelia

Patients with symptomatic Chiari I malformation, with or without syringomyelia, are universally considered for surgery, unless other overriding medical reasons are prohibitive. The controversy surrounds the management of asymptomatic patients with Chiari I malformation, without syringomyelia, and this is largely due to the poorly charted natural history of the disease. There are no prospective studies outlining the natural history of hindbrain hernia and syringomyelia. A recently published retrospective series of pediatric patients with asymptomatic Chiari I malformation and no syringomyelia who were followed up for several years showed that most patients did not deteriorate with time (66).

A completely asymptomatic patient with Chiari I malformation without syringomyelia can be managed at first conservatively and followed closely. The controversy centers on what constitutes asymptomatic hindbrain hernia. In most patients who can give history themselves, on close questioning there is clear evidence of cough-induced headache or occipital pain. Some even admit to arm pain on exertion. In small children, motor developmental delay of mild degree is frequently seen in both arm dexterity and fluency of walking. All such cases should be seen as symptomatic patients and considered for treatment. Other more subtle symptoms and signs such as drop attacks or eye signs can go unnoticed. There is a spectrum of symptom intensity, and the doctor's response is relevant to his expertise in the field.

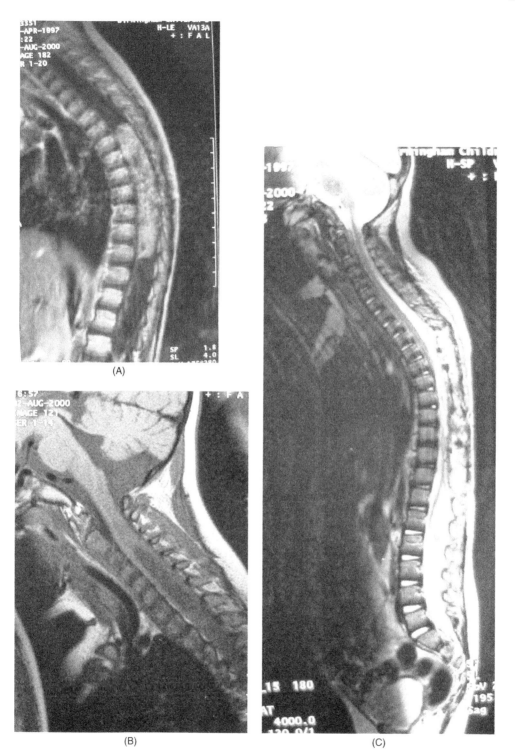

Figure 4 Spinal MR scans of a 3-year-old girl who presented with a new limp of the right leg. (**A**) Sagittal T1W scan with intravenous contrast injection. A large intramedullary tumor, contrast enhancing, is seen in the mid and lower thoracic region, extending over 7 spinal segments. Large syringomyelia cavities are seen above and below the tumor. (**B**) Sagittal T1W scan of the posterior fossa and the cervical and upper thoracic spine. The syringomyelia cavity is extending cranially up to the level of C3. (**C**) Postoperative T2W sagittal scan. The tumor has been removed and the syringomyelia cavity has disappeared.

Similarly, the natural history of untreated syringomyelia is not charted conclusively. Syringomyelia if untreated usually follows a progressive course over a number of years in most patients, although the time spectrum that such a deterioration occurs in not well defined. The neurological function of arms and legs can deteriorate if the syringomyelia cavity continues to extend, and such patients may end up quadriplegic. The cavity may extend both cranially and caudally, causing damage to the surrounding parenchyma of the spinal cord. Long-standing syrinx provokes gliosis formation in the cavity walls and the surrounding cord, which can cause progressive axonal loss (14,67). Even though surgical treatment may lead to radiologic improvement or complete resolution of the syrinx cavity, this is often not associated with clinical improvement. The syringomyelia cavity can reach the upper cervical cord and medulla, syringobulbia; it may destroy neurological function in the arms and eventually affect the function of the lower brain stem, producing respiratory paralysis and death.

A small number of patients with untreated Chiari I–related syringomyelia remain stable over long periods, years at times, with no neurophysiological abnormalities even in the presence of a large syrinx. In such patients, especially children, it is difficult to advise on risk from sports and other intense activities. It is difficult to postulate on the risk of sudden neurological deterioration, although such a complication is well documented. The development of abnormal nerve conduction studies already indicates compromise of neuronal tissue and commonly directs towards surgical treatment.

Indications for Surgical Treatment

- In patients with Chiari I malformation with or without syringomyelia, the presence of symptoms and clinical findings relevant to either of the conditions constitutes an indication surgical treatment with craniovertebral decompression. Similarly, a tense syrinx occupying the cervical cord, even if asymptomatic, merits surgical treatment, as it potentially threatens the medulla and vital neurological functions. On the other hand, the patient with a small, two level cavity and with no symptoms relating to the syrinx, can be watched with repeat MR scans annually.
- The presence of scoliosis in children with Chiari I malformation and syringomyelia even in the absence of other neurological symptoms requires surgical treatment with craniovertebral decompression to stabilize the progress of scoliosis (68–71). Most orthopedic surgeons would not contemplate surgical correction of the scoliosis in the presence of untreated hindbrain hernia and syringomyelia, as the risk of postoperative paraplegia or quadriplegia is significant.
- Patients with posttraumatic syringomyelia in general merit early surgery to avoid progressive neurologic deterioration.
- In patients with dysraphic states, the syringomyelia rarely constitutes a problem and an indication for surgery and often it remains unchanged after successful cord untethering. Nevertheless, the presence of cord tethering due to untreated diastematomyelia or spinal lipoma in association to neurological symptoms and/or signs necessitates the relevant untethering procedure.
- Patients with spinal cord tumors usually require surgical treatment for their tumor. Successful tumor excision commonly leads to reduction of the syringomyelia cavity (Fig. 4). Re-enlargement of the cavity after initial successful treatment commonly implies tumor recurrence.
- Patients with spinal arachnoid cysts and syringomyelia commonly require surgical excision of the cyst.
- Patients with postinflammatory syringomyelia present particular difficulties because commonly they have significant neurological deficits from their condition even before syringomyelia develops, and it is not always easy to appreciate if the development of radiological syringomyelia is associated with the onset of new symptoms. When a clear link is established between radiological and clinical deteriorations, surgery should be pursued. If such a clear link is not apparent, a period of observation and six-monthly repeat scanning may be preferable.

SURGICAL MANAGEMENT OF HINDBRAIN HERNIA–CHIARI I MALFORMATION

It is established principle that surgical management of hindbrain hernia should involve craniovertebral decompression, aiming to remove the block of CSF flow in the region of the foramen magnum due to the prolapsed tonsils (13,14,20,23,31,72–77). Syringopleural or syringosubarachnoid shunts should not be used as primary treatment, because they have a very poor success rate in the presence of an operative subarachnoid block, which acts as a filling mechanism for the syringomyelia (67).

Controversy still exists on whether the arachnoid matter should be opened or not during craniovertebral decompression. Both techniques have very similar success rate of around 80% (72). Apart from the bony compression that the occipital bone is exerting on the prolapsing cerebellum at the region of the foramen magnum, a dominant factor contributing to the block in CSF circulation is the arachnoiditis and severe adhesions, which are usually the result of the long-standing tonsillar herniation and impaction. Failure to divide such adhesions is a potential source of recurrence. Another source of potential failure when leaving the arachnoid intact is an unrecognized tear, which can lead to formation of a subdural collection of CSF in the region of the foramen magnum. Recently, intraoperative ultrasound scanning (US) has been used to decide on the need to open the arachnoid. This has been employed widely, but it appears that the absence of intraoperative flow of CSF at the region of the foramen Magendie may be an indication for opening the arachnoid membrane (78).

Another controversial issue is the use of dural graft to enlarge the cisterna magna. The published results are similar for both grafting and nongrafting techniques. Adhesion formation around the graft can trigger recurrence of CSF block in the region of the cisterna magna, especially in young children who tend to regrow part of the removed foramen magnum. The use of foreign material as a graft has a higher risk of infective complications and recurrent adhesion formation. Instead fascia lata or pericranium appears to be better tolerated. On the other hand, nongrafting is associated with higher risk of need for repeat surgery (14,23,26,73).

The postoperative complication rate for craniovertebral decompression is low. Wound infection, meningitis, subdural hematoma, urinary tract infection, and thromboembolic complications have all been observed at a low rate. CSF leak seems to be slightly higher when a dural graft has not been employed during craniovertebral decompression. A state of sterile meningitis affects a significant number of patients after craniovertebral decompression, more often when the arachnoid has been opened, and is usually self-limiting after the first few days, occasionally requiring a short course of steroids. Perioperative mortality is rare. A very small percentage of patients suffer catastrophic complications such as posterior fossa hematoma, transverse sinus thrombosis, and brainstem infarction due to posterior inferior cerebellar artery damage. Cerebellar sagging or slump has been reported as delayed side effect of craniovertebral decompression. It was more common in the 1980s and early 1990s and presented with combination of intractable headaches and lower cranial nerve signs. In recent years, there has been a tendency for smaller occipital craniectomy, which appears to have reduced the incidence of this complication.

Surgical Management of Posttraumatic Syringomyelia

The current treatment of posttraumatic syringomyelia includes decompressive laminectomy, subarachnoid space reconstruction by adhesiolysis, opening up of the subarachnoid pathways past the fracture site, and the formation of a surgical meningocele (3,4,6–10,79,80). This results in collapse of the syrinx in 80% of patients. Syringosubarachnoid and syringopleural shunts have been widely used in the 1970s and 1980s with encouraging early results, but recently their long-term effectiveness has been questioned (67,81–85). Infection of the drain, as well as mechanical problems, has been reported. The drain functions for some time, the cord collapses around it, and the draining holes become occluded by gliotic tissue. Subsequently, the syrinx refills if the filling mechanism has not been addressed surgically. The use of drains now has little place in the initial management of syringomyelia. The technique of omental graft transposition has been tried and did not offer any substantial benefits, hence it has been abandoned (86).

Surgical Management of Recurrent Syringomyelia

Early recurrence of syringomyelia after initial reduction following successful surgery calls for reexploration of the craniovertebral junction and extensive dissection of the adhesions in the regions of all the foramina of the fourth ventricle (75,87). This surgical strategy is associated with an average success rate (60%). Surgical variations include the use of stents in the foramen of Magendie to avoid recurrent adhesions, which have been reported to offer good long-term control of the syringomyelia. If that fails, then as a last measure a syringopleural shunt could be attempted, with only a 40% chance of success. Overall, patients with recurrent syringomyelia and/or recurrent arachnoiditis in the region of the foramen magnum pose significant challenge on their long-term management, and they do not have good long-term outcome, as they continue to deteriorate over a number of years.

Recurrent posttraumatic syringomyelia after initially successful surgical treatment requires repeat exploration of the fracture site and adhesiolysis. This procedure tends not to have good long-term success. Similarly, recurrent postinflammatory syringomyelia pauses formidable surgical challenges, as the results of repeat surgery are not rewarding. If repeat adhesiolysis fails, as a last measure a syringopleural shunt can be attempted, with limited chances of success.

Management of the Associated Hydrocephalus

Traditionally, hydrocephalus when present should be treated first, before a craniovertebral decompression. Often, initial ventricular shunting reduces the size of syrinx cavity but rarely reverts the presence of Chiari I malformation and almost never avoids the need for craniovertebral decompression. Recently, endoscopic third ventriculostomy has been used to treat hydrocephalus with good results on syringomyelia resolution (88). In patients with hydrocephalus, a ventriculoperitoneal shunt and syringomyelia that have been controlled well, development of recurrent enlargement of the syringomyelia cavity implies shunt obstruction until proven otherwise. Shunt revision should be performed first before any other strategy is contemplated.

Treatment Outcome

Up to 80% of patients with Chiari I–related syringomyelia experience clinical and/or radiological improvement after craniovertebral decompression. Following successful treatment many symptoms improve with a varying pattern. Headaches associated with Chiari I malformation and most other neurological symptoms improve well. Established neurological deficits such as sensory loss and weakness, muscle wasting, and severe lower cranial nerve palsies improve little or none at all. Increased tone or hyperreflexia and established spasticity from syringomyelia improves little and not uncommonly other surgical options have to be employed (e.g., intrathecal Baclofen).

In paraplegics, loss of pain sensitivity leads to other problems, particularly if the motor system is intact and the patient uses the arms energetically. Trophic changes may supervene in skin or joints. Multiple burns, and a tendency to self-mutilation affecting the intellectually challenged, have been observed. The fingers may become coarsely thickened and painless hands may be damaged by a wheelchair. Damage to joints that have lost pain sensation may be severe. Such damaged joints are called neuropathic or Charcot joints. About half of them are painful. In the shoulder, the head of the humerus may rapidly absorb. Around the elbow the joint tends to become overgrown with massive osteophytes, limitation of movement is common. Paraplegic patients have increased risk of developing cervical spondylosis, possibly related to increased use of their arms as a result of the paraplegia.

Up to 15% of the patients do not experience radiological resolution of the syringomyelia after adequate surgical treatment. Most of them end up having reexploration of the craniovertebral junction and it appears that in most of them there are residual arachnoid adhesions at the region of the foramen of Magendie, division of which appears to lead to radiological improvement of syringomyelia.

A significant number of patients continue to deteriorate clinically, despite radiological improvement after surgery. It is believed that progressive gliosis around the syrinx walls may be responsible for the continued deterioration.

Intracranial Hypertension and Syringomyelia

Intracranial hypertension may be more common among patients with isolated Chiari I malformation than previously realized, especially children. Routine systematic detailed ophthalmoscopy can detect papilledema, which if left untreated can cause blindness. There have been reports of an incidence of up to 13% of papilledema in patients with hindbrain hernia with or without syringomyelia and some patients may have raised intracranial hypertension without papilledema (89,90). The incidence of intracranial hypertension in the absence of papilledema remains unknown and may well be more frequent than initially thought.

REFERENCES

1. Abbe R, Coley WB. Syringomyelia, operation—exploration of cord—withdrawal of fluid—exhibition of patient. J Nerv Mental Dis 1892; 19:512–520.
2. Heiss JD, Patronas N, DeVroom HL, et al. Elucidating the pathophysiology of syringomyelia. J Neurosurg 1999; 91:553–562.
3. Barnett HJM, Botterell EH, Jousse AT, et al. Progressive myelopathy as a sequel to traumatic paraplegia. Brain 1966; 89:159–173.
4. Edgar RE, Quail P. Progressive post-traumatic cystic and non-cystic myelopathy. Br J Neurosurg 1994; 8:7–22.
5. Frankel HL. Ascending cord lesion in the early stages following spinal injury. Paraplegia 1969; 6:111–118.
6. Lyons BM, Brown DJ, Calvert JM, et al. The diagnosis and management of post traumatic syringomyelia. Paraplegia 1987; 25:340–350.
7. Rossier AB, Foo D, Shillito J, et al. Posttraumatic cervical syringomyelia. Brain 1985; 108:439–461.
8. Shannon N, Symon L, Logue V, et al. Clinical features, investigation and treatment of post-traumatic syringomyelia. J Neurol Neurosurg Psychiatry 1981; 44:35–42.
9. Williams B, Terry AF, Jones HWF, et al. Syringomyelia as a sequel to traumatic paraplegia. Paraplegia 1981; 19:67–80.
10. Williams B. Post-traumatic syringomyelia, an update. Paraplegia 1990; 28:296–313.
11. Milhorat TH, Capocelli AL, Anzil AP, et al. Pathological basis of spinal cord cavitation in syringomyelia: Analysis of 105 autopsy cases. J Neurosurg 1995; 82:802–812.
12. Milhorat TH, Miller JI, Johnson WD, et al. Anatomical basis of syringomyelia occurring with hindbrain lesions. Neurosurgery 1993; 32:748–754.
13. Oldfield EH, Muraszko K, Shawker TH, et al. Pathophysiology of syringomyelia associated with Chiari I malformation of the cerebellar tonsils. Implications for diagnosis and treatment. J Neurosurg 1994; 80:3–15.
14. Williams B. Syringomyelia. Neurosurg Clin N Am 1990; 1:653–685.
15. Bertram CD, Brodbelt AR, Stoodley MA. The origins of syringomyelia: Numerical models of fluid/structure interactions in the spinal cord. J Biomech Eng 2005; 127(7):1099–1109.
16. Carpenter PW, Berkouk K, Lucey AD. Pressure wave propagation in fluid-filled co-axial elastic tubes. Part 2: Mechanisms for the pathogenesis of syringomyelia. J Biomech Eng 2003; 125(6):857–863.
17. Chang HS, Nakagawa H. Hypothesis on the pathophysiology of syringomyelia based on simulation of cerebrospinal fluid dynamics. J Neurol Neurosurg Psychiatry 2003; 74:344–347.
18. Cho KH, Iwasaki Y, Imamura H, et al. Experimental model of posttraumatic syringomyelia: The role of adhesive arachnoiditis in syrinx formation. J Neurosurg 1994; 80:133–139.
19. Anderson NE, Willoughby EW, Wrightson P, et al. The natural history of syringomyelia. Clin Exp Neurol 1986; 22:71–80.
20. Attenello FJ, McGirt MJ, Gathinji M, et al. Outcome of Chiari-associated syringomyelia after hindbrain decompression in children: Analysis of 49 consecutive cases. Neurosurgery 2008; 62:1307–1313.
21. Badie B, Mendoza D, Batzdorf U. Posterior fossa volume and response to suboccipital decompression in patients with Chiari I malformation. J Neurosurg 1995; 37:214–218.
22. Di Lorenzo N, Fortuna A, Guidetti B. Craniovertebral junction malformations. Clinicopathological findings, long-term results, and surgical indications in 63 cases. J Neurosurg 1982; 57:603–608.
23. Durham SR, Fjeld-Olenec K. Comparison of posterior fossa decompression with and without duraplasty for the surgical treatment of Chiari malformation Type I in pediatric patients: A meta-analysis. J Neurosurg Pediatrics 2008; 2:42–49.
24. Dyste GN, Menezes AH, VanGilder JC. Symptomatic Chiari malformations. An analysis of presentation, management, and long term outcome. J Neurosurg 1989; 71:159–168.
25. Fenoy AJ, Menezes AH, Fenoy KA. Craniocervical junction fusions in patients with hindbrain herniation and syringohydromyelia. J Neurosurg Spine 2008; 9:1–9.

26. Hayhurst C, Richards O, Zaki H, et al. Hindbrain decompression for Chiari–syringomyelia complex: An outcome analysis comparing surgical techniques. Br J Neurosurg 2008; 22:86–91.

27. Menezes AH. Chiari I malformations and hydromyelia-complications. Pediatr Neurosurg 1991–1992; 17:146–154.

28. Menezes AH. Honoured guest presentation: Lifetime experiences and where we are going: Chiari I with syringohydromyelia controversies and development of decision trees. Clin Neurosurg 2005; 52:297–305.

29. Milhorat TH, Chou MW, Trinidad EM, et al. Chiari I malformation redefined: Clinical and radiographic findings for 364 symptomatic patients. Neurosurgery 1999; 44:1005–1017.

30. Payner TD, Prenger E, Berger TS, et al. Acquired Chiari malformations: Incidence, diagnosis, and management. Neurosurgery 1994; 34:429–434.

31. Tubbs RS, McGirt MJ, Oakes WJ. Surgical experience in 130 pediatric patients with Chiari I malformations. J Neurosurg 2003; 99:291–296.

32. Williams B, Sgouros S, Nenji E. Cerebrospinal fluid drainage for syringomyelia. Eur J Pediatr Surg 1995; 5 (suppl I):27–30.

33. Batzdorf U. Primary spinal syringomyelia. Invited submission from the joint section meeting on disorders of the spine and peripheral nerves, March 2005. J Neurosurg Spine 2005; 3(6):429–435.

34. Holly LT, Batzdorf U. Syringomyelia associated with intradural arachnoid cysts. J Neurosurg Spine 2006; 5(2):111–116.

35. Mauer UM, Freude G, Danz B, et al. Cardiac-gated phase-contrast magnetic resonance imaging of cerebrospinal fluid flow in the diagnosis of idiopathic syringomyelia. Neurosurgery 2008; 63:1139–1144.

36. Ball MJ, Dayan AD. Pathogenesis of syringomyelia. Lancet 1972; 2:799–801.

37. Fischbein NJ, Dillon WP, Cobbs C, et al. The "presyrinx" state: A reversible myelopathic condition that may precede syringomyelia. AJNR AM J Neuroradiol 1999; 20:7–20.

38. Goh S, Bottrell CL, Alken AH, et al. Presyrinx in children with Chiari malformations. Neurology 2008; 71:351–356.

39. Levy EI, Heiss JD, Kent MS, et al. Spinal cord swelling preceding syrinx development. Case report. J Neurosurg 2000; 92(suppl 1):93–97.

40. Gardner JW. Hydrodynamic mechanism of syringomyelia: Its relationship to myelocele. J Neurol Neurosurg Psychiatry 1965; 28:247–259.

41. Gardner WJ, Angel J. The mechanism of syringomyelia and its surgical correction. Clin Neurosurg 1959; 6:131–140.

42. Milhorat TH, Johnson WD, Miller JI, et al. Surgical treatment of syringomyelia based on magnetic resonance imaging criteria. Neurosurgery 1992; 31:231–245.

43. Williams B, Page N. Surgical treatment of syringomyelia with syringopleural shunting. Br J Neurosurg 1987; 1:63–80.

44. Williams B. A critical appraisal of posterior fossa surgery for communicating syringomyelia. Brain 1978; 101:223–250.

45. Williams B. Simultaneous cerebral and spinal fluid pressure recordings. Cerebrospinal dissociation with lesions at the foramen magnum. Acta Neurochir 1981; 59:123–142.

46. Sansur CA, Heiss JD, DeVroom HL, et al. Pathophysiology of headache associated with cough in patients with Chiari I malformation. J Neurosurg 2003; 98(3):453–458.

47. Kakoulas B. Pathology of spinal injuries. Central Nerv Syst Trauma 1984; 1:117–129.

48. Samii M, Klekamp J. Surgical results of 100 intramedullary tumours in relation to accompanying syringomyelia. Neurosurgery 1994; 35:865–873.

49. Nyland H, Krogness KG. Size of posterior fossa in Chiari Type 1 malformation in adults. Acta Neurochir 1978; 40:233–242.

50. Nishikawa M, Sakamoto H, Hakuba A, et al. Pathogenesis of Chiari malformation: A morphometric study of the posterior cranial fossa. J Neurosurg 1997; 86:40–47.

51. Stovner LJ, Bergan U, Nilsen G, et al. Posterior cranial fossa dimensions in the Chiari I malformation: Relation to pathogenesis and clinical presentation. Neuroradiology 1993; 35:113–118.

52. Tubbs RS, Wellons JC III, Smyth MD, et al. Children with growth hormone deficiency and Chiari I malformation: A morphometric analysis of the posterior cranial fossa. Pediatr Neurosurg 2003; 38:324–328.

53. Sgouros S, Kountouri M, Natarajan K. Posterior fossa volume in children with Chiari malformation Type I. J Neurosurg 2006; 105(2 Suppl Pediatr):101–106.

54. Sgouros S, Kountouri M, Natarajan K. Skull base growth in children with Chiari malformation type I. J Neurosurg 2007; 107(3 Suppl Pediatr):188–192.

55. Chumas PD, Armstrong DC, Drake JM, et al. Tonsillar herniation: The rule rather than the exception after lumboperitoneal shunting in the pediatric population. J Neurosurg 1993; 78:568–573.

56. Duddy MJ, Williams B. Hindbrain migration after decompression for hindbrain hernia: A quantitative assessment using MRI. Br J Neurosurg 1991; 5:141–152.
57. Milhorat TH. Classification of syringomyelia. Neurosurg Focus 2000; 8(3):E1.
58. Meadows J, Kraut M, Guarneri M, et al. Asymptomatic Chiari Type I malformations identified on magnetic resonance imaging. J Neurosurg 2000; 92:920–926.
59. Armonda RA, Citrin CM, Foley KT, et al. Quantitative cine-mode magnetic resonance imaging of Chiari I malformations: An analysis of cerebrospinal fluid dynamics. Neurosurgery 1994; 35:214–224.
60. Baledent O, Gondry-Jouet C, Stoquart-Elsankari S, et al. Value of phase contrast magnetic resonance imaging for investigation of cerebral hydrodynamics. J Neuroradiol 2006; 33(5):292–303.
61. McGirt MJ, Nimjee SM, Floyd J, et al. Correlation of cerebrospinal fluid flow dynamics and headache in Chiari I malformation. Neurosurgery 2005; 56:716–721.
62. McGirt MJ, Nimjee SM, Fuchs HE, et al. Relationship of cine phase-contrast magnetic resonance imaging with outcome after decompression for Chiari I malformation. Neurosurgery 2006; 59(1):140–146, discussion 140–146.
63. Wetjen NM, Heiss JD, Oldfield EH. Time course of syringomyelia resolution following decompression of Chiari malformation Type I. J Neurosurg Pediatrics 2008; 1:118–123.
64. Anderson NE, Frith RW, Synek VM. Somatosensory evoked potentials in syringomyelia. J Neurol Neurosurg Psychiatry 1986; 49:1407–1410.
65. Kakigi R, Shibasaki H, Kuroda Y, et al. Pain-related somatosensory evoked potentials in syringomyelia. Brain 1991; 114:1871–1889.
66. Novegno F, Caldarelli M, Massa A, et al. The natural history of the Chiari Type I anomaly. J Neurosurg Pediatrics 2008; 2:179–187.
67. Sgouros S, Williams B. A critical appraisal of drainage in syringomyelia. J Neurosurg 1995; 82:1–10.
68. Arai S, Ohtsuka Y, Moriya H, et al. Scoliosis associated with syringomyelia. Spine 1993; 18:1591–1592.
69. Bhangoo R, Sgouros S. Scoliosis in children with Chiari I-related syringomyelia. Childs Nerv Syst 2006; 22:1154–1157.
70. Ghanem IB, Londono C, Delalande O, et al. Chiari I malformation associated with syringomyelia and scoliosis. Spine 1997; 22:1313–1317.
71. Ono A, Suetsuna F, Ueyama K, et al. Surgical outcomes in adult patients with syringomyelia associated with Chiari malformation type I: The relationship between scoliosis and neurological findings. J Neurosurg Spine 2007; 6(3):216–221.
72. Hoffman CE, Souweidane MM. Cerebrospinal fluid related complications with autologous duraplasty and arachnoid sparing in type I Chiari malformation. Neurosurgery 2008; 62(3 suppl 1):156–160.
73. Munshi I, Frim D, Stine-Reyes R, et al. Effects of posterior fossa decompression with and without duraplasty on Chiari malformation-associated hydromyelia. Neurosurgery 2000; 46:1384–1390.
74. Rhoton AL. Microsurgery of Arnold–Chiari malformation in adults with and without hydromyelia. J Neurosurg 1976; 45:473–483.
75. Sacco D, Scott RM. Reoperation for Chiari malformations. Pediatr Neurosurg 2003; 39:171–178.
76. Sahuquillo J, Rubio E, Poca MA, et al. A surgical technique for the treatment of Chiari I malformation and Chiari I/Syringomyelia complex—Preliminary results and Magnetic Resonance Imaging quantitative assessment of hindbrain migration. Neurosurgery 1994; 35:874–884.
77. Yundt KD, Park TS, Tantuwaya VS, et al. Posterior fossa decompression without duraplasty in infants and young children for treatment of Chiari malformation and achondroplasia. Pediatr Neurosurg 1996; 25:221–226.
78. Milhorat TH, Bolognese PA. Tailored operative technique for Chiari Type I malformation using intraoperative color Doppler ultrasonography. Neurosurgery 2003; 53:899–906.
79. Klekamp J, Batzdorf U, Samii M, et al. Treatment of syringomyelia associated with arachnoid scarring caused by arachnoiditis or trauma. J Neurosurg 1997; 86:233–240.
80. Sgouros S, Williams B. Management and outcome of post-traumatic syringomyelia. J Neurosurg 1996; 85:197–205.
81. Barbaro NM, Wilson CB, Gutin PH, et al. Surgical treatment of syringomyelia. Favorable results with syringoperitoneal shunting. J Neurosurg 1984; 61:531–538.
82. Batzdorf U, Klekamp J, Johnson JP. A critical appraisal of syrinx cavity shunting procedures. J Neurosurg 1998; 89:382–388.
83. Lesoin F, Petit H, Thomas CE, et al. Use of the syringoperitoneal shunt in the treatment of syringomyelia. Surg Neurol 1986; 25:131–136.
84. Padovani R, Cavalo M, Gaist G. Surgical treatment of syringomyelia: Favorable results with syringo-subarachnoid shunting. Surg Neurol 1989; 32:173–180.

85. Tator CH, Meguro K, Rowed DW. Favourable results with syringosubarachnoid shunts for treatment of syringomyelia. J Neurosurg 1982; 56:517–523.

86. Sgouros S, Williams B. A critical appraisal of pediculated omental graft transposition in progressive spinal cord failure. Br J Neurosurg 1996; 10:547–553.

87. Tubbs RS, Webb DB, Oakes WJ. Persistent syringomyelia following pediatric Chiari I decompression: Radiological and surgical findings. J Neurosurg 2004; 100(Suppl Pediatr 5):460–464.

88. Hayhurst C, Osman-Frah J, Das K, et al. Initial management of hydrocephalus associated with Chiari malformation Type I–syringomyelia complex via Endoscopic third ventriculostomy: An outcome analysis. J Neurosurg 2008; 108:1211–1214.

89. Poca MA, Sahuquillo J, Ibanez J, et al. Intracranial hypertension after surgery in patients with Chiari I malformation and normal or moderate increase in ventricular size. Acta Neurochir Suppl 2002; 81:35–38.

90. Sgouros S, Willshaw H. Intracranial hypertension associated with Chiari I malformation. Childs Nerv Syst 2006; 22:1053–1054.

Surgery for Chiari I Malformation and Syringomyelia

John J. Oró

The Chiari Care Center, Neurosurgery Center, The Medical Center of Aurora, Aurora, Colorado, U.S.A.

The decision to offer surgical treatment to a person harboring CM I is based on (*i*) an appropriate clinical presentation, (*ii*) exclusion of conditions presenting in a similar fashion, (*iii*) the impact of the symptoms on the quality of life, and (*iv*) the findings on imaging studies. The goals of surgery are (*i*) establishment of normal or near-normal cerebrospinal fluid flow at the craniocervical junction and (*ii*) decompression of the neural tissues. The techniques used should minimize the surgical risks.

According to Ellenbogen et al. (1), over 20 different operations for CM I have been described. The most commonly used approach includes removal of bone from the subocciput (the bone below the external occipital protuberance or inion), a C1 laminectomy, opening of the dura matter, and the suturing of a patch graft. However, many surgical variations exist and no consensus has developed.

SURGICAL CASE

Before reviewing the variations and their rationale, let us consider treatment of a person with a Chiari I malformation with 14 mm of tonsillar herniation and crowding at the craniocervical junction.

After induction of general anesthesia, the patient is positioned prone on the surgical table with the head supported using a three-pin head holder. Hair is clipped from the midline at the back of the head and the area is prepped in a sterile fashion. An incision is created in the midline extending from the inion to the C2 level.

The muscles are separated in the midline exposing the subocciput and the arch of C1. Using surgical bone instruments, bone is removed from the subocciput including the posterior margin of the foramen magnum. The arch of the C1 vertebra is also removed.

The exposed dura matter is then opened in a Y-shaped fashion revealing the transparent arachnoid membrane and the cerebellar tonsils. The arachnoid membrane is opened and fine arachnoid bands extending to the tonsils or spinal cord are sectioned with microinstruments. The degree of tonsillar crowding is then evaluated (Fig. 1).

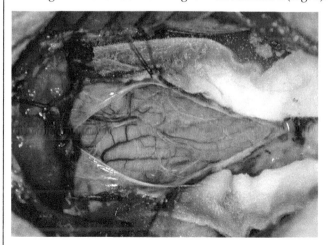

Figure 1 Craniovertebral decompression. After craniectomy the dura and the arachnoid have been opened to expose the prolapsed cerebellar tonsils.

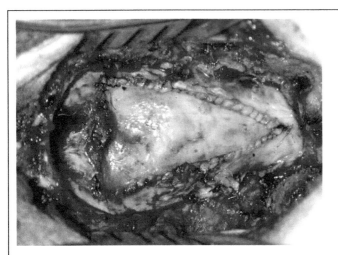

Figure 2 After decompression of the craniovertebral junction, the dura is closed with a graft, which is sutured water tight.

If the intradural space at the craniocervical junction remains crowded following dural opening, the tips of one or both tonsils can be shrunk using a bipolar cautery forceps. Care is taken to avoid cauterization of the tonsillar surfaces that will come in contact with the dura or each other following closure.

When a syrinx is present, the author believes it is important to separate the tonsils and evaluate the foramen of Magendie, the midline outlet of the fourth ventricle. If a veil (a retained rhombic roof) is found covering the outlet, it is sectioned with microinstruments. High microscopic visualization is used to avoid brainstem injury.

A patch graft is then sewn to the edges of the open dura in order to expand the intradural space (Fig. 2). The author's choice is autogenous pericranium obtained through a small linear incision just above the inion.

Although the benefit of performing a cranioplasty has not been proven, it may be of benefit. The author uses a customized titanium mesh plate to cover the upper two-thirds of the decompression (Fig. 3). The suboccipital musculature previously reflected can now be sutured to the plate for a more natural wound closure.

Both wounds are then closed. Patients are usually discharged on the second postoperative day (day 3 in the hospital), although some may need an additional day or two.

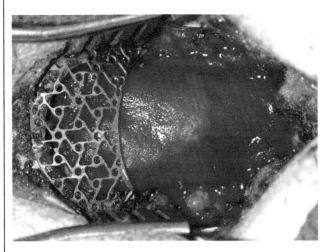

Figure 3 A titanium mesh plate can be used to cover the upper two-thirds of the decompression.

SURGICAL VARIATIONS

While the above case demonstrates one approach to the posterior fossa decompression procedure, many variations exist.

Size of Bony Decompression

The appropriate size of the posterior fossa decompression described in the literature varies widely. Too much bone removal risks cerebellar slump. Too little bone removal can result in decreased benefit. Customization based on the extent of herniation, the degree of compression, and the anatomy of the region is important. In 2003, Milhorat and Bolognese (2) described tailoring the operative technique using intraoperative ultrasonography.

Should the Dura Be Opened?

Since the earliest surgical reports, posterior fossa decompression for CM I has included opening of the dura matter. Advantages include a wider decompression and the ability to perform intradural procedures such as the release of arachnoid adhesions and shrinkage of the cerebellar tonsils.

In 2000, Munshi et al. (3) reported the results of surgery in 23 patients with duraplasty compared with 11 patients undergoing an extradural approach (bony decompression without duraplasty). Of the extradural patients, 73% improved, 1 developed a superficial wound infection, and 2 required reoperation with duraplasty. Of those undergoing duraplasty, 87% improved, 2 developed CSF leak, and 1 developed aseptic meningitis.

In 2008, Hayhurst et al. (4) reported 16 patients with CM I with or without syringomyelia treated with extradural decompression. Headaches resolved in only 50% of the patients and dysesthetic pain and weakness did not improved in 60%. The authors suggest "that bone decompression should only be reserved for patients with isolated headache."

Should the Arachnoid Be Opened?

At times, only the dura matter is open, leaving the arachnoid membrane intact. The advantages of not opening the arachnoid include a lower risk of pseudomeningocele, external CSF leak, meningitis, and surgical adhesions.

The advantages of opening the arachnoid include the ability to lyse adhesions, shrink the cerebellar tonsils as needed, and evaluate for a "veil" over the foramen of Magendie in cases with syringomyelia.

Shrinkage or Resection of the Tonsils

As noted by Alden et al. in 2001 (5), tonsillar shrinkage or resection has been advocated "as a way to improve the volume mismatch and to increase communication between the fourth ventricle and the spinal compartment." "No neurological deficit has been demonstrated as a result of tonsillar resection; however, the exact function of this structure is largely unknown."

The case against tonsillar shrinkage or resection includes the finding that the cerebellar tonsils can reshape and ascend following decompression. In addition, although the function of the tonsils is unknown, our understanding of the cerebellum is changing and recent evidence suggests that the cerebellum contributes to such cognitive processes as working memory, multitasking, and word finding.

Should the Dura Be Closed or Left Open?

Duddy and Williams (6) and Krieger et al. (7) advocate leaving the dura open and closing only the muscle and skin layers. However, Alden et al. (5) notes "Other authors have emphasized that duraplasty is essential for the prevention of scar formation and recurrent symptoms." Regardless of the choice, the presence of subarachnoid blood should be minimized because it can result in adhesions and hydrocephalus.

Graft Material for Duraplasty

Among the most troublesome complications of Chiari surgery is cerebrospinal fluid (CSF) leak. A persistent leak can lead to a collection of spinal fluid within the tissues of the neck, called a pseudomeningocele. This pocket of fluid, sometimes quite large, can crowd the foramen magnum resulting in recurrence of symptoms. If not repaired, the duraplasty may adhere to the neural tissues. If severe enough, this scarring is difficult, if not impossible, to treat and can lead to life-long symptoms. If spinal fluid leaks through the skin, meningitis can occur and also cause arachnoid scarring.

Neurosurgeons have used a variety of graft materials for duraplasty with varying success. Synthetic materials include polyesterurethane, polyglactin 910 mesh, and expanded polytetrafluoroethylene (ePTFE). Biological options include bovine pericardium, porcine small intestinal submucosa, collagen matrix, and autograft pericranium (external periosteum).

Breakdown and perforation have been noted in polyglactin mesh and collagen matrix. A number of Chiari specialists rely primarily on autogenous pericranium, although good to excellent results have also been reported with ePTFE (8,9).

What Type of Sealant?

Not all neurosurgeons use a dural sealant as part of the duraplasty procedure. However, a sealant may reduce risk of CSF leak. Several types of sealants have been used. Absorbable hemostatic agents such as oxidized cellulose hemostat or collagen hemostat can be coated with small amount of the local wound blood to create a blood patch. Synthetic absorbable dural sealants include polyethylene glycol hydrogel and fibrin glue.

Should a Cranioplasty Be Performed?

Traditionally, posterior fossa decompression has been performed without cranioplasty (closure of the bony defect). However, cranioplasty can provide protection from injury, reduction of "soft spot" headache, and a rigid surface for attachment of the suboccipital muscles.

Cranioplasty materials include autograft bone, hydroxyapatite, and methylmethacrylate. Demineralized bone matrix is not recommended because it turns to scar. Recently, preformed titanium plates have been developed that simplify the cranioplasty procedure. Fenestrations within the plates allow suturing of the suboccipital muscles to the plate.

By care, experience, and careful observation of results, neurosurgeons can refine their technique to improve outcome and decrease surgical risks.

REFERENCES

1. Ellenbogen RG, Armonda RA, Shaw DW, et al. Toward a rational treatment of Chiari I malformation and syringomyelia. Neurosurg Focus 2000; 8(3):E6.
2. Milhorat TH, Bolognese PA. Tailored operative technique for Chiari type I malformation using intraoperative color ultrasonography. Neurosurgery 2003; 53(4):899–906.
3. Munshi I, Frim D, Stine-Reyes R, et al. Effects of posterior fossa decompression with and without duraplasty on Chiari malformation-associated hydromyelia. Neurosurgery 2000; 46(6):1384–1390.
4. Hayhurst C, Richards O, Zaki H, et al. Hindbrain decompression for Chiari-syringomyelia complex: An outcome analysis comparing surgical techniques. Br J Neurosurg 2008; 22(1):86–91.
5. Alden TD, Ojemann JG, Park TS. Surgical treatment of Chiari I malformation: Indications and approaches. Neurosurg Focus 2001; 11(1):E2.
6. Duddy MJ, Williams B. Hindbrain migration after decompression for hindbrain hernia: A quantitative assessment using MRI. Br J Neurosurg 1991; 5(2):141–152.
7. Krieger MD, McComb JG, Levy ML. Toward a simpler surgical management of Chiari I malformation in a pediatric population. Pediatr Neurosurg 1999; 30(3):113–121.
8. Attenello FJ, McGirt MJ, Garcés-Ambrossi GL, et al. Suboccipital decompression for Chiari I malformation: outcome comparison of duraplasty with expanded polytetrafluoroethylene dural substitute versus pericranial autograft. Childs Nerv Syst 2009; 25(2):183–190.
9. Messing-Jünger AM, Ibáñez J, Calbucci F, et al. Effectiveness and handling characteristics of a three-layer polymer dura substitute: A prospective multicenter clinical study. J Neurosurg 2006; 105(6):853–858.

19 | Idiopathic Intracranial Hypertension

Caroline Hayhurst
Department of Neurosurgery, The Walton Centre for Neurology and Neurosurgery, Liverpool, U.K.

Alison Rowlands
Department of Ophthalmology, North Cheshire NHS Trust, Warrington, U.K.

Fiona Rowe
Division of Orthoptics, University of Liverpool, Liverpool, U.K.

A variety of names exist for the pathological entity that was originally called pseudotumor cerebri over a century ago. It is a condition defined by the presence of pathologically raised intracranial pressure in the absence of dilated ventricles or intracranial mass lesion with normal CSF composition. The underlying mechanism of raised intracranial pressure without manifestations of a focal lesion or focal deficit remains incompletely understood. Therefore many different concepts for etiology, investigation, and management have evolved over the years. The ultimate treatment of this elusive condition overlaps among neurologist, ophthalmologist, and neurosurgeon.

HISTORICAL PERSPECTIVES

The technical developments that led to the definition of the concept of idiopathic intracranial hypertension (IIH) were the invention of the ophthalmoscope in 1851 and the introduction of the technique of lumbar puncture by Quincke in 1891. The syndrome, originally named meningitis serosa, was first described by Quincke in 1893 (1,2). Quincke described a mixed group of patients with raised intracranial pressure without a focal mass lesion, but with a variety of etiological factors including head injury, pregnancy, and otitis media. In addition, several of the patients he described presented with a reduced level of consciousness or focal deficits, which would preclude a diagnosis of IIH today. Similarly, Nonne further described patients who presented with features of raised intracranial pressure consistent with tumor, but who were subsequently demonstrated not to have a mass lesion and all recovered spontaneously (3). He coined the term pseudotumor cerebri. These reports and others linking raised intracranial pressure with papilledema to middle ear infection, termed otitic hydrocephalus, predate radiological imaging studies.

The introduction of neuroradiological investigations such as venography and ventriculography in the 1930s led to the exclusion of cases with ventriculomegaly and a clear underlying mechanism of development of hydrocephalus. In 1937, Dandy described 22 cases of raised intracranial pressure without brain tumor with normal ventriculography, all of whom recovered following subtemporal decompression (4).

Following the frequent observations of an IIH-like syndrome, following middle ear infection and transverse sinus thrombosis, Ray and Dunbar (5) reported two cases of "pseudotumor cerebri" who showed evidence of obstruction of the superior saggital sinus on sinography, thus introducing the mechanism of venous outflow obstruction to the debate on etiology, whereas early reports had focused on a disorder of CSF dynamics. Subsequently, Foley introduced the term benign intracranial hypertension to denote patients with intracranial hypertension without ventricular abnormality or focal neurological signs with marked papilledema and normal CSF constituents (6). He divided his cases into those secondary to dural sinus thrombosis following ear disease and those with no history of preceding infection. In summary, the development of neuroradiological techniques shifted the balance of thought regarding the pathophysiology of IIH away from obstruction of CSF flow due to the absence of ventricular dilatation and towards a primary disorder of cerebral venous blood flow. Increased brain water content was also held

Table 1 Modified Dandy Criteria for IIH (13,18)

Symptoms and signs of raised ICP (headache, vomiting, visual obscurations, and papilledema)
No localizing signs (except false localizing signs such as VI nerve palsy)
No reduction in consciousness
Normal CT/MRI with no evidence of dural sinus thrombosis
ICP >250 mm H_2O with normal CSF constituents
No other cause of raised ICP found

---

responsible when biopsy specimens taken at the time of subtemporal decompression provided histological evidence of edema (7). However MR studies fail to demonstrate increased water content consistently in IIH.

Foley's term benign intracranial hypertension is inaccurate as the sequelae of the untreated disease are far from benign. Buchheit et al. (8) introduced the term IIH to denote a specific syndrome with no identifiable cause. Dandy, in his original description of the syndrome, set out the common diagnostic features and these became known as the Dandy criteria (4), which have subsequently been updated most notably by Digre and Corbett (9) and Friedman and Jacobson (10). These modified Dandy criteria must be met for the condition to be termed IIH (Table 1). In addition, the term pseudotumor cerebri syndrome has been introduced to encompass a syndrome with a common mode of presentation and treatment and a variety of known etiological mechanisms (11). Johnston et al. proposed a classification of primary pseudotumour ceribri syndrome (PTCS), which is IIH and secondary PTCS (secondary to cranial venous outflow obstruction or abnormal CSF constituents) (11).

EPIDEMIOLOGY

The incidence of IIH is 1 to 3 per 100,000 population per year (12,13). The condition is between 4 and 10 times more common in women, particularly women between the ages 15 to 44 when it is strongly associated with obesity. The incidence rises to 21 per 100,000 population per year in this subgroup. The condition is rare in populations where obesity is not prevalent. IIH is also seen in children; however, the female preponderance and association with obesity are not consistently present in this age group. Although the condition can be seen in any age group, the peak incidence is in the third decade of life (14). Familial cases of IIH have been reported (8,15). The disease may present, worsen, or recur with pregnancy.

PATHOPHYSIOLOGY

Despite extensive research into the underlying causative disease mechanism, no unifying theory exists. Even which intracranial subcompartment is affected (CSF, blood, or brain parenchyma) is disputed. Evidence of venous outflow obstruction in patients with IIH, combined with the fact that CSF drainage, either intermittent or continuous relieves symptoms, points to CSF outflow obstruction as the final common pathway in the pathophysiology of the disease. Why in some cases this mechanism leads to hydrocephalus and in others IIH is not clear?

Although the term IIH implies there is no single identifiable etiological agent, many associated conditions and putative causal factors have been observed in those diagnosed with IIH, leading to possible pathogenetic mechanisms (Fig. 1). However, evidence for a true secondary syndrome would require that treatment or reversal of the associated condition relieved the symptoms of raised intracranial pressure. There is no strong evidence that this is the case. IIH is strongly associated with female sex and obesity. Weight loss and bariatric surgery have both been demonstrated to alleviate symptoms and reduce papilledema. Conversely, rapid weight gain is associated with relapses. Sleep apnea (Pickwickian syndrome) may also lead to symptoms and signs of IIH.

In approximately 10% of patients overall there is an identifiable underlying causal agent (Table 2). However, Johnston and Paterson (14) demonstrated that 48% of patients in their series had some etiological factor, although this figure is lower when only adult females are included.

The relationship between venous outflow obstruction and IIH was originally described following septic thrombosis of the transverse sinus following middle ear infection. All causes of sinus obstruction may lead to papilledema and raised intracranial pressure, including sinus

Interference with cerebral venous outflow and disorders of cerebral vascular dilatation	Disordered membrane transport mechanisms	Dysfunction of the arachnoid villi
(1) Intracranial venous sinus obstruction Mastoiditis Otitis, sinusitis Trauma Blood dyscrasias with thrombosis Oral contraceptives	(1) Endocrine dysfunction Obesity Pregnancy Menarche Addison's disease Hypoparathyroidism Steroid therapy and its withdrawal	(1) Blockage by increased protein in CSF Guillain Barre syndrome Spinal cord tumor
(2) Extracranial cerebral venous obstruction Thrombosis of superior vena cava Block dissection of neck Mediastinal tumor	(2) Hypervitaminosis A	(2) Dysfunction of microtubular system of arachnoid villi
(3) Cerebral venous stasis Oral contraceptives Endocrine dysfunction as in pregnancy and menarche	(3) Tetracycline therapy	
(4) Cerebral vascular dilatation due to CO_2 retention Extreme obesity, Pickwickian syndrome Chronic obstructive pulmonary disease Respiratory paralysis	(4) Postinfectious state	
Vascular engorgement and increased cerebral blood volume	Brain edema	Reduced CSF absorption
Through autoregulatory vasodilatation	Increased intracranial pressure Headache Papilledema Idiopathic intracranial hypertension	

Figure 1 Schematic outline of possible mechanisms in the pathogenesis of IIH

obstruction by tumor, elevated pressure due to arteriovenous fistulae, and thrombosis secondary to a hypercoagulable state (protein C and S deficiency, systemic malignancy, SLE, and Factor V Leiden mutation). Extracranial obstruction to venous outflow may occur following radical neck dissection or thrombosis following the use of indwelling central venous lines.

There is a clear link between the ingestion of certain medications and exogenous substances and the onset of an IIH-like syndrome. The strongest evidence exits for excess of vitamin A and for tetracycline and related antibiotics. Vitamin A may be ingested in foodstuffs such as liver, in vitamin A–related compounds used in the treatment of skin diseases, and as all-transretinoic acid used in the treatment of leukemia. Interestingly, prolonged use of corticosteroids can cause IIH, despite the observation that use of steroid can alleviate symptoms. Withdrawal of the medication or substance responsible usually leads to resolution of symptoms.

CLINICAL FEATURES

Headache is the most common symptom of IIH, occurring in over 90% of cases. Headache is usually generalized but is nonspecific in nature and quality. Although there can be increased severity with any type of Valsalva maneuver, headache can also be migrainous in nature.

In large case series of patients with IIH after headache, visual disturbance is the most common symptom, occurring in 35% to 60% of cases (14,16). Visual symptoms range from blurring of vision to progressive and in some cases rapid loss of visual acuity or rapid field loss. Wall and George (17) found a 96% incidence of visual field defects in 50 patients with IIH at presentation. Permanent visual loss can occur in up to 20% of cases (18). Transient visual obscurations, typically associated with coughing or straining, occur frequently. Dizziness, nausea, and vomiting may occur but alterations in consciousness do not typically occur.

Table 2 Etiological Agents

1. Venous outflow obstruction
    Dural venous sinus compression or obstruction
    Dural arteriovenous fistula
    Traumatic
    Septic thrombosis of dural venous sinus
    Occlusion of internal jugular vein
2. Hematological
    Coagulopathy with sinus thrombosis
    Anemia
    Leukemia
    Polycythemia
Myeloma
    POEMS
3. Endocrine/metabolic
    Hypothyroidism
    Hyperadrenalism
    Addison's disease, Cushing's syndrome
    Hypoparathyroidism, pseudohypoparathyroidism
    Acromegaly
    Pregnancy
    Polycystic ovary syndrome
    Turner's syndrome
    Renal disease
4. Exogenous substances
    Vitamin A
    Steroids
    Tetracycline and related antibiotics
    Nalidixic acid
    Carbidopa, levodopa
    Amiodarone
    Oral contraceptives
    Phenytoin
    Danazol
    Lithium

It is increasingly recognized that headache may be the sole symptom, with the absence of any visual disturbance or papilledema but with elevated CSF pressure that responds to treatment. Therefore, IIH becomes a component of the differential diagnosis of chronic migraine and chronic daily headache (Table 3).

IIH may also present with atypical features such as CSF rhinorrhea (19,20), facial pain (21), and hemifacial spasm (22). False localizing signs such as VIth nerve palsy or IVth nerve palsy, with torticollis in children, may be seen.

Table 3 Presenting Symptoms of IIH

Common
    Headache
    Visual loss
    Visual obscurations
    Diplopia
    Nausea and vomiting
    Tinnitus
Atypical
    CSF rhinorrhea
    Facial pain
    Hemifacial spasm

INVESTIGATIONS

The role of investigation in IIH serves to exclude an underlying lesion and document visual dysfunction, in addition to confirming the diagnosis of IIH by demonstrating raised CSF pressure by lumbar puncture. As stated in the modified Dandy criteria, a diagnosis of IIH requires demonstration of normal or small ventricles with no mass lesion, raised ICP, and normal CSF constituents. Therefore, the minimum requirements are cranial imaging and lumbar puncture. Magnetic resonance imaging with contrast-enhanced sequences and CSF flow studies has superseded CT as the imaging modality of choice. The addition of MR angiography and venography will demonstrate any associated vascular malformation. It is mandatory to exclude venous sinus thrombosis in all patients. MR venography may demonstrate a patent but narrowed venous sinus. Formal angiography or retrograde venography is reserved for those with an abnormal vascular tree on initial MRI studies. The majority of imaging studies are normal; however, a small proportion may demonstrate slit ventricles, enlarged optic nerve sheaths, or an empty sella (23).

Lumbar puncture should be performed in the lateral decubitus position, and as stated in the modified Dandy criteria, an opening pressure greater than 250 mm H_2O is defined as abnormal (9). Pressures between 200 and 250 mm H_2O are nondiagnostic. Moreover, patients with chronic daily headache, or anxious patients, may have an erroneously high isolated opening pressure due to an accompanying Valsalva. In addition, it has been reported that 42% of obese asymptomatic females have opening pressures of greater than 250 mm H_2O (24). In both these cases, continuous intracranial pressure monitoring by using an intraparenchymal fiberoptic or intraventricular transducer may demonstrate persistently raised pressure or abnormal pressure waves. Similarly, CSF infusion studies for measurement of CSF absorption have been used to demonstrate increased resistance to CSF outflow in IIH; however, this is not a uniform finding and is therefore not diagnostic in isolation but has proved to be useful in treatment evaluation, particularly of shunt function.

VISUAL ASSESSMENT

Detailed neuro-opthalmological assessment should be undertaken serially in all patients. Clinical examination reveals papilledema in almost all cases; however, as previously stated, its absence does not exclude the diagnosis. Fundoscopy may demonstrate bilateral, unilateral, or asymmetrical swelling of the optic nerve head (Fig. 2). There may be associated disc hyperemia, engorged retinal veins, or frank pre-papillary hemorrhages. Stages of papilledema include early, acute, chronic, and vintage (Figs. 3 to 6). Secondary vascular changes may eventually produce a secondary optic atrophy (Fig. 7).

Simple edema is the one predominant feature of papilledema. This shows itself by a separation of the elements of the normal tissues by fluid that contains no cells and has little tendency to coagulate. It is in the disc that edema produces most change. The fluid lying among the nerve fibers and in the anterior layers of the lamina cribrosa separates and stretches these

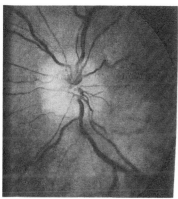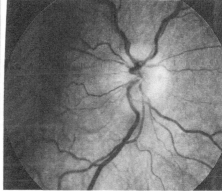

Figure 2 Asymmetric papilledema.

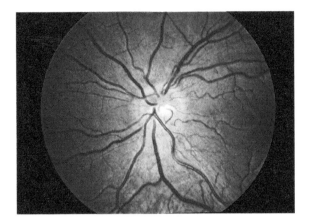

Figure 3 Early papilledema.

elements until these seem to form only a meshwork, in the interstices of which the fluid lies. The disc is thus increased in size in every diameter. As the disc swells lateral wards, it displaces the retina, either raising it up from the pigment layer or throwing it into a series of folds that run concentric with the edge of the disc. As the swelling increases, the axial bundles are lifted upwards and inwards so as to narrow the physiological pit and the filling in of this is completed by the edema, which raises the inner limiting membrane from the central vessels.

Optic disc swelling further compromises the low pressure, predominantly venous, fine blood supply to the prelaminar region and initiates a vicious circle of edema, congestion, and further edema. The vascular changes on the nerve head are therefore secondary to and not the cause of the disc edema. The vascular changes in papilledema consist mainly of venous and capillary congestions. The larger veins in the disc are dilated. In the zone of the swollen disc, which corresponds to the anterior layers of the lamina cribrosa, there are numerous small dilated venules and capillaries. Evidence of vascular congestion is afforded by the hemorrhages, which may occur everywhere on the disc and in the retina in its immediate neighborhood. These are most frequently seen as striate hemorrhages along the nerve fiber layers. Hemorrhages on the disc and in the peripapillary region remain one of the diagnostic features of papilledema.

Signs of chronic papilledema (gliosis, pallor, hard exudates, and optociliary shunt vessels) have been associated with permanent visual field loss. Hayreh suggested that the chronic atrophic changes seen in the optic disc in patients with papilledema may be due to chronic ischemia secondary to compromise of the prelaminar arterial blood supply (25).

Opthalmological investigations include detailed fundoscopy, preferably using a slit-lamp and/or direct ophthalmoscope. Optic nerve swelling must be differentiated from optic drusen or pseudopapilledema secondary to hypermetropia and other causes of optic nerve swelling, such as optic neuritis or malignant hypertension. It should be noted that hypoxia or sleep pnoea syndromes can produce optic disc swelling in the absence of raised intracranial pressure.

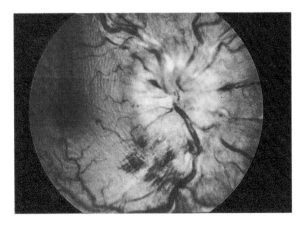

Figure 4 Acute papilledema.

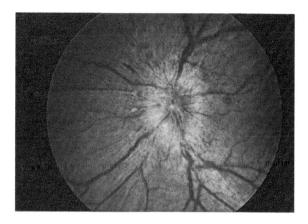

Figure 5   Chronic papilledema.

Accurate assessment of progression of papilledema changes can be done using confocal scanning tomography.

Visual loss has been related to the papilledema noted with raised ICP, and visual field defects are classically those relating to a disorder of the optic nerve head. The visual loss of IIH is not, however, due to papilledema alone. The visual field defect associated with papilledema is an enlarged blind spot. Other visual field defects of IIH relate to pathology of the anterior optic nerve. Where there is transmission of CSF to the optic nerve sheath in cases of raised ICP, this places pressure on the optic nerve with resultant axoplasmic stasis. It is the pressure on the optic nerve (the anterior optic nerve in particular where it adjoins the globe) and the resultant axoplasmic stasis of nerve conduction that results in the visual field defects associated with the raised ICP of this condition. The use of confocal scanning laser ophthalmoscopy for evaluation of papilledema quantitates the magnitude of swelling and monitors resolution (26). The data obtained has provided further insight into optic nerve compliance with the effects of raised ICP. It had a high sensitivity for detecting small changes in disc volumes and correlates closely with visual field change in the short term. As such it provided an indication of therapeutic failure by detecting stable or increasing disc volume (27). However, decreasing volume may indicate not only resolution of papilledema but secondary optic atrophy, so accompanying fundoscopy and visual field assessment remain essential.

Measurement of visual function is essential in the evaluation of patients with IIH. When assessing visual function in patients with IIH, visual acuity, peripheral, and central fields should all be sequentially recorded (28,29). In this condition, loss of visual function is the only serious complication and may occur early or late in its course (29). Visual loss is insidious and often asymptomatic for long periods of time and visual disaster can only be anticipated by monitoring the visual fields and acuity. The low incidence of the symptom of visual loss is undoubtedly due to the gradual deterioration of vision that often spares central vision until late in the

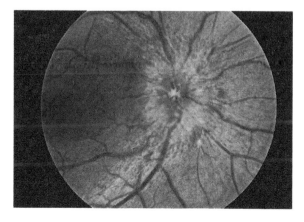

Figure 6   Vintage papilledema.

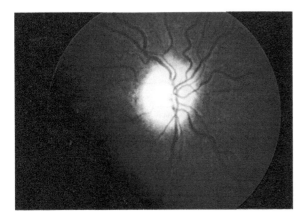

Figure 7 Optic atrophy.

course of the illness. The frequency of subclinical visual loss underscores the need for thorough ophthalmological examination with perimetry. The level of visual acuity or appearance of the optic nerve head (stage of papilledema) often do not indicate the state of visual function and visual acuity usually remains normal in patients with papilledema except where the condition is of long standing (30) or where edema extends into the central 10 degrees of the visual field.

Visual field testing is most sensitive to identifying visual impairment in IIH. Recommended perimeters for quantitative assessment of visual fields include the Humphrey field analyzer (Carl Zeiss International, Dublin, CA) and Goldmann perimeter (Haag Streit International, Koeniz, Switzerland). The latter is no longer in production but despite this, it continues to be used extensively for neurological evaluation of visual fields. It is currently being replaced by the Octopus 900 (Haag Streit International).

The Humphrey automated perimeter provides a sensitive and highly precise assessment of the visual field (Fig. 8). It is a single unit, fully automatic, computerized, projection perimeter. It uses projected stimuli, which can be varied over a range of more than 51 dB, providing a static threshold assessment of the field of vision. A projection device presents the stimulus at points in the visual field specified by the program selected, which typically includes a central 30-degree assessment.

The Goldmann perimeter is a spherical projection perimeter with a system permitting direct registration of the target position. The target for determining the differential threshold of light sensor in central and peripheral parts of the visual field is projected on to the inside of the sphere. The Goldmann predominantly uses kinetic perimetry in which a mobile target of fixed luminosity is used with which positions of equal sensitivity are plotted perpendicularly to the limits of the expected visual fields or isopters through the free movement of the target in all directions (Fig. 9).

The Octopus 900 provides a 90-degree full field projection perimetry with a range of 47 dB. It is a combination manual and automated perimeter with computerized projection (Fig. 10).

The visual field defects noted with IIH relate to optic nerve head pathology and are most frequently documented within the central 30 degrees of the visual fields. The types of field defects in IIH are typically similar to those found in patients with glaucoma apart from an enlarged blind spot (28,31) (Fig. 11). These nerve fiber bundle defects include inferior nasal defects (32), arcuate defects, concentric constrictions (6,28,33), generalized depression of the visual field, and cecocentral scotomas (6) (Figs. 12 and 13). When bundles of nerve fibers are damaged at the optic disc by papilledema, the visual field supplied by the fibers loses its sensitivity and the result is a scotoma or a localized depression. Typically, the first nerve fiber bundles affected are those entering the upper or lower pole of the optic disc. As a result, paracentral scotomas appear within an arcuate region around fixation, or there is a depression in the nasal field of vision, or both. Less commonly, localized loss of tissue on the nasal side of the optic disc will produce a temporal wedge, a wedge-shaped region of reduced sensitivity with its apex at the physiologic blind spot (34).

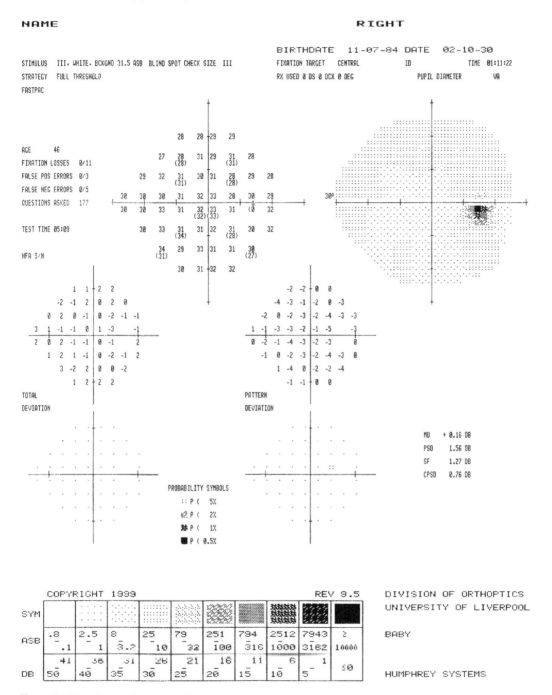

Figure 8   Humphrey perimetry result: normal.

The earliest field defects noted tend to be nasal loss, especially inferonasal steps and constriction of either peripheral or central isopters. Occasionally, arcuate defects and scotomas in the central 30 degrees (especially on automated testing) are seen as early findings. Smith and Baker found in their study that the most common field abnormality was a generalized

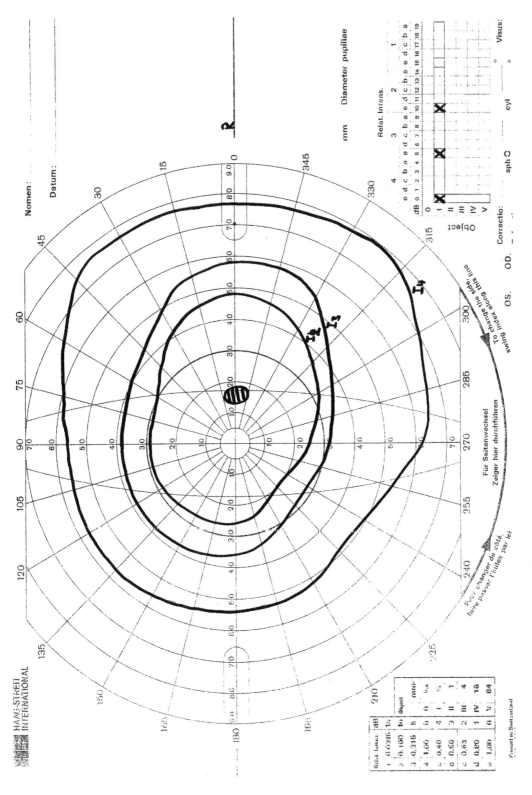

Figure 9 Goldmann perimetry result: normal.

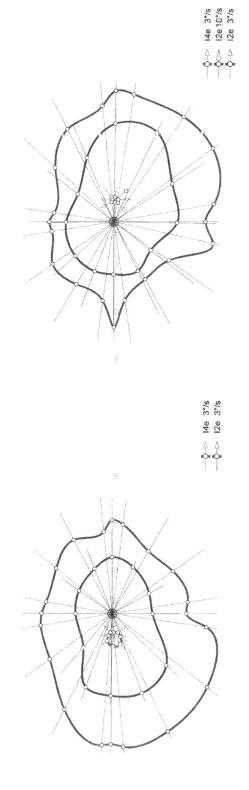

Figure 10 Octopus perimetry result: normal.

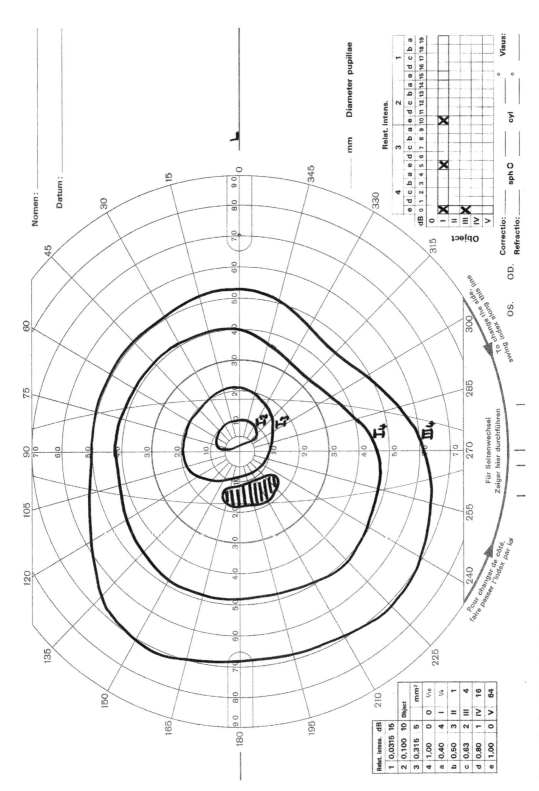

Figure 11 Enlarged blind spot.

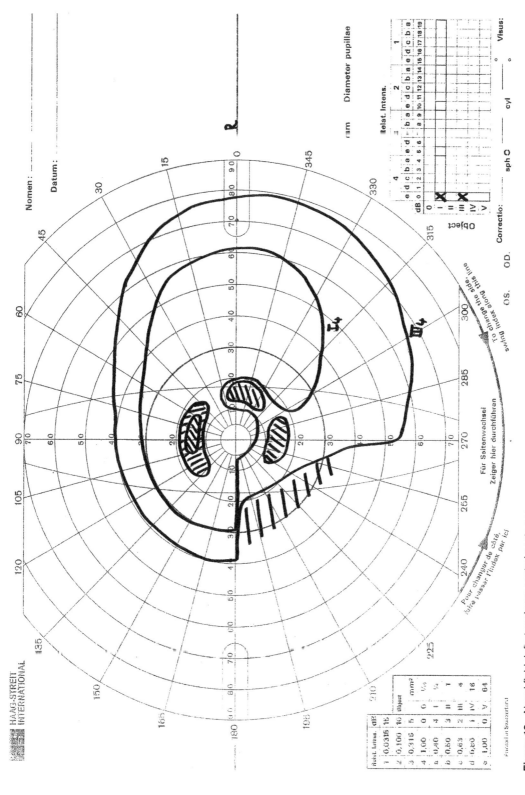

Figure 12 Nasal field defect and paracentral scotomas.

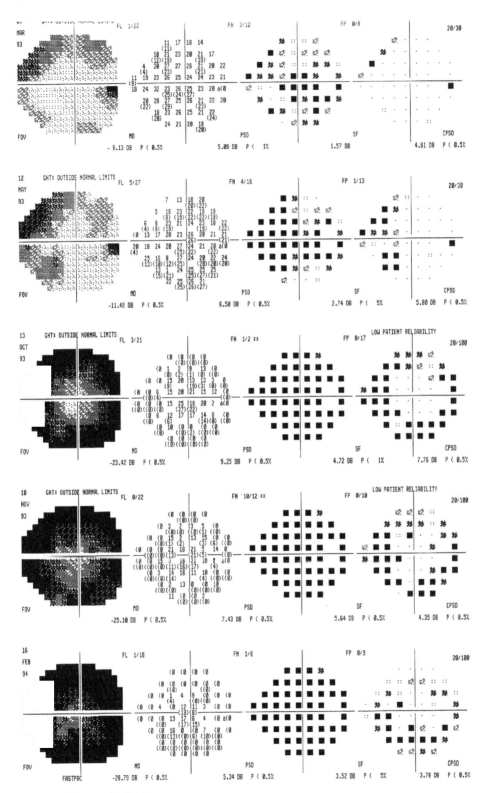

Figure 13 Progressive field loss.

Table 4 Incidence of Visual Loss and Serious Visual Deficit

References	Visual loss (%)	Serious visual loss (%)
Dandy (1937) (4)	22.7	4.5
Lysak and Svien (1966) (33)	28	4.3
Johnston and Paterson (1974) (14)	14.5	4
Vasilouthis and Uttley (1976) (87)	21.4	7
Rush (1980) (28)	32	11
Corbett, Savino, Thompson, et al. (1982) (29)	49	25
Orcutt, Page, and Sanders (1984) (88)	49	10.3
Wall and George (1987) (36)	77.5	21
Sorenson, Krogsaa, and Ojemis (1988) (89)	16.6	4
Wall and George (1991) (17)	96	22
Rowe and Sarkies (1999) (39)	86	6

Serious visual loss defined as visual field loss of greater than 50% and/or visual acuity levels of less than 6/36.

depression that was present in 19 eyes (35). This was followed in frequency by infranasal loss, paracentral defects, arcuate scotomas, temporal wedge defects, and altitudinal loss.

Visual loss, due to optic nerve atrophy, is the most serious complication of papilledema in IIH. The incidence of visual field defects ranges up to 96% (36–38). The incidence of permanent serious visual loss has been reported in up to 25% of cases in single studies (Table 4). Many publications do not involve documenting visual function serially over a period of time using sensitive testing strategies and therefore may have also missed visual deficits unnoticed by the patients themselves. The wide range of incidence of visual loss and severe visual loss reflects the ascertainment bias and the sensitivity of tests used for the assessment of visual function. Detection of asymptomatic visual loss is also of importance. Rowe and Sarkies reported that at initial visual assessment, 53% of patients were not aware of their visual field defects, which were of minimal to moderate degree (39). Throughout the follow-up period, 66.7% of the visual field defects were minimal or mild and unlikely to have been noticed by the patient. This further demonstrates the necessity for visual monitoring to detect visual loss, particularly that of an insidious nature.

TREATMENT

The treatment of IIH varies depending on the identification of an underlying cause and the clinical features, whether it is isolated headache or visual failure as the predominant symptom. Where venous outflow obstruction has been excluded as a cause of IIH, the management algorithm demonstrated in Figure 14 outlines the treatment options. It should be noted that no intervention for IIH is supported by Class 1 evidence and a Cochrane Review of 2007 failed to find any published studies of intervention suitable for inclusion in a systematic review (40).

Treatment of Venous Outflow Obstruction

The association of IIH and venous sinus abnormalities has been known since the 1950s; however, there has been a resurgence of interest in venous outflow obstruction as a cause of IIH following the expanding use of endovascular techniques. Marks et al. first reported the use of intracranial venous stenting for transverse sinus stenosis in a patient presenting with pulsatile tinnitus in 1994 (41). Subsequently, multiple case series have described the successful treatment of intractable IIH with venous stenting. In the setting of intracranial hypertension secondary to sinus thrombosis, the management of the venous outflow obstruction is well defined and includes systemic anticoagulation, thrombolysis, and venous stent placement. However, it appears that there are some cases of primary IIH where there is sinus narrowing with compromise of venous outflow as demonstrated by an intraluminal pressure gradient across the stricture. The role of venous stenting in these cases is uncertain. Indeed King et al. (42) suggested that the venous stenosis may be a direct result of compression from raised intracranial pressure and not vice versa, as CSF drainage has been shown to reduce the venous pressure gradient in some but not in all cases. However, there are a total of 30 cases of refractory IIH treated with stenting of the transverse sinus reported in the literature (43–48). Of these patients

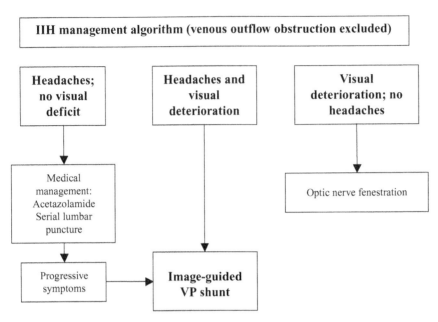

Figure 14   Algorithm for management of IIH.

there was improvement or complete resolution of symptoms in 24. Reported complications include acute subdural hematoma in one patient and transient hearing loss on the stented side in four patients. Intraluminal thrombosis secondary to stenting has also been reported (46) and systemic anticoagulation followed by antiplatelet therapy is required.

In summary, all patients with IIH should have MR venography to exclude venous sinus thrombosis and identify any sinus stenosis (most commonly of the transverse sinus). Where a stenotic venous segment is suspected, retrograde cerebral venography combined with intraluminal pressure measurements should be performed. Venous stenting in such cases may provide an alternative and curative treatment option to CSF diversion, but there is as yet no data to confirm long-term efficacy.

Medical Management

In the absence of visual loss, it is appropriate to pursue medical treatment with the aim of relief of headaches. In some patients, the condition is self-limiting and no treatment is required. The majority of patients are obese and weight loss has been shown to reduce symptoms and result in resolution of papilledema. However, to achieve this, a significant weight loss of up to 10% of body weight is required (49,50). Such weight loss is difficult to achieve and sustain, therefore advocating weight loss often fails as a treatment of IIH.

Acetazolamide, a carbonic anhydrase inhibitor, is the most commonly used agent for treatment of IIH. This drug reduces the CSF production by decreasing sodium ion transport across the choroidal epithelium. Acetazolamide was originally shown to significantly reduce CSF production in humans by Rubin et al. in 1966 (51). Side-effects are common, including acroparesthesia, altered taste, and depression. In addition, acetazolamide has a teratogenic effect in animals (52,53) and should be avoided in pregnancy. When used alone acetazolamide has been demonstrated to be effective in 46.7% to 47.1% of cases (11,54). Cases where acetazolamide alone is effective tended to be those with mild symptoms and resolution occurred after three months of the treatment. Other diuretics, such as furosemide, are less effective in reducing CSF production but may be used where acetazolamide is not tolerated. There is no widely accepted standard for the length of treatment with acetazolamide and it is often dictated by the clinical response. There are no contraindications to prolonged treatment with acetazolamide, if the side effects are tolerated.

Serial lumbar punctures to drain CSF may be used. It is proposed that in addition to temporary reduction in ICP, repeated lumbar punctures create a dural sieve, allowing continued CSF egress and sustained reduction in ICP. However, repeated lumbar punctures are poorly tolerated in most patients, and in obese patients lumbar puncture is difficult, often requiring fluoroscopic guidance.

Surgical Management

Surgical intervention is indicated where medical management fails to relieve intractable headaches or if there is progressive visual deficit. In addition, urgent surgical intervention is required where there is sudden acute visual deterioration.

CSF shunting procedures provide rapid and effective reduction in intracranial pressure. However, as with all shunt procedures, the incidence of shunt malfunction is high. In the majority of patients with IIH, the ventricles are normal size or even slit-like. Therefore, the lumbar theca has been the favored proximal drainage site for many years. Standard lumboperitoneal shunts may be valveless or incorporate a distal slit valve or integrated differential pressure valves aimed to prevent overdrainage in the upright position. Lumboperitoneal shunting is an effective means of symptom control in IIH. A large series of shunted patients with IIH reported by Johnston et al. (11) describes 91 (30.8%) patients shunted as the primary treatment or at the time of failure of medical therapy. Seventy of the shunts were lumboperitoneal; the rest comprising cisterna magna to right atrium shunts. High-pressure headache was relieved in all cases, as was in papilledema. Two (2.2%) patients lost visual function at the time of shunt malfunction. McGirt et al (55) report 42 patients treated with LP or VP shunts for intractable headache, demonstrating symptom recurrence despite a functioning shunt in 19% at 12 months and 48% by 36 months. Complications of lumboperitoneal shunts are not insignificant and include not only obstruction, infection and overdrainage as with all CSF diversion techniques, but also radiculopathy, catheter migration, acquired Chiari 1 malformation (Fig. 15) and syringomyelia (56–63). In the series reported by Johnston et al. (11) there were a total of 269 shunt revisions. 60.4% of the cohort required at least one shunt revision. In addition, of the 70 LP shunts, 7 (10%) required revision for symptomatic acquired Chiari 1 malformation. The published series from our institution describes 17 patients with IIH treated with lumboperitoneal shunts for progressive visual deterioration or intractable headaches despite medical management. 14 patients (82%) required at least one shunt revision, most commonly due to shunt migration (64). In the series of McGirt

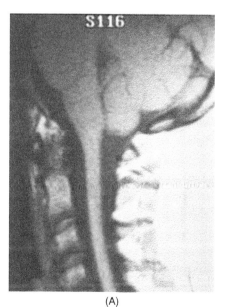 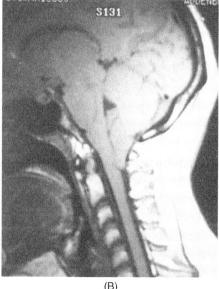

(A)   (B)

Figure 15 Acquired Chiari I malformation.

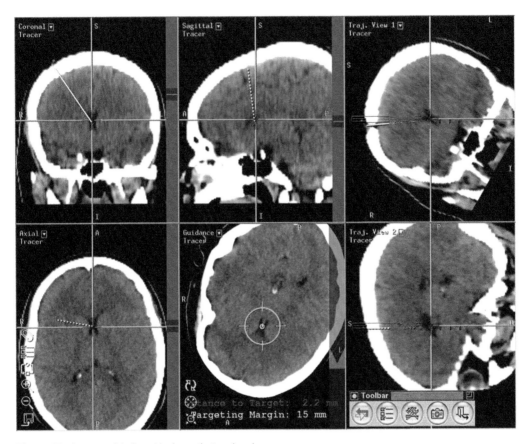

Figure 16   Image-guided ventricular catheter planning.

et al., 86% of LP shunts were revised due to malfunction compared to 44% of VP shunts at
two years (55). The increasing use of stereotaxy has led to increased interest in ventriculoperitoneal shunt placement for IIH in an attempt to avoid the inherent problems of LP shunts. The
use of both frame-based and frameless stereotaxy has been described (55,65–67), with a lower
overall shunt failure rate than is described for LP shunts. However, until recently neuronavi-
gated ventricular catheter placement required rigid head fixation or a frame-based procedure,
both undesirable in shunt surgery. The introduction of noninvasive electromagnetic navigation
allows real-time navigation of the ventricular catheter tip to a preplanned intraventricular target point. The use of electromagnetic neuronavigation to place ventricular catheters in IIH has
been reported (68,69). In our institution, since 2004 we have routinely adopted electromagnetic
image-guided VP shunt placement as the procedure of choice in IIH where medical therapy has
failed. Using the Medtronic Axiem™ system (Medtronic Navigation Inc., Louisville, CO), the
ventricular catheter is placed using the EM stylet as a trocar into the largest CSF space, usually
the frontal horn (Figs. 16 and 17). Additional operative time is minimal and head fixation or
separate incisions for the reference frame are not required. Although shunt failure still occurs,
there are no complications related to ventricular access, and the specific complications to LP
shunts of migration and acquired Chiari malformation are avoided. One criticism of any form
of CSF shunting is that IIH is a potentially self-limiting condition and that treatment with a
long-standing implant may be unnecessary.

Historically, subtemporal decompression played a significant role in reducing ICP prior to
the introduction of CSF diversion techniques. However, unilateral subtemporal decompression
on the nondominant temporal fossa still has a role where CSF shunting has failed to alleviate symptoms despite a functioning shunt. Complications include epilepsy, focal neurological
deficit, and meningitis.

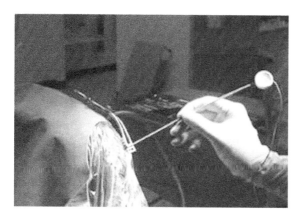

Figure 17 Electromagnetic-guided ventricular catheter placement.

Optic Nerve Sheath Fenestration

Optic nerve sheath fenestration is a procedure that may be employed for preventing impending blindness from papilledema. Optic nerve sheath fenestration was first described by DeWecker in 1872 (70) and then by Carter in 1887 (71). Management of visual loss secondary to papilledema remains the primary indication for optic nerve sheath fenestration and is advocated before serious visual loss has occurred. Optic nerve sheath fenestration has been found effective for reversing visual loss and protecting the optic nerve from further damage.

The aim of the procedure is to produce an opening within the optic nerve sheath by excising a portion of the sheath or by multiple slit incisions. The most frequently used approach is via a medial conjunctival peritomy with disinsertion of the medial rectus. Access is gained to the optic nerve sheath just posterior to the globe. The major technical problem is being able to spread apart the ciliary vessels lying on the optic nerve sheath. Damage to these vessels not only hinders surgical access through hemorrhage but is likely to cause optic disc and choroidal infarction. Sometimes it is difficult to be certain that the subarachnoid space has been entered, particularly if the nerve sheath has been incised obliquely, but usually incision of the sheath is accompanied by a gush of CSF.

Lateral approach to the nerve involves either a lateral orbitotomy or access without bone removal via a lateral canthotomy or via an upper eyelid skin crease incision. Some surgeons prefer a lateral approach because this approach is more direct and perpendicular to the optic nerve than the medial orbitotomy (72,73). Anderson and Flaharty (74) found that the need for reoperations can be considerably reduced by the lateral approach. A large segment of dura mater and arachnoid is completely removed by means of the lateral approach, which bares the optic nerve and allows the easy egress of CSF. The medial approach may have a lower incidence of postoperative pupillary abnormalities due to the temporal location of the ciliary ganglion and avoidance of transient lateral rectus paresis compared with the lateral orbitotomy (75–78). Although exposure may be greater, particularly with the lateral orbitotomy, the major disadvantage of the lateral approach is the risk to the temporal ciliary vessels with the potentially more serious visual loss if they are damaged. Because the axons of the retinal ganglion cells in the macula traverse the temporal aspect of the optic nerve, damage to these axons may be more likely with a lateral orbital approach (73). Similarly, because choroidal blood supply to the macula is temporal, catastrophic visual loss may be more likely with the lateral than the medial approach. Optic nerve sheath fenestration may also be performed via a craniotomy or an endoscopic endonasal approach.

In most cases, unilateral surgery produces only ipsilateral effects, therefore bilateral procedures are required. Spoor et al. (75,76) found that patients with nerves decompressed early in the course of acute papilledema have much better recovery of vision than those with chronic atrophic papilledema and severe visual loss. Signs of improvement are usually apparent within one week of the operation. Subsidence of venous engorgement occurs initially, followed by a decrease in the height of the edematous disc. Absorption of exudates and hemorrhages on the surface of the disc begin at a later stage. Kaye et al. (79) and Kilpatrick et al. (80) have reported continued high readings on postoperative ICP monitoring, despite papilledema resolution, suggesting that clinical improvement following optic nerve fenestration is independent of a reduction in intracranial pressure overall.

Optic nerve sheath fenestration carries a risk of permanent visual loss as a result of intraoperative axonal or vascular damage (81). Other complications include transient asymmetry of the pupil, probably from trauma to posterior ciliary nerves, and suppurative keratitis Ocular motility problems are common but usually transient (82). The proposed mechanism for production of diplopia following optic nerve fenestration is vertical muscle bruising from the traction sutures, placed at the superior and inferior recti insertions, which resolves spontaneously. Although diplopia is a transient phenomenon following optic nerve sheath fenestration, it is a feature that patients should be warned of before obtaining consent for surgery.

A review of published visual outcome following optic nerve sheath fenestration in 423 eyes of 252 patients demonstrated improved visual fields in 72% patients, with 11% patients having worse visual acuity or fields post-operatively (83).

OUTCOME

Independent of which treatment method is employed, follow-up studies of patients with IIH demonstrate an average duration of symptoms of three months (11,28,30,84). Even without treatment the majority show improvement within a few months (85). A small proportion of patients have a protracted course with symptoms for 12 months or longer (29,86). Recurrence of symptoms may occur in up to 10% of patients (11,29,31).

In terms of visual outcome alone, Rowe and Sarkies (38) demonstrated visual field loss at final assessment in 75% of patients using Goldmann perimetry and 56% patients using Humphrey perimetry. Wall and George (17), in a similar study of visual outcome, noted visual field defects in 51% of eyes using Goldmann perimetry and 72% of eyes using Humphrey perimetry. However, despite such a high rate of detection of field defects, in both studies these defects were mild with the patients unlikely to be aware of the defect. Rowe and Sarkies demonstrated normal visual fields in 43% of cases, with a further 40% with mild field deficit only at final assessment (38). Recent weight gain has been shown to be a risk factor for poor visual outcome (17). Patients who present with visual loss are unlikely to have a good visual outcome.

CONCLUSION

The pathophysiology of IIH is incompletely understood and it is clear that a proportion of patients have a secondary pseudotumor cerebri syndrome with a known etiological agent. However, common to both is the threat of visual failure and poor quality of life. In addition, the management algorithm is shared by both conditions.

IIH may be self-limiting in some patients, and treatment is directed at relief of intractable headaches and to prevent catastrophic visual loss. A number of treatment methods exist, with no single intervention demonstrating superior efficacy. However, overall the prognosis for symptom resolution and normal visual function are good.

REFERENCES

1. Quincke H. Meningitis serosa. Sammi klin Vortr, Leipzig, No 67; Inn Med 1893; 23:655.
2. Quincke H. Uber Meningitis serosa und verwande Zustande. Dtsch Zeit f Nervenheil 1897; 9:140–168.
3. Nonne M. Uber Falle vom Symtptomkomplex "tumor cerebri" mit Ausgang in Heilling (Pseudotumor Cerebri); uber letal verlaufene Falle von "Pseudotumor Cerebri" mit Sektionsbefund. Dtsch Zeit f Nervenheil 1904; 27:169–216.
4. Dandy WE. Intracranial pressure without brain tumor: Diagnosis and treatment. Ann Surg 1937; 106(4):492–513.
5. Ray BS, Dunbar HS. Thrombosis of the dural venous sinuses as a cause of pseudotumor cerebri. Ann Surg 1951; 134(3):376–386.
6. Foley J. Benign forms of intracranial hypertension; toxic and otitic hydrocephalus. Brain 1955; 78(1): 1–41.
7. Joynt RJ, Sahs AL. Brain swelling of unknown cause. Neurology 1956; 6(11):801–813.
8. Buchheit WA, Burton C, Haag B, et al. Papilledema and idiopathic intracranial hypertension. N Engl J Med 1969; 280(17):938–942.

9. Digre KB, Corbett J. Idiopathic intracranial hypertension (pseudotumor cerebri): A reappraisal. Neurologist 2001; 7:2–67.

10. Friedman DI, Jacobson DM. Diagnostic criteria for idiopathic intracranial hypertension. Neurology 2002; 59(10):1492–1495.

11. Johnston I, Owler B, Pickard JD. Pseudotumor cerebri syndrome: Pseudotumor Cerebri, Idiopathic Intracranial Hypertension, Benign Intracranial Hypertension, and Related Conditions. Cambridge, MA: Cambridge University Press, 2007:69–78.

12. Radhakrishnan K, Ahlskog JE, Cross SA, et al. Idiopathic intracranial hypertension (pseudotumor cerebri). Descriptive epidemiology in Rochester, Minn., 1976 to 1990. Arch Neurol 1993; 50(1):78–80.

13. Durcan FJ, Corbett JJ, Wall M. The incidence of pseudotumor cerebri. Population studies in Iowa and Louisiana. Arch Neurol 1988; 45(8):875–877.

14. Johnston I, Paterson A. Benign intracranial hypertension. I. Diagnosis and prognosis. Brain 1974; 97(2):289–300.

15. Fujiwara S, Sawamura Y, Kato T, et al. Idiopathic intracranial hypertension in female homozygous twins. J Neurol Neurosurg Psychiatry 1997; 62(6):652–654.

16. Round R, Keane JR. The minor symptoms of increased intracranial pressure: 101 patients with benign intracranial hypertension. Neurology 1988; 38(9):1461–1464.

17. Wall M, George D. Idiopathic intracranial hypertension. A prospective study of 50 patients. Brain 1991; 114 (Pt 1A):155–180.

18. Gutgold-Glen H, Kattah JC, Chavis RM. Reversible visual loss in pseudotumor cerebri. Arch Ophthalmol 1984; 102(3):403–406.

19. Clark D, Bullock P, Hui T, et al. Benign intracranial hypertension: A cause of CSF rhinorrhoea. J Neurol Neurosurg Psychiatry 1994; 57(7):847–849.

20. Owler BK, Allan R, Parker G, et al. Pseudotumour cerebri, CSF rhinorrhoea and the role of venous sinus stenting in treatment. Br J Neurosurg 2003; 17(1):79–83.

21. Hart RG, Carter JE. Pseudotumor cerebri and facial pain. Arch Neurol 1982; 39(7): 440–442.

22. Benegas NM, Volpe NJ, Liu GT, et al. Hemifacial spasm and idiopathic intracranial hypertension. J Neuroophthalmol 1996; 16(1):70.

23. Wessel K, Thron A, Linden D, et al. Pseudotumor cerebri: Clinical and neuroradiological findings. Eur Arch Psychiatry Neurol Sci 1987; 237(1):54–60.

24. Hannerz J, Greitz D, Ericson K. Is there a relationship between obesity and intracranial hypertension? Int J Obes Relat Metab Disord 1995; 19(4):240–244.

25. Hayreh SS. Optic disc edema in raised intracranial pressure. V. Pathogenesis. Arch Ophthalmol 1977; 95(9):1553–1565.

26. Trick GL, Vesti E, Tawansy K, et al. Quantitative evaluation of papilledema in pseudotumor cerebri. Invest Ophthalmol Vis Sci 1998; 39(10):1964–1971.

27. Mulholland DA, Craig JJ, Rankin SJ. Use of scanning laser ophthalmoscopy to monitor papilloedema in idiopathic intracranial hypertension. Br J Ophthalmol 1998; 82(11):1301–1305.

28. Rush JA. Pseudotumor cerebri: Clinical profile and visual outcome in 63 patients. Mayo Clin Proc 1980; 55(9):541–546.

29. Corbett JJ, Savino PJ, Thompson HS, et al. Visual loss in pseudotumor cerebri. Follow-up of 57 patients from five to 41 years and a profile of 14 patients with permanent severe visual loss. Arch Neurol 1982; 39(8):461–474.

30. Guidetti B, Giuffre R, Gambacorta D. Follow-up study of 100 cases of pseudotumor cerebri. Acta Neurochir (Wien) 1968; 18(4):259–267.

31. Weisberg LA. Benign intracranial hypertension. Medicine (Baltimore) 1975; 54(3):197–207.

32. Dersh J, Schlezinger NS. Inferior nasal quadrantanopia in pseudotumor cerebri. Trans Am Neurol Assoc 1959; 84:116–118.

33. Lysak WR, Svien HJ. Long-term follow-up on patients with diagnosis of pseudotumor cerebri. J Neurosurg 1966, 25(3):284–287.

34. Buchanan TA, Hoyt WF. Temporal visual field defects associated with nasal hypoplasia of the optic disc. Br J Ophthalmol 1981; 65(9):636–640.

35. Smith TJ, Baker RS. Perimetric findings in pseudotumor cerebri using automated techniques. Ophthalmology 1986; 93(7):887–894.

36. Wall M, George D. Visual loss in pseudotumor cerebri. Incidence and defects related to visual field strategy. Arch Neurol 1987; 44(2):170–175.

37. Wall M, Conway MD, House PH, et al. Evaluation of sensitivity and specificity of spatial resolution and Humphrey automated perimetry in pseudotumor cerebri patients and normal subjects. Invest Ophthalmol Vis Sci 1991; 32(13):3306–3312.

38. Rowe FJ, Sarkies NJ. Assessment of visual function in idiopathic intracranial hypertension: A prospective study. Eye 1998; 12(Pt 1):111–118.

39. Rowe FJ, Sarkies NJ. Visual outcome in a prospective study of idiopathic intracranial hypertension. Arch Ophthalmol 1999; 117(11):1571.

40. Lueck C, McIlwaine G. Interventions for idiopathic intracranial hypertension. Cochrane Database Syst Rev 2007; (3):CD003434.

41. Marks MP, Dake MD, Steinberg GK, et al. Stent placement for arterial and venous cerebrovascular disease: Preliminary experience. Radiology 1994; 191(2):441–446.

42. King JO, Mitchell PJ, Thomson KR, et al. Manometry combined with cervical puncture in idiopathic intracranial hypertension. Neurology 2002; 58(1):26–30.

43. Owler BK, Parker G, Halmagyi GM, et al. Pseudotumor cerebri syndrome: Venous sinus obstruction and its treatment with stent placement. J Neurosurg 2003; 98(5):1045–1055.

44. Ogungbo B, Roy D, Gholkar A, et al. Endovascular stenting of the transverse sinus in a patient presenting with benign intracranial hypertension. Br J Neurosurg 2003; 17(6):565–568.

45. Rajpal S, Niemann DB, Turk AS. Transverse venous sinus stent placement as treatment for benign intracranial hypertension in a young male: Case report and review of the literature. J Neurosurg 2005; 102(suppl. 3):342–346.

46. Higgins JN, Cousins C, Owler BK, et al. Idiopathic intracranial hypertension: 12 cases treated by venous sinus stenting. J Neurol Neurosurg Psychiatry 2003; 74(12):1662–1666.

47. Owler BK, Parker G, Halmagyi GM, et al. Cranial venous outflow obstruction and pseudotumor Cerebri syndrome. Adv Tech Stand Neurosurg 2005; 30:107–174.

48. Metellus P, Levrier O, Fuentes S, et al. Endovascular treatment of idiopathic intracranial hypertension. Analysis of eight consecutive patients. Neurochirurgie 2007; 53(1):10–17.

49. Johnson LN, Krohel GB, Madsen RW, et al. The role of weight loss and acetazolamide in the treatment of idiopathic intracranial hypertension (pseudotumor cerebri). Ophthalmology 1998; 105(12):2313–2317.

50. Kupersmith MJ, Gamell L, Turbin R, et al. Effects of weight loss on the course of idiopathic intracranial hypertension in women. Neurology 1998; 50(4):1094–1098.

51. Rubin RC, Henderson ES, Ommaya AK, et al. The production of cerebrospinal fluid in man and its modification by acetazolamide. J Neurosurg 1966; 25(4):430–436.

52. Scott WJ, Schreiner CM, Hirsch KS. Unique pattern of limb malformations associated with carbonic anhydrase inhibition. Prog Clin Biol Res 1983; 110(Pt A):423–429.

53. Bell SM, Schreiner CM, Resnick E, et al. Exacerbation of acetazolamide teratogenesis by amiloride and its analogs active against Na^+/H^+ exchangers and Na^+ channels. Reprod Toxicol 1997; 11(6):823–831.

54. Youroukos S, Psychou F, Fryssiras S, et al. Idiopathic intracranial hypertension in children. J Child Neurol 2000; 15(7):453–457.

55. McGirt MJ, Woodworth G, Thomas G, et al. Cerebrospinal fluid shunt placement for pseudotumor cerebri-associated intractable headache: Predictors of treatment response and an analysis of long-term outcomes. J Neurosurg 2004; 101(4):627–632.

56. Eggenberger ER, Miller NR, Vitale S. Lumboperitoneal shunt for the treatment of pseudotumor cerebri. Neurology 1996; 46(6):1524–1530.

57. Wang VY, Barbaro NM, Lawton MT, et al. Complications of lumboperitoneal shunts. Neurosurgery 2007; 60(6):1045–1048; discussion 1049.

58. Chumas PD, Armstrong DC, Drake JM, et al. Tonsillar herniation: The rule rather than the exception after lumboperitoneal shunting in the pediatric population. J Neurosurg 1993; 78(4):568–573.

59. Chumas PD, Kulkarni AV, Drake JM, et al. Lumboperitoneal shunting: A retrospective study in the pediatric population. Neurosurgery 1993; 32(3):376–383; discussion 383.

60. Hart A, David K, Powell M. The treatment of 'acquired tonsillar herniation' in pseudotumour cerebri. Br J Neurosurg 2000; 14(6):563–565.

61. Johnston I, Jacobson E, Besser M. The acquired Chiari malformation and syringomyelia following spinal CSF drainage: A study of incidence and management. Acta Neurochir (Wien) 1998; 140(5):417–427; discussion 427–428.

62. Padmanabhan R, Crompton D, Burn D, et al. Acquired Chiari 1 malformation and syringomyelia following lumboperitoneal shunting for pseudotumour cerebri. J Neurol Neurosurg Psychiatry 2005; 76(2):298.

63. Sullivan LP, Stears JC, Ringel SP. Resolution of syringomyelia and Chiari I malformation by ventriculoatrial shunting in a patient with pseudotumor cerebri and a lumboperitoneal shunt. Neurosurgery 1988; 22(4):744–747.

64. Karabatsou K, Quigley G, Buxton N, et al. Lumboperitoneal shunts: Are the complications acceptable? Acta Neurochir (Wien) 2004; 146(11):1193–1197.

65. Maher CO, Garrity JA, Meyer FB. Refractory idiopathic intracranial hypertension treated with stereotactically planned ventriculoperitoneal shunt placement. Neurosurg Focus 2001; 10(2):E1.

66. Abu-Serieh B, Ghassempour K, Duprez T, et al. Stereotactic ventriculoperitoneal shunting for refractory idiopathic intracranial hypertension. Neurosurgery 2007; 60(6):1039–1043; discussion 1043–1044.
67. Woodworth GF, McGirt MJ, Elfert P, et al. Frameless stereotactic ventricular shunt placement for idiopathic intracranial hypertension. Stereotact Funct Neurosurg 2005; 83(1):12–16.
68. Azeem SS, Origitano TC. Ventricular catheter placement with a frameless neuronavigational system: A 1-year experience. Neurosurgery 2007; 60(4 suppl 2):243–247; discussion 247–248.
69. Rodt T, Koppen G, Lorenz M, et al. Placement of intraventricular catheters using flexible electromagnetic navigation and a dynamic reference frame: A new technique. Stereotact Funct Neurosurg 2007; 85(5):243–248.
70. DeWecker L. On incision of the optic nerve in cases of neuroretinitis. Int Ophthalmol Cong Rep 1872; 4:11–12.
71. Carter R. Case of swollen optic disc in which the sheath of the optic nerve was incised behind the eyeball. Proc Med Soc Lond 1887; 10:290.
72. Tse DT, Nerad JA, Anderson RL, et al. Optic nerve sheath fenestration in pseudotumor cerebri. A lateral orbitotomy approach. Arch Ophthalmol 1988; 106(10):1458–1462.
73. Kersten RC, Kulwin DR. Optic nerve sheath fenestration through a lateral canthotomy incision. Arch Ophthalmol 1993; 111(6):870–874.
74. Anderson RL, Flaharty PM. Treatment of pseudotumor cerebri by primary and secondary optic nerve sheath decompression. Am J Ophthalmol 1992; 113(5):599–601.
75. Spoor TC, Ramocki JM, Madion MP, et al. Treatment of pseudotumor cerebri by primary and secondary optic nerve sheath decompression. Am J Ophthalmol 1991; 112(2):177–185.
76. Spoor TC, McHenry JG, Shin DH. Optic nerve sheath decompression with adjunctive mitomycin and Molteno device implantation. Arch Ophthalmol 1994; 112(1):25–26.
77. Sergott RC, Savino PJ, Bosley TM. Modified optic nerve sheath decompression provides long-term visual improvement for pseudotumor cerebri. Arch Ophthalmol 1988; 106(10):1384–1390.
78. Hupp SL, Buckley EG, Byrne SF, et al. Posttraumatic venous obstructive retinopathy associated with enlarged optic nerve sheath. Arch Ophthalmol 1984; 102(2):254–256.
79. Kaye AH, Galbraith JE, King J. Intracranial pressure following optic nerve decompression for benign intracranial hypertension. Case report. J Neurosurg 1981; 55(3):453–456.
80. Kilpatrick CJ, Kaufman DV, Galbraith JE, et al. Optic nerve decompression in benign intracranial hypertension. Clin Exp Neurol 1981; 18:161–168.
81. Plotnik JL, Kosmorsky GS. Operative complications of optic nerve sheath decompression. Ophthalmology 1993; 100(5):683–690.
82. Riordan-Eva P. Optic nerve sheath fenestration. Curr Med Literature (Ophthalmic) 1994; 4:67–73.
83. Feldon SE. Visual outcomes comparing surgical techniques for management of severe idiopathic intracranial hypertension. Neurosurg Focus 2007; 23(5):E6.
84. Boddie HG, Banna M, Bradley WG. "Benign" intracranial hypertension. A survey of the clinical and radiological features, and long-term prognosis. Brain 1974; 97(2):313–326.
85. Bradshaw P. Benign intracranial hypertension. J Neurol Neurosurg Psychiatry 1956; 19(1):28–41.
86. Rabinowicz IM, Ben-Sira I, Zauberman H. Preservation of visual function in papilloedema observed for 3 to 6 years in cases of benign intracranial hypertension. Br J Ophthalmol 1968; 52(3):236–241.
87. Vassilouthis J, Uttley D. Benign intracranial hypertension. Clinical features and diagnosis using CT and treatment. Surgi Neurol 1979;12:389– 392.
88. Orcutt JC, Page NGR, Sanders MD. Factors affecting visual loss in benign intracranial hypertension. Ophthalmology 1984; 91:1303–1312.
89. Sorensen PS, Krogsaa B, Gjerris F. Clinical course and prognosis of pseudotumor cerebri. A prospective study of 24 patients. Acta Neurologica Scandinavica 1988; 77:164–177.

Pseudotumor and Obesity

Harold L. Rekate

Pediatric Neurosciences, Barrow Neurological Institute, St. Joseph's Hospital and Medical Center, Phoenix, Arizona, U.S.A.

Pseudotumor cerebri (PC), which is also called benign intracranial hypertension (BIH), is a condition in which intracranial pressure (ICP) is above the normal in the absence of abnormalities of the brain on imaging studies. An increasing number of studies have described PC without papilledema (1–3). However, most patients diagnosed with this condition are found to have papilledema, and some have had severe visual loss and even blindness (4,5). The consensus is that the only neurologic abnormalities that can be ascribed to PC are damage to the optic nerves and unilateral or bilateral abducens palsies. Recently, an encephalopathic condition associated with chronically increased ICP has been described (6). In most patients, however, the management of PC is equivalent to the management of a severe headache disorder.

PATHOPHYSIOLOGY OF PC IN OBESE PATIENTS?

What causes PC? In our early work linking research into the pathophysiology of hydrocephalus with a mathematical model based on computer simulations, we postulated that PC would result from either increased pressure in the superior sagittal sinus (SSS), the end terminus for cerebrospinal fluid (CSF) absorption, or it would develop from an obstruction to CSF outflow at the arachnoid villi associated with an increase in the stiffness or turgor of the brain (7,8). For two reasons increased sagittal sinus pressure was considered the single underlying mechanism for both conditions. First, for CSF to be absorbed, a pressure gradient of about 5 mm Hg is needed between the cortical subarachnoid space and the SSS. Second, increasing sagittal sinus pressure would also increase the turgor of the brain by increasing cerebral blood volume.

To test this hypothesis, we measured venous and intracranial venous sinus pressure in patients with PC. In our first report of 10 patients with documented PC, 5 were obese and 5 were of normal body habitus (9). In the nonobese patients, sagittal sinus pressure was elevated above normal and a gradient was present within the venous pathways. This gradient was usually at the level of the junction of the transverse and sigmoid sinuses, but it also occurs at the level of the jugular foramen. In our five severely obese patients (all women), the problem was related to elevated pressure in the right atrium being transmitted into the intracranial venous system (9). This pattern of elevated intracranial venous sinus pressure in all patients with PC has now been confirmed in our practice in 150 investigations.

Right atrial pressure is a reflection of atmospheric pressure. Therefore, we use 5 mm Hg as the upper limit of normal in patients undergoing venographic pressure measurements. Measurements higher than 10 mm Hg indicate significant difficulties related to PC. Our studies in laboratory animals have documented a substantial pressure gradient between the intracranial compartment and pressure in the SSS until very high ICP is reached by the infusion of artificial CSF (10,11). Based on concurrent measurements of ICP in patients undergoing retrograde venographic pressure measurements, there is a demonstrable pressure gradient of 5 to 10 mm Hg from the intracranial compartment to the pressure in the sagittal sinus. These observations are supported by the work of Portnoy et al. (12,13). Intracranial venous pressure is predictive of ICP in all patients studied in this way. From the right atrium to the SSS, obese patients have documented a 5 to 10 mm Hg increase in venous pressure.

Based partially on this work, Owler et al. have suggested that thin patients with PC who have a documented pressure differential within the cerebral venous sinuses be treated with venous stenting and documented the effectiveness of this technique in the resolution of PC (14). This form of treatment is being pursued in several other centers (15).

The largest studies on the relationship between PC and obesity have been performed by Sugerman and his colleagues at the Medical College of Virginia. They found that morbid obesity leads to a cascade of events, including increased intraabdominal pressure, increased intrathoracic pressure, and increased right heart–loading pressure (16,17). Known differences in the distribution of fat between men and women (apple vs. pear distribution) may explain why PC is so much more common in women than in men. This group also published the results of treatment of PC using a pneumatic suction device that decreases intra-abdominal pressure and relieves the symptoms of PC (18).

DIAGNOSIS OF OBESITY-RELATED PC

There is considerable variation in the diagnosis of and treatment philosophy for PC, especially in the obese population. Headaches are so common in humans that there is a predictable reluctance to pursue these problems when patients seek treatment. The brain is often imaged, and when the findings are negative no further evaluation is recommended. The diagnosis is suspected when the patient is seen by a neurologist who detects papilledema or when the patient begins to experience visual loss and is diagnosed by an ophthalmologist.

Papilledema, headaches, visual loss, and negative imaging of the intracranial compartment lead to lumbar puncture and subsequently to diagnosis. Unfortunately, there are no signs or easy tests to perform other than lumbar puncture to obtain the information needed for diagnosis. Lumbar puncture in the obese is daunting. The needle is often near the full extent of its length, and multiple attempts may be necessary to cannulate the subarachnoid space. At this point, the patient is in pain, severely anxious, and finds it difficult to relax. In this situation measurements of lumbar pressure are often unreliable. Often, the measured ICP may be higher than the actual ICP in obese anxious patients.

We have found it useful to have a radiologist perform the procedure fluoroscopically. After the patient is premedicated with an anxiolytic drug, the lumbar puncture needle is passed under fluoroscopic guidance. Once CSF is flowing freely, the patient must be turned to a lateral decubitus position to obtain a careful manometric determination of ICP. Pressure measurements from prone patients are subject to being elevated by the increased pressure generated by pressure on the pendulous abdomen.

In subtle or confusing cases, particularly when invasive treatments are contemplated, it is often advisable to monitor ICP. In patients with abrupt visual loss, a lumbar drain can be placed into the spinal subarachnoid space to release CSF and to monitor ICP while deciding on more definitive treatment. In most cases, ICP is monitored with a subdural/subarachnoid transducer or an intraparenchymal monitor. ICP can then be recorded for several days to elucidate the dynamics in individual patients.

It is our policy to perform retrograde measurements of intracranial venous pressure in all patients with PC (Fig. 1). We believe that it is essential to determine if the problem is unequivocally related to obesity. In overweight patients, particularly women, it is often assumed that their intracranial hypertension is caused by their obesity. This is not always true. Patients whose body mass index is less than 40 are less likely to have PC. Their obesity is unrelated to their intracranial hypertension if venous structures exiting the brain are constricted. This distinction is crucial because the conditions are treated differently. If patients' right atrial pressure is normal, weight loss will have no effect on ICP. If their body mass index is less than or equal to 35 and their right atrial pressure is higher than 8 mm Hg, then PC is caused by their obesity.

TREATMENT OF OBESITY-RELATED PC

Since the condition of PC was first recognized, its treatment has revolved around corticosteroids, intermittent lumbar puncture, and acetazolamide. Corticosteroids are known to lower ICP, and their use is a good way to protect patients from acute visual loss. However, patients who are placed on corticosteroids gain weight, which is a terrible complication for those with obesity-related PC. Steroids also lower resistance to infection, impair wound healing, and lead to acne. These medications may be acceptable for the acute management

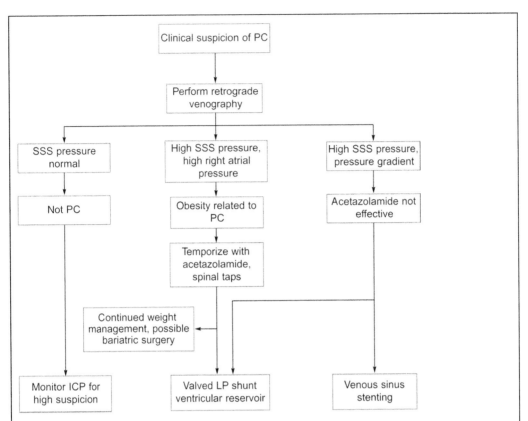

Figure 1 Algorithm for the diagnosis and management of patients who have or might have pseudotumor cerebri. *Abbreviations*: PC, pseudotumor cerebri; SSS, superior sagittal sinus; LP, lumboperitoneal. *Source*: Courtesy of Barrow Neurological Institute.

of PC. However, PC is a chronic disease and its long-term management with steroids should be avoided.

Performing a lumbar puncture lowers ICP briefly. Humans usually replace their entire volume of CSF three times each day. Therefore, the 30 to 50 mL of CSF removed during a spinal tap is replaced within about eight hours. The needle passed through the dura may leave a hole that leaks for a short time. Such leakage may lead to resolution of symptoms for a prolonged but unpredictable period. This scenario is desirable to lower ICP for a few days. However, it is not an effective treatment for an extended period.

Acetazolamide (Diamox™) has been used to treat PC with some success. This medication, a carbonic anhydrase inhibitor, decreases CSF production 50% to 70% and can decrease ICP in patients with obesity-related PC (19).

In our practice, retrograde measurements of dural venous pressure and ICP have clarified the mechanisms of action of acetazolamide on ICP in patients with PC. The use of acetazolamide does not decrease ICP in patients whose PC is unrelated to obesity. Three obese patients with documented significant increases in ICP, who underwent retrograde measurement of their dural sinus pressure, were found to have normal right atrial and sagittal sinus pressures. Measurements obtained 7 to 10 days after they discontinued the use of the acetazolamide documented clear-cut increases in right atrial, intracranial venous, and sagittal sinus pressures. The cause of PC in the obese is right atrial hypertension. Treatment with acetazolamide is linked to decreases in right atrial pressure and effective treatment of such PC.

Unfortunately, many patients are unable to tolerate effective doses of acetazolamide because of its side effects. Dizziness, balance difficulties, and light-headedness are common.

Renal stones have been reported. Furthermore, the expectation of response to treatment among treating physicians is low, and this effective treatment may be abandoned too early in carefully selected patients.

Overall, the surgical management of PC is difficult and is associated with many failures and complications. Which patients with this diagnosis should undergo therapy is controversial? Most patients are managed with acetazolamide, regardless of whether they are obese, and they intermittently undergo spinal taps when their symptoms are worst. Visual loss and diplopia are the two objective problems associated with PC, and patients must be followed carefully to prevent irreversible visual loss. In the absence of a threat to vision, there is little reason to intervene urgently. Trials of medication are often all that is needed to manage the headaches. However, long-term management of this chronic condition with narcotic medication must be avoided. This therapy leads to an independent headache disorder that does not respond to manipulation of ICP. A discussion of the medical management of headaches in the context of PC is beyond the scope of this discussion and my personal expertise. Referral to a neurologist or neuro-ophthalmologist with expertise in these matters is usually necessary.

When vision is threatened or medical management of the severe headache disorder fails, definitive treatment is warranted. In patients with only obesity-related PC, acetazolamide rapidly and effectively lowers right atrial pressure and therefore sagittal sinus pressure and ICP. Unless significant vision has already been lost or the papilledema is so severe that such a loss can be expected, the first course of action should be the use of 500 mg of acetazolamide two to three times per day. As discussed above, patients need to be warned of the side effects. After 4 to 7 days, another spinal tap should be performed to measure ICP to confirm that the medical management is effective. This strategy usually significantly delays the need for surgical intervention. In these cases, we strongly recommend the use of the retrograde venographic measurement of venous pressures to document right atrial hypertension. The knowledge thus acquired provides a stronger position from which to make treatment decisions.

The first advantage is the realization that the PC is caused by obesity through a mechanism that increases intra-abdominal, intrathoracic, and right atrial pressure and that lowering these pressures will resolve the PC. In all but the most severe cases, the use of acetazolamide at the time PC is diagnosed markedly ameliorates the condition while definitive treatment is pursued. In the case of obesity-related PC, definitive treatment means weight loss. In patients whose body mass index is higher than 35, a 15% loss of body weight will likely markedly improve their condition.

In my experience, almost all patients with PC have been made aware of the relationship between their obesity and their PC. Few if any, however, have been counseled about the need to lose weight to manage their PC. The first step therefore is to recommend a program leading to weight loss. For patients who have recently gained considerable weight, as is often the case after delivery of a baby, weight loss by diet and exercise may be all that is needed to "cure" the PC. Weight loss should be pursued under the supervision of a program for weight loss. Data show that diet/weight loss programs can lead to sustained effective weight loss in some patients.

Most severely obese patients with PC have repeatedly tried diets and weight loss programs with partial and short-lived success. For such patients, bariatric surgery with intestinal bypass may be the best and only permanent solution to this vexing problem. Sugerman et al., whose pioneering work on the health effects of obesity and the effect of bariatric surgery on the patient's health, have shown that many complications related to obesity, including PC, resolve with surgical management of weight loss (20,21). Our work has documented decreases in right atrial pressure in patients with obesity-related PC, leading to shunt-independent arrest of the PC (22).

PALLIATION OF OBESITY-RELATED PC

As stated, definitive management of obesity-related PC derives from direct treatment of the obesity itself. Most patients require intestinal bypass surgery, and the subject should be introduced at the time of the initial diagnosis. In patients with mild papilledema, I recommend documentation of ICP using lumbar puncture. Patients begin on acetazolamide to improve the situation while definitive treatment related to weight loss is pursued. In patients with severe papilledema, particularly in those with documented visual loss, I recommend placement of a temporary lumbar drain. A drain leads to the ability to lower ICP and to protect vision. At this point administration of acetazolamide is begun. ICP routinely stabilizes with no further need to drain CSF. If this occurs, the drain can be removed. The medication is continued while the patient loses weight. If the acetazolamide is ineffective in lowering ICP significantly or if the side effects preclude its long-term use, other forms of therapy must be considered. So far, however, we have encountered no patient with obesity-related PC (i.e., documented to be due to right atrial hypertension) whose complaints have not markedly improved or temporarily resolved completely with the use of acetazolamide.

In centers with skilled oculoplastic ophthalmologists, optic nerve sheath fenestration is a viable option for the palliative management of PC. This operation was originally designed to prevent optic nerve ischemia by opening the sheath that encases it within the orbit. It involves entering the orbit through a scleral incision and making an incision in the dural sleeve that encases the nerve. How the procedure protects the nerve from injury is unclear and may involve multiple factors. However, it is thought to decrease pressure on the nerve, thereby preventing ischemic damage. Another proposed mechanism is supported by some MRI data. That is, the subarachnoid space herniates into the orbit, and fenestration of the optic sheath drains CSF into the periorbitum, thereby lowering ICP (23). More work is needed to define the mechanism whereby sheath fenestration relieves the papilledema that causes visual loss. The effectiveness of the nerve sheath fenestration partially seems to depend on the experience of the oculoplastic ophthalmologist. Relatively high complication rates, including visual field disturbances and visual loss, have been reported and both optic nerves need to be fenestrated frequently (24).

A second option for palliative treatment is CSF shunting. PC increases venous pressure and the volume of venous blood in the brain. The total volume of CSF in the cortical and spinal subarachnoid spaces also increases. Lowering pressure in the subarachnoid spaces decreases ICP and protects vision. If ICP can be normalized, there is a reasonable chance that the severe headache disorder can also be ameliorated.

In PC, all of the CSF compartments communicate with each other. Theoretically, therefore, it should be possible to shunt any compartment to drain all of the other compartments. CSF cannot exit the cortical subarachnoid space due to increased pressure in the venous sinuses. Consequently, if shunting to the lateral ventricles is performed, CSF in the other compartments must return to that ventricle to pass through the shunt. As CSF is drained from the lateral ventricle, the septum pellucidum tends to rest on the head of the caudate nucleus, restricting flow from the third ventricle to the lateral ventricle.

This phenomenon is the substrate for postshunt ventricular asymmetry (25). It also tends to cause the ventricles to collapse around the ventricular catheter. Intermittent or permanent occlusion of the ventricular catheter results. To avoid this problem, procedures that access the CSF in the cortical subarachnoid space are preferable to ventricular shunts. In PC, shunts that access the subarachnoid space and the ventricles include lumboperitoneal shunts and shunts to the cisterna magna (22,26–29).

Extraventricular shunts are associated with their own difficulties, especially in obese patients. The failure rate of lumboperitoneal shunts is high and they are difficult to assess (30). In children, lumboperitoneal shunts lower lumbar thecal pressure, leading to herniation of the cerebellar tonsils, a condition also known as an acquired Chiari malformation (31,32). All patients reported in these two papers were infants with valveless lumboperitoneal shunts. Our experience with valved lumboperitoneal shunts in children with slit ventricle syndrome has shown no tendency for this problem to occur.

LP shunts are routinely performed in a lateral decubitus position by using a 14-gauge Tuohy needle for insertion of the proximal catheter. We use programmable valves to normalize ICP in these sensitive patients. We prefer the Codman Hakim Programmable valve with Siphonguard™ (Codman Corp., Raynham, MA), which can be obtained with a flat bottom to prevent its rotation and to allow it to be programmed.

These programmable valves limit some of the usual options for shunting. The Siphonguard™ can be used to prevent overdrainage, and gravity-compensating devices can be used in association with programmable valves to prevent overdrainage. However, devices that contain a diaphragm mechanism for controlling siphoning, such as the Strata Valve™ (Medtronic Corporation, Minneapolis, MN), cannot be used because the overdrainage in LP shunts is not caused by siphoning but by upstream hydrostatic pressure keeping the valve open when the patient is erect.

The placement of peritoneal catheters in obese patients in the lateral decubitus position is also associated with problems. There is a tendency to place the abdominal incision too near the flank. This position makes it difficult to find the peritoneum and makes suturing the posterior sheath very difficult. The problem often leads to the peritoneal catheter pulling out into the subcutaneous tissue and shunt failure. To place peritoneal catheters adequately in morbidly obese patients, it is often necessary to obtain the help of abdominal surgeons who have experience with laparoscopy. Even after laparoscopic placement, peritoneal catheter malposition and distal failure are relatively common problems.

How can one tell whether a lumboperitoneal shunt is working adequately? As stated, measuring ICP by lumbar puncture in very obese patients is difficult and the result is difficult to interpret. The patient is often anxious, and the pressure is often high due to increased intra-abdominal pressure. Some of this difficulty can be avoided by using a reservoir on the valve mechanism. To enable the valve to be reprogrammed and to access the reservoir if necessary, the valve should be placed superficially in the subcutaneous tissue of the back. If it is unclear if the shunt is working and there is no ventricular reservoir to allow accurate measurement of ICP, we tend to inject indium-111 bound to albumin into the thecal sac and scan the abdomen. The radiologist can usually follow the flow of the tracer into the abdomen. If a lumboperitoneal shunt is working, the tracer should be present within the bladder within two hours.

We have found it extremely beneficial to implant a ventricular access device or reservoir into the lateral ventricle at the time a lumboperitoneal shunt is placed. To do so, the use of frameless stereotaxy is essential. The reservoir allows ICP to be measured and the function of the valve to be tested. It also serves as a guide for changing the valve settings in patients with programmable valves. Manometric measurements of ICP are accurate and allow instantaneous assessment of shunt function in the context of PC. In complicated cases whose management is difficult, a butterfly needle can be inserted transcutaneously and affixed to the scalp for prolonged monitoring of ICP to enable fine tuning of ICP dynamics.

Some patients, such as those with spinal stenosis or a hindbrain herniation as in Chiari I and II malformations, are poor candidates for lumboperitoneal shunts. For the reasons discussed above, the need to access the cortical subarachnoid space in these patients remains. Many neurosurgeons prefer to avoid lumboperitoneal shunting because of previous difficulties assessing function and recurrent failures. For such patients, we recommend the use of a cisterna magna to lateral ventricle to peritoneal shunt.

Johnston has recommended that PC patients be routinely treated with cisterna magna to peritoneal shunting. We have found it difficult to shunt to the posterior fossa or craniovertebral junction for several reasons. The valve tends to end up in the muscular folds of the neck. It is difficult to include a tapping reservoir, and these shunts tend to break due to excessive movement in that region. Because of these problems, combined with our desire to have a tapping reservoir in the lateral ventricle, we no longer shunt directly to the cisterna magna, except to connect to a lateral ventricle shunt (22,28). As described in our previous reports of this technique, there are some specific technical considerations associated with performing the procedure. Lumbar catheters must be used for the cisterna magna catheter. Otherwise, typical ventricular catheters end up resting on a nerve root or brainstem causing severe pain or neurologic or cranial nerve deficits.

CONCLUSION

Obesity-related PC is a chronic condition caused by the obesity with which it is related. This condition is much more common in women than in men and, if untreated, can lead to blindness. To treat this condition, the patient's obesity must be treated (Fig. 1). If PC is recognized early and the causative obesity is managed aggressively (e.g., with bariatric surgery), the likelihood of the patient living a normal life is excellent. If the documented cause of the PC is obesity, the condition is chronic and potentially lifelong, requiring a huge outlay of energy and healthcare resources to manage.

REFERENCES

1. Marcelis J, Silberstein SD. Idiopathic intracranial hypertension without papilledema. Arch Neurol 1991; 48(4):392–399.
2. Mathew NT, Ravishankar K, Sanin LC. Coexistence of migraine and idiopathic intracranial hypertension without papilledema. Neurology 1996; 46(5):1226–1230.
3. Winner P, Bello L. Idiopathic intracranial hypertension in a young child without visual symptoms or signs. Headache 1996; 36(9):574–576.
4. Liu GT, Volpe NJ, Schatz NJ, et al. Severe sudden visual loss caused by pseudotumor cerebri and lumboperitoneal shunt failure. Am J Ophthalmol 1996; 122(1):129–131.
5. Varelas PN, Spanaki MV, Rathi S, et al. Papilledema unresponsive to therapy in Pickwickian syndrome: Another presentation of pseudotumor cerebri? Am J Med 2000; 109(1):80–81.
6. Kaplan CP, Miner ME, McGregor JM. Pseudotumour cerebri: Risk for cognitive impairment? Brain Inj 1997; 11(4):293–303.
7. Rekate HL. The usefulness of mathematical modeling in hydrocephalus research. Childs Nerv Syst 1994; 10(1):13–18.
8. Rekate HL. The slit ventricle syndrome: Advances based on technology and understanding. Pediatr Neurosurg 2004; 40(6):259–263.
9. Karahalios DG, Rekate HL, Khayata MH, et al. Elevated intracranial venous pressure as a universal mechanism in pseudotumor cerebri of varying etiologies. Neurology 1996; 46(1):198–202.
10. McCormick JM, Yamada K, Rekate HL, et al. Time course of intraventricular pressure change in a canine model of hydrocephalus: Its relationship to sagittal sinus elastance. Pediatr Neurosurg 1992; 18(3):127–133.
11. Olivero WC, Rekate HL, Chizeck HJ, et al. Relationship between intracranial and sagittal sinus pressure in normal and hydrocephalic dogs. Pediatr Neurosci 1988; 14(4):196–201.
12. Portnoy HD, Branch C, Castro ME. The relationship of intracranial venous pressure to hydrocephalus. Childs Nerv Syst 1994; 10(1):29–35.
13. Portnoy HD, Castro ME. Elevated cortical venous pressure in hydrocephalus. Neurosurgery 1993; 32(1):151
14. Owler BK, Parker G, Halmagyi GM, et al. Pseudotumor cerebri syndrome: Venous sinus obstruction and its treatment with stent placement. J Neurosurg 2003; 98(5):1045–1055.
15. Higgins JN, Cousins C, Owler BK, et al. Idiopathic intracranial hypertension: 12 cases treated by venous sinus stenting. J Neurol Neurosurg Psychiatry 2003; 74(12):1662–1666.
16. Sugerman HJ. Effects of increased intra-abdominal pressure in severe obesity. Surg Clin North Am 2001; 81(5):1063–1075.
17. Sugerman HJ. Increased intra-abdominal pressure and cardiac filling pressures in obesity-associated pseudotumor cerebri. Neurology 1997; 49(2):507–511.
18. Sugerman HJ, Felton WL III, Sismanis A, et al. Continuous negative abdominal pressure device to treat pseudotumor cerebri. Int J Obes Relat Metab Disord 2001; 25(4):486–490.
19. Milhorat TH, Hammock MK, Fenstermacher JD, et al. Cerebrospinal fluid production by the choroid plexus and brain. Science 1971; 173(994):330–332.
20. Sugerman HJ, Felton WL III, Salvant JB Jr, et al. Effects of surgically induced weight loss on idiopathic intracranial hypertension in morbid obesity. Neurology 1995; 45(9):1655–1659.
21. Sugerman HJ, Felton WL III, Sismanis A, et al. Gastric surgery for pseudotumor cerebri associated with severe obesity. Ann Surg 1999; 229(5):634–640.
22. Nadkarni T, Rekate HL, Wallace D. Resolution of pseudotumor cerebri after bariatric surgery for related obesity. Case report. J Neurosurg 2004; 101(5):878–880.
23. Hamed LM, Tse DT, Glaser JS, et al. Neuroimaging of the optic nerve after fenestration for management of pseudotumor cerebri. Arch Ophthalmol 1992; 110(5):636–639.
24. Goh KY, Schatz NJ, Glaser JS. Optic nerve sheath fenestration for pseudotumor cerebri. J Neuroophthalmol 1997; 17(2):86–91.

25. Rekate HL, Williams FC Jr, Brodkey JA, et al. Resistance of the foramen of Monro. Pediatr Neurosci 1988; 14(2):85–89.
26. Johnston IH, Duff J, Jacobson EE, et al. Asymptomatic intracranial hypertension in disorders of CSF circulation in childhood–Treated and untreated. Pediatr Neurosurg 2001; 34(2):63–72.
27. Lee MC, Yamini B, Frim DM. Pseudotumor cerebri patients with shunts from the cisterna magna: Clinical course and telemetric intracranial pressure data. Neurosurgery 2004; 55(5):1094–1099.
28. Nadkarni TD, Rekate HL. Treatment of refractory intracranial hypertension in a spina bifida patient by a concurrent ventricular and cisterna magna-to-peritoneal shunt. Childs Nerv Syst 2005; 21(7):579–582.
29. Rekate HL, Wallace D. Lumboperitoneal shunts in children. Pediatr Neurosurg 2003; 38(1):41–46.
30. Burgett RA, Purvin VA, Kawasaki A. Lumboperitoneal shunting for pseudotumor cerebri. Neurology 1997; 49(3):734–739.
31. Chumas PD, Armstrong DC, Drake JM, et al. Tonsillar herniation: The rule rather than the exception after lumboperitoneal shunting in the pediatric population. J Neurosurg 1993; 78(4):568–573.
32. Chumas PD, Kulkarni AV, Drake JM, et al. Lumboperitoneal shunting: A retrospective study in the pediatric population. Neurosurgery 1993; 32(3):376–383.

Lumboperitoneal Shunts in the Treatment of Benign Intracranial Hypertension

Konstantina Karabatsou

Department of Neurosurgery, The Walton Centre for Neurology and Neurosurgery, Liverpool, U.K.

Benign intracranial hypertension (BIH) continues to be a rather perplexing condition, whose pathophysiology and underlying causative factors are poorly understood by the neuroscientists around the world. The lack of proper understanding of the condition has historically led to several treatment strategies, but none so far has been widely accepted as the treatment of choice.

Approximately 10% to 15% of patients with BIH will be refractory to medical management and will eventually require some form of surgical intervention.

Lumboperitoneal shunting has traditionally been the most common procedure in the surgical management of BIH. There is little doubt that the placement of lumboperitoneal shunt is an effective method providing a rapid resolution of the symptoms as long as it remains patent and functional.

Our experience combined with the experience from other centers worldwide has showed that although the lumboperitoneal shunts have excellent results in the short-term management of patients with BIH, their results tend to be short lived. These patients eventually will require further surgical intervention in the long term (1–3). The major disadvantage of the lumboperitoneal shunt is the frequent need for revision and subsequent high failure rate. The most common complication is shunt obstruction, which in the majority of them is due to blockage of the peritoneal catheter. Other problems include migration or fracture of the catheter, radiculopathy, infection, and arachnoiditis.

Overdrainage of the shunt can initially cause low-pressure headaches, which can progress to tonsillar herniation with significant and potentially devastating consequences. The development of Chiari malformation following placement of lumboperitoneal shunt is more common than was previously thought, especially in children and young adults, as it can now be detected more easily with the widespread use of MRI (4). The incorporation of a valve mechanism to the shunting device could potentially decrease the development of tonsillar herniation.

There is also a strong argument that delayed shunt malfunction can occur leading to development of raised intracranial pressure symptoms, which can go unrecognized till they finally turn to be harmful for the patient. Whether shunting induces a shunt-dependence state or a feature inherent to this particular condition is difficult to speculate.

The use of ventriculoperitoneal shunt seems to be associated with lower risk of shunt obstruction and shunt revision. The presence of small ventricles, which is commonly the rule in patients with BIH, should not preclude the placement of a VP shunt, as nowadays it is possible to overcome this with the use of stereotactic, frameless image guidance systems, and more recently electromagnetic field–based navigation systems (5). There is always the potential risk of brain injury and epilepsy associated with ventriculoperitoneal shunts, but a careful placement of a shunt under guidance should minimize the risk of these mishaps.

Although there are no randomized controlled trials comparing the efficacy and durability of ventriculoperitoneal shunts versus lumboperitoneal shunts, there is a growing body of evidence in favor of the use of ventriculoperitoneal shunts. The wide availability of frameless navigation systems allows the safe and accurate placement of shunts in most cases.

There have recently been some reports supporting the use of endoluminar venous sinus stenting in the treatment of patients diagnosed with venous sinus obstruction following retrograde cerebral venography and manometry. The concept behind this seems very attractive but its long-term results and applicability remain to be validated.

There is still a lot to be learnt about the pathophysiology of this complex condition, which might change its management in the future. A better understanding of the etiology and natural history might enable us to address the causative factors directly and provide us with advanced and efficient new management modalities.

Until then the lumboperitoneal shunts will have a role to play in the management of patients with BIH with intractable headache and visual deterioration when medical management has failed.

However, in accordance with our experience, we would favor the placement of ventriculoperitoneal shunt in the treatment of such patients, provided navigation systems are available for the safe placement of the ventricular catheter, particularly when the size of the ventricles is small.

REFERENCES

1. Karabatsou K, Quigley G, Buxton N, et al. Lumboperitoneal shunts: Are the complications acceptable? Acta Neurochir (Wien) 2004; 146(11):1193–1197.
2. McGirt M, Woodworth G, Thomas G, et al. Cerebrospinal fluid shunt placement for pseudotumor cerebri-associated intractable headache: Predictors of treatment response and an analysis of long-term outcomes. J Neurosurg 2004; 101:627–632.
3. Rosenberg ML, Corbett JJ, Smith C, et al. Cerebrospinal fluid diversion procedures in pseudotumor cerebri. Neurology 1993; 43:1071–1072.
4. Chumas P, Kulkarni A, Drake JM, et al. Lumboperitoneal shunting: A retrospective study in the pediatric population. Neurosurgery 1993; 32(3):376–383.
5. Tulipan N, Lavin P, Copeland M. Stereotactic ventriculoperitoneal shunt for idiopathic intracranial hypertension: Technical note. Neurosurgery 1998; 43:175–177.

Venous Outflow Obstruction and Venous Sinus Thrombosis in Idiopathic Intracranial Hypertension

Pietro Spennato, Giuseppe Cinalli, Claudio Ruggiero, and Maria Consiglio Buonocore

Department of Pediatric Neurosurgery, Santobono Children's Hospital, Naples, Italy

The presence of an obstruction to venous outflow at the level of dural sinuses is nowadays the most accredited hypothesis for intracranial hypertension. CSF is absorbed in the superior sagittal sinus (SSS) at the level of the pacchionian granulations, carried by pressure gradient between CSF pressure and venous pressure in the SSS, which normally is 0 to 4 mm Hg. When venous pressure is higher, a higher CSF pressure is necessary to drive bulk flow of CSF across the meninges. As resistance to venous drainage increases, brain turgor also increases (1,2). Thereafter ventricular dilatation, as expected in case of high CSF pressure, is not possible because of the presence of a not "compliant" brain in a nonexpansive skull, unlike in young children with open sutures, in which intracranial venous hypertension and the resultant increase in ICP may lead to progressive head enlargement, with dilation of ventricles and subarachnoid spaces (3,4) [Fig. 1(A) to 1(C)].

Many authors have postulated theories incorporating elevated intracranial venous pressure as an underlying component of pseudotumor cerebri (PTC). However, to date, only few investigators have identified reliable structural abnormalities seen consistently on imaging studies or necropsy that would help explain the disease.

In 1951, Ray and Dunbar (5) performing sagittal sinus venography in four patients with PTC found thrombosis in the posterior half of the SSS or in the dominant transverse sinus. Their technique involved inserting a catheter into the anterior SSS through a burr-hole. Two of these patients had a history of peripheral thrombophlebitis and one had mastoiditis. The presence of anatomic abnormalities of the venous sinuses had not been universally observed in cases of "*idiopathic* intracranial hypertension"; indeed, nowadays, "thrombosis in a dural sinus" is a criterion of exclusion from the diagnosis.

King et al. (6) performed cerebral venography and manometry in nine patients with idiopathic intracranial hypertension. Using angiographic catheters passed into the intracranial venous sinuses through the jugular veins, they consistently recorded venous hypertension in the SSS and proximal transverse sinuses, with a significant drop in venous pressure at the level of the lateral third of the transverse sinus. This abnormality was not anatomically justified by the venography. The appearance of the transverse sinus on venography varied from smooth tapered narrowing to discrete intraluminal filling defects that resembled mural thrombi. They also found that the gradient could be eliminated by reducing CSF pressure with the removal of CSF through cervical puncture. Venous hypertension was not recorded in two patients in which intracranial hypertension was secondary to drugs (minocycline). Their conclusion was that poorly understood forms of venous pathology such as congenital stenosis should be implicated in the etiology.

Different results had been achieved by Karahalios et al. (7), who performed cerebral venography and manometry in 10 patients: in five, they identified dural venous outflow obstruction ("*secondary* PTC") and in the remaining five normal venous anatomy ("*idiopathic* PTC"). Dural sinus pressure was measured during venography: patients with obstruction tended to have a high pressure gradient across the obstruction, with high pressure proximally and lower pressure distally. Patients with no obstruction had elevated right atrial pressures as well as elevated venous sinus pressures. According to that study, PTC, whether

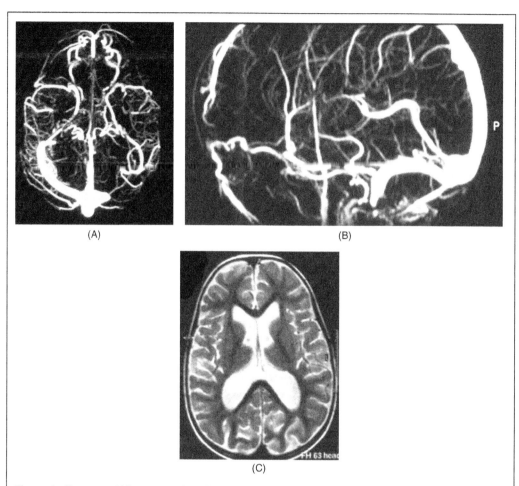

(A)   (B)

(C)

Figure 1 Two-year old boy presenting with progressive macrocrania and papilledema. Angio MRI showed complete block at the origin of left transverse sinus and at the transverse–sigmoid junction on the right side, with persistence of a small middle occipital sinus (**A**) and (**B**). Mild ventricular dilatation with enlarged subarachnoid spaces are evident (**C**).

secondary to intracranial venous outlet obstruction or idiopathic, may have increased venous pressure as its final common pathway. In patients with venous outflow obstruction, the resistance to venous drainage generates the elevated venous backpressure. Patients without outflow obstruction (idiopathic PTC) had elevated central systemic venous pressure, which may be transmitted up through the jugular veins and paravertebral plexus to the sinuses. To explain the elevated central systemic venous pressure in their idiopathic cases, Karahalios et al. (7) proposed different hypotheses, all linked to obesity—a constant finding in their series. Obesity-related cardiomyopathy can lead to congestive heart failure and a subsequent increase in central venous pressure. Obesity can lead also to sleep apnea or increased work in breathing, which in turn leads to respiratory acidosis, right-sided heart failure, and thus increased central venous pressure. Sugerman et al. (8) have suggested that carbon dioxide retention in these patients may lead to increased ICP. Finally, increased systemic venous pressure may be secondary to an increase in intra-abdominal pressure, which in turn leads to increased pleural pressure and decreased venous return from the brain to the heart. According to this theory, the effectiveness of diuretics as medical treatment should be explained not only with their ability to decrease CSF production, but also with their ability to decrease central plasma volume and hence venous pressure.

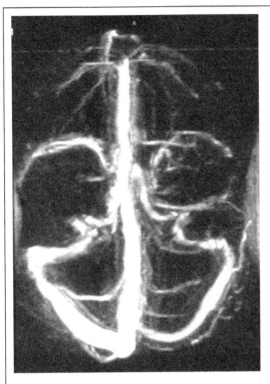

Figure 2 Angio MRI. Normal venous outflow. Although some signal void are evident in the lumen of both sigmoid sinuses, the outline of the sinuses is always present without narrowing or images of complete block. No significant collateral circulation is visible.

In the last decade, magnetic resonance imaging (MRI) and magnetic resonance venography (MRV) have largely replaced catheter angiography for examining the venous system in patients suspected of having IIH to exclude venous sinus thrombosis (Fig. 2). With respect to the SSS, MRV provides images that are generally regarded as diagnostic and easy to interpret (9). On the contrary the transverse sinuses are difficult to evaluate, because of wide variations in radiological appearances inviting confusion between normal anatomical variants and disease (10). The signal in phase-contrast MRV mainly comes from the bulk movement of protons (in blood) within a range of velocities chosen by the operator. A segment of signal void in a sinus implies that flow velocities over that segment are outside the range prescribed in the study ("*flow gaps*") (Fig. 2). This does not necessarily mean thrombosis, and it may not necessarily be abnormal—that is, arachnoid granulations might cause a local alteration of blood flow around them. However, it raises the possibility of stenosis or occlusion (11). Sometimes significant collateral circulation can be observed around the stenosis or the occlusion (Fig. 3). This collateral circulation obviously develops to bypass the obstruction and could be a significant factor in the stabilisation or long-term resolution of some clinical conditions.

Imaging studies that examined the venous outflow of the brain in IIH have inconsistently demonstrated stenoses or anomalies in the transverse dural sinuses (12,13). In a recent paper, Higgins et al. (11) reviewed MRVs from 20 patients with idiopathic intracranial hypertension and compared them with MRVs from a control group of 40 asymptomatic volunteers, matched for age and sex. They found that the lateral sinuses presented a range of appearances with significant different distributions in the two groups ($p = 0.001$). Bilateral lateral sinus flow gaps were seen in 13 of 20 patients with idiopathic intracranial hypertension. The large majority of controls had strong uniform signal from at least one lateral sinus, and usually from both. In no control cases flow gaps were seen on both sides. The authors explained these results, in disagreement with previous studies, with the strict criteria that they have adopted to enrol the healthy controls: all the controls had no history of recurrent headache or other symptoms/signs attributable to cranial venous involvement ("*super-controls*"), whereas in previous series it had been considered as "healthy controls," also subjects investigated for headache.

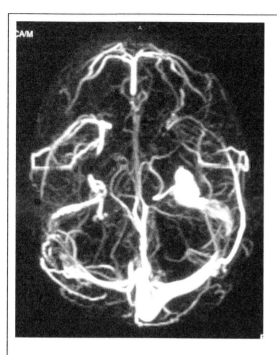

Figure 3 Complete block of both lateral sinuses, bypassed by significant collateral circulation, more evident at the level of the right lateral sinus.

This discrepancy can be also explained with the technique used during evaluation. Time-of-flight MR venography (TOF MRV) has been the most popular technique of MR venography despite its limitations, specifically the artifactual signal loss that occurs at predictable locations in the venous system due to in-plane flow and turbulence (12,14). The transverse and sigmoid sinuses are locations in the dural venous sinuses routinely plagued by such artefacts. Also with the traditional digital subtraction angiography, which is usually performed in two static planes, it is difficult to fully appreciate the transverse sigmoid junctions. In the past, cerebral arteriography was performed to exclude other pathologies and not specifically to interrogate the venous system; thus, subtle venous outflow findings were likely overlooked (12).

Farb et al. recently developed a new technique of MR venography: autotriggered elliptic-centric-ordered three-dimensional gadolinium-enhanced MR venography (ATECO MRV), which has been shown to be superior to TOF techniques due to its flow insensitivity and decreased artifactual signal loss (12). With this technique they found bilateral sinovenous stenoses in 27 of 29 patients with IIH and in only 4 of 59 control patients. This study indicates that patients with PTC have dural venous sinuses that are anatomically different than those of normal controls: consistent flow abnormality without radiologically confirmed thrombus had been found in more than 90% of patients. Interestingly, the location of the stenotic regions demonstrated in this study matches the location of the pressure gradients, recorded in the study of King et al. (distal transverse sinus) (6). Farb et al. (12) encountered two types of dural narrowing: the "long smooth tapered narrowing," indicating an extraluminal compressive stenosis (Fig. 4) and the "acutely marginated apparent intraluminal filling defect," indicating an enlarged, partially obstructing, intraluminal arachnoid granulation [Fig. 5(A) to 5(D)].

All these studies confirm that narrowing of the distal transverse sinuses and elevated venous sinus pressure are related to the disease process; however, whether this is primary cause, a contributory factor, or a secondary phenomenon is uncertain. In the first case a dural sinus stenosis should be postulated as primary cause of a PTC (fixed stenosis) (6). In this theory the resulting chronic low-grade venous hypertension is in turn transmitted to the CSF to cause elevated pressure. In this setting reconstruction of the venous lumen with endovascular stents would be effective in lowering intracranial hypertension. This procedure has been used effectively several times, but seems not to be efficient in all cases (15). The

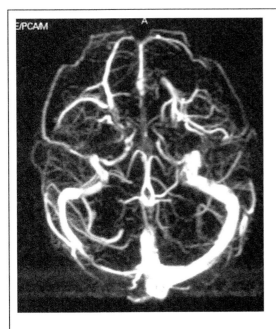

Figure 4 Seven-year-old boy admitted with a seven-day history of headache and vomiting with papilledema. Note the long smooth tapered narrowing of the right lateral sinus.

exact nature of the stenosis is not known: an occult venous sinus thrombosis or vasculitis may cause an obstruction or stricture of the transverse sinus. Large arachnoid granulations may cause anatomical obstruction of the venous sinuses if they enlarge. Heterotopic brain or brain hernias may be also the cause of transverse sinus obstruction (16).

Alternatively, narrowing of the venous sinuses may be secondary to another unknown primary event, such as edematous brain or dysfunctional CSF flow unrelated to venous obstruction (dynamic stenosis) (17). As the pressure increases, according to the Monroe–Kellie doctrine, the vascular compartment and dural sinuses will be compressed (18).

However, a third hypothesis should be considered: a primary (unknown) abnormality, present over a variable period of time prior to patient presentation, induces slowly stretch and collapse of the dural walls of the transverse sinuses yielding to the extralumenal pressure. As the distal transverse sinus continues to narrow, it eventually exceeds a threshold and creates a flow limiting *dynamic* stenosis and resultant pressure gradient. This results in a surge in intracranial pressure that brings the patient to presentation. The anatomy of the distal transverse sinus in some way likely predisposes it to this phenomenon (12). The observation with MRI and MR venography of reversibility of the sinus stenosis following CSF diversion procedures supports the second and the third hypotheses (19,20) [Fig. 6(A) and 6(B)].

In summary, as suggested by Rekate in a recent editorial (21), in all patients with PTC, an increased dural venous pressure is measurable. In most of these patients—including patients with anatomical venous constriction, dural thrombosis, or obesity-related right atrial hypertension—the increase in venous sinus pressure causes PTC. It seems likely that there are a number of patients in whom there is an increase in ICP that causes the increased venous pressure by changing the geometry of the dural venous sinuses. The system therefore reflects a positive feedback loop in which geometric changes in the dural venous sinuses lead to increased venous sinus pressure. This increased venous sinus pressure in turn leads to increased ICP, which leads to further distortion of the dural venous sinuses and so on. It does not matter at which point the perturbation begins. What is not known is whether placement of a venous stent could break the positive feedback loop.

Other conditions, which increase venous pressure may lead to intracranial hypertension, have been reported. These include dural arteriovenous fistulae (22), carotid-cavernous fistulae (23), iatrogenic disruption of venous drainage (after acoustic neuroma resection (24), radical neck dissection (25)), catheter-induced subclavian vein thrombosis (26), venous sinus compression by tumors (e.g., meningiomas) (27), and acute lymphocytic leukemia.

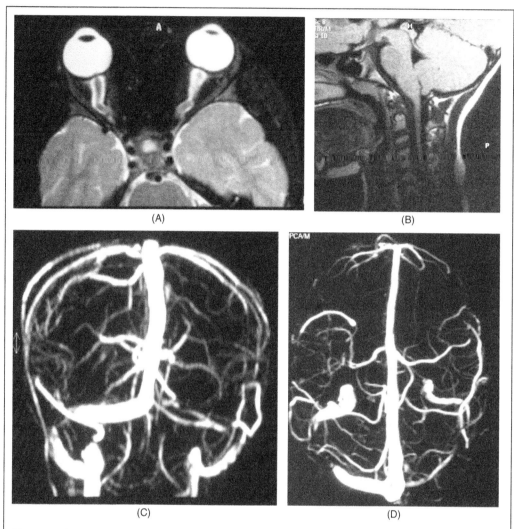

Figure 5 Eight-year-old girl presenting with headache, papilledema, and diplopia. MRI showed enlargement of the CSF spaces around the optic nerve (**A**), herniation of cerebellar tonsils to C1 level (**B**). Angio MRI showed a complete stop of the right transverse sinus (**C**) and long smooth tapered narrowing of the left lateral sinus (**D**).

DURAL VENOUS SINUS THROMBOSIS

Dural venous sinus thrombosis, often associated with otitis or other craniofacial infections, has long been recognized as being associated with intracranial hypertension, so that some early investigators had considered dural sinus thrombosis as the cause of pseudotumor (5) [Fig. 7(A) and 7(B)]. However, on the basis of the modern modified Dandy criteria, dural sinus thrombosis should be excluded as diagnostic criteria for *idiopathic* intracranial hypertension. Therefore, dural venous sinus thrombosis should be considered a *secondary pseudotumor syndrome* (28).

Nowadays only 10% of dural venous sinus thrombosis can be attributed to infection due to the widespread use of antibiotics (29,30). Among the numerous noninfective medical conditions, congenital thrombophilia is the most frequent, particularly the increased resistance to activated protein C with factor V Leiden mutation and the 20210 G to A mutation of the prothrombin gene (29). However, despite the continuing description of new causes, the proportion of cases of unknown etiology remains between 20% and 35% (29).

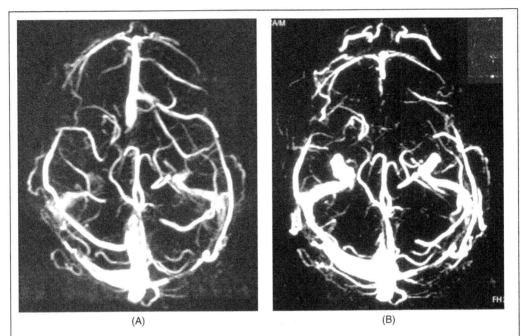

Figure 6 Thirteen-year-old boy with a history of obesity and drastic diet allowing recent loss of 7 kg in one month. The patient presenting with frontal headache, neck pain, vomiting, diplopia, and papilledema with retinal hemorrhages. Angio MRI showed severe narrowing of both lateral sinuses (**A**). After medical treatment and two lumbar punctures at one-month interval, Angio MRI performed eight months after (**A**) shows recanalization of the right transverse sinus and significant collateral circulation at the level of the left transverse sinus (**B**).

Some authors have hypothesized that *idiopathic* intracranial hypertension should be long-term chronic sequela of previous macroscopic sinus venous thrombosis, or the effect of an unrecognised non occlusive venous cerebral thrombus (12,31,32). To support this hypothesis, in a recent paper De Lucia et al. (31), comparing a group of 17 adults affected by "*idiopathic* intracranial hypertension" (no radiographic evidence of thrombosis) with healthy controls, observed an hypercoagulable state in the patients' group. In detail, the number of subjects with protein C deficiency was significantly higher in patients than in controls. Moderate-to-high titers of anticardiolipin antibodies (β_2-glycoprotein type I) were found in 8 out of

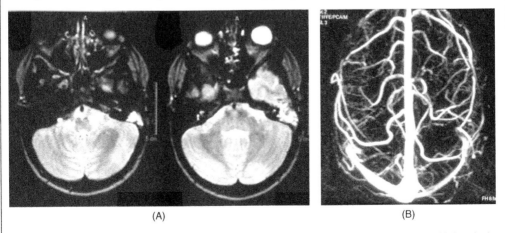

Figure 7 Eight-year-old boy with a one-year history of recurring left mastoiditis, presenting with headache, diplopia, and papilledema. MRI showed evidence of previous mastoid infections (**A**) and complete blockage of both transverse sinuses (**B**).

17 patients. Increased plasma levels of prothrombin fragment 1+2, fibrinopeptide A (FPA), and PAI-1 were demonstrated in the patients group. Gene polymorphisms for factor V Leiden mutation, prothrombin mutation 20210 A/G, MTHFR 677 C/T, PAI-1 4G/5G, ACE I/D were detected in 13 patients.

Presentation of dural venous sinus thrombosis is variable: acute onset, often associated with focal signs, is typical of obstetric and infectious etiology, subacute (duration of two days to one month) or chronic (duration of greater than one month) onset is frequently observed in inflammatory diseases and in coagulation disorders (29). The chronic pattern of onset is typically characterized by isolated intracranial hypertension and may be mistaken for idiopathic intracranial hypertension, if appropriate investigations are not performed. MRI, in combination with MR angiography, is currently the modality of choice for the diagnosis and follow-up (29,33). The advantage of MRI is direct visualization of the clot in the sinus. It can show also the associated cerebral lesions. The clot can have different appearances based on the duration of the thrombosis. At a very early stage (<5 days), the occluded vessels appear isointense on T1 MRI and hypointense on T2 MRI. This is the only time when MRI gives a false-negative result. It can be corrected with MRA, which shows the missing sinus. After about five days, due to the conversion of oxyhemoglobin to methemoglobin, the thrombus becomes hyperintense, first on T1 and later on T2 MRI. After the first month, MRI patterns are variable because the thrombosed sinus can either remain totally or partially occluded or can recanalize and return to normal. In the majority of cases, there is an isointensity on T1 and hyperintensity on T2 MRI. At six months, abnormalities persist in about two-thirds of cases (29). Helical CT venography has been developed recently as an excellent tool to detect cranial venous thrombosis (34). Frequent abnormalities are filling defects, sinus wall enhancement, abnormal collateral venous drainage, and tentorial enhancement. CT venograms may be easier to interpret and have fewer artifacts than MRA. They may be especially helpful in the very acute or late stages, when MRI can be misleading (29). Also in case of dural venous thrombosis, lumbar puncture remains useful to measure and decrease intracranial pressure if it is elevated and threatening vision. The CSF composition is often abnormal.

Treatment of dural venous thrombosis, which should be started as soon as the diagnosis is established, consists of reversing the underlying cause when known, use of antithrombotics, control of seizures, and control of intracranial hypertension, with same protocol as for idiopathic intracranial hypertension (29).

VENOUS SINUS STENTING AND OTHER ENDOVASCULAR TREATMENTS

As discussed above, venous hypertension is considered an important pathogenetic factor (or cofactor) in inducing intracranial hypertension in patients with PTC. On modern neuroimaging, narrowing or stenosis at the level of the lateral portion of the transverse sinuses is frequent findings, especially in children. Recently, attempts to treat these stenoses with endovascular techniques have been reported, often with conflicting results. Endovascular treatments include thrombolytic therapy, balloon venoplasty, and venous sinus stent placement. In cases of venous sinus thrombosis, thrombolytic therapy has been effective in relieving venous sinus obstruction. Although some cases of idiopathic intracranial hypertension have been successfully treated with anticoagulation (5), usually thrombolysis fails (7,6,16). Balloon venoplasty may be more useful but has been shown to be often ineffective, because of high risk of restenosis (7,16).

Venous sinus stent has the advantage of reduction of recurrences. In the series of Higgins et al. (11), 12 patients who met criteria for diagnosis of IIH underwent stenting of a stenosis in the transverse sinus. Patients were heparinized during the procedure; this was subsequently converted to low-dose aspirin after eight weeks. Following the procedure, five patients became asymptomatic, two improved, and five remained unchanged. The authors were not able to define the exact role of stenting in the management of patients with idiopathic intracranial hypertension. However, they suggested to reserve stenting to cases refractory to conventional therapies.

Owler et al. (35) performed direct retrograde cerebral venography and manometry in nine patients with PTC. They distinguished patients with "venogenic" and "nonvenogenic" PTC and recommended stenting to patients, in which morphological obstruction of the venous transverse sinus and pressure gradient across the stenosis had been demonstrated. They treated with stenting four patients: in all headache rapidly improved; vision improved in three, but one in which it remained poor despite normalized CSF pressures. They concluded that "patients with PTC should be evaluated with direct retrograde cerebral venography and manometry because venous transverse sinus obstruction is probably more common than is currently appreciated. In patients with a lesion of the venous sinuses, treatment with an endoluminal venous sinus stent is a viable alternative for amenable lesions."

SECONDARY PSEUDOTUMOR IN CHILDREN

In children, especially in younger children, an identifiable cause can be found with high frequency: in one series including only children younger than six years, the etiology was identified in 84% of patients (36). The most frequent had been middle ear infection, accounting for about 30% (37,38)."Minor" head trauma may also lead to intracranial hypertension, secondary to thrombosis of sagittal, sigmoid or transverse sinus (34). It has been reported in the history of 5% to 20% of pediatric patients (37,38). Pediatric PTC has been associated with some endocrine conditions, such as menarche, hypoparathyroidism, and thyroid replacement (37,38). Stronger association, however, is with both corticosteroid treatment and cessation or reduction of treatment (38). In the first case, PTC supervenes after a prolonged course [average 2½ months in one series (39)], while, when it results from reduction or cessation of corticosteroids, it can appear acutely (38). Among medications, minocycline, often prescribed in the treatment of acne, and nalidixic acid had been most frequently reported to be the cause of PTC in children. The appearance of intracranial hypertension does not appear to be a dose-related phenomenon: it can supervene immediately after the initiation of therapy or only after the patient has been on the antibiotic for months (38). PTC has been recognized in malnourished children and immediately upon renourishing malnourished children (38). Pathogenesis of intracranial hypertension is unclear. The possibility of dural venous thrombosis cannot be excluded, as well as vitamin A deficiency (or intoxication during renourishing) (38).

REFERENCES

1. Rekate HL. Brain turgor (Kb): Intrinsic property of the brain to resist distortion. Pediatr Neurosurg 1992; 18:257–262.
2. Rottenberg DA, Foley KM, Posner JB. Hypothesis: The pathogenesis of pseudotumor cerebri. Med Hypotheses 1980; 6:913–918.
3. Bateman GA, Smith RL, Siddique SH. Idiopathic hydrocephalus in children and idiopathic intracranial hypertension in adults: Two manifestations of the same pathophysiological process? J Neurosurg 2007; 107(suppl 6):439–444.
4. Cinalli G, Sainte-Rose C, Kollar EM, et al. Hydrocephalus and craniosynostosis. J Neurosurg 1998; 88:209–214.
5. Ray BS, Dunbar HS. Thrombosis of the dural venous sinuses as a cause of "pseudotumor cerebri." Ann Surg 1951; 134:367–386.
6. King JO, Mitchell PJ, Thomson KR, et al. Cerebral venography and manometry in idiopathic intracranial hypertension. Neurology 1995; 45:2224–2228.
7. Karahalios DG, Rekate HL, Khayata MH, et al. Elevated intracranial venous pressure as a universal mechanism in pseudotumor cerebri of varying etiologies. Neurology 1996; 46:198–202.
8. Sugerman HJ, Felton WL III, Salvant JB Jr, et al. Effects of surgically induced weight loss on idiopathic intracranial hypertension in morbid obesity. Neurology 1995; 45:1655–1659.
9. Vogl TJ, Bergman C, Villringer A, et al. Dural sinus thrombosis: Value of venous MR angiography for diagnosis and follow up. Am J Radiol 1994; 162:1191–1198.
10. Lee AG, Brazis PW. Magnetic resonance venography in idiopathic pseudotumor cerebri. J Neuroophthalmol 2000; 20:12–13.
11. Higgins JNP, Gillard JH, Owler BK, et al. MR venography in idiopathic intracranial hypertension: unappreciated and misunderstood. J Neurol Neurosurg Psychiatry 2004; 75:621–625.

12. Farb RI, Vanek I, Scott JN, et al. Idiopathic intracranial hypertension: The presence and morphology of sinovenous stenosis. Neurology 2003; 60:1418–1424.

13. Johnston I, Kollar C, Dunkley S, et al. Cranial venous outflow obstruction in the pseudotumour syndrome: Incidence, nature and relevance. J Clin Neurosci 2002; 9:273–278.

14. Ayanzen RH, Bird CR, Keller PJ, et al. Cerebral MR venography: Normal anatomy and potential diagnostic pitfalls. AJNR Am J Neuroradiol 2000; 21:74–78.

15. Higgins JNP, Cousins C, Owler BK, et al. Idiopathic intracranial hypertension: 12 cases treated by venous sinus stenting. J Neurol Neurosurg Psychiatry 2003; 74:1662–1666.

16. Kollar C, Parker G, Johnston I. Endovascular treatment of cranial venous sinus obstruction resulting in pseudotumor syndrome. Report of three cases. J Neurosurg 2001; 94:646–651.

17. Corbett JJ. Increased intracranial pressure: Idiopathic and otherwise. J Neuroophthalmol 2004, 24:103–105.

18. Greitz D, Wirestam R, Franck A, et al. Pulsatile brain movement and associated hydrodynamics studied by magnetic resonance phase imaging. The Monro–Kellie doctrine revisited. Neuroradiology 1992; 34:370–380.

19. Higgins JNP, Pickard JD. Lateral sinus stenoses in idiopathic intracranial hypertension resolving after CSF diversion. Neurology 2004; 62:1907–1908.

20. Rohr A, Dorner L, Stingele R, et al. Reversibility of venous sinus obstruction in idipathic intracranil hypertension. AJNR Am J Neuroradiol 2007; 28:656–659.

21. Rekate HL. Hydrocephalus and idiopathic intracranial hypertension. J Neurosurg 2007; 107(suppl 6):435–438.

22. Cognard C, Casasco A, Toevi M, et al. Dural arteriovenous fistulas as a cause of intracranial hypertension due to impairment of cranial venous outflow. J Neurol Neurosurg Psychiatry 1998; 65:308–316.

23. Halbach VV, Hieshima GB, Higashida RT, et al. Carotid cavernous fistulae: Indications for urgent treatment. AJR Am J Roentgenol 1987; 149:587–593.

24. Vijayan N. Postoperative headache in acoustic neuroma. Headache 1995; 35:98–100.

25. Marr WG, Chambers RG. Pseudotumor cerebri syndrome: Following unilateral radical neck dissection. Am J Ophthalmol 1961; 51:605–611.

26. Birdwell BG, Yeager R, Whitsett TL. Pseudotumor cerebri: A complication of catheter-induced subclavian vein thrombosis. Arch Intern Med 1994; 154:808–811.

27. Marr WG, Chambers JW. Occlusion of the cerebral dural sinuses by tumor simulating pseudotumor cerebri. Am J Ophthalmol 1966; 61:45–49.

28. Binder DK, Horton HC, Lawton MT, et al. Idiopathic intracranial hypertension. Neurosurgery 2004; 54:538–552.

29. Crassard I, Bousser MG. Cerebral venous thrombosis. State of the art. J Neuroophthalmol 2004; 24:156–163.

30. Southwick FS, Richardson EP Jr, Swartz MN. Septic thrombosis of the dural venous sinuses. Medicine 1986; 65:82–106.

31. De Lucia D, Napolitano M, Di Micco P, et al. Benign intracranial hypertension associated to blood coagulation derangements. Thromb J 2006; 4:21.

32. Sussman J, Leach M, Greaves M, et al. Potentially prothrombotic abnormalities of coagulation in benign intracranial hypertension. J Neurol Neurosurg Psychiatry 1997; 62:229–233.

33. Padayachee TS, Bingham JB, Graves MJ, et al. Dural sinus thrombosis: Diagnosis and follow-up by magnetic resonance angiography and imaging. Neuroradiology 1991; 33:165–167.

34. Casey SO, Alberico RA, Patel M. Cerebral CT venography. Radiology 1996; 198:163–170.

35. Owler BK, Parker G, Halmagyi GM, et al. Pseudotumor cerebri syndrome: Venous sinus obstruction and its treatment with stent placement. J Neurosurg 2003; 98:1045–1055.

36. Couch R, Camfield PR, Tibbles JAR. The changing picture of pseudotumor cerebri in children. Can J Neurol Sci 1985; 12:48–50.

37. Dhiravibulya K, Ouvrier R, Johnston I, et al. Benign intracranial hypertension in childhood: Review of 23 cases. J Paediatr Child Health 1991; 27:304–307.

38. Lessell S. Pediatric pseudotumor cerebri (idiopathic intracranial hypertension). Surv Ophthalmol 1992; 37:155–166.

39. Walker AE, Adamkiewicz JJ. Pseudotumor cerebri associated with prolonged corticosteroid therapy: Report of 4 cases. JAMA 1964; 188:779–784.

20 | Arachnoid Cysts

Concezio Di Rocco
Department of Pediatric Neurosurgery, Catholic University Medical School, Rome, Italy

Mateus Dal Fabbro
Division of Neurosurgery, State University of Campinas, Campinas, Brazil

Gianpiero Tamburrini
Department of Pediatric Neurosurgery, Catholic University Medical School, Rome, Italy

INTRODUCTION

Arachnoid cysts are benign congenital lesions more frequently encountered in children. According to the literature, 60% to 80% of these malformations are diagnosed in patients under the age of 16 years (1), the largest proportion of them in the first two years of life (2). Although these lesions are reported to have an incidence of 1% of intracranial space occupying lesions in most reports (2), studies based on neuroimaging or autopsy observations in large series indicate lower incidence ranging from 0.17 (3) to 0.3% (4). Males are affected approximately twice more than females. Arachnoid cysts can be found anywhere along the cerebrospinal axis, including the spinal spaces, although with a lower frequency in this compartment.

Arachnoid cysts should be differentiated from other congenital conditions such as dilated cisterns, arachnoid pouches, sacs, diverticula, and also porencephalic cavities, which communicate with the normal arachnoid spaces or the ventricular system. Similarly, other noncongenital arachnoidal lesions developed subsequently to traumatic, hemorrhagic, or infectious events should not be classified as arachnoid cysts, and for this reason are not discussed in this chapter.

Several aspects regarding the pathogenesis and the natural history of arachnoid cysts have not been well clarified yet, and are still a matter of debate. More importantly, there is still much controversy concerning the optimum treatment, if any required, as these cysts are frequently diagnosed incidentally on the basis of routine prenatal ultrasonography, or after birth by computer-assisted tomography (CT) or magnetic resonance imaging (MRI) performed for other reasons, generally minor head trauma, macrocrania, developmental delay, and epilepsy. For example, in a recent report arachnoid cysts were found in 7 instances in a sample of 3000 subjects submitted to cranial CT scan for head trauma (5), constituting the second most common pathological incidental finding after the group of 8 tumors of different histopathologic types.

As arachnoid cysts are benign, noninfiltrative lesions, the signs and symptoms when present arise from the compression exerted by the cyst over neighboring neurovascular structures, or from intracranial hypertension (ICH), either resultant directly from cyst expansion or secondary to obstructive hydrocephalus. Hence, the clinical presentation and evolution, and consequently the treatment, vary mainly in relation to the topographic localization of the cysts within the cerebrospinal axis. Therefore, it is reasonable to classify these cysts according to this topographic localization, and discuss each category separately in terms of clinical presentation and surgical treatment. We also report a brief review on the latest information about the pathogenesis of the arachnoid cysts, as this is uniformly valid, regardless of the topography. Lastly, some general particularities are also discussed.

PHYSIOPATHOGENESIS OF ARACHNOID CYSTS

The congenital nature of arachnoid cysts is suggested by the observation of a high incidence in the pediatric population (1,2), the concomitance with other congenital malformations (heterotopias, absence of the Sylvian vein, agenesis of the corpus callosum) (2), and the occasional occurrence in siblings (2,6) or in genetic disorders as neurofibromatosis type 1 (NF1), glutaric aciduria type 1 (GAT1), Down syndrome, mucopolysaccharidosis (7), and oculopharyngeal muscular dystrophy (8). Nevertheless, spontaneous postnatal development of this kind of lesion has been documented (9).

Arachnoid cysts are believed to originate from a minor anomaly in the development of the endomeninges that results in duplication or splitting of the arachnoid membrane (1,2). Their structure is very similar to the normal arachnoid, been distinguished from this by presenting split membranes, hyperplasic arachnoid cells and a thick layer of collagen in the cyst wall, and by the absence of traversing trabecular processes within the cyst (10,11).

The mechanisms involved in their expansion are not well understood, and the theories intended to explain it are not uniformly accepted. Three are the most popular: (*i*) the presence of an osmotic gradient between the cyst contents and the subarachnoid space, which would favor fluid influx to the cyst. This theory fails mostly because the cyst fluid constitution is very similar and isosmotic to the cerebrospinal fluid (CSF) (2). Besides, slow movement of fluid between the cyst and the subarachnoidal space, which would prevent the existence of any osmotic gradients, have been demonstrated in a considerable number of patients, either intra-operatively or from CT cisternographies with intrathecal metrizamide. (*ii*) The unidirectional valve (ball-valve, slit-valve) hypothesis, where a small communication between the cyst and the subarachnoidal space would permit only one-way fluid movement toward the cyst. Cerebrospinal fluid influx would occur due to a pressure gradient resultant of arterial or venous pulsations in the subarachnoidal space, and a valve mechanism probably constituted of an arachnoid fold would prevent fluid egress, resulting in progressive fluid accumulation inside the cyst ultimately. This hypothesis is supported by MRI and cine-mode MRI studies, as well as by endoscopic direct observations. (*iii*) Hypothesis of fluid secretion by the cyst wall cell lining, where it is postulated that the cyst walls themselves produce fluid, consequently explain the cyst growth in cases of complete exclusion of the cystic cavity from the CSF circulation. This theory is strongly supported by structural and ultrastructural analysis of the cyst wall architecture (2,12), but here also controversy is present because these findings were not uniformly confirmed (13). These structural characteristics regard the similarity of the cyst cell lining to subdural and arachnoid granulations neurothelium, with the presence of intercellular clefts with sinusoid dilations, desmosomal intercellular junctions, pinocytotic vesicles, multivesicular bodies, lysosomal structures, basal lamina, and microvilli on the luminal surface, findings altogether consistent with fluid secretion (2,10,14).

TOPOGRAPHIC CLASSIFICATION OF ARACHNOID CYSTS

Topographic classification of arachnoid cysts is consistent with the anatomical distribution of these lesions, which correspond to the physiological cisternal spaces, a feature that further supports their maldevelopmental origin. Table 1 summarizes the classification of arachnoid cysts according to their distribution within the cerebrospinal axis. Sylvian fissure arachnoid cysts (SACs) are the most frequent, followed by sellar regions, median posterior fossa, and cerebral convexity (Table 2).

Sylvian Fissure Arachnoid Cysts

General Characteristics
In the pediatric population 35% to 67% of the arachnoid cysts are located in the Sylvian fissure region (1,2), but this is also the most common localization in adults. Some disagreement exists in the literature concerning the nomenclature, as these lesions were variably defined as middle

Table 1 Topographic Classification of Arachnoid Cysts

Supratentorial cysts	Infratentorial cysts	Spinal cysts
Sylvian	Cerebellar hemisphere	Extradural
Sellar region	Midline vermis/cisterna magna	Intradural
Cerebral convexity	Cerebellopontine angle	
Interhemispherical	Retroclival	
Quadrigeminal plate	Intraventricular	
Intraventricular		

Table 2 Arachnoid Cysts: Topographic Distribution
in the Pediatric Population (%)

Location	%
Supratentorial	77
Sylvian	34
Sellar region	15
Cerebral convexity	15
Interhemispherical	8
Quadrigeminal plate	5
Infratentorial	23
Median	17.5
Cerebellar hemisphere	5
Retroclival	0.5

fossa ACs or temporal ACs. We consider Sylvian fissure AC the most appropriate definition, as these cysts typically open the fissure, spreading the frontal from the temporal lobes, and completely exposing the middle cerebral artery (MCA), the insula or, even the intracranial segment of the internal carotid artery (ICA) when reaching large dimensions. There is a slight predilection for the left side; male-to-female ratio is approximately 3:1 (2,7). Bilateral cysts are very rare and are frequently associated to some genetic disorder, as NF1 or GAT1. The last condition is important to be adequately recognized because any simple surgical procedure can carry disproportionately high risks for these patients. Thus, to avoid unexpected complications, it is advisable to always have a preoperative genetic evaluation when in presence of bilateral SACs.

Clinical Presentation
The most frequent symptom is headache, often mild, present in up to 62% of the patients (15), followed by epileptic seizures, contralateral motor weakness, and mild proptosis. Macrocrania or focal cranial bulging is common findings in small infants. Other possible clinical findings are mental impairment or developmental delay in 10% of the cases (7), and attention deficit/hyperactivity disorder less frequently. Facial pain and decreased visual acuity have also been reported (2). Subdural hematomas or hygromas complicating SACs are more frequent in adults, but can be encountered occasionally in children as well. Hydrocephalus, generally communicating, is present in approximately 10% of these cases (16).

Diagnosis
CT scans and MRI show a sharply defined extra-axial nonenhancing space occupying lesion with signal intensity equal to that of CSF (17) in the middle fossa, usually enlarging the Sylvian fissure, showing mass effect varying from slight compression of the temporal lobe to ipsilateral ventricular system compression and midline brain shift. Bone abnormalities such as thinning and bulging or the temporal squama and anterosuperior displacement of the greater and lesser sphenoid wings can be present. Based on the image findings, these cysts are classified in three categories (18): Type 1, when the cyst has small dimensions, a biconvex or semicircular shape and is limited to the anterior middle fossa (Fig. 1); type 2, the most common one (1), when the cyst is medium-sized, often triangular or quadrangular shaped, occupying the anterior and middle parts of the temporal fossa, frequently showing mild to moderate mass effect (Fig. 2); and type 3, the most severe form, when the cyst occupies the middle fossa almost entirely, with prominent mass effect, usually associated with an atrophic temporal lobe (Fig. 3). CT cisternography with metrizamide allows further evaluation of the cyst communications with the subarachnoidal space by showing early cyst enhancement, late enhancement, or nonenhancement in the cases of noncommunicating cysts, but not absolutely associated with type 1, type 2, and type 3 cysts. When prolonged intracranial pressure recordings are utilized in differentiating normal and hypertensive cysts, unfortunately type 2 cysts may exhibit either normal or increased intracystic pressures (6). Consequently, this type of examination is scarcely useful in identifying those lesions that may or may not benefit from surgical treatment, differently from type 1 and

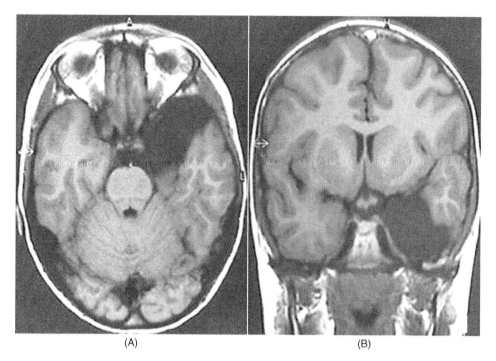

Figure 1 T1 axial (**A**) and coronal (**B**) MR scans of a left type 1 Sylvian arachnoid cyst; the cyst involves only the anterior third of the middle cranial fossa; it displaces the left temporal pole posteriorly and superiorly.

type 3 cysts. Indeed, type 1 nearly always are characterized by normal pressures, whereas type 3 by abnormal high values. The same considerations may apply to other functional examinations, namely, SPECT, which may reveal both normal and hypometabolic cerebral parenchyma in relation to type 2 cysts. Conventional angiography, CT, and MRI angiography are not usually employed for the diagnosis or preoperative evaluation, but typically show the deviation of the ipsilateral MCA trunk and branches by a nonvascularized lesion. Additionally, some small abnormal arteries can be depicted occasionally running on the cyst walls and are considered as the probable cause of the hemorrhagic complications often observed. Differential diagnosis

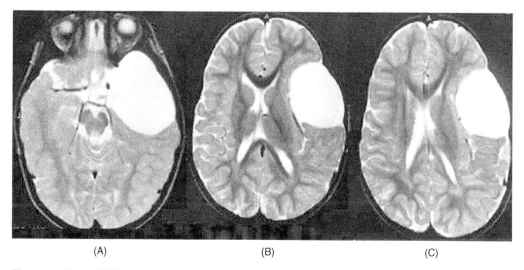

Figure 2 T2 axial MR images of a left type 2 Sylvian arachnoid cyst; the cyst involves the anterior two-thirds of the middle cranial fossa, enlarges the Sylvian fissure, and compresses the left lateral ventricle.

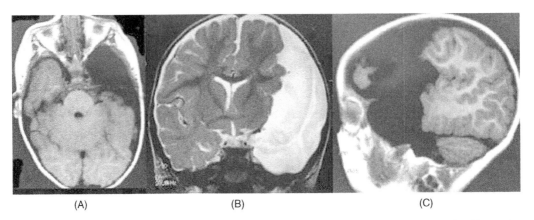

(A)   (B)   (C)

Figure 3   T1 axial (**A**), T2 coronal (**B**), and T1 sagittal MR images of a left type 3 Sylvian arachnoid cyst; the cyst occupies the middle cranial fossa entirely and has a suprasylvian extension with midline shift and significant compression of the adjacent neural structures.

mainly includes porencephalic cysts, distinguished on imaging by the absence of compressive effects over the adjacent structures and by the presence of communication with the lateral cerebral ventricles. Epidermoid tumors are another differential diagnosis, but these are very rare in this location and can be distinguished easily by means of different patterns on FLAIR and diffusion-weighted MRI sequences.

Treatment

The indications for surgical intervention in SACs are far from reaching a consensus, mainly because of the high rate of failure of the surgical procedures either in decreasing the cysts' dimensions in image controls or in achieving significant clinical improvements, as well as by the somewhat high incidence of complications. As an overall rule, asymptomatic, incidental SACs should not undergo surgery, except in the rare situation of progressive cyst enlargement, or in large cysts where MRI depicts signals of previous bleedings. The real incidence of intracystic or subdural hemorrhage as a complication of minor head trauma in asymptomatic children is unknown, but it is certainly not high enough to justify prophylactic surgical interventions, especially in cases of type 1 or type 2 cysts. Instead, the presence of macrocrania or localized cranial bulging in small infants is an indication for surgical treatment in order to avoid progressive deformities and possible interference with brain development. Surgery is also indicated in the presence of documented ICH (19) and focal neurologic deficits attributable to the cyst, like contralateral motor weakness, as well as neuropsychological developmental delay and intractable focal epilepsy, provided that there is consistency with the cyst localization by means of neurophysiologic evaluations. Mild headache or benign forms of epilepsy are not a strong indication for surgery, and each of these cases should be individually analyzed before taking any decision, a period of observation being highly advisable in which the response to an adequate conservative treatment can be carefully appreciated.

Surgical Considerations

The objective of the surgical treatment is a reduction in the cyst dimensions in order to resolve ICH and/or the compression over surrounding parenchyma. There are three surgical options for the treatment of SACs. (*i*) Craniotomy for cyst fenestration and partial resection of the cyst walls, where as wide as possible communications with the basal cisterns are performed and the nonadherent portions of the walls are resected. This is considered the most physiological treatment, as the partial resection of the cyst walls would at least theoretically lead to a decrease in the fluid production, and opening communications with the basal cisterns would allow CSF to circulate, leading ultimately to a decrease in the cyst volume. The literature reports a success rate of up to 79% with this procedure (1). The most frequent complications are subdural hygromas, depending on a CSF fistula between the subarachnoid and the subdural

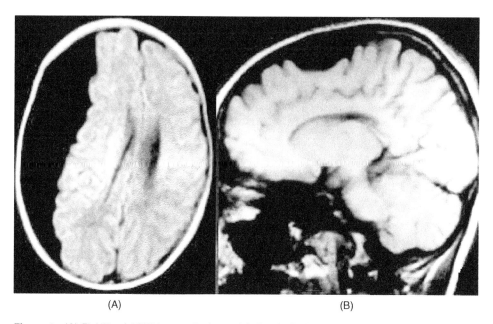

Figure 4 (**A**) FLAIR axial MR image of a huge right hemispheric convexity arachnoid cyst. Note the significant midline shift and compression of the right cerebral hemisphere. (**B**) T1 sagittal MR view of a small frontal paramedian convexity arachnoid cyst; the cyst compresses and enlarges the adjacent cerebral parenchyma.

spaces, which are observed in about 6% of the operated patients (19), but even deaths and major neurological deficits have also been reported (20). (*ii*) Cyst shunting, for example, to the peritoneal cavity (cystoperitoneal shunt), is a simple and less-invasive procedure that provides expressive volumetric cyst reduction, but as drawbacks has the higher risk of infection, the high rate of shunt malfunction requiring revisions, and shunt dependence (2,19). (*iii*) Endoscopic cyst fenestration, which combines the advantages of a more physiologic treatment with a less-invasive procedure, but obviating a shunt device. The principles of this technique are the same as those of craniotomy, except that with the endoscopic technique no cyst wall resection is performed. However, the results of endoscopic and microscopic cyst fenestration in terms of complications and success rates are comparable, although the endoscopic series are still too small. In both techniques efforts should be made in performing wide communications with the basal cisterns, because suboptimum communications are considered as the main cause of failure. In summary, cyst fenestration either with the open or the endoscopic technique is the first choice in the treatment of these patients, as it is the most physiologic approach to the pathology. Shunting should be avoided or reserved for specific cases after failure of the fenestration techniques.

Cerebral Convexity Arachnoid Cysts

General Characteristics
This group accounts for approximately 10% of all arachnoid cysts in children and comprises two different and somewhat heterogeneous categories: hemispherical cysts, more common, and focal cysts, very rare. Hemispherical ACs are large lesions that usually cover all or a great part of one hemisphere surface [Fig. 4(A)] and are thought to be a maximal evolution of a Sylvian fissure AC (2). Consequently, they could be classified as grade IV Sylvian ACs.
    The second category of cerebral convexity ACs constitutes a discrete group of focal lesions, with generally small dimensions, and presents the almost unique feature among cranial ACs of lacking direct relations or contiguity with any CSF cistern [Fig. 4(B)]. Whether these cysts present a different physiopathologic basis is a matter of speculation, but this is not supported by anatomopathological studies, which confirm their similarity with ACs in any other location.

Clinical Presentation

Hemispherical ACs usually present with macrocrania, often asymmetric, the affected side being larger. Other less common symptoms are epilepsy and headache in older children (2). Focal ACs are generally discovered in the evaluation of a focal cranial bulging and may also be associated with epilepsy, although infrequently. Focal neurological signs are remarkably absent in both forms of convexity cysts and this is an important clinical information to be considered in the differential diagnosis of other lesions such as low-grade tumors and chronic subdural hematomas, which are frequently associated with focal neurological deficits such as hemiparesis.

Diagnosis

Skull plain radiographs of patients of hemispherical ACs can show an asymmetric cranial vault and bone thinning on the affected side, while with the focal lesions a circumscribed thinned bone bulging may be evidenced. CT scan confirms these bone abnormalities and further depicts their fluid content with the same signal of CSF. Hemispherical cysts are always accompanied by relevant mass effect of variable intensity, from ipsilateral ventricular compression to remarkable midline brain shift. Focal cysts instead are usually small and show minimal or absent mass effect over the brain parenchyma. CT alone can establish the definitive diagnosis, but MRI is usually employed in order to provide further details important to the differential diagnosis. In fact MRI is the best diagnostic tool due to the abundance of furnished details that not only minimize the possibility of misdiagnosis but also help in planning the surgical strategy. MRI typically shows a sharply demarcated subdural, noninvasive, and nonenhancing lesion, which exerts variably compressive effects over the brain. Additionally, it shows the anatomical relationships of the cyst with eloquent cortical areas or superficial veins, permitting the surgeon to preview possible difficulties and so plan more accurately the ideal surgical approach.

The main differential diagnoses of hemispherical ACs are chronic subdural hematomas or hygromas. On CT scan, the presence of adjacent cranial bone thinning or bulging, indicating a longstanding lesion, or a more irregular, wedged aspect of the cyst internal walls, which is mainly determined by the cyst extensions through an enlarged and deformed Sylvian fissure, puts forth the diagnosis of an arachnoid cyst rather than a chronic subdural hematoma, in which bony abnormalities are absent and the internal membrane in contact with the cortex is more regular, convex shaped. MRI satisfactorily overcomes the limitations of CT scan in providing a more definite diagnosis, since the former characteristically depicts signals of blood metabolites in chronic hematomas, enabling easy distinction from the typical CSF signal of ACs.

Regarding focal convexity cysts, the differential diagnoses are mainly low-grade gliomas, or less frequently bony lesions with intracranial cystic extensions like granulomas or dermoid cysts. However, thanks to MRI high specificity to different fluid contents, and the richness of furnished anatomical details, none of these lesions pose significant diagnostic problems, especially with the aid of spectroscopy and diffusion sequences.

Treatment

The indications for the surgical treatment of hemispherical ACs follow the same principles of those of Sylvian ACs. Therefore, asymptomatic lesions should not be submitted to surgery, unless MRI shows signals suggestive of previous intracystic bleedings. However, when facing such voluminous lesions with mass effect, the decision-making process may be difficult for the neurosurgeon. One should keep in mind that cyst involution after surgery frequently is not as significant as it would be desired and that surgery might bring unnecessary risks for an asymptomatic patient in which the intracranial environment is adequately balanced. On the other hand, symptomatic patients with symmetric or asymmetric macrocrania, or drug-resistant epilepsy, should undergo surgery in order to alleviate the ICH or eliminate the compressive effects of the lesion. Conversely, mild symptomatic patients with headache or satisfactorily controlled epilepsy should undergo surgery only in case of confirmed elevated intracranial pressure by means of invasive monitoring. Focal convexity ACs respond better to surgical treatment.

Surgical Considerations

Hemispherical ACs are challenging to the surgeon. Responses to craniotomy for partial cyst resections and fenestrations to the basal CSF cisterns are variable, both in terms of cyst reduction and clinical improvement, associated with high rate of complications such as subdural hygromas. Such results could be explained by the failure of the cerebral hemisphere to reexpand enough to occupy the residual huge and long-existing cavity. Endoscopic fenestrations of hemispherical ACs have been reported anecdotally, but constitute an emerging option. Hence, at present, the best accepted surgical procedure is shunting, generally to the peritoneal cavity. Here, the use of programmable valves is advisable, because these allow a more accurate control of cyst drainage, permitting a gradual cyst reduction that minimizes the incidence of complications such as subdural fluid collections and consequently decreases the necessity of reoperations for valve change (21). Furthermore, programmable valves are more prone to be removed in a later phase in selected patients, thus minimizing the undesired lifelong shunt dependence. Nevertheless, it must be pointed out that the risks of infection or mechanical complications characteristic of shunts are present and represent an important drawback of the technique.

Focal cerebral convexity ACs are best treated by craniotomy and resection of the nonadherent cyst walls. In fact, the superficial position and small-to-moderate dimensions of these cysts make them particularly suitable to craniotomy, which generally results in marked cyst reduction or even resolution, with low risks, provided adequate standard microsurgical techniques are employed.

Sellar Region Arachnoid Cysts

General Characteristics

Arachnoid cysts localized in the sellar region are divided into two categories: intrasellar and suprasellar cysts. Intrasellar cysts generally harbor small dimensions, but can occasionally present some suprasellar extension with optic chiasm compression. These lesions are found almost exclusively in adults, whereas the suprasellar cysts are typically diagnosed in childhood, where 87% of these lesions are found (2). The suprasellar region constitutes the second most common site of ACs in children, accounting for approximately 15% of them, 78% of which are recognized in the first year of life (2). There is also a slight male predominance with a ratio of approximately 1.5:1. These lesions are believed to originate as a defect in the arachnoid membranes in the confines of the Liliequist membrane and the prepontine-interpeduncular cisterns (22,23), what has motivated some authors to name them as prepontine. However, as these cysts mostly occupy the suprasellar cistern, compressing superiorly the optic chiasm and the floor of the third ventricle, suprasellar ACs is the most widely accepted definition (Fig. 5).

Clinical Presentation

Suprasellar ACs are frequently symptomatic, mainly because of the high association with hydrocephalus, which can be found in up to 100% of the cases (1). Macrocrania, psychomotor delay, and other manifestations of ICH, such as vomiting and irritability, are the usual presenting clinical symptoms and signs (2,23,24). Visual impairment, consisting of either acuity or field deficits are found in approximately one-third of patients (23). Endocrine symptoms, such as growth retardation and precocious puberty, can occasionally lead to the diagnosis of these lesions as well (2). A further rare but typical clinical manifestation is the bobble-head doll syndrome (BHDS), which can be encountered in children usually younger than 10 years who harbor lesions extending into the third ventricle (25). This syndrome is characterized by continuous 2 to 3 Hz back-and-forth movements (bobbing) of the head, involving in some cases also the trunk and arms. It worsens with walking and excitement and typically disappears during sleep. Symptoms may not resolve after surgical treatment, depending possibly on the duration of the symptomatic period prior to surgery (25).

Diagnosis

CT scans show a distorted and enlarged suprasellar cistern with compressive effects over the adjacent structures, often associated with supratentorial hydrocephalus. CT cisternography with metrizamide delineates the late or nonenhanced cyst, but can give just a few anatomical

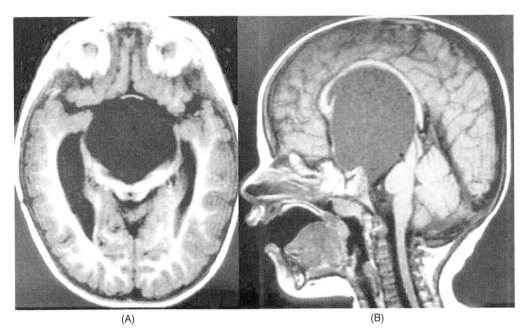

(A)   (B)

Figure 5 Inversion recovery T1 axial (**A**) and T1 sagittal (**B**) MR images of a suprasellar arachnoid cyst. Note the symmetrical enlargement of the cerebral peduncles (**A**), the posterior displacement of the brainstem (**A, B**), and the extension of the cyst from the sellar region up to the roof of the lateral ventricles (**B**).

details. MRI is the method of choice, as it is able to depict the exact extensions of the lesion, which often reaches moderate-to-large dimensions, extending laterally toward the temporal lobes, posteriorly into the interpeduncular and prepontine cisterns, and superiorly, typically elevating the floor of the third ventricle. This last aspect may render the diagnosis difficult even with MRI, because the lesion may be misinterpreted as a dilated third ventricle, due to the extreme thinness of the third ventricle floor (23). Noncommunicating hydrocephalus is almost uniformly present, and it ensues by one of two mechanisms: obstruction of the foramina of Monro by superior expansion of the lesion through the third ventricle or obstruction of the aqueduct of Sylvius due to ventral compression of the midbrain by the lesion occupying the interpeduncular cistern.

Differential diagnosis is mainly a dilated third ventricle, as mentioned above, from which it can be distinguished by the presence in the suprasellar ACs of verticalized optic chiasm and mammilary bodies, and a ventrally flattened pons, as postulated by Wang et al. (23). Other differential diagnoses are Rathke cleft cysts, optic or hypothalamic cystic gliomas, and epidermoid cysts. Rathke cleft cysts present generally small dimensions and frequently harbor an intrasellar component and dishomogeneous MRI signals. Gliomas and epidermoid cysts can also be successfully differentiated on the basis of adequate appreciation of different MRI sequences, as ACs are nonenhancing, avascular, noninfiltrative, and characteristically show signals identical to CSF.

Treatment

Suprasellar ACs are almost always symptomatic by either direct compression on optic–hypothalamic structures or because of hydrocephalus. Thus, the surgical treatment is often necessary as soon as the diagnosis is established, in order to avoid further visual, developmental, or endocrine deficits, and/or cranial deformities. Since the introduction of the neuroendoscopic techniques, these have superceded other surgical options like open craniotomy for cyst resection or cyst shunting, favored by the almost uniform presence of hydrocephalus and by employing the same approaches used for the endoscopic third ventriculostomy, providing ultimately overall good results with a low complication rate (23,24).

Surgical Considerations

Because of their relatively recent introduction in the clinical practice, the endoscopic techniques for the treatment of suprasellar arachnoid cysts are still not standardized. Cystoventriculocisternotomy seems to provide the best results and currently is the technique most frequently employed. The procedure consists in entering the cyst superiorly through the ventricles, establishing communication between the cyst and the third ventricle, and then perforating the inferior cyst walls in order to communicate it widely with the basal cisterns as well (e.g., interpeduncular and prepontine cisterns). This allows free CSF circulation through the third ventricle, the cyst, and the basal cisterns that leads to both volumetric cyst reduction and resolution of hydrocephalus. Other successful endoscopic techniques have been described, such as the electrocoagulation shrinkage of the cyst walls inside the third ventricle, with the advantage of eliminating the redundant cyst walls that could later lead to aqueduct obstruction (24). Although it seems more physiologic, this technique carries the risk of coagulating in the proximity of hypothalamic structures.

No significant inadvertent vascular lesion has been reported with the endoscopic treatment of suprasellar arachnoid cysts, but injury to the basilar artery is the most serious complication to be avoided because of proximity to the basilar apex. The most frequent complications are endocrine dysfunctions and oculomotor deficits. Failure of the treatment of the cyst or associated hydrocephalus requiring shunting occurs in approximately 13% of patients (24), mainly in those who had been treated already using shunt devices prior to surgery, especially for a long period.

Interhemispheric Fissure Arachnoid Cysts

General Characteristics

Interhemispheric fissure arachnoid cysts are rare lesions, accounting approximately for 8% of all intracranial ACs (2), although higher incidences were also reported (26), especially in surgical series (27). These lesions are frequently diagnosed in early childhood, indeed 80% of them within the first year of life. Such a high rate is explained because approximately 30% of interhemispheric ACs are diagnosed by means of routine prenatal echography. Another 25% of the cases are diagnosed early in the neonatal period, also prompted by prenatal echography that detects hydrocephalus requiring further postnatal investigation, which leads to the correct identification of the adjacent interhemispheric arachnoid cyst (27). Males significantly outnumber females in an approximate 4:1 ratio (27). Interhemispheric fissure ACs generally show large dimensions when diagnosed, although not infrequently symptoms are mild or absent. There are two varieties of interhemispheric fissure ACs: median interhemispheric and parasagittal cysts. The former are uniformly associated with some degree of corpus callosum dysgenesis, varying from partial to complete agenesis (Fig. 6). The causal relationship of these findings has not been well established yet, but it is thought that the early mechanical interference of the cyst on the corpus callosum would lead to its defective formation in the embryonic period (2,28). Median interhemispheric cysts are frequently associated with hydrocephalus, resulting either from obstruction of the foramina of Monro by the compression of the third ventricle by the cyst, or due to aqueduct extrinsic constriction by the frequent posterior cystic extensions that reach the quadrigeminal plate cistern. Parasagittal cysts are slightly more common, and instead are not associated with callosal malformations. These lesions are unilateral and wedge-shaped, due to the presence of the intact midline falx, and are less frequently associated with hydrocephalus.

Clinical Presentation

The two different categories of interhemispheric fissure ACs do not differ significantly in clinical manifestations. The most frequent finding in both is macrocrania, encountered in approximately 80% of the patients (27), followed by localized cranial bulging or cranial asymmetry, although not as evident as in Sylvian fissure or cerebral convexity cysts. In approximately 30% (27,29) of patients some degree of developmental delay can be detected, usually mild or moderate, and it is apparently more associated with the median interhemispheric variety, suggesting some role of the callosal dysgenesis in the neurocognitive deficit. Ocular movement disorders may also be found in a minority of patients. Symptoms are not frequent, epilepsy as well as symptoms

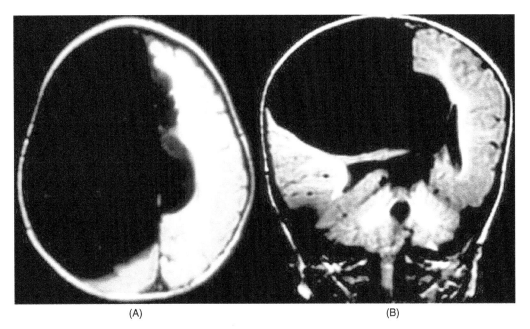

(A)   (B)

Figure 6 Gradient echo T1 axial (**A**) and fast spin echo T1 coronal (**B**) MR scans of a huge interhemispheric arachnoid cyst; the cyst is associated with a complete agenesis of the corpus callosum and an almost complete agenesis of the right cerebral hemisphere (**A**); it compresses the residual adjacent neural structures significantly (**A**, **B**), displacing the midline structures and the left lateral ventricle contralaterally (**B**).

related to ICH, such as irritability, hypoactivity or vomiting are seen in approximately 15% of the cases. Focal neurological deficits are almost uniformly absent to the point that their presence supports the differential diagnosis of porencephalic cysts that can be confirmed by adequate neuroimaging studies.

Diagnosis

Diagnosis is established by means of CT scans and MRI, which allow the cyst classification as median interhemispheric or parasagittal types. Both imaging studies show an extra-axial lesion with fluid contents characteristically equal to CSF. MRI gives more anatomic details: it is superior in delineating the callosal dysgenesis and also other abnormalities less-frequently associated, such as cortical heterotopias (29). According to the topographic localization of interhemispheric fissure ACs in relation to the corpus callosum, these lesions can be further classified as anterior, medium, or posterior. The anterior variety often reaches the lamina terminalis cistern. The medium located cysts can occasionally reach the ambiens cistern, especially in the parasagittal location. Finally, the posterior cysts, which are more common, frequently harbor extensions to the quadrigeminal cistern and less commonly have some infratentorial component.

The most important differential diagnoses of median interhemispheric ACs are cysts associated with callosal agenesis, which may be encountered in 25% of the patients with prosencephaly type I-C. In fact, the overall knowledge of cysts associated with callosal agenesis is evolving, but it is still confusing and controversial, making frequently difficult the differentiation of these cysts from interhemispheric ACs. These difficulties can be overcome by carefully studying the ventricles, as although hydrocephalus may be present in both conditions, in prosencephalic patients a superior distention of the third ventricle roof from below and an indentation of the superiorly located cyst by the falx can be often depicted, whereas median interhemispheric ACs are usually not indented because of the falcine hypoplasia. Furthermore, in contrast to interhemispheric ACs, in prosencephaly I-C the occipital horns of the lateral ventricles are disarranged and barely recognizable. The last distinguishing feature is the basal ganglia characteristics, which are usually fused in prosencephalic patients, while normally separated in the midline in interhemispheric ACs.

Making the differential diagnosis of parasagittal ACs with other cystic lesions of glial, ependymal, or choroidal nature may also be difficult. A valuable tool is the appreciation of the pattern of intravenous contrast enhancement, which is typically absent in ACs. The presence of the falx cerebri limiting the contralateral expansion of the parasagittal AC is also helpful for the distinction. In more difficult cases, CT scan with intrathecal metrizamide should be employed, as this shows the delayed enhancement of the arachnoid cyst and the nonenhancement of lesions of other nature. Nevertheless, problems for the correct diagnosis may remain in cases of noncommunicating ACs.

Treatment

As most interhemispheric ACs are diagnosed in neonates, the surgical treatment is almost always advised. The basic objective is to not only avoid or minimize neuropsychomotor delay, but also progressive macrocrania or cranial deformities. A conservative attitude can be adopted in asymptomatic children with small cysts, provided a close follow-up is undertaken. This picture is somewhat different in older asymptomatic children, where developmental delay is not an issue, allowing a conservative approach to be adopted more easily. Nevertheless, as mentioned above, interhemispheric cysts are typically lesions of small infants and show moderate-to-large dimensions, thus the conservative treatment may be regarded as almost an exceptional option.

Surgical Considerations

Regardless of location, either median or parasagittal, interhemispheric ACs are best treated by means of open surgery. This surgical approach allows partial cyst resection and the establishment of communications with the basal cisterns. Cysts that are located anteriorly are usually communicated with the lamina terminalis cistern and cysts that are more posteriorly located with the quadrigeminal or ambiens cistern. Finally, cysts that are not directly contiguous with any CSF cistern may be communicated with the lateral or third ventricles, depending on their topography and the thickness of the ventricular walls as assessed by preoperative neuroimaging. The response to open surgery is usually satisfactory, with postoperative cyst reduction and clinical improvement in the majority of the patients (27). When cysts recur, a second craniotomy may be attempted, depending on the intraoperative findings at the first operation. The most frequent complication is subdural hygroma. Extracranial shunting procedures should be reserved for repeated failures of cyst resection and fenestration.

Recently, neuroendoscopic procedures have been employed for the treatment of interhemispheric ACs, where endoscopic communications with the ventricular system have been performed (29). Good results have been obtained, although failures requiring a second procedure and complications such as subdural collections have been described as well. Ventricular shunting alone may be considered in cases where hydrocephalus is prominent and the cyst harbors small dimensions, but surgeons and families of patients must be aware of the possibility of cyst expansion after the ventricular shunting, which may require further treatment.

Quadrigeminal Plate Arachnoid Cysts

General Characteristics

Arachnoid cysts occupying the quadrigeminal plate cistern are very rare lesions. Indeed just a few cases have been described in the literature. Nevertheless, most of the reported cases were found in the pediatric age, but differently from other locations, here there is some predominance of females (2). These cysts are frequently associated with noncommunicating hydrocephalus due to third ventricle or aqueductal compression. Quadrigeminal cistern ACs can extend superiorly to the posterior interhemispheric fissure, inferiorly compressing the superior cerebellar vermis, or laterally to the ambiens cisterns (2) (Fig. 7).

Clinical Presentation

Quadrigeminal ACs are often symptomatic lesions, mainly due to the high association with hydrocephalus, which may lead to developmental delay or symptoms of ICH, such as irritability,

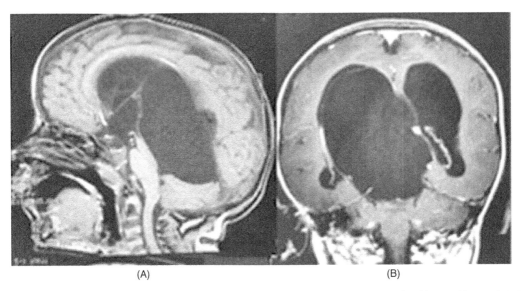

(A)   (B)

Figure 7   T1 sagittal (**A**) and coronal (**B**) MR scans of a large quadrigeminal plate arachnoid cyst with associated hydrocephalus; the quadrigeminal plate is compressed anteriorly, and the posterior wall of the roof of the third ventricle is displaced upwards (**A**). In the coronal view (**B**) note the extension of the cyst inside the right lateral ventricle and the contralateral displacement of the interventricular septum.

vomiting, and tense fontanels. The most frequent finding in children is macrocrania, but a variety of other signs may be present. These are related either with hydrocephalus, tectal plate compression, or cerebellar vermis dysfunction. Some examples are papilledema, pupillary asymmetry or pupillary reflex abnormalities, gaze abnormalities such as Parinaud syndrome (although remarkably rare if compared to neoplastic lesions), trochlear nerve deficits, nystagmus, and also ptosis, retractional nystagmus, and gait ataxia. More rarely auditive deficits and limb weakness have also been reported (30).

Diagnosis
When reaching large dimensions, these lesions may be diagnosed in the prenatal period by means of ultrasonography. For the postnatal investigation, MRI is the diagnostic method of choice, as it provides a detailed assessment of the cyst extensions and its anatomical relationships. The image characteristics are those typical of arachnoid cysts, that is, a nonenhancing, noninfiltrative CSF-containing lesion. When reaching large dimensions, quadrigeminal ACs may be partly infratentorial and partly supratentorial. Differential diagnoses are the rare tectal plate cysts, which are benign lesions that differ from ACs because they are intra-axial lesions, and thus harbor different features that can be successfully addressed by MRI. The most important feature is that these lesions push backwards the tectal plate, rather than dislocating and flattening it anteriorly as do quadrigeminal cistern ACs (31). Quadrigeminal cistern ACs must also be distinguished from diverticular extensions of the third ventricle through the suprapineal recess, which may be present with massive hydrocephalus (2). Other conditions such as postinflammatory subarachnoid pouches or dilated cisterns associated with posterior fossa tumors also enter in the differential diagnosis of quadrigeminal cysts ACs and can be difficult to distinguish even with MRI (2). Lastly, tumors of the pineal region such as germinomas, teratomas, pinealomas, and others that extend to the quadrigeminal cistern do not pose significant problems for the differential diagnosis, because these generally harbor at least some solid, enhancing component, and moreover can have their contiguity with the posterior walls of the third ventricle easily assessed by MRI, allowing a clear differentiation of the typical extra-axial situation of ACs.

Treatment
As they are commonly symptomatic, these cysts often require surgical treatment with the objective of resolving the compressive effects of the lesion over the neighboring neurovascular structures. Rare asymptomatic patients should be treated conservatively.

Surgical Considerations
The deep location of quadrigeminal cistern ACs and the proximity to such important structures as the midbrain, the trochlear nerves, and the major deep cerebral veins make the surgical approach to quadrigeminal cistern ACs challenging. Craniotomy for microsurgical approach to these cysts provides good results, but risks associated with such invasive procedure, such as excessive surgical manipulation of important neurovascular structures and massive blood loss cannot be underestimated, especially when operating on small children. Furthermore, failure in resolving the hydrocephalus often requires an additional ventricular shunt. Cyst shunting is not a good option because contact of the catheter with the neighboring structures may result in significant postoperative complications.

The proximity to the third ventricle or to the trigone and occipital horns of the lateral ventricles in large quadrigeminal cistern ACs makes these lesions especially suitable to endoscopic treatment, rendering this the best surgical alternative for the moment. This technique consists in entering the lateral ventricles anteriorly and, by assuming an anteroposterior trajectory, in reaching the posterior aspects of the third or lateral ventricles and then establishing communications between the ventricles and the cyst. Additionally, a third ventriculocisternostomy is performed, allowing also the resolution of the hydrocephalus and thus obviating ventricular shunting procedures. In fact, a recent report on the endoscopic transventricular approach on seven patients with quadrigeminal cistern ACs, including six children, has demonstrated good results with a low rate of complications and five of six children shunt free postoperatively (32). Possible complications include postoperative CSF collections, transient disturbance of eye movements, and hydrocephalus decompensation. Nevertheless, it must be reminded that although endoscopic approaches are less invasive, the risk of inadvertent damage to neurovascular structures is still present, and for this reason all care should be taken in order to avoid complications as massive venous bleeding, which could be disastrous, especially during an endoscopic approach where prompt hemorrhage control cannot be achieved easily.

Posterior Fossa Arachnoid Cysts

General Characteristics
Approximately 25% of all arachnoid cysts in children are located in the posterior fossa (2). In adults, these are much less frequent. Males may slightly outnumber females (2,33). Posterior fossa ACs are divided into two main categories according to their topography: (*i*) retrocerebellar, the most common variety, and (*ii*) cerebellopontine angle (CPA) arachnoid cysts, very rare, especially in children. Retrocerebellar ACs are further divided into midline ACs, which are those that push anteriorly the cerebellar vermis, spreading the cerebellar hemispheres (Fig. 8), and lateroposterior ACs, those located mainly over one cerebellar hemisphere between this and the occipital dura-mater and bone. Other less-common locations are the retroclival region, the fourth ventricle, and the arachnoid space over the superior cerebellar vermis, below the tentorium and posterior to superior medullary velum. ACs encountered in these latter locations are very rare, and so the scanty available knowledge provided by anecdotal reports does not allow them to be discussed as separate categories, nor their clinical behavior to be adequately delineated. The rationale outlined for the treatment of ACs in other locations will be applicable to the management of these rare lesions.

Clinical Presentation
Symptoms differ according to the cyst localization in the posterior fossa. Retrocerebellar cysts are frequently symptomatic, often associated with hydrocephalus. The most frequent findings are macrocrania or neurodevelopmental delay, and symptoms are usually those associated with ICH, such as vomiting and irritability. Occasionally, a localized bulging in the occipital squama may be the clue for the diagnosis of a posterior fossa AC in an otherwise normal child.

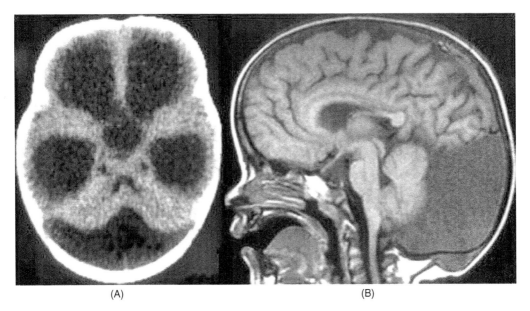

(A)   (B)

Figure 8 **(A)** CT scan of a retrocerebellar arachnoid cyst with secondary hypertensive triventricular dilatation; the persistence of the vermian structures is a differentiating sign from the Dandy–Walker complex. **(B)** T1 sagittal MR scan of a different case of retrocerebellar arachnoid cyst. Note the slightly different signal of the CSF inside the cyst due to its exclusion from the CSF pathways; no sign of ventricular dilatation is evident.

On the other hand, cysts located in the CPA angle, much more rare, may be associated with auditory deficits, tinnitus, or trigeminal neuralgia. Such symptoms are easier to interpret in an adult and difficult to be identified in a child. Hydrocephalus may be present in large-sized cysts, and motor deficits due to brain stem compression are exceptionally rare, as are facial nerve deficits.

The rare cysts located within the fourth ventricle tend to mimic the so-called "false-arrested hydrocephalus" in children or normotensive hydrocephalus in adults (34).

Diagnosis
Similarly to arachnoid cysts of other regions, posterior fossa ACs are diagnosed by CT scan and MRI as an extra-axial, noninfiltrative, and nonenhancing cystic lesion with fluid content signal equal to CSF. These cysts show variable compressive effects over the cerebellum, the fourth ventricle, and even the brainstem in cases of CPA cysts and may be associated with noncommunicating hydrocephalus.

Differential diagnoses of ACs located in the CPA are mainly epidermoid cysts. Anatomic details displayed by MRI are very helpful in making the distinction between these lesions, because epidermoids tend to engulf rather than displace the neighboring neurovascular structures as ACs typically do. Signal patterns found especially in FLAIR and diffusion-weighted sequences are also very valuable in depicting epidermoids as lesions with contents different from CSF (35,36).

Cystic astrocytomas and hemangioblastomas accounted previously for some difficulty in the differential diagnosis of lateroposteriorly located ACs, but since the introduction of MRI and with the continuous evolution of this technique, these difficulties are overcome and distinction among these lesions can easily be performed now.

Much more problematic is the distinction between midline retrocerebellar ACs from Dandy–Walker malformations and variants, megacisterna magna, or Blake's pouch cysts, as all these are CSF-containing malformations and differentiation must be based strictly on anatomical characteristics. Classical Dandy–Walker malformations do not pose significant problems, as they are characterized by a posterior cyst that communicates widely with a dilated fourth ventricle through a partially, with an upward orientation, or a totally lacking cerebellar vermis, in an enlarged posterior fossa with high-positioned tentorium and torcula (2,33,37). The differential diagnosis with the so-called Dandy–Walker variants, the Blake's pouches, and megacisterna magna is challenging. The entity of Dandy–Walker variant is not defined clearly, much controversy is still present and some authors have proposed abandoning this terminology (37). The best accepted definition concerns situations where vermian hypogenesis is present, and so the posterior cyst communicates with the fourth ventricle, but the posterior fossa is normally sized. Problems for the correct diagnosis are present when the vermian hypogenesis is minimal and thus hardly identified even with MRI. Megacisterna magna is also a matter of discussion and confusion, but it concerns a grossly larger cisterna magna, not associated with vermis hypogenesis, in a normal sized posterior fossa. Some advocate that a large number of lesions diagnosed as either Dandy–Walker variants or Megacisterna magna are indeed Blake's pouch cysts (37). These cysts are in turn diverticular extensions of the fourth ventricle through an imperforated foramen of Magendie, which occupy the cisterna magna posteriorly. Although much more common in the topography of the foramen of Magendie, these cysts may also be originated from the foramina of Luschka, extending laterally to the CPA and so constituting a rare differential diagnosis of lesions in this region as well. Differently from ACs, the walls of Blake's pouch cysts have an ependymal lining instead of meningothelial cells characteristic of ACs. Although the cyst wall architecture cannot be addressed by neuroimaging, the use of paramagnetic intravenous contrast media allows the identification of choroid plexus that usually accompany the ependyma, and so extends into the cyst cavity, a feature that definitely rules out ACs, because these lesions have typically no communication with the fourth ventricle and thus cannot contain choroid plexus inside (37). In fact, the position of the choroid plexus may be an important clue for the correct diagnosis and differentiation of these posterior midline lesions (37). Nevertheless, the demonstration of a communication between the fourth ventricle and the posterior cyst remains the key feature for the adequate distinction of these malformations from a midline retrocerebellar AC. CT cisternography and flow-sensitive MRI (38) are important tools to be employed for this purpose.

Treatment

Except for small- or medium-sized lesions in asymptomatic patients, posterior fossa ACs should be treated surgically, mainly because most are diagnosed in small children with macrocrania due to an associated hydrocephalus. CPA ACs, although rare, are often symptomatic when encountered, thus requiring surgical treatment as well.

Surgical Considerations

As in the other locations, the surgical options available for the treatment of midline retrocerebellar ACs are craniotomy for partial cyst excision and fenestration to the basal cisterns, endoscopic fenestration, and cyst shunting. Open surgery has provided good results, but often leads to postoperative hydrocephalus or its decompensation in those patients in whom it was already present, due to postoperative scar formation and obstruction of fourth ventricle outflow. For this reason, shunting remains a good option, either combined or not with ventricular shunting, although carrying always the inherent risks of infection, malfunction, and dependence. Endoscopic fenestration is a less-invasive alternative, but due to the small number of cases, benefits over open surgery have not been clearly demonstrated yet.

For the treatment of posterolateral retrocerebellar ACs, open surgery for the resection of the nonadherent parts of the cyst walls is preferred. This procedure generally provides cyst volumetric reduction and cerebellar reexpansion, restores normal CSF flow in the decompressed fourth ventricle, and is less prone to hydrocephalic complications, since the cyst is noncontiguous with the fourth ventricle outflow structures.

Cerebellopontine angle ACs are best treated with neuroendoscopic techniques. The deep location of these cysts and the close anatomical relationship with important neurovascular structures such as cranial nerves and arteries of the posterior circulation make rigid endoscopes the most suitable tools for the surgical approach to these lesions. The endoscope provides a good exposure of the cyst, allowing the performance of multiple fenestrations to the posterior fossa CSF cisterns through a minimally invasive approach, thus avoiding excessive manipulation of such important neurovascular structures. CPA cyst shunting is not recommended in order to avoid contact of the catheter with the cranial nerves, which could lead to postoperative pain or deficits.

Spinal Arachnoid Cysts

General Characteristics
Arachnoid cysts may be located rarely in the spinal compartment. The incidence is somewhat higher in male subjects, and approximately 50% are found in the pediatric age, affecting usually adolescents. Overall incidence of spinal arachnoid cysts peaks in the second decade of life (39,40,41). The midthoracic spine is more frequently involved, followed by the thoracolumbar, lumbosacral, and cervical regions (42). Spinal ACs are divided into two categories: intradural and extradural ACs. Intradural ACs are very rare and are believed to arise from alterations of the arachnoid trabeculae (2,43). These are encountered generally in the posterior spinal canal, although may be rarely found in lateral or anterior positions within the canal, this being a nearly exclusive feature of spinal ACs of the pediatric population (43,44).

Extradural ACs are more common and are thought to result from diverticular extensions of the arachnoid through defective areas of the dura mater, usually in the region where the nerve root dural sleeve joins the dural sac (2,39,44). These cysts extend extradurally compressing the spinal cord, but usually leave behind a pedicle that connects them with the spinal subarachnoid space. Nevertheless, extradural cysts where such communications were not found have been reported as well (44). Less commonly these lesions may also be found in the posterior midline (2).

Clinical Presentation
Most of the spinal ACs are asymptomatic. When present, symptoms usually have subtle onset over months or years before the diagnosis is established. The signs and symptoms show some consistency with the affected spinal level, but there is not a direct, linear relation as it could be expected. The symptomatology covers a wide range of clinical manifestations: low back pain, perineal pain, micturition urgency or more pronounced sphincteric deficits, and neurogenic bladder, which are more frequent in lumbosacral lesions; radicular pain, sensitive disturbances, or muscular weakness such as flaccid paraparesis may be found in association with thoracolumbar lesions; radicular pain, dysesthesia, or spastic paraparesis in midthoracic lesions; and tetraparesis or Horner syndrome in cervical region ACs. Noteworthy is that although these lesions are more often posteriorly located, motor symptoms are much more frequent than are sensitive symptoms. Furthermore, especially in the extradural variety, symptoms are often fluctuating, worsening during the performance of Valsalva maneuvers that are frequently employed in daily activities like physical exertion, coughing, straining, and sneezing (2,39). Sudden onset of symptoms was also reported in association with minor traumatic events or physical exertion (2,39,44).

Diagnosis
Plain radiographs may show indirect signals of an AC, especially in the extradural variety, such as bone erosion, intervertebral foramen enlargement, interpedicle distance widening, and bone scalloping (2,39). These X-ray abnormalities generally are not encountered with intradural ACs. Major spine abnormalities such as kyphosis or scoliosis may be rarely present. MRI is the diagnostic method of choice, as it is able to show a lesion with fluid contents isointense to CSF and depicts exactly its extensions and relations with the nerve roots. The major limitation of MRI is in detecting the pedicle of extradural ACs, which is better accomplished by thin slices CT scan with intrathecal metrizamide and 3D reconstruction. Cine-mode MRI seems to be promising to overcome this MRI limitation (39).

Differential diagnosis of intradural ACs is cystic tumors or postinflammatory cystic cavities, but either condition usually do not pose significant difficulties if the presence of contrast enhancement or infiltrative characteristics is adequately appreciated. Extradural ACs must be differentiated from other congenital cystic lesions such as neuroepithelial, neurenteric, and teratoid cysts (2), as well as from synovial cysts.

Treatment

Asymptomatic spinal ACs do not require treatment, but close clinical and neuroimaging follow-up is advisable in order to allow early detection of eventual symptoms prior to their evolution to any significant neurological deficit. In the presence of motor or sphincteric deficits, surgical treatment is mandatory. For other symptomatic ACs, such as in those patients with painful complaints or dysesthesias, surgery is also recommended because conservative treatment often leads to incomplete relief.

Surgical Considerations

The surgical treatment of choice for both intradural and extradural varieties is resection of the cyst. Laminotomy is always preferred in order to avoid postoperative instability or progressive deformity. In the treatment of intradural ACs, total cyst resection may not be feasible due to the presence of pial adhesions. In these situations, the removal of the nonadherent portions of the cyst and its communication with the spinal subarachnoid space are considered appropriate, providing good results. If the cyst recurs, another surgical exploration may be considered before indicating shunting procedures, which in turn also provide good results, but carry always the risks of shunt malfunction and infection.

Similarly, extradural spinal ACs are best treated by surgical excision. A good cleavage plane is usually present allowing total cyst resection, closure of the cyst pedicle, and repair of the adjacent dural defect, with excellent results. When total cyst resection is not possible due to adhesions and the pedicle cannot be identified, cyst marsupialization to the peridural space is a good alternative.

Regardless of type or level, patients' response to the surgical treatment is usually good, with a high rate of partial or even total recovery of the neurological deficits postoperatively. The deficits most difficultly recovered are those related to sphincteric disturbances.

CONCLUDING REMARKS

It is clear that knowledge regarding the pathogenesis and the clinical behavior of arachnoid cysts is still incomplete, and several questions remain open. Probably for this reason, the treatment options have not reached an optimal status yet, although several advances have been achieved, enabling the neurosurgeon to be confident in surgery as an effective treatment for these patients. Grouping these cysts by similarities and differences among them provides the means for increasing the comprehension of the pathology, allowing the achievement of a more clear rationale that shall guide ultimately to the most adequate treatment.

On the other hand, genetics have evolved rapidly in the last two decades to point that different genetic conditions associated with arachnoid cysts have been recognized. In parallel, thanks the standardization and evolution of prenatal routine echographic techniques, a significant and growing number of cases has been diagnosed intra-uterus, allowing prompt neonatal evaluation and early treatment if necessary. Besides the important achieved benefits that relate to the prevention of progressive neurological deterioration by means of early neonatal interventions, these achievements together permitted the pathology to be surely recognized as congenital, an important certainty that was lacking until some years ago.

On clinical grounds, a lot of advances have been achieved in the last decade. Continuous evolution of MRI has provided several gains, as arachnoid cysts are now rarely misdiagnosed for other lesions. Cine-mode and cardiac-gated flow-sensitive MRI sequences are new and promising techniques that are proving to be very useful in the correct characterization of these cysts, their communication with physiologic CSF cavities, and in elucidating thus important elements necessary for the decisions concerning the most adequate treatment. Moreover, neuroimaging provides satisfactorily all the important details required for an adequate preoperative surgical planning. CT scan with intrathecal metrizamide, a very valuable tool for the study of arachnoid cysts until now, probably will be progressively substituted by these less-invasive MRI modalities, provided their efficacy and growing accuracy will be confirmed in the future.

Finally, the surgical treatment of arachnoid cysts is still challenging and is a matter of controversy and debate. Although the overall response to surgical procedures is good, especially if compared with some decades ago, complications are still present, and the frequent need of a second or subsequent procedure is a significant negative aspect. Programmable valves are already a conquest, and their evolution will probably be helpful in the future, especially for the treatment of those large cysts where cerebral reexpansion is not expected. Nevertheless, the most promising surgical modality at this moment is endoscopy, which appears to provide a more physiologic approach to the pathology, as does open surgery, but with much less invasiveness. The continuous refinement of the endoscopic instruments and auxiliary tools, together with the continuous evolution of the endoscopic techniques that accompany the growing experience of the neurosurgical community, may allow endoscopic techniques in the future to assume the standard role played today by the microsurgical techniques in the treatment of arachnoid cysts. Hopefully, the continuous evolution of the surgical modalities and techniques and the other mentioned fields will provide treatments that best fit patients' individual characteristics, so minimizing morbidity, mortality, and ultimately improving the quality of life.

REFERENCES

1. Kang JK, Lee KS, Lee IW, et al. Shunt-independent surgical treatment of middle cranial fossa arachnoid cysts in children. Childs Nerv Syst 2000; 16:111–116.
2. Di Rocco C. Arachnoid cysts. In: Youmans JR, ed. Neurological Surgery. Philadelphia, PA: WB Saunders, 1996:967–994.
3. Hume Adams J, Corsellis J, Duchen L. Malformations of the nervous system. In: Greenfield J, Hume Adams J, Corsellis J, Duchen L, eds. Greenfield's Neuropathology. New York: Edward Arnold, 1984:426–427.
4. Katzman GL, Dagher AP, Patronas NJ. Incidental findings on brain magnetic resonance imaging from 1000 asymptomatic volunteers. JAMA 1999; 282:36–39.
5. Eskandary H, Sabba M, Khajehpour F, et al. Incidental findings in brain computed tomography scans of 3000 head trauma patients. Surg Neurol 2005; 63:550–553; discussion 553.
6. Sinha S, Brown JI. Familial posterior fossa arachnoid cyst. Childs Nerv Syst 2004; 20:100–103.
7. Gosalakkal JA. Intracranial arachnoid cysts in children: A review of pathogenesis, clinical features, and management. Pediatr Neurol 2002; 26:93–98.
8. Jadeja KJ, Grewal RP. Familial arachnoid cysts associated with oculopharyngeal muscular dystrophy. J Clin Neurosci 2003; 10:125–127.
9. Struck AF, Murphy MJ, Iskandar BJ. Spontaneous development of a de novo suprasellar arachnoid cyst. Case report. J Neurosurg 2006; 104:426–428.
10. Miyagami M, Tsubokawa T. Histological and ultrastructural findings of benign intracranial cysts. Noshuyo byori 1993; 10:151–160.
11. Rengachary SS, Watanabe I. Ultrastructure and pathogenesis of intracranial arachnoid cysts. J Neuropathol Exp Neurol 1981; 40:61–83.
12. Di Trapani G, Di Rocco C, Pocchiari M, et al. Arachnoid cysts in children: Ultrastructural findings. Acta Neuropathol (Wien) 1981; 7:392–395.
13. Schachenmayr W, Friede RL. Fine structure of arachnoid cysts. J Neuropathol Exp Neurol 1979; 38:434–446.
14. Go KG, Houthoff HJ, Blaauw EH, et al. Arachnoid cysts of the sylvian fissure. Evidence of fluid secretion. J Neurosurg 1984; 60:803–813.
15. Mazurkiewicz-Beldzinska M, Dilling-Ostrowska E. Presentation of intracranial arachnoid cysts in children: Correlation between localization and clinical symptoms. Med Sci Monit 2002; 8:CR462–CR465.
16. Levy ML, Meltzer HS, Hughes S, et al. Hydrocephalus in children with middle fossa arachnoid cysts. J Neurosurg 2004; 101:25–31.
17. Osborn AG, Preece MT. Intracranial cysts: Radiologic–pathologic correlation and imaging approach. Radiology 2006; 239:650–664.
18. Galassi E, Tognetti F, Gaist G, et al. CT scan and metrizamide CT cisternography in arachnoid cysts of the middle cranial fossa: Classification and pathophysiological aspects. Surg Neurol 1982; 17:363–369.
19. Tamburrini G, Caldarelli M, Massimi L, et al. Subdural hygroma: an unwanted result of Sylvian arachnoid cyst marsupialization. Childs Nerv Syst 2003; 19:159–165.
20. Borges G, Fernandes YB, Gallani NR. Brainstem hemorrhage after surgical removal of arachnoid cyst of the Sylvian fissure: A case report. Arq Neuropsiquiatr 1995; 53:825–830.
21. Germano A, Caruso G, Caffo M, et al. The treatment of large supratentorial arachnoid cysts in infants with cyst-peritoneal shunting and Hakim programmable valve. Childs Nerv Syst 2003; 19:166–173.
22. Fitzpatrick MO, Barlow P. Endoscopic treatment of prepontine arachnoid cysts. Br J Neurosurg 2001; 15:234–238.

23. Wang JC, Heier L, Souweidane MM. Advances in the endoscopic management of suprasellar arachnoid cysts in children. J Neurosurg 2004; 100:418–426.
24. Sood S, Schuhmann MU, Cakan N, et al. Endoscopic fenestration and coagulation shrinkage of suprasellar arachnoid cysts. Technical note. J Neurosurg 2005; 102:127–133.
25. Hagebeuk EE, Kloet A, Grotenhuis JA, et al. Bobble-head doll syndrome successfully treated with an endoscopic ventriculocystocisternostomy. J Neurosurg 2005; 103:253–259.
26. Pascual-Castroviejo I, Roche MC, Martinez Bermejo A, et al. Primary intracranial arachnoidal cysts. A study of 67 childhood cases. Childs Nerv Syst 1991; 7:257–263.
27. Caldarelli M, Di Rocco C. Surgical options in the treatment of interhemispheric arachnoid cysts. Surg Neurol 1996; 46:212–221.
28. Menezes AH, Bell WE, Perret GE. Arachnoid cysts in children. Arch Neurol 1980; 37:168–172.
29. Cinalli G, Peretta P, Spennato P, et al. Neuroendoscopic management of interhemispheric cysts in children. J Neurosurg 2006; 105:194–202.
30. Hayashi T, Kuratomi A, Kuramoto S. Arachnoid cyst of the quadrigeminal cistern. Surg Neurol 1980; 14:267–273.
31. Kumar K, Malik S, Schulte PA. Symptomatic spinal arachnoid cysts: Report of two cases with review of the literature. Spine 2003; 28:E25–E29.
32. Gangemi M, Maiuri F, Colella G, et al. Endoscopic treatment of quadrigeminal cistern arachnoid cysts. Minim Invasive Neurosurg 2005; 48:289–292.
33. Erdincler P, Kaynar MY, Bozkus H, et al. Posterior fossa arachnoid cysts. Br J Neurosurg 1999; 13:10–17.
34. Korosue K, Tamaki N, Fujiwara K, et al. Arachnoid cyst of the fourth ventricle manifesting normal pressure hydrocephalus. Neurosurg 1983; 12:108–110.
35. Dutt SN, Mirza S, Chavda SV, et al. Radiologic differentiation of intracranial epidermoids from arachnoid cysts. Otol Neurotol 2002; 23:84–92.
36. Liu P, Saida Y, Yoshioka H, et al. MR imaging of epidermoids at the cerebellopontine angle. Magn Reson Med Sci 2003; 2:109–115.
37. Nelson MD Jr, Maher K, Gilles FH. A different approach to cysts of the posterior fossa. Pediatr Radiol 2004; 34:720–732.
38. Yildiz H, Yazici Z, Hakyemez B, et al. Evaluation of CSF flow patterns of posterior fossa cystic malformations using CSF flow MR imaging. Neuroradiology 2006; 48:595–605.
39. Choi JY, Kim SH, Lee WS, et al. Spinal extradural arachnoid cyst. Acta Neurochir (Wien) 2006; 148:579–585; discussion 585.
40. Dastur HM. The radiological appearances of spinal extradural arachnoid cysts. J Neurol Neurosurg Psychiatry 1963; 26:231–235.
41. Neo M, Koyama T, Sakamoto T, et al. Detection of a dural defect by cinematic magnetic resonance imaging and its selective closure as a treatment for a spinal extradural arachnoid cyst. Spine 2004; 29:E426–E430.
42. Cloward RB. Congenital spinal extradural cysts: Case report with review of literature. Ann Surg 1968; 168:851–864.
43. Lee HJ, Cho DY. Symptomatic spinal intradural arachnoid cysts in the pediatric age group: Description of three new cases and review of the literature. Pediatr Neurosurg 2001; 35:181–187.
44. Liu JK, Cole CD, Sherr GT, et al. Noncommunicating spinal extradural arachnoid cyst causing spinal cord compression in a child. J Neurosurg 2005; 103:266–269.

21 | Colloid Cysts

Philippe Decq
Service de Neurochirurgie, Hôpital Henri Mondor, Créteil, France

Hieronymus Damianus Boogaarts
Department of Neurosurgery, Radboud Universiteit Nijmegen, Medical Centre, Nijmegen, The Netherlands

INTRODUCTION

Colloid cysts are histologically benign tumors that represent between 0.5% and 2% of all intracranial neoplasms. These are mostly located at the anterior part of the third ventricle and are able to produce occlusion of the foramina of Monro with resultant obstructive biventricular hydrocephalus. Because of their obstructive nature, colloid cysts can cause rapid neurological deterioration and even sudden death. On the other hand, neurological and neuropsychological deficits can be observed in patients without increased intracranial pressure (1). The vast majority of colloid cysts reported in the literature is symptomatic and were therefore treated.

Since Dandy's first surgical approach to a colloid cyst in 1921 several treatment modalities have been developed (2). Generally, these are divided into two categories: open surgical removal and percutaneous aspiration procedures. Apart from these treatments, simple shunting of CSF without removal of the cyst has been described. This chapter reviews different aspects of the colloid cysts reviewing the natural history of these tumors and focusing on treatment modalities with special attention to the endoscopic procedure.

EPIDEMIOLOGY

As colloid cysts can be asymptomatic like in Cushing's case, the exact incidence rate of these histological benign tumors is difficult to determine (3). Modern imaging techniques lead to the diagnosis of an increasing number of asymptomatic colloid cysts. The prevalence of colloid cysts is estimated at 1 in 8500 persons based on autopsy series and series of patients who underwent MR neuroimaging (4). The incidence of symptomatic colloid cysts in a defined population in Finland during a 14.5-year period was registered as 3.2 new cases per one million head of population per annum, corresponding to 2% of all cerebral tumors (5). Vandertop calculates about one symptomatic case per million person-years (4). Age at diagnosis ranges from intrauterine diagnosed till the age of 75 (6,7). The mean age at diagnosis in symptomatic cysts is in the fourth or fifth decade of life in series over 30 patients (5,8–15). Although colloid cysts are presumed to be congenital, only a minority is reported in children (16,17). Large series describe a male predominance; this is confirmed by our series of 49 patients with 29 males. The reason for this unequal distribution remains unknown (18,19).

PATHOLOGY AND PATHOPHYSIOLOGY

Colloid cysts are usually found attached to the roof of the anterior part of the third ventricle. It can be located also more posteriorly in the third ventricle; other locations have been described also such as the lateral ventricles, septum pellucidum, fourth ventricle, or prepontine region (11,20–30), but are extremely rare. Multiple locations, paired or even triple cysts have been described in literature (19,31). The size of the cyst is reported from only several millimeters up to 9 cm in diameter (19,32).

The different names given to the cysts (colloid cyst, neuroepithelial cysts, neurenteric cyst, primary actinomycoma) reflect the uncertainty about their origin (33–35). Generally, there are two different hypotheses. Historically, a neuroepithelial origin, including origin from the choroid plexus, ependyma, and embryonic paraphysis is suggested. The second hypothesis suggests a nonneural endodermal origin (36). The latter hypothesis is in accord with most available morphological data and is therefore accepted by most authorities. Although most colloid cysts are incidental findings, several familial cases are described suggesting an autosomal recessive inheritance with variable penetrance in only rare cases (11,18,37).

Symptoms are related to enlargement of the cysts. Occlusion of the foramen of Monroe can result in obstructive hydrocephalus. Also compression of nearby structures like the fornix can give symptoms. Because of its pendular attachment to the tela choroidea, intermittent symptomatology might occur, first postulated by Sjovall in 1910 (38). The cyst may enlarge due to production of colloid material, and often signs of inflammation are found (11). Bleeding is another mechanism of cyst enlargement (14,39,40). This sudden increase in size is related to serious neurological deficit; it is not known which cysts are more prone to bleed. Sudden deterioration in patients with colloid cysts is rare; it is often preluded by intermittent, vague, or misdiagnosed symptoms (29,41). This period rarely lasts less than 24 hours (29). The exact mechanism of rapid deterioration is not known; it can be related to the above-mentioned CSF outflow obstruction. It can also be the cause of venous infarction caused by postural kinking of the proximal internal cerebral veins (42). A third hypothesis suggests local compression of the wall of the third ventricle, thus compromising cardiovascular regulatory centers in the hypothalamus [see comment (4)]. As suggested by Hamlat et al. the mechanism in such cases is a multifactorial and dynamic process in which increased sagittal sinus pressure might play a central role (24). Acute deterioration might be provoked by lumbar puncture.

CLINICAL PRESENTATION

The spectrum of symptomatology in patients with colloid cysts is large, and there are no pathognomical signs (12,19). The mean duration of symptoms in a recent report of about one year reflects this and the difficulty in early diagnosis (43). Kelly distinguished three categories of presentation: headache as the main problem in the first group, a progressive or fluctuating dementia with or without symptoms of raised intracranial pressure only in the second group, and a third group of paroxysmal attacks with complete freedom from all symptoms in between. Probably, the distinction between the groups is not so strict and combinations are possible. Headache is the most presenting symptom as presented in a review of 939 patients (72%) (5). The duration, location, and character of the headache are variable, but often have an increasing intensity occurring in combination with other symptoms. The occurrence of "classical" postural headache is probably overestimated. Other symptoms include, nausea and vomiting, visual deficit, gait disturbances, seizures, short-term memory deficit, symptoms known as triad occurring in normal pressure hydrocephalus, and psychiatric symptoms. CSF leakage as presenting symptom in patients with colloid cysts without cranial trauma is rare (15,44). Sudden death is, as mentioned before, rare and lumbar puncture might be a precipitating factor (40,45). Reports of other precipitating factors are head trauma and an airplane flight (29,46).

NEURORADIOLOGY

CT imaging of colloid cysts mostly reveals a homogeneous well-defined rounded mass at the foramina of Monro, often slightly hyperdense with respect to the brain, but might occasionally be hypodense or isodense to it [Fig. 1(A)] (47–50). Some colloid cysts can show mild-to-moderate enhancement, a ring-like pattern of enhancement is rarely observed (47,48,51,52). Calcifications can be noted in a minority (48). Hydrocephalus, sometimes in combination with periventricular hypodensities, is common and found in 70% to 100% of the cases (48,53). On MR imaging, colloid cysts have a varied appearance but are usually homogeneously hyperintense on T1-weighted images and hypointense on T2-weighted images [Fig. 1(B) and (C)]. The central portion of colloid cyst can be low in T2 signal intensity, probably related to cholesterol esters [Fig. 1(D)] (54,55). The hypointensity on T2-weighted images may predict difficulty of aspiration during stereotactic or endoscopic procedures (56).

MANAGEMENT

The ideal management of colloid cysts remains controversial. Since the introduction of neuroendoscopy, a promising alternative to open surgical methods developed, although long-term results are not yet available. With the advent of computed tomography and particularly MRI the management of incidental, asymptomatic, colloid cysts became an issue (57). Our knowledge about the natural course should guide our treatment of asymptomatic cysts. Different surgical

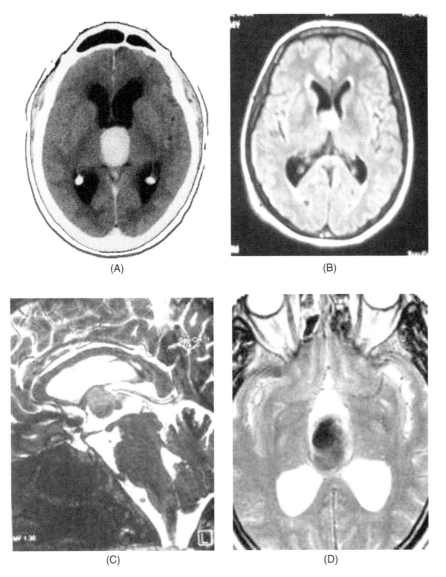

(A)   (B)

(C)   (D)

Figure 1 (**A**) Noncontrast CT showing hyperdense colloid cysts; (**B**) MR, axial view; (**C**) MR saggital view; and (**D**) axial T2-weighted MRI with hypodense colloid cyst.

modalities are considered and the results of neuroendoscopic removal since 1994 in our center (Henri Mondor) are reported.

Natural History
The natural history of these histological benign tumors has not been clearly elucidated (58). Although some can be followed without any increase in size and remain asymptomatic, the thread of acute obstructive biventricular hydrocephalus with even subsequent sudden death remains a subject of numerous reports (40). Characterization of different risk profiles have been attempted to identify patients at risk for brisk neurological decline. Patients sustaining acute neurological deterioration related to colloid cysts tend to be younger than patients undergoing surgery for colloid cysts. The mean age of operated patients was in their fifth decade; conversely reviewed cases of colloid cysts associated with sudden death is in their second or third decade. Thus, patients with colloid cysts and headaches now rarely go undiagnosed if they seek medical

attention, whereas patients who do develop acute hydrocephalus tend to be young and probably have not had prior neurological symptoms.

According to Pollock et al., the natural history of colloid cyst of the third ventricle is related to the interaction of the rate of cyst growth, the development of CSF obstruction, and the fact that most colloid cysts stop enlarging as the patient ages (59). They discern three classes of patients. Class I patients are asymptomatic with slow cyst growth and a cyst that stops enlarging before causing CSF obstruction. In class II patients, the cyst growth is more gradual initially, causing some amount of CSF obstruction and ventricular dilatation, with no or only slight symptoms, but stops before causing CSF blockage, rendering the patient asymptomatic despite having enlarged ventricles. Adapting brain characteristics remain intracranial pressure normal despite the presence of ventriculomegaly. Class III patients have rapidly enlarging cysts, with CSF obstruction occurring before the cyst stops growing, and the patient becomes symptomatic. The latter category is more likely to have cysts with increased signal on T2-weigthed magnetic resonance images compared with patients in Classes I and II colloid cyst—probably related to a more liquid cyst content, reflecting ongoing expansion. It has to be noted that cyst growth can also occur due to intralesional hemorrhage (38). Spontaneous rupture of a colloid cyst is also reported (60). Besides growth, a cyst can also diminish in size spontaneously (61).

Conservative Treatment

The vast majority of reported cases of colloid cyst are symptomatic, therefore requiring treatment. The option of conservative treatment depends on two factors: first, the imaging characteristics of the lesion should be consistent with those of a colloid cyst; second, the risk of acute deterioration should be much lower than treatment-related complications. The risk of complications from different surgical modalities can be abstracted from reported series, but the risk and risk factors of asymptomatic cysts are much more difficult to quantify. The proposed natural course, as discussed above, gives some indication of cysts that should be treated. Pollock considers Class I and II patients, of whom in the latter category 50% was symptomatic, safe to follow with serial neuroimaging. The size of the cyst has been reported as an absolute indicator for removal. Kondziolka manages asymptomatic colloid cysts of less than 5 mm in diameter conservatively. According to him colloid cysts of more than 5 mm in diameter should be operated on whether they are symptomatic or not (62). In his updated series, he managed six asymptomatic patients with incidentally discovered small cysts (<7 mm) successfully for periods of 3 to 7 years (53). Others report that diagnosed colloid cysts measuring over 1 cm should be resected because sudden death has not been reported as having been caused by colloid cyst measuring less than this dimension (4,24). Again it should be noted that the risk of acute deterioration of colloid cysts is very low and is often preluded by vague or misdiagnosed symptoms rarely shorter than 24 hours, making patient information of paramount importance. Camacho et al. reported 24 patients (mean age 52 years) with colloid cysts in whom no surgery was recommended with a mean follow-up interval of 19 months, the most common symptoms were headache and anxiety/nervousness. Most of these patients had normal ventricles (71%) (8). Asymptomatic cyst should be monitored frequently (at least annually) and patients should report symptomatology without delay. In summary, the following remarks can be made: small (less than 1 cm in diameter) asymptomatic cyst without related hydrocephalus can be managed safely conservatively. If related hydrocephalus is present or the cyst tends to enlarge on subsequent neuroimaging, risk of deterioration and surgical risk should be balanced taking into account the clinical condition of the patient and personal preferences.

Shunt Placement

Shunting as the primary treatment for colloid cyst is only advised for patients not capable of undergoing extensive surgery. Although sometimes effective, shunt placement has several drawbacks. First, the danger of acute symptoms remains, but is now related to shunt obstruction, also shunt infection can occur. Camacho et al. describes five patients who were shunted elsewhere as primary treatment who experienced all malfunction (8). Second, shunt placement should be bilateral or a septostomy must be performed. Third, shunting only resolves symptoms related to hydrocephalus, continuing mass effect on the fornix could cause severe irreversible memory deficit. The cyst can continue to grow causing compression of cardiovascular centers and subsequent acute life threatening symptoms. Shunting as only treatment, like conservative treatment, gives no histological results but can be performed in old patient with ventriculomegaly and normal pressure hydrocephalus symptoms.

Percutaneous Aspiration

Stereotactic Aspiration
Stereotactic aspiration of colloid cysts is reported to be a valuable surgical method. Initially, freehand aspiration without resection was described by Gutierrez-Lara et al. in 1975 (63). Bosch et al. were the first to describe stereotactic aspiration, which they used in four patients. Although others reported success with this minimal-invasive treatment, there are several drawbacks (48,64–69). A small, mobile cyst or a cyst with a tough outer capsule might be difficult to aspirate for it can slide away from the needle. Second, high viscosity of the cyst content can make aspiration difficult. Hypodense cyst on preoperative CT scanning tends to be of low viscosity making aspiration successful. Unfortunately, the majority (70%) of the colloid cysts are hyperdense. Third, because of puncture only, and leaving the capsule, high recurrence rates are reported (70). Finally, several complications, probably related to the blindness of the procedure, have been described like memory disorders and hemorrhage (70,71).

Neuroendoscopic Removal
Endoscopic aspiration of colloid cyst was first reported by Powell et al. in 1983 (50). Since then numerous reports on endoscopic treatment appeared (13,72–80) (Fig. 2). The advantages reported are shorter operating time, lower complication rate related to smaller cortical incision, and lower risk of a seizure disorder. Although the new technique seems promising, several remarks have to be made: endoscopic removal of colloid cysts requires a learning curve and should therefore be done by experienced neurendoscopists (78). The recurrence rate has been a matter of concern because total removal seems difficult. However, in certain cases complete removal is reported (80,81). Also, complete removal was reported by Horvath (82) by using a biportal approach. Some authors question whether the cyst capsule should be removed completely (73,78). Generally, the follow-up is short due to its relatively recent introduction but longer follow-up is available as time goes by.

Neurendoscopic removal at Hospital Henri Mondor: Results and technique
From January 1994 till June 2006, 49 consecutive patients underwent endoscopic surgery for colloid cyst of the third ventricle. Twenty women and 29 male patients, ranging in age from 20 to 76 years (mean 40.9), presented with following symptoms: headache (82%), nausea or vomiting (47%), memory deficit (45%), mental status changes (24%), gait disturbances (24%), visual deficit (20%), and comatose (8%). Duration of symptoms varied from several days to 10 years of intermittent headaches. Seven patients were already known with a colloid cyst, two by incident, one patient had an ischemic cerebrovascular stroke without permanent deficit, the other recurrent sinusitis for which a CT was performed. Five patients were previously operated on their colloid cyst at another institution (four stereotactic puncture, one transcortical transventricular approach). Internal shunting was performed in four patients at another institution, and two patients received an emergency external drain at our institution. Internal shunts were externalized for ventricular augmentation prior to operation. The cyst diameter ranged from 7 to 50 mm (mean 17.4). Under endotracheal general anesthesia, a 4-cm linear skin incision is made parallel to the midline, 4 cm laterally and 4 cm in front of the coronal suture. After performing a 1-cm diameter burr hole, the dura is incised and the neuroendoscope (Decq Neuroendoscope; Karl Storz, Tuttlingen, Germany) introduced. In 10 procedures the ventricles were not large enough to allow safe freehand-guided introduction of the neuroendoscope, therefore stereotactic guidance was used. In other procedures, the neuroendoscope was introduced into the ventricle under freehand guidance. The entrance side was chosen taking into account ventricular size and extension of the cyst. Operating time ranged from 35 to 240 minutes (mean 88.6 minutes) depending on the viscosity of the colloid material, the diameter of the foramen of Monro, and the position of the cyst. A pellucidostomy was performed in three patients and an endoscopic

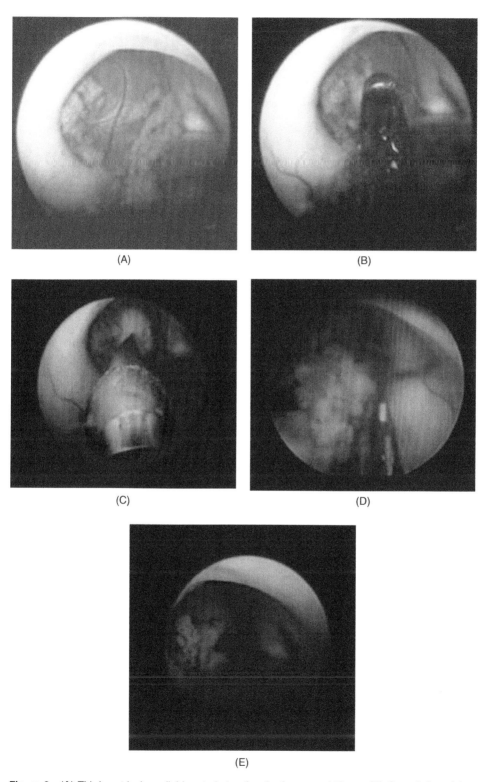

Figure 2 (**A**) Third ventricular colloid cyst obstructing the foramen of Monro. (**B**) Coagulation of the outer wall of the colloid cyst. (**C**) Puncturing the cyst with subsequent aspiration of its contents. The transparent cannula permits monitoring of the aspiration. (**D**) Opening of the cyst wall with microscissors. (**E**) Coagulation and removal of remnants.

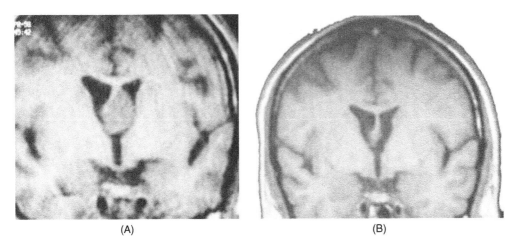

(A)   (B)

Figure 3   (A) Preoperative coronal T1-weighted coronal MRI. (B) Postoperatively after 1.5 years, MRI shows neither rest nor obstruction of the foramina of Monro.

third ventriculostomy was performed in six patients. Two patients required reinternalization of their previous externalized shunts, and five patients had temporary EVD placement (one because of small perioperative bleeding, two because of postoperative hydrocephalus related to aseptic and septic meningitis, two as escape mechanism). One patient required postoperative permanent shunting because of gait disturbances related to hydrocephalus. Postoperative complications were aseptic meningitis (pleocytosis without any identified organism) in five patients, and bacterial meningitis was successfully treated by antibiotics in one patient. One patient experienced permanent memory deficit, after a rapid neurological decline preoperatively requiring emergency shunting. One patient had a pulmonary embolism; one patient had a superficial wound infection, requiring antibiotic treatment. A transient hemiparesis was noted in one patient without clear cause. One patient had an asymptomatic subdural hematoma, which resolved spontaneously. A postoperative seizure was noted in one patient, two weeks after surgery. No patient had a permanent seizure disorder.

Clinical follow-up postdischarge was available in 48 of 49 patients, with a mean of 4.2 years, ranging from 70 days to 11.1 years. Of the 49 patients, 48 were available for imaging follow-up (MR in all but two, one because of a pacemaker, the other because of refusal). Immediate (within 14 days) imaging follow-up was done in 10 patients. Postdischarge imaging was done in 48 patients; mean imaging follow-up time was of 3.9 years (range 42 days till 11.1 years) after the operation. The postoperative MR appearances were divided into three categories: (A) no cyst or membrane visible; (Fig. 3) (B) free floating membrane, with content similar to CSF on MRI; (Fig. 4) and (C) residual cyst with content different from CSF on MRI. Twenty-three cases had no visible remnant. Two patients had a free-floating membrane (group B) and twenty-three patients had a remnant (group C). From the latter group two patients were reoperated, one of them being operated for the third time. Reoperations went without complications, leaving in one patient a membrane (group B) and in the patient operated three times a small rest cyst (group C). In 39 patients sequential imaging was available, imaging characteristics remained stable in 29 patients, it declined in three (one C to A, two C to B), and increased in seven (three A to C, four B to C). The reason for changing characteristics is not known—in some it might be the natural history, in others suboptimal imaging with thick slices might be the cause. A standardized follow-up (spatial and temporal) would probably elucidate this question.

Preoperative imaging was available for evaluation in 39 patients; hydrocephalus (Evans' index $\geq$ 0.30) was present in all with a mean of 0.43, ranging from 0.30 to 0.54. In 37 patients, both pre- and postoperative imaging were available; Evans' index went from a mean from 0.43 to 0.36.

Table 1 gives an overview on reports of endoscopic colloid cyst removal. In nine studies published in the last decade, including ours, removal was clearly assessed and evaluable. Of

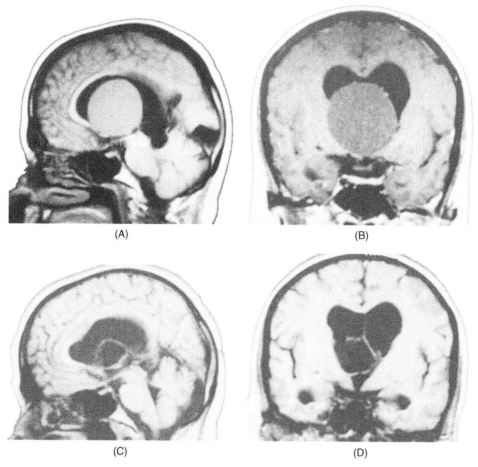

Figure 4 (**A**, **B**) Preoperative MRI of the largest colloid cyst of our series [(**A**) sagittal view, (**B**) coronal view]. (**C**, **D**) Postoperative view showing free floating membrane with pseudocyst content similar to CSF.

204 evaluable patients total or near total removal was possible in 60%. In 10 of 216 patients (4.6%) reoperation was needed.

OPEN SURGICAL REMOVAL

Transcortical–Transventricular Approach

Since the initial report of Dandy the transcortical transventricular approach has been routinely used and permits radical removal (84). As operative techniques improved during the last half of the 20th century, mortality and morbidity have declined over the years. In an extensive review from 1858 to 1996, Hernesniemi et al. reported decline in mortality rate in macrosurgery era from 19% to 1.4% in the microsurgery era. Cabbell and Ross (1996) and Solaroglu et al. (2004) reported no mortality in 18 and 26 patients, respectively (43,85). The reported morbidities since 1996 are given in Table 2. The complication classically reported for this approach is the occurrence of postoperative epilepsy, present in 11 of 118 cases (9.3%). Other complications include memory deficit due to fornix transection (86), meningitis (3.3%), and wound infection among others. Total removal was possible in 87 of 88 reported cases (98.8%). This approach has not been recommended in patients with no hydrocephalus (5,87). Charalampaki et al. describe an endoscope-assisted transcortical–transventricular removal of colloid cysts of the third ventricle with total removal in all (100%) (88).

Table 1 Results of Endoscopic Colloid Cyst Removal

Studies	No. of cases	Clinical relevant complications	Initial total or near total endoscopic removal (A + B)	Reoperation	Follow-up
(75)	10	1 septic meningitis, 1 intraoperative bleeding, 1 stitch granuloma, 1 mispuncture of the ventricle	3 (30%)	1	19 mo (2–47)
(77)	7	Right basal ganglia infarction, short-term memory loss	7 (100%)	0	nr
(72)	13	3 transient memory deficit, 2 hydrocephalus requiring postop shunt placement	9 (69%)	1	48 mo (6 mo to 7 yr)
(76)	14	1 transient memory deficit, transient hemiparesis	11 (78%)	0	25 mo (3–38)
(80)	18	1 transient memory deficit, 2 aseptic meningitis	18 (100%)	0	32 mo (8–52 mo)
(78)	12	1 transient memory deficit	Nr (satisfactory in 11)	2	25 mo (173 wk)
(79)	12	1 transient memory deficit	8 (67%)	0	56 mo (12–93 mo)
(74)	20	1 permanent memory deficit, 1 aseptic meningitis, 3rd cranial nerve palsy, unconsciousness, psychosis, shunt infection, revision, salt wasting syncrome	17 (85%)	1	64 mo (1 to 10 yr)
(13)	61	1 septic meningitis, 1 temporary hemiparesis, 1 communicating hydrocephalus, 3 early intraventricular hemorrhages, 1 trajectory hematoma	23 (38%)	3	32 mo (1–132 mo)
(83)	49	5 aseptic meningitis, 1 bacterial meningitis, 1 seizure, 1 pulmonary embolism, 1 superficial wound infection, 1 transient hemiparesis, 1 asymptomatic subdural hematoma	26 (54%)	2	48 mo (42 days to 10.5 yr)

Free-floating membrane, with content similar to CSF on MRI.
Abbreviations: A, removal; B, no cyst or membrane visible; Nr, not reported.

Table 2 Results of Transcortical–Transventricular Removal Series Since 1996

Studies	No. of cases	Clinical relevant complications	Initial total or near total removal (A + B)	Reoperation	Follow-up
(85)	18	1 Bone flap resorption, shunt infection, subdural hygroma, transient cognitive and memory deficits, subgaleal fluid collection	17 (94%)	0	Nr
(53)	20	1 temporary heminaresis, 1 seizure 5 mo postop	20 (100%)	0	52 mo (0.5 to 11 yr)
(89)	8	1 pulmonary embolism; died, 1 infection, 1 mild hemiparesis, 1 transient impairment of consciousness	8 (100%)	0	46 mo (0–92 mo)
(9)	30	8 Seizures, 2 intracerebral hematoma, 4 CSF leak, 3 meningitis, 2 wound infection, 2 shunt blockage	Nr	Nr	Nr
(90)	16	Meningitis, closed CSF fistula	16 (100%)	0	42 mo (9–121 mo)
(43)	26	2 seizure, 1 wound infection	26 (100%)	0	46 mo (8 mo to 6.5 yr)

Free floating membrane, with content similar to CSF on MRI.
Abbreviations: A, removal; B, no cyst or membrane visible; Nr, not reported.

Table 3 Results of Interhemispheric Transcallosal Approach Since 1996

Studies	No. of cases	Clinical relevant complications	Initial total or near total removal (A + B)	Reoperation	Follow-up
(5)	31	1 Meningitis, 1 brain abscess, 1 hemiparesis, 1 shunt operation, 1 transient memory deficit, 1 wound infection, 1 right parietal venous hemorrhagic infarction, 1 chronic subdural hematoma	31 (100%)	0	52 mo (2 mo to 14.5 yr)
(14)	23	4 transient confusion and/or memory deficit, 1 mutism	23 (100%)	0	Nr
(11)	34	6 infection (of whom 4 bone flap removal), 6 neurological deficit, 4 seizures, 3 reoperation (1 CSF leak, 1 chronic subdural hematoma, 1 cyst not found) 1 endocrinological, 1 other	34 (100%)	1	70
(9)	62	4 cortical venous infarcts with associated varying grades of limb weakness, 3 injury thalamostriate vein and pericallosal artery, 4 CSF leak, 2 meningitis, 2 wound infection	Nr	Nr	Nr

Free floating membrane, with content similar to CSF on MRI.
Abbreviations: A, removal; B, no cyst or membrane visible; Nr, not reported.

Interhemispheric Transcallosal Approach

The interhemispheric transcallosal approach provides natural planes for dissection to the anterior part of the third ventricle through a callosal section. The cyst is accessed to the midline via the septum and directly to its attachment. This approach avoids cortical incision and theoretically thereby should not lead to the possible complication of epileptic seizures; however, practically the risk of epilepsy after this approach is also about 5% (91). Other complications such as venous infarction due to bridging vein damage or short-term memory deficit due to damage to the fornices (14,77,86,92,) might occur. Infrequent reported complications are damage to the pericallosal artery, superior longitudinal sinus thrombosis, diffuse subarachnoid hemorrhage, transient left hemiparesis, disconnection syndrome, and mutism due to bilateral retraction of the gyrus cingularis (91,93–96). Hernesniemi reported on transcallosal removal of 31 patients and also gave an extensive review of transcallosal removal. In his review, mortality in the macrosurgery era was 5.5% (only 18 patients of whom 1 died), which declined to 3.7% (4 of 106) in the microsurgical era. Review of the literature since his report is summarized in Table 3. Total or near total removal is possible in all (100%) reported cases.

CONCLUSION

Symptomatic colloid cysts of the third ventricle should be treated. Total removal of colloid cysts can best be accomplished with the microsurgical approach (98.8%). The risk of seizure disorder is not negligible. Neuroendoscopy permits removal in 60% with no mortality and low morbidity, especially a low risk of seizure disorder. Because both treatment modalities have pros and cons, the definite choice is also related to the experience of the neurosurgeon.

REFERENCES

1. Lobosky CM, Vangilder GC, Damasio AR. Behavioral manifestations of third ventricular colloid cysts. J Neurol Neurosurg Psychiatry 1984; 47:1075–1080.
2. Wilkins RH, Dott NM, Dandy WF. Neurosurgical Classics-XXIV. J Neurosurg 1964; 21:892–905.
3. Fulton JF. Harvey Cushing, a biography. Springfield, IL: Charles C Thomas, 1946.
4. de Witt Hamer PC, Verstegen MJ, De Haan RJ, et al. High risk of acute deterioration in patients harboring symptomatic colloid cysts of the third ventricle. J Neurosurg 2002; 96:1041–1045.
5. Hernesniemi J, Lievo S. Management outcome in third ventricular colloid cysts in a defined population: A series of 40 patients treated mainly by transcallosal microsurgery. Surg Neurol 1996; 45:2–14.
6. Gaertner HJ, Prager B, Himkel GK. Colloid cyst of the third ventricle with XYY-syndrome. J Hirnforsch 1993; 34(4):555–560.
7. Romani R, Niemelä M, Korja M, et al. Dizygotic twins with a colloid cyst of the third ventricle: case report. Neurosurgery 2008; 63:E1003.
8. Camacho A, Abernathey CD, Kelly PJ, et al. Colloid cyst: Experience with the management of 84 cases since the introduction of computed tomography. Neurosurgery 1989; 24:293–700.
9. Desai KI, Nadkarni TD, Muzumdar DP, et al. Surgical management of colloid cysts of the third ventricle—A study of 105 cases. Surg Neurol 2002; 57:295–304.
10. Schroeder HW, Gaab MR. Endoscopic resection of colloid cysts. Neurosurgery 2002; 51(6):1441–1444.
11. Jeffree RL, Besser M. Colloid cyst of the third ventricle: A clinical review of 39 cases. J Clin Neurosci 2001; 8:328–331.
12. Kelly R. Colloid cysts of the third ventricle: Analysis of 29 cases. Brain 1951; 74:23–65.
13. Longatti P, Godano U, Gangemi M. Cooperative study by the Italian neuroendoscopy group on the treatment of 61 colloid cysts. Childs Nerv Syst 2006; 22:1263–1267.
14. Mathiesen T, Grane P, Lindgren L, et al. Third ventricle colloid cysts: A consecutive 12-year series. J Neurosurg 1997; 86:5–12.
15. Nitta M, Smon L. Colloid cysts of the third ventricle. A review of 36 cases. Acta Neurosurg 1985; 76:99–104.
16. Macdonald RL, Humphreys RP, Rutka JT, et al. Colloid cysts in children. Pediatr Neurosurg 1994; 20:169–177.
17. Maqsood AAR, Devi IB, Mohanty A, et al. Third ventricular colloid cysts in chlidren. Pediatr Neurosurg 2006; 42:147–150.
18. Partington MW, Bookalil AJ. Familial colloid cyst of the third ventricle. Clin Genet 2004; 66:473–475.
19. Witzig EP. Etude statistique du kyste colloide du troisieme ventricule (pretendu kyste de la paraphyse). Serie anatomo-clinique de 75 cas. Acta Neurol Belg 1982; 82:281–299.

20. Bertalanffy H, Kretzschmar H, Gilsbach JM, et al. Large colloid cyst in lateral ventricle simulating brain tumour. Case report. Acta Neurochir (Wien) 1990; 104:151–155.
21. Christiaens JL, Cousin R, Dhellemmes P, et al. Kyste colloïde intrasellaire. Neurochirurgie 1976; 22:649–651.
22. Ciric I, Zivin I. Neuroepithelial (colloid) cyst of the septum pellucidum. J Neurosurg 1975; 43:69–73.
23. Efkan CM, Attar A, Ekinci C, et al. Neuroepithelial (colloid) cyst of the parietal convexity. Acta Neurochir (Wien) 2000; 142:1167–1168.
24. Hamlat A, Pasqualini E, Askar B. Hypothesis about the physiopathology of acute deterioration and sudden death caused by colloid cysts of the third ventricle. Med Hypotheses 2004; 63:1014–1017.
25. Jan M, Zeze VB, Velut S. Colloid cyst of the fourth ventricle: Diagnostic problems and pathogenic considerations. Neurosurgery 1989; 24(6):939–942.
26. Jaskolski DJ, Wrobel-Wisniewska G, Papierz W, et al. Colloid-like cyst located in the prepontine region. Surg Neurol 2003; 60:260–264.
27. Killer HE, Flammer J, Wicki B, et al. Acute asymmetric upper nasal quadrantanopsia caused by a chiasmal colloid cyst in a patient with multiple sclerosis and bilateral retrobulbar neuritis. Am J Ophthalmol 2001; 132:286–288.
28. Maurice-Williams RS, Wadley JP. Paired colloid cysts of the third and lateral ventricles. Br J Neurosurg 1998; 91:128–131.
29. Ryder WJ, Kleinscmidt-Demaster BK, Keller TS. Sudden deterioration and death in patients with benign tumors of the third ventricle area. J Neurosurg 1986; 64:216–223.
30. Shima T, Ishikawa S, Okada Y, et al. "Colloid cyst" of the lateral ventricle–Report of a case. No Shinkei Geka 1976; 4(8):791–797.
31. Shuangshoti S, Phisitbutr M, Kasantikul V, et al. Multiple neuroepithelial (colloid) cysts: association with other congenital anomalies. Neurology 1997; 27(6):561–566.
32. Shuangshoti S, Netsky MG. Neuroepithelial (colloid) cysts of the nervous system. Further observations on pathogenesis, location, incidence, and histochemistry. Neurology 1966; 16:887–903.
33. Bengtson BP, Hedeman LS, Bauserman SC. Symptomatic neuroepithelial (colloid) cysts of the third ventricle. A unique case report in nontwin brothers. Cancer 1990; 66:779–785.
34. Graziani N, Dufour H, Figarella-Branger D, et al. Do the suprasellar neurenteric cyst, the Rathke cleft cyst and the colloid cyst constitute a same entity? Acta Neurochir 1995; 133:174–180.
35. Powers JM, Dodds HM. Primary actinomycoma of the third ventricle—The colloid cyst. A histochemical and ultrastructural study. Acta Neuropathol 1977; 37:21–26.
36. Takahiro T, Hruban RH, Carson BS, et al. Colloid cysts of the third ventricle: Immunohistochemical evidence for nonneuroepithelial differentiation. Hum Pathol 1992; 23:811–816.
37. Joshi SM, Gnanalingham KK, Mohaghegh P, et al. A case of familial third ventricular colloid cyst. Emerg Med J 2005; 22:909–910.
38. Sjovall E. Über eine Ependymcyste embryonalen Charakters (Paraphyse?) im dritten Hirnventrikel mit lipochromer Veranderungen mit autreten vo Halbondkorperchen. Beitr Pathol Anat 1910; 47: 248.
39. Beems T, Menovsky T, Lammens M. Hemorrhagic colloid cyst. Case report and review of the literature. Surg Neurol 2006; 65:84–86.
40. Malik GM, Horoupian DS, Boulos RS. Hemorrhagic (colloid) cysts of the third ventricle and episodic neurologic deficits. Surg Neurol 1980; 13:73–77.
41. Buttner A, Winkler PA, Eisenmenger W, et al. Colloid cyst of the third ventricle with fatal outcome: A report of two cases and review of the literature. Int J Legal Med 1997; 110:260–266.
42. Parkinson D. Colloid cysts. J Neurosurg 2002; 97:1249 [Comment].
43. Solaroglu I, Beskonakli E, Kaptanoglu E, et al. Transcortical–transventricular approach in colloid cysts of the third ventricle: Surgical experience with 26 cases. Neurosurg Rev 2004; 27:89–92.
44. Kane PJ, Mendelow AD, Keoch AJ, et al. Cerebrospinal fluid rhinorrhoea associated with colloid cyst. Short report. Br J Neurosurg 1991; 5:317–320.
45. Kava MP, Tullu MS, Deshmukh CT, et al. Colloid cyst of the third ventricle: A cause of sudden death in a child. Indian J Cancer 2003; 40:31–33.
46. Cultrera F, Parisi G, Platania N, et al. Neurological deterioration after head trauma in patients with colloid cysts of the 3rd ventricle. J Neurosurg Sci 2004; 48:67–70.
47. Ganti SR, Antunes JL, Louis KM, et al. Computed tomography in the diagnosis of colloid cysts of the third ventricle. Radiology 1981; 138:385–391.
48. Hall WA, Lundsford LD. Changing concepts in the treatment of colloid cysts: An 11-years experience in the CT era. J Neurosurg 1987; 66:186–191.
49. Hine AL, Chui MS. Hypodense colloid cyst of the third ventricle. Can Assoc Radiol J 1987; 38:288–291.
50. Powell MP, Torrens MJ, Thomson JLG, et al. Isodense colloid cysts of the third ventricle: A diagnostic and therapeutic problem resolved by ventriculoscopy. Neurosurgery 1983; 13:234–237.

51. Bullard D, Osborne D, Cook W. Colloid cyst of the third ventricle presenting as a ring-enhancing lesion on computed tomography. Neurosurgery 1982; 11:790–791.

52. Sener RN, Jinkins JR. Case report. CT of intrasellar colloid cyst. J Comput Asssist Tomogr 1991; 15(4):671–672.

53. Kondziolka D, Lunsford LD. Microsurgical resection of colloid cysts using stereotactic transventricular approach. Surg Neurol 1996; 46:485–492.

54. Amaro D, Castillo M, Chen H, et al. Colloid cyst of the third ventricle: Imaging–pathologic correlation. AJNR Am J Neuroradiol 2000; 21:1470–1477.

55. Maeder PP, Holtas SI, Basibuyuk LN, et al. Colloid cysts of the third ventricle: Correlation of MR and CT findings with histology and chemical analysis. AJNR Am J Neuroradiol 1990; 11:575–581.

56. EL Khoury C, Brugieres P, Decq P, et al. Colloid cyst of the third ventricle: Are MR imaging patterns predictive of difficulty with percutaneous treatment? Am J Neuroradiol 2000; 21:489–492.

57. Camacho A, Abernathey CD, Kelly PJ, et al. Colloid cysts: experience with the management of 84 cases since the introduction of computed tomography. Neurosurgery 1989; 24(5):693–700.

58. Pollock BE, Huston J III. Natural history of asymptomatic colloid cysts of the third ventricle. J Neurosurg 1999; 91:364–369.

59. Pollock BE, Shreiner SA, Huston J III. A theory on the natural history of colloid cysts of the third ventricle. Neurosurgery 2000; 46(5):1077–1083.

60. Motoyama Y, Hashimoto H, Ishida Y, et al. Spontaneous rupture of a presumed colloid cyst of the third ventricle. Neurol Med Chir (Tokyo) 2002; 42:228–231.

61. Hattab N, Freger P, Tadie M, et al. Taitement des kystes colloïdes du 3e ventricule par dérivation ventriculaire. Neurochirurgie 1990; 36:129–131.

62. Kondziolka D, Lunsford LD. Stereotactic techniques for colloid cysts: roles of aspiration, endoscopy, and microsurgery. Acta Neurochir Suppl 1994; 61:76–78.

63. Gutierrez-Lara F, Patino R, Hakim S. Treatment of tumors of the third ventricle: A new and simple technique. Surg Neurol 1975; 3:323–325.

64. Apuzzo MLJ, Clandrasoma PT, Zelman V. Computed tomographic guidance stereotaxis in the management of lesions of the third ventricular region. Neurosurgery 1984; 15:502–508.

65. Bosch DA, Rahn T, Backlund ED. Treatment of colloid cysts of the third ventricle by stereotactic aspiration. Surg Neurol 1978; 9:15–18.

66. Donauer E, Moringlane JR, Ostertag CB. Colloid cyst of the third ventricle. Open operative approach or stereotactic aspiration? Acta Neurochir 1986; 83:24–30.

67. Kondziolka D, Lunsford LD. Stereotactic management of colloid cysts: Factors predicting success. J Neurosurg 1991; 75:45–51.

68. Mohadjer M, Teshmar E, Mundinger F. CT-stereotactic drainage of colloid cysts in the foramen of Monro and the third ventricle. J Neurosurg 1987; 67:220–223.

69. Rivas JJ, Lobato RD. CT-assisted stereotactic aspiration of colloid cysts of the third ventricle. J Neurosurg 1985; 62:238–243.

70. Mathiesen T, Grane P, Lindquist C, et al. High recurrence rate following aspiration of colloid cysts in the third ventricle. J Neurosurg 1993; 78:748–752.

71. Peragut JC, Riss JM, Farnarier P, et al. Kystes colloïdes du 3è ventricule, scanner IRM et ponction stéréotaxique. A propos de 9 observations. Neurochirurgie 1990; 36:122–128.

72. Abdou SM, Cohen AR. Endoscopic treatment of colloid cysts of the third ventricle. Technical note and review of the literature. J Neurosurg 1998; 89:1062–1068.

73. Decq P, Le Guerinel C, Brugieres P, et al. Endoscopic management of colloid cysts. Neurosurgery 1998; 42(6):1288–1294.

74. Hellwig D, Bauer BL, Schulte M, et al. Neuroendoscopic treatment for colloid cysts of the third ventricle: The experience of a decade. Neurosurgery 2003; 52:525–533.

75. Kehler V, Brunori A, Gliemroth J, et al. Twenty colloid cysts – comparison of endoscopic and microsurgical management. Minim Invasive Neurosurg 2001; 44(3):121–127.

76. King WA, Ullman JS, Frazee JG, et al. Endoscopic resection of colloid cysts: Surgical considerations using the rigid microscope. Neurosurgery 1999; 44(5):1103–1111.

77. Lewis AI, Crone KR, Taha J, et al. Surgical resection of third ventricle colloid cysts. Preliminary results comparing transcallosal microsurgery with endoscopy. J Neurosurg 1994; 81:174–178.

78. Rodziewicz GS, Smith MV, Hodges CJ. Endoscopic colloid cyst surgery. Neurosurgery 2000; 46(3):655–662.

79. Schroeder HWS, Gaab MR. Endoscopic resection of colloid cysts. Neurosurgery 2002; 51:1441–1445.

80. Teo C. Complete endoscopic removal of colloid cysts: Issues of safety and efficacy. Neurosurg Focus 1999; 6(4):e9.

81. Gaab MR, Schroeder HW. Neuroendoscopic approach to intraventricular lesions. J Neurosurg 1998; 88:496–505.

82. Horvath Z, Vetö F, Balás I, et al. Complete removal of colloid cyst via CT-guided stereotactic biportal neuroendoscopy. Acta Neurochir (Wien) 2000; 142(5):539–545.
83. Decq P, Le Guerinel C, Sakka L, et al. Endoscopic surgery of third ventricle lesions. Neurochirurgie 2000; 46(3):286–294 (French).
84. Dandy WE. Case reports of colloid cysts in the third ventricle (group I). In: Benign Tumors in the Third Ventricle of the Brain: Diagnosis and Treatment. Baltimore, MD: Williams and Wilkins, 1933: 4–37.
85. Cabbell KL, Ross AD. Stereotactic microsurgical craniotomy for the treatment of third ventricular colloid cysts. Neurosurgery 1996; 38(2):301–307.
86. Aggleton JP, Mcmackin D, Carpenter J, et al. Differential cognitive effects of colloid cysts in the third ventricle that spare or compromise the fornix. Brain 2000; 123:800–815.
87. Cetinalp E, Ildan F, Boyar B, et al. Colloid cyst of the third ventricle. Neurosurg Rev 1994; 17:135–139.
88. Charalampaki P, Filippi R, Welschehold S, et al. Endoscope-assisted removal of colloid cysts of the third ventricle. Neurosurg Rev 2006; 29:72–79.
89. Kehler U, Brunori A, Gliemroth J, et al. Twenty colloid cysts—Comparison of endoscopic and microsurgical management. Minim Invasive Neurosurg 2001; 44:121–127.
90. Barlas O, Karadereler S. Stereotactically guided microsurgical removal of colloid cysts. Acta Neurochir (Wien) 2004; 146(11):1199–1204.
91. Gokalp HZ, Yuceer N, Arasil E, et al. Colloid cyst of the third ventricle. Evaluation of 28 cases of colloid cysts of the third ventricle operated on by transcortical transventricular (25 cases) and transcallosal/transventricular (3 cases) approaches. Acta Neurochir 1996; 138:45–49.
92. Apuzzo ML, Chandrasoma PT, Cohen D, et al. Computed imaging stereotaxy: experience and perspective related to 500 procedures applied to brain masses. Neurosurgery 1987; 20(6):930–937.
93. Garido E, Fahs GR. Cerebral venous and sagittal sinus thrombosis after transcallosal removal of a colloid cyst of the third ventricle: Case report. Neurosurgery 1990; 26:540–542.
94. Rabb CH, Apuzzo MLJ. Transcallosal approach to the third ventricle. In: Schmidek HH, Sweet WH, eds. Operative Neurosurgical Techniques, Indications, Methods and Results, 3rd ed. Philadelphia, PA: Saunders Publishers, 1995:715–723, chap. 54.
95. Stoodley MA, North JB, Reilley PL, et al. Short report. False aneurysm following intracranial surgery. Br J Neurosurg 1994; 8:599–602.
96. Yamanaka K, Iwai Y, Nakajima H, et al. Multiple brain hemorrhages after removal of a giant colloid cyst of the third ventricle. Neurol Med Chir (Tokyo) 1998; 38:24–27.

22 | Tumor-Related Hydrocephalus

Paul Chumas, Daniel Crimmins, and Atul Tyagi
Department of Neurosurgery, Leeds General Infirmary, Leeds, U.K.

Pediatric patients with brain tumors usually present with   signs and symptoms of raised intracranial pressure, which is often a consequence of tumor-related hydrocephalus. Hydrocephalus occurs in this situation because pediatric tumors are usually large, tend to arise in the midline, and cause obstruction of the ventricular system. In adults, obstructive, tumor-related hydrocephalus is far less common, but communicating hydrocephalus secondary to carcinomatosis does occur relatively frequently. While the treatment of the tumor itself is obviously the primary concern for the surgeon and patient alike, the abnormal CSF dynamics are important as they may result in significant morbidity and delay the delivery of adjuvant therapies. The aim of this chapter is to review the management of tumor-related hydrocephalus in both adults and children.

MANAGEMENT OF PEDIATRIC TUMOR-RELATED HYDROCEPHALUS

General Concepts

Historically, children with brain tumors were diagnosed late and were often dehydrated and emaciated from vomiting and lack of nutrition at the time of presentation. With the advent of shunts in the 1950s, it became routine practice to insert a shunt to control the raised ICP and allow the child to improve before undertaking any tumor surgery. With CT and later MRI, this delay in diagnosis fortunately has been reduced and, as a result of this and the recognition of the problems associated with shunts, there has been a change in the management of tumor-related hydrocephalus. Today, we usually work on the basis that if the tumor can be successfully dealt with, the underlying hydrocephalus will subsequently spontaneously resolve. The surgeon's aim is to safely facilitate this spontaneous resolution by temporizing—with "permanent treatment" only being resorted to when necessary. In general, hydrocephalus due to tumors that are distorting the ventricular system but not actually growing within the ventricular system are relatively easily achieved by solely removing the tumor. However, tumors, which are located largely within the ventricular system, have a higher chance of requiring either temporary or permanent treatment.

Unfortunately, there are very few studies that have specifically looked at the problems associated with tumor-related hydrocephalus—with these patients usually being included in larger series of hydrocephalic patients. Nonetheless, it is clear that shunting patients with tumor-related hydrocephalus is associated with an increased risk of shunt malfunction and infection compared to shunting in nontumor patients. The main risk factors for infection are the use of an EVD, multiple surgical procedures, and CSF leak (1,2). Patients who require a feeding gastrostomy or who have a tracheostomy are also at increased risk of a shunt infection (3). Some have recommended shunting these patients in the lateral position and tunneling the peritoneal catheter down the back rather than across the chest in order to have the shunt tubing as far as possible from the tracheostomy site.

The early shunt malfunction problems seen in patients with tumor-related hydrocephalus are usually related to cellular debris (tumor or blood). To date, there is no good evidence that any particular make or type of shunt is superior to any other in dealing with tumor-related hydrocephalus. Another, perhaps largely theoretical, risk is of the spread of tumor via the shunt (4,5). Although filters have been designed to try and avoid this, these were associated with significant rates of shunt obstruction and have been abandoned largely. In fact, shunt-related spread of this kind is very rare, which probably reflects the fact that the immune system outside the CNS is very capable of dealing with the shedding of a small number of tumor cells.

With the widespread acceptance of endoscopy over the last two decades, the surgeon has a greater choice of treatment options (6). Endoscopy may also give the surgeon the opportunity to obtain a tissue diagnosis at the same time as treating the hydrocephalus or allow the surgeon to drain a tumor cyst into the ventricular system. Even when a shunt is required, endoscopy may be of value as it may help simplify the treatment of the hydrocephalus—for example, fenestrating the septum pellucidum in cases of bilateral foramen of Monro obstruction so that only a single shunt is required to drain both lateral ventricles.

However, it should be remembered also that the presence of enlarged ventricles may actually assist the surgeon during the removal of certain tumors (e.g., intraventricular tumors) and therefore this aspect needs to be taken into account when deciding when and how to treat the hydrocephalus and the tumor.

The surgeon therefore needs to carefully consider the following:

(a) Does the clinical state of the child necessitate emergency treatment and if so what (EVD, third ventriculostomy ± biopsy, shunt ± other endoscopic procedure, or tumor removal)?
(b) What is the surgical plan for the tumor? In particular, is the intention to try and remove the tumor and see if the hydrocephalus will resolve spontaneously?
(c) In those patients who are to undergo a biopsy only or no tumor surgery—what is the best long-term treatment option?
(d) If the aim is to remove the tumor—how long will the hydrocephalus take to resolve and what temporizing measures will be required to get the patient through this period until his or her own absorption is adequate? Is it possible to minimize the side effects of the abnormal CSF dynamics during this period (CSF leak, pseudomeningocele, etc.)?
(e) In patients with persistent abnormal CSF dynamics after tumor removal, is the hydrocephalus still "obstructive" or is it now partially "communicating" due to the presence of blood, infection, and/or cellular debris? If it is "obstructive" at what level is the block now and is ETV an option?

Perhaps the most important point to remember when treating this group of patients is that the tumor and the hydrocephalus are interrelated and so the management should mirror this. It is also important to remember that while it is often possible to treat the hydrocephalus by just removing the tumor, this should not be at the expense of increased morbidity. In particular, these children will frequently present with papilledema and their vision needs to be carefully monitored. Although their vision might continue to deteriorate despite our best efforts, it is important that the surgeon is sure that any raised ICP has been adequately dealt with—a child who has lost vision but in whom the surgeon has managed to avoid inserting a shunt is not a success.

Having discussed these general points, we will now review tumor-related hydrocephalus by site.

Supratentorial Tumors

The most common tumors to cause hydrocephalus in the supratentorial compartment are craniopharyngiomas, chiasmatic/hypothalamic tumors, thalamic tumors, intraventricular tumors (e.g., choroid plexus tumors, giant cell astrocytomas, colloid cysts), and large hemispheric tumors causing midline shift and hence obstruction of the ventricular system. As mentioned above, the hydrocephalus in the latter group is usually successfully treated by tumor removal alone. However, in young children (younger than 1 year of age), the absorption pathways may not be as well developed and some of these children may require a shunt to control their raised ICP.

Craniopharyngiomas are perhaps one the most difficult tumors to deal with in neurosurgery. From the perspective of this chapter the important issues are the treatment of any associated hydrocephalus and the possible treatment options of any craniopharyngioma cysts that are accessible through the ventricular system. Children with craniopharyngiomas frequently have endocrine, visual and hypothalamic problems. In addition, often they have had radiotherapy or multiple operations. All of these factors interact and result in cognitive deficits—however, hydrocephalus has been found to be an independent risk factor for cognitive problems (7). From the visual perspective, these patients tolerate raised ICP particularly poorly and should not be allowed to lose visual function from a potentially treatable cause. Therefore the importance of good control of the hydrocephalus in this group of patients cannot be stressed enough.

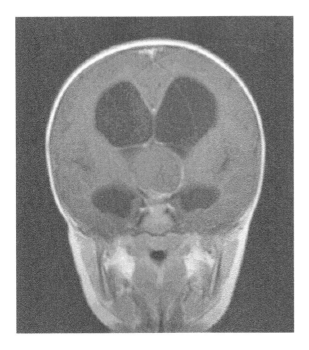

Figure 1 Suprasellar/third ventricular cranio-pharyngioma. Hydrocephalus initially treated by endoscopic aspiration of the cyst.

When hydrocephalus develops in these patients, it is usually due to third ventricular obstruction (Fig. 1). If there is a large cyst bulging up into the third ventricle, then consideration should be given to an endoscopic fenestration of the cyst ($\pm$ biopsy and insertion of access device). Often, this will result in resolution of the hydrocephalus with release of pressure on the optic chiasm and give the surgeon time to plan the definitive treatment of the tumor. An additional bonus of draining the cyst in this fashion is that it results in the cyst becoming more accessible from below at the time of open resective surgery.

When the hydrocephalus develops as a result of solid or cystic tumor pushing up the floor of the third ventricle, it may be necessary to consider insertion of a shunt. Consideration will have to be given as to whether both ventricles can be drained by one ventricular catheter or whether it is necessary to insert bilateral shunts or fenestrate the septum pellucidum.

Hypothalamic/chiasmatic tumors are a very variable group of tumors both clinically and radiologically. The role of tumor surgery in this group of patients is controversial and patients with progressive disease (clinical or radiological) now receive chemotherapy as first line treatment in many centers. Only large tumors will produce hydrocephalus (by compressing the anterior third ventricle) (Fig. 2), and as this is in patients in whom visual function is already compromised, the need to limit periods of raised ICP is obvious.

The treatment of any associated hydrocephalus is by shunting—with endoscopy only playing a potential role in taking a biopsy and fenestrating the septum. One shunt complication particularly associated with these tumors is the formation of ascites, which can be very problematic (8).

Thalamic tumors may present also with hydrocephalus (Fig. 3), particularly if they are bilateral (9). Often the obstruction is posterior enough to allow consideration of an ETV. If a biopsy is to be considered at the same time, then it is necessary to use either a flexible scope or a rigid scope; in the latter case be prepared to make two burr holes. The first burr hole is placed in the standard position for an ETV (on the coronal suture) with a second burr hole placed further anteriorly so that the surgeon has a straight trajectory backwards through the foramen of Monro to the tumor. It is usually not possible with a rigid scope to get back far enough from a standard ETV burr hole to biopsy lesions at the back of the third ventricle without damaging the fornix or cause bleeding from either the choroid plexus or the thalamostriate vein. Although we use a rigid scope routinely for undertaking ETVs, we prefer to use a flexible scope if we are aiming to combine this with a biopsy. We have also found that a GI endoscopy biopsy capsule gives

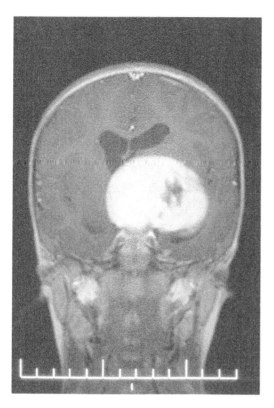

Figure   2 Hypothalamic/chiasmatic   pilomyxoid astrocytoma.

larger specimens than the standard kit provided for neuroendoscopy. The chance of getting a "positive" biopsy is increased if tumor is visible and not covered by ependyma. As the main aim is to treat the hydrocephalus, we advise that the ETV be undertaken before the biopsy—in case there is bleeding from the tumor and visibility is lost. This is also true of pineal region tumors

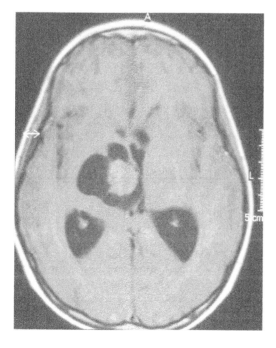

Figure 3   Right thalamic pilocytic astrocytoma.

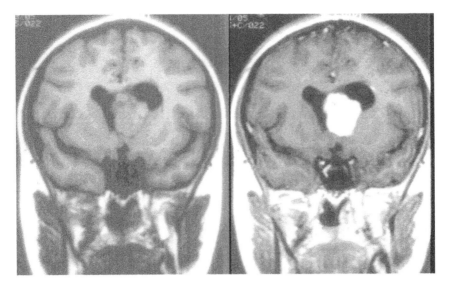

Figure 4 Subependymal giant cell tumor causing hydrocephalus in a child with tuberous sclerosis complex. The hydrocephalus resolved after removal of the tumor.

Intraventricular tumors are relatively rare and include choroid plexus tumors, meningiomas, giant cell astrocytomas (SEGAs) (Fig. 4), and colloid cysts (already dealt with in the previous chapter). The treatment of any associated hydrocephalus (or loculated ventricle) follows the principles outlined above under "general concepts." In particular, it is important to consider the timing of any shunt insertion in order not to lose the surgical working space provided by the dilated ventricle, which will help at the time of tumor removal.

Choroid plexus tumors are associated with a high rate of shunt requirement postexcision. This is only rarely thought to be due to overproduction of CSF and more to do with problems with absorption due to cellular debris. Treatment of intraventricular tumors is excision, and the hydrocephalus in general will settle spontaneously in the case of meningiomas, SEGAs, and colloid cysts.

Infratentorial Tumors

We will discuss in this section pineal, cerebellar, and brain stem tumors. The most common group is the "cerebellar tumors" and this and the pineal tumors usually present with hydrocephalus. Patient recovery after posterior fossa surgery is frequently adversely affected by CSF complications.

Pineal region tumors are a pathologically diverse group of tumors and their definitive treatment depends upon the exact histological nature of the tumor and whether the tumor is "secreting" (AFP/B-HCG) or not. The associated hydrocephalus is due to obstruction of the aqueduct (Fig. 5), and the surgeon's initial aims should be to obtain blood and CSF for tumor markers to treat the hydrocephalus and to obtain a tissue diagnosis. Endoscopy often allows the surgeon to achieve all these aims during the same procedure (Fig. 6) and is now recognized as an important aid to the management of these tumors (10,11). As these tumors are located at the back of the third ventricle, the same technical points that were described above for the endoscopic management of thalamic tumors apply. In addition, it is important to remember to collect the CSF for markers and cytology as soon as the ventricle is cannulated and before any irrigation has occurred. Ideally, a tumor biopsy would be undertaken only if the blood and CSF markers were negative but in reality, the first time that CSF is usually available is at the time of endoscopy, and therefore it seems reasonable to collect CSF, perform an ETV, and attempt a biopsy at the same time (and in that order). The success rate for the ETV to control the hydrocephalus in this group of patients is of the order of 94% with a histological diagnosis reached in 94% of patients. The overall complication rate was 11% with no mortality or permanent morbidity (12). Our diagnostic rate for endoscopic biopsy of pineal tumors is

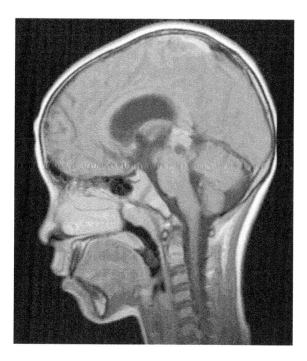

Figure 5 Pineal germinoma. Hydrocephalus managed by endoscopic third ventriculostomy and biopsy.

78%, which compares well with that in the literature (78–100%). The less attractive alternative to an endoscopic procedure is to offer a shunt or an EVD to deal with the hydrocephalus and to undertake a stereotactic biopsy or open procedure in order to obtain a tissue diagnosis.

Tectal plate tumors are a distinct subgroup of pineal region tumors that usually present with longstanding hydrocephalus as evidenced by a large head circumference. These tumors are histologically usually low-grade gliomas and have an indolent course. Providing the clinical and radiological findings are characteristic, these patients very rarely require any form of treatment for the tumor (even biopsy) other than observation. In view of the large head, placing a shunt in these patients is associated with a significant risk of overdrainage and subdural collections. The fact that after ETV, the ventricular size tends to change less, means that the risk of symptomatic

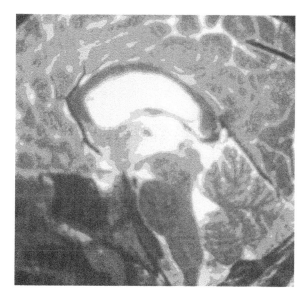

Figure 6 Tectal glioma (presumed). Hydrocephalus treated by endoscopic third ventriculostomy.

subdurals is far lower after ETV than after shunt surgery. The expected success rate after ETV in this group of patients is of the order of 80% to 100% (13). However, it should be remembered that it is necessary for the ETV to work indefinitely, and there have been a number of cases reported in the literature of late rapid deterioration many years after an ETV (14). For this reason, we prefer insertion of an access device at the time of the ETV so that it can be used for emergency drainage of CSF at peripheral hospitals or even in the community. Likewise, we feel that patients and caregivers need to understand that their hydrocephalus is never "cured" but merely controlled and if they develop symptoms, then it is necessary to seek attention urgently. It is important to remember that the risk of sudden late deterioration after ETV is probably no different than the risk of death associated with shunt malfunction (approximately 1%).

Cerebellar tumors

In children the most common tumors growing into or arising from the fourth ventricle are medulloblastomas (off the inferior vermis) (Fig. 7) and ependymomas. In contrast, the most common cerebellar hemispheric tumors are pilocytic astrocytomas. As already mentioned, patients with hemispheric and fourth ventricular tumors usually present with tumor-related hydrocephalus—however, unless the diagnosis has been particularly delayed, it is relatively uncommon for emergency treatment of the hydrocephalus to be required. In the majority of patients, it is possible to commence steroids and plan for surgery on the next available list. At the time of the operation, some surgeons will routinely place an EVD, while others may just place a burr hole (for potential use if the patient deteriorates on the ward), while still others elect not to place a burr hole at all. It should be remembered that EVD placement is not without risks of its own—including infection, failure to cannulate the ventricle, hematomas, etc.. In fact the placement of a frontal EVD prior to or during posterior fossa surgery in 15 children who had surgery in the sitting position was associated with extradural hematomas in 5, all of which needed surgical evacuation (15).

At the time of the posterior fossa surgery, it is important to try and limit the amount of blood spilling into the ventricular system (especially up the aqueduct and into the third ventricle) and to irrigate profusely at the end of the procedure. It is also important to try and prevent a CSF leak or pseudomeningocele formation by trying to achieve as good a dural closure as possible and to replace the bone flap (16). A further important layer of coverage can be achieved by leaving a cuff of occipital musculature on the bone at the beginning of the procedure, thus allowing the occipital muscles to be reattached at the end without a gap at the top through which CSF may escape. A pressure bandage is used in the postoperative period by many surgeons

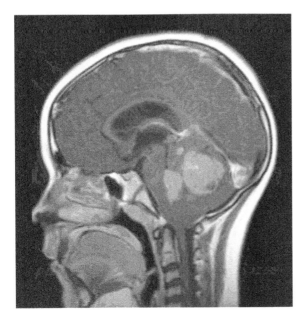

Figure 7 Posterior fossa medulloblastoma. Hydrocephalus treated by resection of tumor alone.

to try and prevent the development of a pseudomeningocele, with variable success. However, the development of a pseudomeningocele in itself is not necessarily a problem and usually this will settle over the next few weeks—although a large pseudomeningocele might cause problems with the fitting of the head mould for radiotherapy. Treatment of a pseudomeningocele depends upon whether there is persisting hydrocephalus or pressure problems and whether these are settling or progressing. Temporary measures include lumbar puncture, lumbar drain, or EVD. Permanent treatment options include ETV, VP shunting, or LP shunting—depending upon the ventricular size. Certainly, because of the risk of infection, if a CSF leak occurs, it should be dealt with urgently. Often this can mean merely placing further sutures; however, if the leak is persistent, then it may be necessary to drain the CSF either temporarily or permanently and the options available are the same as those for the treatment of a pseudomeningocele.

The chances of requiring permanent treatment for hydrocephalus after a tumor is removed from within the fourth ventricle are far higher than for tumors located within the cerebellar hemisphere—where the tumor merely distorts the fourth ventricle. It would therefore appear that operating on a tumor within the fourth ventricle is an independent risk factor that may result in failure of opening of the normal CSF pathways after tumor removal. The cause of this is almost certainly multifactorial and probably includes cellular debris (tumor and blood), resulting in an element of "communicating hydrocephalus" along with fourth ventricle out-flow obstruction as a result of postoperative inflammatory changes. It is therefore important in hemispheric tumors to try and avoid entering either the ventricle or the cisterna magna unless absolutely necessary. Overall, the risk of requiring a permanent CSF diversionary procedure is historically reported to be 40% for midline fourth ventricular tumors and almost 0% for hemispheric tumors (17). Other risk factors for persisting hydrocephalus reported in the literature include the presence of a CSF leak, pseudomeningocele formation, extent of resection, infection, the use of a dural substitute, and a child younger that two years of age (17,18). Of these, the first two risk factors likely reflect abnormal CSF dynamics rather than being causative—although obviously a CSF leak may result in a CSF infection. Though hydrocephalus has been proposed as a risk factor for cerebellar mutism, there is no evidence for it and it is more likely due to type and size of tumor (19,20).

In an attempt to further reduce the need for shunt insertion after posterior fossa tumor surgery, the Paris group proposed the concept of performing an ETV prior to the posterior fossa surgery (15). In a nonrandomized, retrospective study, they showed that 22 of 82 (27%) patients with posterior fossa tumors treated in a standard fashion (with steroids and a perioperative EVD) had postoperative symptomatic hydrocephalus requiring treatment and 16 (20%) needed a shunt. In contrast, only 4 of 67 (6%) patients with posterior fossa tumors in whom a preoperative ETV was undertaken required a permanent shunt. These authors also felt that these patients had a "smoother perioperative period." The main criticism to this proposal has been that it subjects all patients with fourth ventricular tumors and hydrocephalus to an ETV when at least 70% would have required no treatment anyway. Other authors have suggested that if the patient has continuing hydrocephalus, an ETV should be attempted in the postoperative period (21). It is clear that a number of unanswered questions therefore remain on this subject. If it can be shown that preoperative treatment of the hydrocephalus by an ETV does result in a "smoother postoperative course" and less CSF-related morbidity, then it might well be worth while considering this procedure on all patients with a posterior fossa tumor. Some technical questions also remain—if the patient has a pretumor resection ETV, then does it make a difference whether the posterior fossa surgery is undertaken in the sitting or prone position? When does the ETV need to be undertaken in relation to the posterior fossa surgery in order to achieve this benefit?

Brainstem tumors consist of diffuse pontine, focal, exophytic, and cervicomedullary tumors. Hydrocephalus is often a fairly late manifestation but as the cause of the hydrocephalus is normally obstruction, consideration should be given to undertaking an ETV. From a technical perspective, there is usually sufficient room to perform an ETV—even in cases of diffuse pontine gliomas where there may appear to be very little room between the pons and the clivus. However, in these cases with possible distortion of the anatomy, it is important on the preoperative imaging to identify the position of the basilar artery. This is feasible with good-quality MR scans.

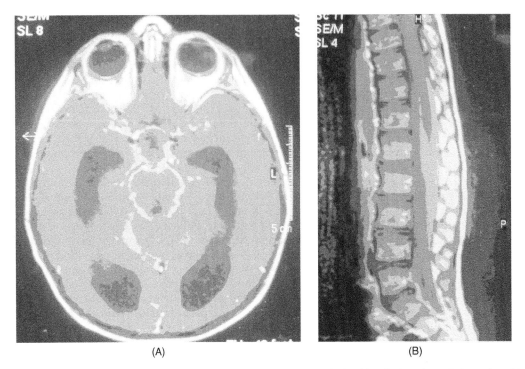

(A)   (B)

Figure 8 Spinal leptomeningeal grade II astrocytoma with hydrocephalus. Ventriculoperitoneal shunt placed to treat hydrocephalus.

Spinal Cord Tumors
Occasionally, the initial presentation of a spinal cord tumor may be with hydrocephalus (Fig. 8). In malignant tumors, the mechanism appears straightforward in which microscopic leptomeningeal seeding can obstruct CSF reabsorption at the level of the basal cisterns or the arachnoid villi. In these cases, the optimal treatment is to insert a shunt (22,23). In benign tumors, the mechanism is thought to be related to altered CSF compartment compliance or increased protein content. Thus, the best treatment is tumor removal thereby restoring the normal compliance and normal CSF protein content (22). A further manifestation of abnormal CSF dynamics seen in some of these patients is the development of a syrinx, which is discussed in another section of this book.

MANAGEMENT OF ADULT TUMOR-RELATED HYDROCEPHALUS
As mentioned earlier, hydrocephalus plays a far smaller role in the management of adult patients with brain tumors than that in children. In general, the considerations given under the pediatric section of this chapter are also applicable to adult patients with tumor-related hydrocephalus. Metastatic tumors are the most common tumors seen in adults and the decision to treat the hydrocephalus (and/or the tumor) needs to be taken after discussion with the patient, the family, and the palliative care team. The hydrocephalus associated with carcinomatosis is due to diffuse leptomeningeal spread, which causes problems with absorption, and if treatment is indicated, the only option is shunting.

Two other groups of patients seen in adult practice but far less commonly seen in pediatric practice are patients with hydrocephalus secondary to vestibular schwannomas [and other cerebellopontine (CP) angle tumors] (Fig. 9) and patients with pituitary tumors. The treatment in these groups is the same as with tumors in similar sites in children. In the case of CP angle tumors in adults, specific care must be taken during tumor surgery to prevent CSF leaks (otorrhea and rhinorrhea). This includes obliteration of communications with mastoid air cells, dural closure, and in some cases prophylactic lumbar drainage postoperatively (24).

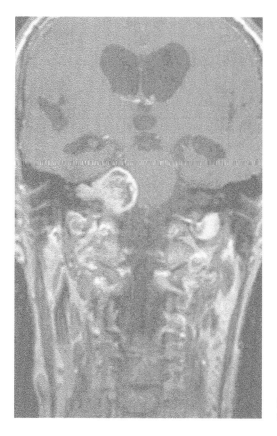

Figure 9 Vestibular schwannoma with hydrocephalus.

REFERENCES

1. Pople IK, Bayston R, Hayward RD. Infection of cerebrospinal fluid shunts in infants: A study of etiological factors. J Neurosurg 1992; 77:29–36.
2. Tuli S, Drake JM. Multiple shunt failures: An analysis of relevant features. Childs Nerv Syst 1999; 15:79.
3. Taylor AL, Carroll TA, Jakubowski J, et al. Percutaneous endoscopic gastrostomy in patients with ventriculoperitoneal shunts. Br J Surg 2001; 88:724–727.
4. Berger MS, Baumeister B, Geyer JR, et al. The risks of metastases from shunting in children with primary central nervous system tumors. J Neurosurg 1991; 74:872–877.
5. Rickert CH. Abdominal metastases of pediatric brain tumors via ventriculo-peritoneal shunts. Childs Nerv Syst 1998; 14:10–14.
6. Kestle J, Cochrane D, Alisharan R. The initial treatment of hydrocephalus: An assessment of surgeons' preference between third ventriculostomy and shunt insertion. Neurol Res 2000; 22:65–68.
7. Thompson D, Phipps K, Hayward R. Craniopharyngioma in childhood: Our evidence-based approach to management. Childs Nerv Syst 2005; 21:660–668.
8. Gil Z, Beni-Adani L, Siomin V, et al. Ascites following ventriculoperitoneal shunting in children with chiasmatic-hypothalamic glioma. Childs Nerv Syst 2001; 17:395–398.
9. Sainte-Rose C, Crimmins D, Grill J. Thalamic gliomas. In: Tonn JC, Westphal M, Rutka J, et al., eds. Neuro-oncology of CNS Tumours, Vol 1, 1st ed. Berlin, Germany: Springer, 2006:363–376.
10. Macarthur DC, Buxton N, Punt J, et al. The role of neuroendoscopy in the management of brain tumours. Br J Neurosurg 2002; 16:465–470.
11. Yamini B, Refai D, Rubin CM, et al. Initial endoscopic management of pineal region tumors and associated hydrocephalus: Clinical series and literature review. J Neurosurg 2004; 100:437–441.
12. Pople IK, Athanasiou TC, Sandeman DR, et al. The role of endoscopic biopsy and third ventriculostomy in the management of pineal region tumours. Br J Neurosurg 2001; 15:305–311.
13. Wellons JC III, Tubbs RS, Banks JT, et al. Long-term control of hydrocephalus via endoscopic third ventriculostomy in children with tectal plate gliomas. Neurosurgery 2002; 51:63–67; discussion 67–68.
14. Drake J, Chumas P, Kestle J, et al. Late rapid deterioration after endoscopic third ventriculostomy: Additional cases and review of the literature. J Neurosurg 2006; 105:118–126.

15. Sainte-Rose C, Cinalli G, Roux FE, et al. Management of hydrocephalus in pediatric patients with posterior fossa tumors: The role of endoscopic third ventriculostomy. J Neurosurg 2001; 95:791–797.

16. Gnanalingham KK, Lafuente J, Thompson D, et al. Surgical procedures for posterior fossa tumors in children: Does craniotomy lead to fewer complications than craniectomy? J Neurosurg 2002; 97:821–826.

17. Culley DJ, Berger MS, Shaw D, et al. An analysis of factors determining the need for ventriculoperitoneal shunts after posterior fossa tumor surgery in children. Neurosurgery 1994; 34:402–407; discussion 407–408.

18. Kumar V, Phipps K, Harkness W, et al. Ventriculo-peritoneal shunt requirement in children with posterior fossa tumours: An 11-year audit. Br J Neurosurg 1996; 10:467–470.

19. Catsman-Berrevoets CE, Van Dongen HR, Mulder PG, et al. Tumour type and size are high risk factors for the syndrome of "cerebellar" mutism and subsequent dysarthria. J Neurol Neurosurg Psychiatry 1999; 67:755–757.

20. Ozgur BM, Berberian J, Aryan HE, et al. The pathophysiologic mechanism of cerebellar mutism. Surg Neurol 2006; 66:18–25.

21. Morelli D, Pirotte B, Lubansu A, et al. Persistent hydrocephalus after early surgical management of posterior fossa tumors in children: Is routine preoperative endoscopic third ventriculostomy justified? J Neurosurg 2005; 103:247–252.

22. Morandi X, Amlashi SF, Riffaud L. A dynamic theory for hydrocephalus revealing benign intraspinal tumours: Tumoural obstruction of the spinal subarachnoid space reduces total CSF compartment compliance. Med Hypotheses 2006; 67:79–81.

23. Rifkinson-Mann S, Wisoff JH, Epstein F. The association of hydrocephalus with intramedullary spinal cord tumors: A series of 25 patients. Neurosurgery 1990; 27:749–754; discussion.

24. Pirouzmand F, Tator CH, Rutka J. Management of hydrocephalus associated with vestibular schwannoma and other cerebellopontine angle tumors. Neurosurgery 2001; 48:1246–1253; discussion 1253–1244.

ETV in the Management of Hydrocephalus Secondary to Pediatric Posterior Fossa Tumors

Christian Sainte-Rose

Pediatric Neurosurgery, Université René Descartes Paris V, Hôpital Necker Enfants Malades, Paris, France

In 1990s, the diffusion of endoscopic third ventriculostomy (ETV) in the management of obstructive hydrocephalus offered a new tool in treatment of hydrocephalus secondary to posterior fossa tumors. Prerequisite of successful ETV is the presence of blockage of the cerebrospinal fluid (CSF) pathway at the level of fourth ventricle outlets or at the aqueduct.

Since its first introduction in the management of hydrocephalus secondary to posterior fossa tumors in 1995 (1), and the confirmation of its efficacy in early 2000s (2), ETV has been utilized increasingly. Theoretically, ETV offers the same advantages of implantation of ventriculoperitoneal shunting, such as rapid normalization of raised ICP, improvement of the patient's general condition, prevention of postoperative ICP elevation, and long-term control of hydrocephalus, without the shunt-related complications. However, subsequent studies did not confirm the initial enthusiasm (2), questioning, above all, the possibility of ETV to provide long-term control of hydrocephalus (3–5). Moreover, considering that ETV is not without risk and that in most patients hydrocephalus can be resolved with surgical removal of posterior fossa tumor alone (6), the role of preoperative ETV remains controversial (3,4).

In 2001, we reviewed 67 ETVs performed before tumor removal in patients with hydrocephalus (9% mild, 31% moderate, 60% severe hydrocephalus). In our series, there were no deaths and no permanent morbidity related to the procedure, a 98.5% rate of immediate symptomatic resolution, and a 94% rate of shunt-free patients after tumor removal (2). Comparing these results with patients with hydrocephalus (26% mild, 38% moderate, 26% severe hydrocephalus) who underwent "conventional treatment" (steroid medication, early surgery, and ventricular drainage) in which the rate of postoperative hydrocephalus was 26.8%, and with patients with no evidence of ventricular enlargement (4.2% of postoperative hydrocephalus), we concluded that ETV had a curative effect on intracranial hypertension and a prophylactic effect by preventing the development of hydrocephalus after tumor removal. Preoperative normalization of CSF hydrodynamics seems to decrease the risk of permanent postoperative impairment of CSF circulation. Hopf et al. (7) and Valenzuela and Trellez (8) have also reported similar good results.

In the series of Ruggiero et al., preoperative treatment of severe hydrocephalus by ETV performed in a group of patients at higher risk of developing postoperative hydrocephalus did not prevent postoperative hydrocephalus in all cases, but reduced the risk of postoperative hydrocephalus in those patients at lower risk (10–15%) (5).

In recent studies (3,4), the low incidence of persistent hydrocephalus following early tumor removal led the authors to believe that the routine use of preoperative ETVs is not justified.

However, the rationale for preoperative ETV does not end with the prevention of delayed postoperative hydrocephalus. It can be used as a real alternative to external ventricular drainage as an emergency procedure on admission, offering immediate resolution of the symptoms of intracranial hypertension and giving time to schedule the tumor surgery. In some situations it is even preferable, offering more physiological CSF drainage, eliminating the risks of CSF infection related to external drainage, and reducing the risks of overdrainage and its possible dangerous consequences for the tumor. Moreover, it protects against acute postoperative hydrocephalus caused by cerebellar swelling as efficiently as external drainage.

Patients with severe symptoms at presentation are also particularly at risk of a worse postoperative course (4). Complications of posterior fossa surgery (above all pseudomeningocele, CSF leak, and acute cerebellar swelling) were significantly lower in the group of patients treated with preoperative ETV than in the control group both in our series than in that of Ruggiero et al. (2,5). In particular, we observed fewer immediate postoperative complications in the group of patients treated with preoperative ETV than the control group treated "conventionally": 25% and 38%, respectively, and a smoother postoperative course and a faster recovery, particularly in tumors adhering to brain stem.

Furthermore, in patients in whom the tumor has spread in the CSF at presentation, an ETV allows chemotherapy to be undertaken prior to tumor excision by controlling hydrocephalus (2). ETV represents the treatment of choice for treating hydrocephalus associated with inaccessible tumors (9).

In conclusion, preoperative ETV should be suggested only in patients with severe hydrocephalus, who otherwise require alternative treatment such as external ventricular drainage, and who are at higher risk to develop post-operative hydrocephalus.

More agreement in the neurosurgical community is present in considering postoperative hydrocephalus obstructive in nature as well as to offer ETV as an alternative to shunt insertion to such patients (2–4).

We performed ETV to manage postoperative hydrocephalus in eight patients with a success rate of 100% (2). Subsequently, Fritsch et al. (3) reported 2 patients, Morelli et al. (4) 6 patients, and Tamburrini et al. (10) 27 patients (of a total of 30) of postoperative hydrocephalus successfully treated by ETV. According to these results, the choice of an ETV to manage hydrocephalus following posterior fossa surgery appears to be justified.

REFERENCES

1. Chumas P, Sainte-Rose C, Cinalli G, et al. III Ventriculostomy in the management of posterior fossa tumors in children. Proceedings of the ISPN congress, Santiago, Chile, 26–29 September 1995. Childs Nerv Syst 1995; 11:540.
2. Sainte-Rose C, Cinalli G, Roux FE, et al. Management of hydrocephalus in pediatric patients with posterior fossa tumors: The role of endoscopic third ventriculostomy. J Neurosurg 2001; 95:791–797.
3. Fritsch MJ, Doerner L, Kienke S, et al. Hydrocephalus in children with posterior fossa tumors: Role of endoscopic third ventriculostomy. J Neurosurg 2005; 103(1 suppl):40–42.
4. Morelli D, Pirotte B, Lubansu A, et al. Persistent hydrocephalus after early surgical management of posterior fossa tumors in children: Is routine preoperative endoscopic third ventriculostomy justified? J Neurosurg 2005; 103(3 suppl):247–252.
5. Ruggiero C, Cinalli G, Spennato P, et al. Endoscopic third ventriculostomy in the treatment of hydrocephalus in posterior fossa tumors in children. Childs Nerv Syst 2004; 20:828–833.
6. Due-Tonnessen BJ, Helseth E. Management of hydrocephalus in children with posterior fossa tumors: Role of tumor surgery. Pediatr Neurosurg 2007; 43:92–96.
7. Hopf NJ, Grunert P, Fries G, et al. Endoscopic third ventriculostomy: An outcome analysis of 100 consecutive procedures. Neurosurgery 1999; 44:795–806.
8. Valenzuela S, Trellez A. Pediatric neuroendoscopy in Chile. Analysis of the first 100 cases. Childs Nerv Syst 1999; 15:457–460.
9. Ray P, Jallo GI, Kim RYH, et al. Endoscopic third ventriculostomy for tumor-related hydrocephalus in a pediatric population. Neurosurg Focus 2005; 19(6):E8.
10. Tamburrini G, Pettorini BL, Massimi L, et al. Endoscopic third ventriculostomy: the best option in the treatment of persistent hydrocephalus after posterior cranial fossa tumour removal? Childs Nerv Syst 2008; 24:1405–1412.

23 | Longstanding Overt Ventriculomegaly in Adult (LOVA)

Shizuo Oi

Division of Pediatric Neurosurgery, Jikei University Hospital Women's & Children's Medical Center, Tokyo, Japan

Satoshi Takahashi

Division of Pediatric Neurosurgery, Jikei University Hospital Women's & Children's Medical Center and Department of Neurosurgery, Keio University School of Medicine, Tokyo, Japan

INTRODUCTION

Longstanding overt ventriculomegaly in adult (LOVA) is a specific form of noncommunicating hydrocephalus that often causes hydrocephalic dementia. It is a unique category of hydrocephalus firstly presented by the senior author in the middle of 1990s (1–4). Before this new category developed, patients with LOVA might have been considered as a part of normal pressure hydrocephalus (NPH) and were treated by shunts, but treatment of patients with LOVA is extremely difficult in terms of their sensitive compliance of brain parenchyma. LOVA patients definitely develop bilateral subdural hematoma when treated by differential pressure valve (DPV) shunts (1), and that is one of the reasons why LOVA should be categorized and every neurosurgeon has to understand what LOVA is.

This chapter describes the clinical features of this unique clinical entity of LOVA with its history, diagnostic criteria, CSF dynamics, treatment modalities, and outcomes with typical illustrative cases with LOVA that we have treated recently.

HISTORY AND TERMINOLOGY OF ADULT HYDROCEPHALUS

Hydrocephalus is a clinicopathological condition of disturbed cerebrospinal fluid (CSF) circulation. A variety of underlying etiology result in hydrocephalus and its classification and terminology are still controversial (summarized in Table 1).

Terminology of "normal pressure hydrocephalus"

The term "normal pressure hydrocephalus (NPH)" (4) was firstly proposed by Hakim and Adams in 1964 and 1965 (5,6). He defined this type of hydrocephalus as a syndrome with specific clinical features as treatable dementia. But he named the clinical entity as NPH from its pathophysiological aspects. This discrepancy of clinical and pathophysiological aspects cause the confusion in the classification of hydrocephalus in the adult at the present time, over 40 years after his initial proposal. As a variety of ICP dynamics has become recognized in NPH patients in accordance with advances in continuous ICP monitoring and the technique of dynamic analyses, a new term, "hydrocephalic dementia" was proposed by Oi in 1998 in order to avoid misleading its pathophysiological aspect (7).

Communicating/Noncommunicating Hydrocephalus and Obstructive/Nonobstructive hydrocephalus

Communicating/noncommunicating hydrocephalus and obstructive/nonobstructive hydrocephalus (8) are another complicated terminology that is easily confused. In the definition of Dandy's communicating/noncommunicating hydrocephalus, the communication of the CSF pathway is between the lateral ventricle and the lumbar subarachnoid space (confirmed by injection of dye into the lateral ventricle and detection by lumbar puncture) (9). On the other hand, the obstruction in the definition is at any region in the major CSF pathway including the ventricular system and entire cistern/subarachnoid space, so that the cause or condition

Table 1 Classification of Hydrocephalus

Objects involved	Category	Subtypes
Patient	Onset	Congenital–acquired
		Fetal–neonatal–infantile–child–adult–geriatric
		Acute–subacute–chronic
	Causes	Primary–secondary, idiopathic
	Underlying lesions	Dysgenetic, posthemorrhagic, post-SAH, post-IVH, post-meningitic, post-traumatic, with brain tumor, with spinal cord tumor, with brain abscess, with arachnoid cyst, with cysticercosis, etc.
	Symptomatology	Macrocephalic–normocephalic–microcephalic
		Occult–symptomatic–overt
		Coma–stupor–dementia
		Hydrocephalus, parkinsonism complex, etc.
Hydrocephalus	Pathophysiology: (1) CSF circulation	Communicating–noncommunicating
		Nonobstructive–obstructive
		External–internal–interstitial
		Isolated compartments: UH, IFV, IRV, ICCD, DCH, DLFV, etc.
	(2) ICP dynamics	High–normal
	Chronology	Slowly progressive–progressive–longstanding–arrested
Treatment	Postshunt	Shunt-dependent–shunt-independent
		Slit-like ventricle–slit ventricle syndrome, etc.

Source: From Ref. 7.

for nonobstructive hydrocephalus is limited to either CSF overproduction by choroid plexus papilloma or CSF malabsorption due to sinus thrombosis (10).

Hydrocephalus Chronology in Adult

It has become clear that the pathophysiology of hydrocephalus does not remain constant but changes with time. Oi proposed the concept of hydrocephalus chronology in adult (HCA) in 1998 (7). In adult patients with secondary hydrocephalus in acute brain diseases, intracranial pressure (ICP) changes dramatically in combination with brain compliance. Oi classified this chronology into five periods (stage I to stage V) (Fig. 1). In this chronology, true NPH may be identified in late stage III and stage IV.

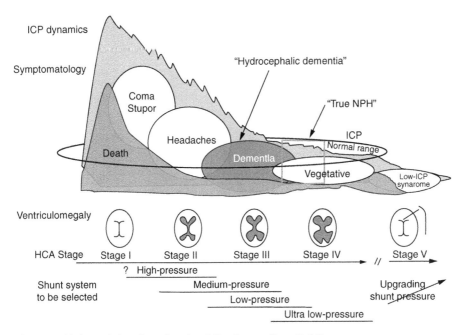

Figure 1 Hydrocephalus chronology in adults. *Source*: From Ref. 7.

History of "Longstanding Overt Ventriculomegaly in Adult (LOVA)"

Hydrocephalus is usually treatable with shunt placement (1–3). The selection of shunt system, mainly in respect of the differential pressures, should be based on the specific ICP dynamics or HCA stage. Recently, adjustable pressure shunt systems are also widely accepted (11–13). In addition to shunt placement, neuroendoscopic procedures including endoscopic third ventriculostomy (ETV) are also an alternative treatment (14,15).

Oi et al. reported a unique category of hydrocephalic state in adult that is extremely difficult to treat with a shunt because of lost compliance of brain parenchyma. Patients with this clinical entity develop bilateral subdural hematoma when treated with shunts (3).

This unique category of hydrocephalus in adults was named "longstanding overt ventriculomegaly in adult (LOVA)." The terminology of LOVA was first proposed by Oi et al. in 1996. Oi et al. reported two patients with spina bifida with marked ventriculomegaly. Both patients were treated with immediate repair of myeloschisis, but no shunt was placed until adolescence. After the CSF shunt procedure, both these patients had problems with shunt dependence and required fine shunt flow regulation.

In 1999, Oi et al. reported application of neuroendoscopic procedure (ETV) to treat patients with LOVA. In this report, neuroendoscopic procedures including ETV were recommended for this clinical entity because management with shunt procedures is definitely associated with postoperative low-ICP syndrome requiring very fine control of the CSF flow. It was hypothesized that hydrocephalic state has progressed very slowly from infancy to adulthood and its symptoms remain subclinical until becoming apparent incidentally. Not only hydrocephalus associated with myeloschisis but also aqueduct stenosis may be underlying etiology for this clinical entity.

In 2000, Oi et al. reported 20 patients with LOVA and reviewed its clinical features and analyzed its specific pathophysiological characteristics (1).

Before the introduction of this new concept of clinical entity, hydrocephalus that should have been considered LOVA has been reported as a part of NPH or noncommunicating hydrocephalus or late onset idiopathic aqueductal stenosis. After introduction of LOVA, some repots on patients with LOVA in terms of its therapeutic modalities and clinical features have been reported (16–19).

Using terminology described above correctly, LOVA is a specific form of noncommunicating hydrocephalus that often causes hydrocephalic dementia.

DIAGNOSTIC CRITERIA AND DIFFERENTIAL DIAGNOSIS IN ADULT HYDROCEPHALUS

Concept and Diagnostic Criteria

The LOVA is a chronological concept of hydrocephalus (Table 2) (1). In the chronology of HCA, it may be identified in late stage II and stage III. It may be summarized as a complex entity with the following compatible subtypes: (*i*) onset may be congenital in origin but becomes manifest during adulthood; (*ii*) the underlying lesion is aqueductal stenosis; (*iii*) symptoms include macrocephaly, increased ICP symptoms, dementia, subnormal IQ, and others; (*iv*)

Table 2   Concept, diagnostic criteria, and treatment of LOVA[a]

Category	Definition
Concept	Chronological entity of progressive hydrocephaly with longstanding ventriculomegaly in adult, most likely starting from infancy
Diagnostic criteria	(1) Overt ventriculomegaly involving the lateral and third ventricles with obliterated cortical sulci on CT/MR imagine
	(2) Clinical symptomes include macrocephaly with or without subnormal IQ, headaches, dementia, gait disturbance, urinary incontinence, vegetative state, akinetic mutism, apathetic consciousness, and parkinsonism
	(3) Neuroimages may demonstrate expanded or destroyed sella turcica as evidence of longstanding ventriculomegaly
Therapeutic specificity	Treatable with shunt, but extremely delicate pressure control such as that provided by a PPV is required; neuroendo-scopic third ventriculostomy is mostly effective

[a] Definitive LOVA applies to patients having the diagnostic criteria of 1 and also 2 and/or 3.
Source: From Ref. 7.

pathophysiological characteristics include noncommunicating CSF circulation and an ICP dynamics that mainly consist of high ICP; (v) the chronology is long term and progressive; (vi) the hydrocephalus becomes arrested after shunt placement or ventriculostomy. What is important is that its progressive clinical symptoms of hydrocephalus are not diagnosed until adulthood, but subclinical hydrocephalus has been present probably from infancy. Significantly expanded or destroyed sella turcica indicates the presence of hydrocephalus from infancy (Fig. 1). And in the two patients described below there was history of macrocephaly in childhood.

Diagnostic criteria proposed by Oi et al. in 2000 are consisted of three characteristics.

1. Overt ventriculomegaly involving the lateral and third ventricles with obliterated cortical sulci on CT/MR imaging.
2. Clinical symptoms include macrocephaly with or without subnormal IQ, headaches, dementia, gait disturbance, urinary incontinence, vegetative state, akinetic mutism, apathetic consciousness, and parkinsonism.
3. Neuroimaging may demonstrate expanded or destroyed sella turcica as evidence of long-standing ventriculomegaly.

Patients meeting the diagnosis of 1 and also 2 and/or 3 are diagnosed as definitive LOVA.

Neuroimaging Studies

Patients with LOVA present severe ventriculomegaly involving the lateral and third ventricles with decreased thickness of cortical mantle and obliterated sulci (1). Dilatation of lateral ventricles is symmetrical with marked enlargement of third ventricle. Skull X-ray films reveal an enlarged or completely destroyed sella turcica with or without digital markings. Sagittal T2-weighted MR images are extremely useful when making diagnoses of LOVA because it shows three signs that characterize the situation, that are vertically expanded third ventricle, empty (phantom) sella (Fig. 2), and aqueduct stenosis (Figs. 3 and 4).

Cardiac-gated cine-MR imaging can be used for proving aqueduct stenosis that is one of the main features of this clinical entity. It usually reveals no significant CSF movements within the aqueduct.

Preoperative 3D CT ventriculography is also applied for showing dilatation of lateral and third ventricles and aqueduct stenosis.

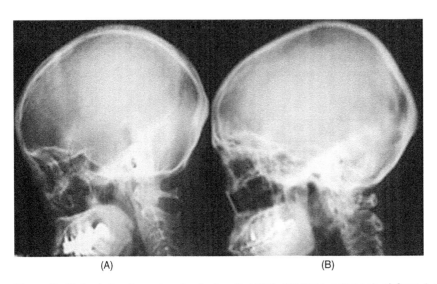

(A)   (B)

Figure 2 Plain skull radiographs of patients with LOVA. (**A**) Plain radiograph of Case 1 showed remarkably destroyed sella turcica. (**B**) Plain radiograph of Case 2 saucer like sella.

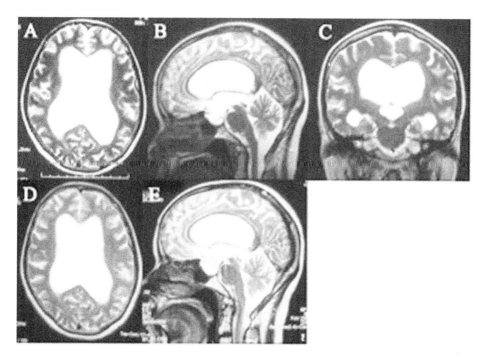

Figure 3 MR images of Case 1. (*Upper row*) Preoperative T2-weighted MR images showing aqueduct stenosis. (*Lower row*) Postoperative T2-weighted MR images showing good CSF flow through the third ventriculostomy stoma.

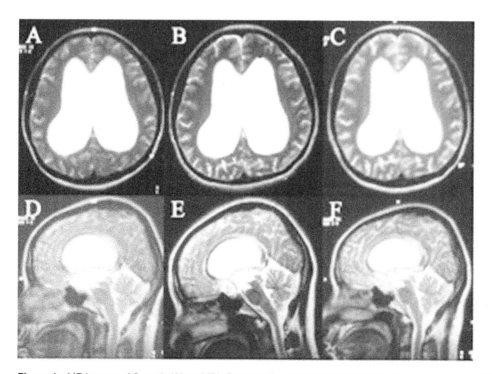

Figure 4 MR images of Case 2. (**A**) and (**D**): Preoperative, T2-weighted MR images showing aqueduct stenosis. (**B**) and (**E**): Three days postoperative, T2-weighted MR images showing satisfactory CSF flow through the ETV stoma. (**C**) and (**F**): One-year postoperative, T2-weighted MR images showing persistent flow through the ETV stoma.

Differential Diagnosis

Differential diagnosis should be made between NPH and late-onset idiopathic aqueductal stenosis (LIAS) (20,21) or aqueductal stenosis (22). To make the diagnosis of LOVA, aqueductal stenosis should be present in sagittal section of T2-weighted MR image. Then secondary aqueductal stenosis caused by brain tumors or arachnoiditis should be ruled out using MR image with intravenous infusion of gadolinium. To differentiate LOVA from LIAS is the most difficult. Aqueduct stenosis in patients with LOVA is from infancy, and that in patients with LIAS is acquired. And LOVA should be distinguished from LIAS, because the ability to absorb CSF is different. To differentiate LOVA from LIAS, radiological findings of enlarged or completely destroyed sella turcica at X-ray or history of macrocephaly in adulthood are of use.

CSF DYNAMICS AND SPECIFIC PATHOPHYSIOLOGY

If the progressive course of a once-arrested hydrocephalus occurs in cases of LOVA, it may be caused by the development of a blockage in the once-reestablished CSF pathway, an impaired alternative pathway, or an increase in CSF production (1).

Clinical features of aqueductal stenosis in adults include a wide variety of symptoms. It has been suggested that longstanding ventriculomegaly may involve skull-base structures, resulting in visual, hormonal, and auditory symptoms. These symptoms and signs may occur as the initial symptoms of LOVA in adulthood. Therefore, the mechanism by which arrested hydrocephalus can be reversed may be based on longstanding slowly progressive high-ICP dynamics reaching a threshold.

Patients with LOVA, when treated with shunts show the therapeutic problems of regulating CSF flow. Because of longstanding severe ventriculomegaly, the involved brain parenchyma has lost its compliance. Also, the craniocerebral disproportion of structures due to macrocephaly presents difficulties. Postoperative subdural hematoma is highly likely when treated with DPV shunt systems. As indicated in the study by Oi et al. in 2000, LOVA usually appears as a high- or very high pressure hydrocephalus when it becomes symptomatic. The shunt system initially chosen should be equipped with a high resistance valve.

In patients with LOVA, absorption of CSF seems to be intact, as ETV is effective as mentioned later.

TREATMENT MODALITIES

Nowadays, neuroendoscopic surgery such as ETV is well-established treatment of choice, but adjustable pressure VP shunt placement is another surgical treatment of choice (1).

Initially, before the treatment modalities for LOVA had been established, medium- or low- pressure DPV were used, but all patients experienced subdural hematoma and underwent reoperation.

Some patients underwent VP shunt using pressure-programmable valve (PPV). In patients in whom PPVs were placed, CSF flow was initially controlled by using the high-pressure range of the shunt pressure setting. After a while, all patients developed the condition of shunt-dependent arrested hydrocephalus.

Neuroendoscopic procedure in the form of ETV has proved to be the best treatment of choice. ETVs are performed according to the protocol described elsewhere. The surgeon's experience in neuroendoscopy is important in achieving good results. Intraoperatively, after ventriculostomy, water-soluble contrast-enhanced material is injected to lateral ventricle, and washed out of the material is observed by CT scanning obtained about 24 hours after surgery (Fig. 5). Most patients improve without need of a subsequent procedure within a few days.

Kiefer et al. reported that newly developed gravitational shunts are equivalent therapeutic options (17–19). For patients with LOVA, it seems much better to undergo ETV, as they can be shunt free. Kiefer et al. mentioned high complication rates associated with ETV, but we believe ETV is very safe surgical strategy, if it is performed by skilled surgeons.

Patients with LOVA are prone to overdrainage, and cautious CSF drainage is required.

OUTCOMES AND LONG-TERM PROGNOSIS

Patients with LOVA treated with ETV improve clinically by various degrees (1). Gait disturbance usually disappears. Urinary incontinence and dementia also disappear in most cases. Patients

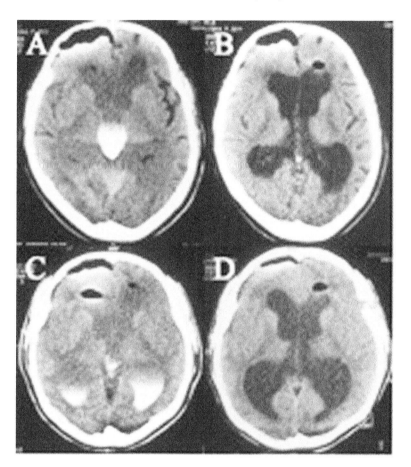

Figure 5　Intraoperative CSF dynamic study. (**A**) and (**B**): CT scanning of Case 1. (**C**) and (**D**): CT scanning of case 2. (**A**) and (**C**) were obtained just after operation showing contrast in the ventricles, and (**B**) and (**D**) were obtained one day postoperative showing clearance of the contrast from the ventricles.

who could not manage their daily life become able to live on their own. The patients treated with ETV usually do not require any further treatment unless the stoma at the floor of third ventricle closes, which seldom occurs (23,24). Clinical improvement of patients with LOVA treated by ETV is fairly good.

Compared to the dramatical clinical improvement seen, ventriculomegaly usually remains radiologically after ETV (Figs. 3 and 4). In patients with LOVA, compliance of brain parenchyma decreases, and only slight ICP decrease that does not reflect in ventricular size is enough for clinical improvement.

To predict the effectiveness the surgical procedure of ETV, intraoperative infusion of water-soluble contrast-enhanced material to ventricular system is extremely useful. As shown in Figure 5, if ETV is performed successfully, the enhanced material washes out within 24 hours.

As for long-term follow-up of the patients, in order to evaluate the effectiveness of ETV, flow void observed in sagittal section of T2-weighted image at the floor of third ventricle is extremely useful to estimate the patency of the pathway (Figs. 3 and 4).

ILLUSTRATIVE CASES

Case 1

This 61-year-old female had been well until six years ago, when the patient had sudden onset of loss of consciousness. The patient was brought to nearby neurosurgical clinic, where diagnosis of hydrocephalus and epilepsy was made. The patient has been noted to have difficulty in walking for one year. Right dragging gait had been deteriorating progressively with small step gait and some short-term memory disturbance in the last few months. Neurological examination revealed mild dementia as well as gait disturbance. The patient had fine tremor on the upper extremities and rigidity with cogwheel phenomenon in the right upper extremity. MRI showed marked ventriculomegaly with aqueduct stenosis [Fig. 3(A) to 3(C)]. Diagnosis of LOVA was made, and the patient underwent ETV under general anesthesia. Intraoperatively, water-soluble contrast material was injected to the lateral ventricle, and wash out of the material was confirmed on CT scanning obtained one day postoperative [Fig. 5(A) and 5(B)]. During the postoperative stay in the hospital, the gait disturbance improved, and the patient became able to walk without difficulty. Only fine tremor on the left upper extremity remained, but it disappeared within one month after discharge. After 18 months of initial surgery, the patient remains in good condition with no complaints. MRI obtained 18 months after surgery shows still ventriculomegaly, as well as flow void at the floor of third ventricle, which indicates patency of the CSF pathway [Fig. 3(D) and 3(E)].

Case 2
A 47-year-old female with progressive gait disturbance and urinary incontinence was referred to our outpatient clinic for evaluation and treatment. The patient's information regarding the perinatal period was unclear, but some difficulty in delivery was reported. On birth, the patient was normocephalic, but the patient's head has been macrocephalic as indicated by size "L" or "LL" for caps. For three years before presentation, the patient has been noted to have progressive balance disturbance and episodic urinary incontinence. The patient also stated deteriorating vision in the last year. Neurological examination revealed gait disturbance with impaired tandem gait. The patient showed no memory disturbance. MRI revealed ventriculomegaly as well as aqueduct stenosis [Fig. 4(A) and 4(D)]. The patient underwent ETV. Intraoperatively, water-soluble contrast material was injected to her lateral ventricle, and wash out of the material was confirmed on CT scanning obtained one day postoperative [Fig. 5(C) and 5(D)]. One month after surgery, the patient became free from symptoms of gait disturbance and urinary incontinence. And six months after ETV, the patient remained free from symptoms.

CONCLUSION
Longstanding overt ventriculomegaly in adults (LOVA) is a unique pathophysiological and chronological change in the brain and skull. Underlying etiology for the clinical entity is probably aqueduct stenosis from infancy. It remains enigmatic why the hydrocephalic state becomes active and progressive in adulthood. Management of hydrocephalus in patients with LOVA is difficult because of lost compliance of the brain. Neuroendoscopic surgery in the form of ETV is a promising procedure to avoid the problems of shunt dependency or overdrainage.

REFERENCES
1. Oi S, Shimoda M, Shibata M, et al. Pathophysiology of long-standing overt ventriculomegaly in adults. J Neurosurg 2000; 92(6):933–940.
2. Oi S, Hidaka M, Honda Y, et al. Neuroendoscopic surgery for specific forms of hydrocephalus. Childs Nerv Syst 1999; 15(1):56–68.
3. Oi S, Sato O, Matsumoto S. Neurological and medico-social problems of spina bifida patients in adolescence and adulthood. Childs Nerv Syst 1996; 12(4):181–187.
4. Oi S. Classification and definition of hydrocephalus: origin, controversy, and assignment of the terminology. In: Cinalli G, Maixner WJ, Sainte-Rose C, ed. Pediatric Hydrocephalus. Milano, Italy: Springer, 2004:95–112.
5. Hakim S. Some Observation on CSF Pressure. Hydrocephalic Syndrome in Adult with "Normal" CSF Pressure: Recognition of a New Syndrome [Spanish]. Thesis No. 957. Bogota, Colombia: Javeriana University School of Medicine, 1964.
6. Adams RD, Fisher CM, Hakim S, et al. Symptomatic occult hydrocephalus with "normal" cerebrospinal-fluid pressure. A treatable syndrome. N Engl J Med 1965; 273:117–126.
7. Oi S. Hydrocephalus chronology in adults: Confused state of the terminology. Crit Rev Neurosurg 1998; 8(6):346–356.
8. Oi S, Di Rocco C. Proposal of "evolution theory in cerebrospinal fluid dynamics" and minor pathway hydrocephalus in developing immature brain. Childs Nerv Syst 2006; 22(7):662–669.

9. Dandy WE. Extirpation of the choroids plexus of the lateral ventricles in communicating hydrocephalus. Ann Surg 1918; 68:569–579.

10. Russell DS. Observation on the Pathology of Hydrocephalus Medical Research Council Special Report Series No. 265. London: His Majesty's Stationary Office, 1949:112–113.

11. Zemack G, Romner B. Seven years of clinical experience with the programmable Codman Hakim valve: a retrospective study of 583 patients. J Neurosurg 2000; 92(6):941–948.

12. Pollack IF, Albright AL, Adelson PD. A randomized, controlled study of a programmable shunt valve versus a conventional valve for patients with hydrocephalus. Hakim-Medos Investigator Group. Neurosurgery 1999; 45(6):1399–1408.

13. Katano H, Karasawa K, Sugiyama N, et al. Clinical evaluation of shunt implantations using Sophy programmable pressure valves: Comparison with Codman-Hakim programmable valves. J Clin Neurosci 2003; 10(5):557–561.

14. Vries JK. An endoscopic technique for third ventriculostomy. Surg Neurol 1978; 9(3):165–168.

15. Di Rocco C, Massimi L, Tamburrini G. Shunts vs endoscopic third ventriculostomy in infants: Are there different types and/or rates of complications? A review. Childs Nerv Syst 2006; 22(12):1573–1589.

16. Canu ED, Magnano I, Paulus KS, et al. Neuropsychophysiological findings in a case of long-standing overt ventriculomegaly (LOVA). Neurosci Lett 2005; 385(1):24–29.

17. Kiefer M, Eymann R, Meier U. Five years experience with gravitational shunts in chronic hydrocephalus of adults. Acta Neurochir (Wien) 2002; 144(8):755–767.

18. Kiefer M, Eymann R, Strowitzki M, et al. Gravitational shunts in longstanding overt ventriculomegaly in adults. Neurosurgery 2005; 57(1):109–119.

19. Kiefer M, Eymann R, Steudel WI, et al. Gravitational shunt management of long-standing overt ventriculomegaly in adult (LOVA) hydrocephalus. J Clin Neurosci 2005; 12(1):21–26.

20. Fukuhara T, Luciano MG. Clinical features of late-onset idiopathic aqueductal stenosis. Surg Neurol 2001; 55(3):132–136.

21. Kelly PJ. Stereotactic third ventriculostomy in patients with nontumoral adolescent/adult onset aqueductal stenosis and symptomatic hydrocephalus. J Neurosurg 1991; 75(6):865–873.

22. Tisell M. How should primary aqueductal stenosis in adults be treated? A review. Acta Neurol Scand 2005; 111(3):145–153.

23. Javadpour M, May P, Mallucci C. Sudden death secondary to delayed closure of endoscopic third ventriculostomy. Br J Neurosurg 2003; 17(3):266–269.

24. Lipina R, Palecek T, Reguli S, et al. Death in consequence of late failure of endoscopic third ventriculostomy. Childs Nerv Syst 2007 [Epub ahead of print].

The Neuropsychological Aspects of Longstanding Overt Ventriculomegaly in Adults

Mohammed Al Jumaily, Conor Mallucci, and Peter Murphy
Department of Neurosurgery, The Walton Centre for Neurology and Neurosurgery, Liverpool, U.K.

Longstanding overt ventriculomegaly in adults (LOVA) is characterized by chronic hydrocephalus associated with gross ventricular dilatation and a head circumference of more than two standard deviations above normal (1). Conceivably, the centers of higher mental functions are subjected to chronic pressure and reorganization within the cerebral cortex, especially in these patients with thin cerebral mantle.

Neuropsychological assessment of patients with LOVA can be performed with the Repeatable Battery for the Assessment of Neuropsychological Status (RBANS) and the Hospital Anxiety and Depression Scale (HADS). Academic and occupational achievements offer an additional indication of neuropsychological status.

1. Repeatable Battery for the Assessment of Neuropsychological Status (RBANS)
   The RBANS is a brief, individually administered test that helps determine the neuropsychological status of adults who have neurological injury or disease. It covers many of the higher mental functions including immediate memory, visuospatial recognition, constructional language, attention, and delayed memory. A score of 100 represents the 50th percentile of the normal distribution of Neuropsychological Status.
2. Hospital Anxiety and Depression Scale (HADS)
   This is a test designed to detect the presence and severity of mild degrees of mood disorder, anxiety, and depression. Scores of 0 to 7 are considered normal, while 8 to 10 are borderline, and 11 or over indicate clinical cases of anxiety and depression.

We tried to explore the neuropsychological characteristics of LOVA patients. Twenty patients, 10 males and 10 females, were reviewed in a special follow-up clinic. They had neuropsychological assessment using the RBANS and the HADS tests. The patients were also interviewed about their academic achievements and occupation.

Results of RBANS: Mean value for total scale was 70.84 (SD: 14.8, range: 45–96); mean value for immediate memory was 75.37 (SD: 18.8, range: 40–109); mean value for visual–spatial and constructional tasks was 81.74 (SD: 18.9, range: 50–121); mean value for language was 81.32 (SD: 15.9, range: 54–111); mean value for attention was 70.42 (SD: 15.9, range: 46–91); mean value for delayed memory was 71.63 (SD: 20.9, range: 40–102). It is clear from the mean scores that the majority of these patients perform poorly on all aspects studied. There is a particular effect on the attention where 100% of patients were below average. With few exceptions, these patients tended to have a poor memory capacity involving both immediate and delayed. It is surprising that the visual–spatial, reconstruction, and language faculties of these patients showed a wide range, with some being well above the general population. Nevertheless, the mean for all three remained below average. There was no significant difference between males and females neuropsychological tests results in this series.

Results of HADS: Mean value for anxiety was 7.10 (SD: 5.8, range: 1–17); mean value for depression was 6.05 (SD: 4.8, range: 0–14). There is wide range in the scores of anxiety and depression. The mean values, however, indicate that these two disorders are not a general characteristic in LOVA patients.

Academic achievements and occupation: Out of the 20 patients only 3 finished university and surprisingly were all nurses! The employment was surprisingly high with 11 (55%) in a job at time of assessment; 4 were unemployed, 3 retired, and 1 was a student.

In patients ventriculomegaly in the context of LOVA, it is reasonable to hypothesize different levels of cerebral reserve to explain cognitive deficits in the presence of severe lesions (2). Longstanding mechanical stress of brain has allowed the adaptation and the functional reorganization of spared structures utilizing its own cerebral reserve. It is thought that considerable neural plasticity has occurred during the LOVA-progression taking place at level of the left occipitotemporal cortex and cerebellum (3), in particular cerebellar modulation in procedural control activities, as the cerebellum appears completely intact (1,5).

In summary, patients with LOVA, although exhibiting a general global cognitive impairment, seem to adapt quite well in the general population regarding employment. They show little anxiety and depression about their relative disability.

REFERENCES

1. Oi S, Shimoda M, Shibata M, et al. Pathophysiology of long-standing overt ventriculomegaly in adults. J Neurosurg 2000; 92:933–940.
2. Canu ED, Magnano I, Paulus KS, et al. Neuropsychophysiological findings in a case of long-standing overt ventriculomegaly (LOVA). Neurosci Lett 2005; 385(1):24–29.
3. Bigler ED. The neuropsychology of hydrocephalus. Arch Clin Neuropsychol 1988; 3:81–100.
4. Ackermann H, Mathiak K, Ivry RB. Temporal organization of "internal speech" as a basis for cerebellar modulation of cognitive functions. Behav Cogn Neurosci Rev 2004; 3:14–22.
5. Hülsmann E, Erb M, Grodd W. From will to action: Sequential cerebellar contributions to voluntary movement. Neuroimage 2003; 20:1485–1492.

24 | Cerebrospinal Fluid Shunts

Spyros Sgouros
Department of Neurosurgery, "Attikon" University Hospital, University of Athens, Athens, Greece

Dimitris Kombogiorgas
Department of Neurosurgery, Birmingham Children's Hospital, Birmingham, U.K.

INTRODUCTION

Cerebrospinal fluid (CSF) shunts are devices that transport CSF from an intracranial production site to an extracranial absorption site. A typical CSF shunt system consists of a proximal catheter, a one-way valve, and a distal catheter. The proximal catheter is inserted in a CSF production site, usually one of the lateral ventricles. The shunt valve controls the CSF flow and the distal catheter transports the CSF to the absorption site, usually the peritoneal cavity or cardiac atrium (Fig. 1). The role of the perfect shunt would be to allow one-way flow of CSF from the head to the absorption site, while always maintaining normal intracranial pressure.

The use of CSF shunts remains a fundamental therapeutic modality in the management of hydrocephalus, which converted that disease from a debilitating disease with poor outcome (1) to a fully treatable disease with good intellectual and physical outcome (2). Knowledge of the manufacture and principles of function of shunts allows neurosurgeons to intelligently select among many types and designs of shunts in each individual case and understand some of their complications.

HISTORY

It is thought that Hippocrates made the first attempt to treat hydrocephalus by ventricular puncture, although actually he may have drained the subdural space (3,4). Ventricular puncture continued to be used in the 18th century (5). In order to avoid infection, closed ventricular drainage was attempted near the end of the 19th century. The fluid was usually diverted to the subcutaneous or subdural spaces (6). Since the turn of 20th century, various intracranial and extracranial spaces have been investigated for draining of CSF, including unusual sites as salivary gland duct, gallbladder, ureter, fallopian tube, thoracic duct, and spinal epidural space (5). The modern era of CSF shunts commenced in 1950s. In 1952, Nulsen and Spitz were first to report the successful use of ventriculojugular shunt using a spring and stainless steel ball valve (7). Holter invented and produced the Holter-valve for his own son in 1955 (8). His design employs a flexible silicon diaphragm and has proven timeless, as it is in use even today in different commercial iterations. Pudenz et al. introduced silicone as a shunt tubing material, which has since become the material of choice for implanted shunts (9). The efforts of these men heralded the beginning of a new era in hydrocephalus management.

In 1970s, first ventriculoatrial (VA) and lumboperitoneal (LP) and subsequently ventriculoperitoneal (VP) shunting procedures became popular for the treatment of hydrocephalus. Ultimately, the VP shunts replaced VA shunts as the standard practice due to the complications of VA shunts (endocarditis, shunt nephritis, pulmonary hypertension), and based on the work of Ames, the peritoneum is proven as the best reabsorption site of CSF (10). Nowadays VA shunts are performed only in patients whose peritoneum has failed, after multiple abdominal operations. Despite improvements in CSF shunt science and technology, the manufacture of a perfect CSF shunt device remains a challenging goal of the scientific and industrial community.

CEREBROSPINAL FLUID DYNAMICS

In order to understand CSF shunt function, some knowledge of fluid dynamics is required. Hydrodynamics (hydro-: "ύδωρ": water) is the scientific study of the motion of fluids, especially noncompressible liquids (i.e., water), under the influence of internal and external forces. Hydrokinetics is the branch of hydrodynamics dealing with the laws of gases or liquids in

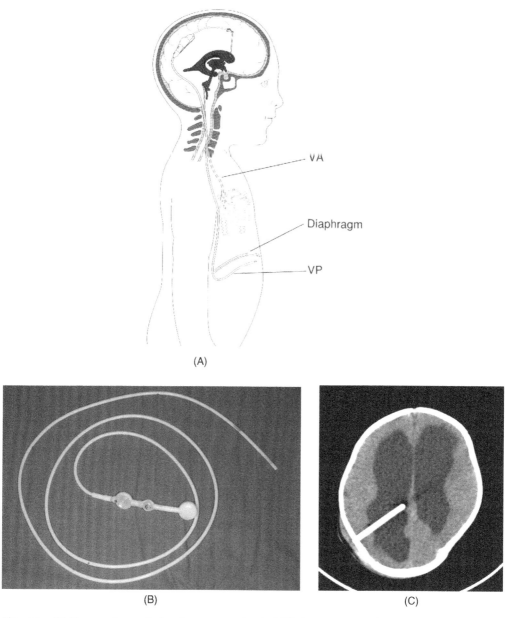

Figure 1 (**A**) Diagram demonstrating the components of a CSF shunt system and their representative positions after implantations. The ventricular catheter is in the right lateral ventricle and the distal catheter is in the right atrium (VA) or the peritoneal cavity (VP). (**B**) A shunt system, without the ventricular catheter, shown before implantation. There is a reservoir, the valve, and the distal catheter. All the components are "glued" together at manufacture-unitized. The whole system is called a two-piece shunt (ventricular catheter + unitized shunt). (**C**) CT scan of the head of a child that had a ventriculoperitoneal shunt inserted. The ventricular catheter is seen in the atrium of the right lateral ventricle. This is the correct ventricular catheter placement.

motion. Pressure, flow, and resistance are important physical concepts relating to hydrocephalus and CSF shunt dynamics (11–14).

The pressure (P) at the bottom of a fluid containing cylinder (such as the shunt tube) is the weight divided by the cylinder's base surface area, which is the product of height, the density of fluid, and the force of gravity as follows: $P = \rho \times h \times g$ (ρ: density of fluid, h: height, g: force of gravity). The flow of fluid (Q) is the quantity of fluid that passes a point during a particular time period and is equal to the pressure difference (DP) between cylinder ends divided by resistance (R), expressed by the mathematical form: $Q = DP/R$. The greater the pressure difference and the lower the resistance, the higher the flow. The resistance of a shunt tubing to flow is described by Poiseuille's law: $R = 8L\mu/\rho gr^4$ (L: length of tube, μ: fluid viscosity, r: inner radius of tube). Its resistance is dependent on many factors including tube diameter, valve geometry, CSF viscosity, temperature, and the presence of turbulence (15). The total resistance for a shunt system is the sum of resistance of the ventricular catheter, the valve, any shunt accessories (i.e., antisiphon device), and the distal catheter (16). A shunt provides a lower-resistance pathway compared to patient's CSF circulation pathway resistance in order to achieve CSF diversion. The pressure gradient (ΔP) driving the flow in a VP shunt system is determined by $\Delta P = \text{IVP} + \text{HP} - \text{OPV} - \text{DCP}$ [IVP: intraventricular pressure, HP ($\rho \times h \times g$): hydrostatic pressure, h: vertical height difference between proximal and distal ends of shunt system, OPV: opening pressure of the shunt valve, DCP: distal cavity pressure, i.e., intra-abdominal pressure in case of VP shunts (6,15)]. Hydrostatic pressure in a patient's shunt will be higher in upright compared to supine position, as the value of height (h) will be larger when upright. Subsequently, the gravity of hydrostatic forces will push CSF out of the head until the pressure in the head will be equal to negative pressure equal to the height of the column of CSF minus the opening pressure of the valve. This phenomenon is well known as siphoning (6,14,15,17). The difference between the various commercial shunt valve designs centers on the mechanism of CSF flow control and its response to the siphoning effect. Nevertheless, in vitro differences between shunt designs do not translate to significant differences in clinical practice, as many comparative studies have shown (18,19).

PRODUCTION OF SHUNT SYSTEM

Shunt manufacturing is a process of assembly of a series of components made from different types of material such as synthetic ruby, plastics, metals, and ceramics. The most commonly utilized material in shunt manufacturing is silicon rubber owing to its biocompatibility, physical properties (hardness, flexibility, elasticity, tensile strength, thermal stability), ease of processing, and wide range of silicon types. Silicon belongs to a category of chemical material named polysiloxanes. The wide range of molecular weights and viscosities in combination with inclusion of other material, that is, vinyl, which modifies certain desired final properties, results in manufacturing a great variety of silicone-made material. Carbon graphite is used for length marking of shunt system. Barium sulfate, bismuth subcarbonate, or tantalum oxide is used as a radiopaque material to allow for shunt system X-ray imaging.

Shunt system production process includes manufacturing of components, cleaning, assembling of components by highly trained personnel, often by hand, according to validated and approved operation steps, assigning of a specific lot number, product testing, final quality inspection, external cleaning operation, packaging, and labeling. All shunt products implanted in humans are covered by international treaties on medical implants, that is, they have approval for human use (FDA approval in the United States; CE marking in Europe) and have to conform to their licensed bench-test specifications, and the factories are subject to strict inspections and quality control. All this makes the final price of shunts high, in comparison to the cost of the raw materials. Commonly, their guarantee is invalidated once the package is opened, in other words their performance once implanted does not have to conform to their bench specifications. Despite that, most manufacturers would perform in vitro test on explanted shunts, purely on scientific interest grounds.

COMPONENTS OF CEREBROSPINAL FLUID SHUNT SYSTEM

Proximal Catheter

The proximal or ventricular catheters are made of silicone rubber. They vary in terms of length, internal and external diameters, tip configuration, shape, stiffness, and marking. They may be straight or preshaped (90° angled catheters and "J" shaped catheter). The length of ventricular catheters usually varies between 15 and 23 cm. The catheter is then cut into appropriate length, commonly 5 to 6 cm. The preshaped catheters or catheters of unitized systems are made in fixed lengths. The holes of ventricular catheter are located at its distal 1 or 2 cm (Fig. 2). The

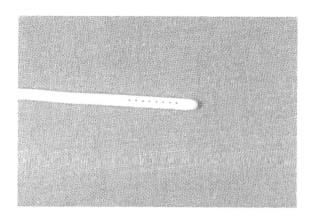

Figure 2 The tip of a new unused ventricular catheter. There are multiple holes in the last 1–2 cm, aimed to reduce the chances of obstruction.

ventricular catheter is provided with a metallic central stylet, which facilitates catheter insertion into the ventricle. There are different shapes of catheter connectors (straight, right angled, "Y" shaped). There are also different types of reservoirs that are attached to the ventricular catheter, mainly to allow the clinician to withdraw a sample of CSF later after shunt implantation. These reservoirs are chambers that are connected between ventricular catheter and shunt valve in order to facilitate stabilization of ventricular catheter and allow CSF sampling in the future. Two varieties are Rickham reservoir and PS medical snap on system [Fig. 1(B)].

In case of LP shunts, there are two types of proximal catheter. The first one, which is most commonly used, is passed through a Tuohy needle into the lumbar subarachnoid space and has an angled open end and several side holes. The second one has a "T" shape end, which is introduced to subarachnoid space after laminectomy but is less likely to migrate.

Shunt Valves

A shunt valve is a mechanical device that regulates CSF flow by opening and closing according to the difference between inlet and outlet pressures. For example, in case of VP shunt the flow through the valve depends on the presence of the difference in pressure between the ventricle and the peritoneal cavity. Opening and closing pressures of a valve are the pressure when valve opens and closes, respectively. They may be different because of a slight change in the mechanical properties of the valves during opening and closing, as valves are made mostly of silicone rubber material, which is deformable, sticky, and not perfectly elastic. This phenomenon is known as hysteresis—it occurs most frequently with slit and miter differential pressure valves (6,11,15) and tends to deteriorate with time due to material fatigue.

Differential Pressure Valves

Differential pressure valves attempt to keep the IVP within predetermined limits, those of valve opening and closing pressure, avoiding IVP to increase too high or decrease too low. When the intraventricular pressure is higher than the valve opening pressure, the valve opens allowing egress of CSF from the ventricle at a rate determined by the resistance of the entire shunt system, until the pressure falls below valve closing pressure resulting in cessation of CSF flow. As the differential pressure across the shunt increases, the mechanism opens up, increasing the surface area through which CSF flows, thus allowing more CSF to flow for approximately the same pressure. A perfect pressure regulator is a device that produces a perfectly horizontal line on a pressure versus flow graph.

In contrast to pressure regulation valves, flow regulation valves try to maintain the same flow rate at any differential pressure. The surface area of the flow-regulating valve decreases in a predetermined fashion to produce a constant flow through the shunt, regardless of the differential pressure. A perfect flow regulation valve produces a straight vertical line on a pressure versus flow graph. In reality, because perfect valves do not exist, most commercially available devices have nonlinear pressure versus flow graphs.

In case of combination of two valves that are placed in series, the total opening pressure will be the sum of opening pressure of each valve. The same is true for the total resistance of a two-valve system. If two valves are placed in parallel, the total opening pressure will be opening pressure of the valve with the lowest opening pressure providing that the proximal and distal ends of the shunt system are at the same level. The total resistance of the system will be $1/R$ total $= 1/R$ valve $1 + 1/R$ valve 2.

There are four types of differential pressure valves:

(a) Slit valves in which there is a slit in a curved rubber layer. The CSF flow arriving from the concave side, if under sufficient pressure, will open the slit in a varying degree based on the upstream pressure. Holter–Hausner valve has the slit valve at the proximal end; Codman Unishunt valve and lumboperitoneal shunt have the slit valves at the distal end of the shunt system. Radionics standard shunt valve has a single membrane silicone in opposition to a Teflon base, acting to create a slit valve in stainless steel housing. More than one set of slits can be used distally to prevent obstruction from accumulating debris inside the catheter adjacent to the slits. Also, slit valves can be used as proximal valves in order to provide an intervening pumping chamber.

(b) Miter valves look like "duck bill" valves, as the orifice ends into two flat horizontally opposed leaflets of silicon. The opening and closing pressures of the valve are related to the mechanical characteristics of the leaflets.

(c) Diaphragm valves have a mobile flexible membrane, which moves in response to pressure differences. The way of movement of the membrane varies among different diaphragm valve subtypes. The membrane may be held by a central piston that moves in a sleeve or surrounds the piston, which acts as the occluder (Fig. 3). Also, in other case, the membrane

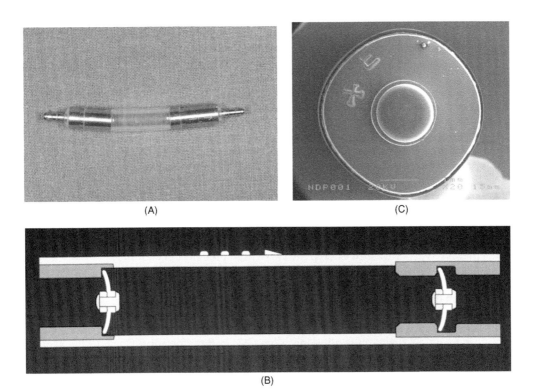

(A)

(C)

(B)

Figure 3 Cylindrical differential pressure valve. (**A**) Late variation of the Holter valve circa 1992, in this example made by PS Medical (now Medtronic Inc), available commercially in this guise until the early 1990s. Later the metal parts were changed for plastic and the medium pressure valve is available even today. (**B**) Diagram representing the structure of the cylindrical DP valve. It has two diaphragm units at each end. *Source*: Courtesy of PS Medical, now Medtronic Inc. The CSF passes circumferentially from the diaphragm rim, in the gap between it, and then the casing that encircles it. (**C**) Scanning electron microscope photograph of the diaphragm unit of a new "unused" cylindrical medium pressure PS Medical DP valve. The structure of the diaphragm is seen. It is secured by a pole in its center, which is attached to the casing further back. The casing is not seen here. The CSF passes all around the free margin of the diaphragm.

can be a dome that deforms under pressure. The opening and closing pressures of the valve are dependent on the stiffness of the material (silicon) of which the membrane is made of.

(d) Spring valves consist of a metallic linear, helical, or circular spring that applies force to a ball located in an occluding orifice (otherwise called ball-in-cone valves). The ball can be metallic, ruby, or sapphire. The spring can apply force to the ball along the axis or tangential to it. The opening and closing pressures of the valve are determined by the stiffness of the spring providing that the sticky forces between the ball and the material around the orifice are negligible.

Differential pressure valves are provided by manufacturers usually in four categories of opening pressure: very low (<1 cm H$_2$O), low (1–4 cm H$_2$O), medium (4–8 cm H$_2$O), and high (>8 cm H$_2$O) pressure.

Flow Control Valves

"Flow control" valves are designed to provide constant flow of CSF over a wide range of pressures by changing the hydrodynamic resistance as the pressure gradient change. In fact, they are differential pressure valves that control the resistance by changing the orifice diameter according to the CSF pressure. Practically, the CSF flow regulation can be achieved by inserting a solid conical cylinder attached to a pressure-sensitive membrane inside a ring (14). The movement of conical cylinder in or out of the ring (orifice) will decrease or increase, respectively, the cross-section surface area of the orifice through which CSF passes. The degree of movement of conical cylinder depends on CSF pressure and its membrane plasticity/stiffness. Flow control valves produce a sigmoid-type flow–pressure curve (6). The best example of "flow control" valves is the Orbis-Sigma OSV valve, introduced in 1987 and now in its second guise (OSVII, Integra Neuroscience, Plainsboro, NJ, U.S.A.), which contains a dome connected to a movable ruby pin with variable profile, which allows a stable flow of CSF of a wide pressure range, while it includes an overflow mechanism in case the CSF pressure becomes too high (Fig. 4). Recently,

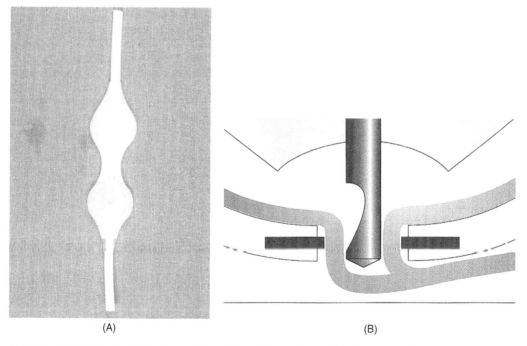

(A) (B)

Figure 4 (**A**) OSV valve (Orbis Sigma Valve, Integra Neuroscience, Plainsboro, NJ, U.S.A.). The upper part of the case is a CSF reservoir. The lower part contains the valve mechanism. The red ruby pinion is seen through the dome attached to its most superior aspect. (**B**) Diagram (reproduced from promotional leaflet of Integra Neuroscience), showing a cut out of the valve mechanism of the valve. The shape of the lateral surface of the mobile pinion allows different CSF flow according to its position, which is influenced by the movement of the dome in response to the ICP.

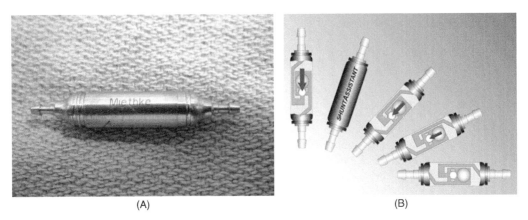

(A)   (B)

Figure 5 (**A**) ShuntAssistant anti-siphon device made by Miethke (Christoph Miethke GmbH & Co KG, Potsdam, Germany). (**B**) Diagram showing the principle of function of ShuntAssistant (reproduced from promotional leaflet of Christoph Miethke GmbH & Co KG). It is a gravitational device containing a large ball, which changes position by gravity and alters the resistance of the device and a smaller ball, which acts as an occluder to prevent retrograde back-flow in the horizontal position.

the OSV valve was also developed in a lower flow setting to suit patients with normal pressure hydrocephalus who may be more prone to chronic subdural hematomas postshunting.

Anti-Siphon Devices

A major breakthrough came in the 1980s, when the syndrome of shunt overdrainage due to "siphoning" was appreciated. "Siphoning" is the rapid loss of CSF from the head in the erect position. Different technological solutions were pursued in order to overcome this. Two main types of devices were developed: the "anti-siphon" or "siphon-control" devices and the "flow control" valves. "Anti-siphon" devices come in different designs, common ones use either a dome to sense atmospheric pressure and apply increased resistance to flow in the erect position (e.g., Delta chamber, Medtronic Inc, Minneapolis, MN, U.S.A.), or gravity-controlled balls, which progressively occlude the CSF passage and increase the resistance to flow, for example, ShuntAssistant (Christoph Miethke GmbH & Co KG, Potsdam, Germany) (Fig. 5) and SiphonGuard (Codman & Shurtleff Inc, Raynham, MA, U.S.A.) (Fig. 6). Most manufacturers have incorporated "differential pressure" valves and anti-siphon devices in single case shunt devices, for example, Delta valve = D.P. diaphragm valve + delta chamber (Medtronic PS Medical) (Fig. 7).

In case of anti-siphon devices with a mobile membrane (20), when siphoning occurs, the pressure inside the shunt becomes negative and then the atmospheric pressure pushes the

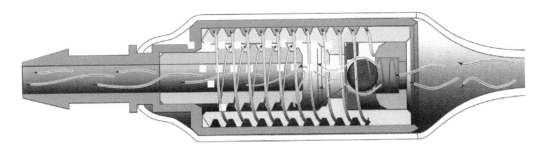

Figure 6 Diagram showing the principle of function of SiphonGuard, an anti-siphon device made by Codman (reproduced from promotional leaflet of Codman & Shurtleff Inc, Raynham, MA, U.S.A.). The position of the ball changes in response to gravity and alters the flow of CSF.

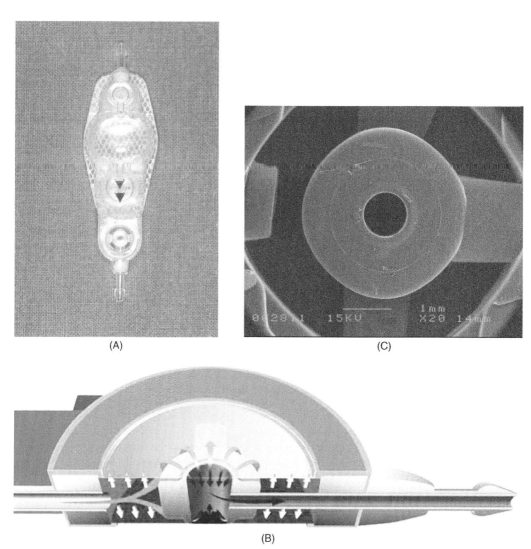

(A)   (C)

(B)

Figure 7 (**A**) Delta valve made by Medtronic (Medtronic Inc, Minneapolis, MN, U.S.A.). The upper part of the case contains a CSF chamber. The middle part contains a differential pressure diaphragm valve, working on the same principle as in Figure 3, but positioned at right angle to the main body of the case. The lower part contains the Delta anti-siphon chamber. (**B**) Diagram showing the principle of function of the Delta chamber (reproduced from promotional material of Medtronic Inc). There are two membranes on either side of a plastic ring. When the siphoning occurs, the membranes are "sucked" on to the ring and occlude its passage of CSF. (**C**) Scanning electron microscopy of an unused Delta chamber, showing the central passage way for CSF.

membrane against the control orifice, increasing the resistance and prevents further siphoning [Fig. 7(B) and 7(C)].

In case of anti-siphon device with gravity-controlled balls, there is an increase of the resistance of the shunt system when the patient is in vertical position by blocking the inlet flow using the balls weight, resulting in reduced flow of CSF through the shunt. When the patient is in horizontal position, the ball no longer blocks the opening and the unit provides substantially less resistance (21) [Fig. 5(B)]. Some gravity-controlled anti-siphon devices (e.g., ShuntAssistant) have titrated settings expressed in centimetes, equivalent to the distance between the right atrium of the heart and the outlet of the peritoneal catheter, representing the height of column of water that they are designed to counteract. Such devices can be implanted either upstream or downstream from the primary valve. The weight of the tantalum ball generates the counterbalance to the hydrostatic pressure in the shunt system according to the patient's posture and is unaffected by changes in subcutaneous pressure.

Positioning of some anti-siphon devices at different locations (or heights) along the course of the shunt will change the negative pressure at which they will start to act, for example, Delta chamber. Subsequently, such anti-siphon devices at the distal end of a shunt or attached to LP shunt will not work (6). It is evident that the neurosurgeon needs to be familiar with the method of action of the anti-siphon device intended to be implanted, in order to utilize it correctly.

Gravity-Actuated Valves

Gravity-actuated valves [Cordis–Hakim–Lumbar valve, Miethke GAV (gravity-assisted valve)] attempt to prohibit or reduce siphoning by increasing opening pressure with the assistance of gravity when a patient sits or stands (15). The Cordis horizontal–vertical valve is used with LP shunt. It has two valves in a series. The first (or inlet) valve is a ball spring valve and does not markedly change resistance with position. The second (or outlet) valve has four balls in a row. The first one is a synthetic ruby ball that sits in a conical seat. The other three stainless steel balls sit on the top of the smaller first ball when the patient is in upright position resulting in high resistance. In the supine position, the balls fall away from the orifice of the valve to allow CSF flow at a low resistance (3,6,15,22). The GAV is a posture-dependent valve. This means that the opening pressure varies depending on the body position of the patient. It consists of a ball-cone valve with a variably predefined opening pressure and a fixed pressure gravitational unit. In order to specify the GAV according to the patient's individual needs, the surgeon determines the opening pressure required for both the horizontal and vertical positions. The unit is composed of a solid titanium body. A spring coil defines the opening pressure of the ball-cone valve. The gravitational unit contains a tantalum ball, which defines the opening pressure of the gravitational unit, and a sapphire ball, which ensures the precise closure of the valve.

Programmable—Adjustable Valves

Programmable valves are differential pressure valves that allow the surgeon to adjust the opening pressure by using an external device. They are, also, called externally adjustable differential pressure valves. In the 1980s, an adjustable valve was produced, the Hakim-Medos "programmable" valve (now called the Codman Hakim programmable valve; Codman & Shurtleff Inc, Raynham, MA, USA), which allowed to adjust the opening pressure setting percutaneously with the help of a magnet system. It offered the facility to change the opening pressure in 18 steps of 10 mm H_2O over a wide range from 30 to 200 mm H_2O and was clinically tested in 1984 (3,22) (Fig. 8).

It was an interesting concept, certainly advanced for its time. It was marketed as "programmable" valve, but it should be referred to better as "adjustable," as the user cannot change its essential functional characteristics, but only its opening pressure, in other words, it only operates one program at different pressure levels. It is a "differential pressure" valve with a ruby ball and seat controlled by a stainless steel spring of adjustable height. Adjustable valves are more expensive than standard differential pressure valves but are well suited for managing difficult or complicated cases such as slit ventricle syndrome, development of subdural collections after shunting of hydrocephalus, and persistent symptoms of hydrocephalus. Also, these are useful in decreasing the size of arachnoid cyst or the ventricles in patients with normal pressure hydrocephalus (23–29).

Recently manufacturers have combined adjustable pressure "differential pressure" valves with anti-siphon devices in a single case. Three notable examples are the Strata valve (30) (Medtronic Inc), an adjustable Delta valve (diaphragm DP valve + Delta chamber) with five pressure settings, and the Miethke Pro-GAV (Christoph Miethke GmbH & Co KG), which combines a ball-in-cone D.P. valve, the opening pressure of which is altered by changing the tension of the spring with a rotor, and a gravity-controlled ball anti-siphon device and the Codman Hakim programmable valve, which has been combined with the Siphonguard in the same case (Codman & Shurtleff Inc). These newer devices offer improved laboratory characteristics but

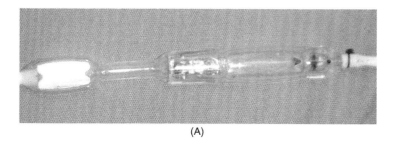

(A)

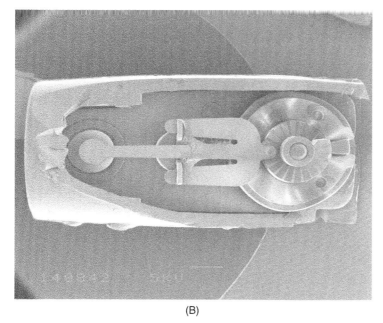

(B)

Figure 8 (**A**): Hakim-Medos programmable valve (Codman & Shurtleff Inc, Raynham, MA, U.S.A.). The part on the left is a CSF reservoir. In the central part is the adjustable valve. (**B**) Scanning electron microscopy of the Medos adjustable valve mechanism. There is a spring mechanism that controls the position of the ruby ball on the left. There is a staircase-like mechanism that rotates and alters the tension on the spring mechanism. This particular valve was removed because of infection. Abnormal material is seen in clumps in the spring mechanism and the "staircase."

have not been available long enough to ascertain their clinical performance. "Flow control" valves have not existed in adjustable guise so far (until early 2009).

Distal Catheters
Distal (peritoneal, vascular, and cardiac) catheters are made from silicon and vary in length between manufacturers. There are two types of peritoneal catheters based on the presence or absence of slit valves at their distal end. The distal catheter is passed through the subcutaneous tissue by using a tunneling device, which is a relatively soft metallic tube with a central trocar.

SHUNTS COMPLICATIONS
Shunting of patients can be affected from numerous types of complications (2,28,31–37) including the following:

1. Mechanical complications as obstruction (Fig. 9), fracture, often associated with calcification and denaturing of the tubing material (Fig. 10), disconnection, malposition of proximal (Fig. 11) or distal shunt catheter, migration of part of the shunt system (e.g., migration of

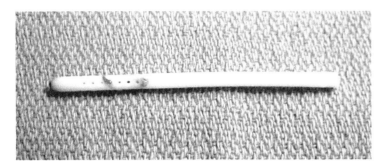

Figure 9 Ventricular catheter removed during an operation for shunt revision. The holes of the catheter are occluded by debris and cellular material.

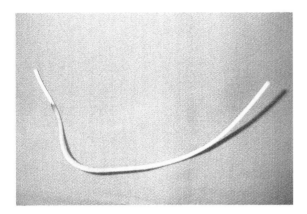

Figure 10 Calcified fractured distal catheter removed during shunt revision. The shunt had been implanted for several years. The calcification is seen on the surface of the tube. This process denatures the material of the catheter and reduces its tensile strength, making it more vulnerable to fracture.

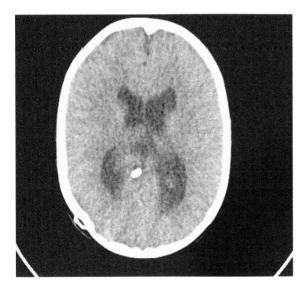

Figure 11 CT scan of a shunted hydrocephalic child who presented with symptoms of raised intracranial pressure a few days after shunt insertion. The ventricular catheter had been malpositioned and its tip is out of the ventricular system, in the brain parenchyma, hence not draining correctly.

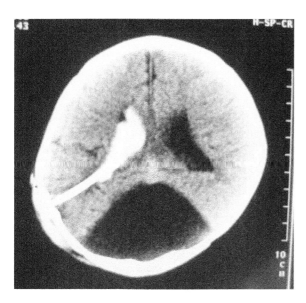

Figure 12 CT scan of the head of a hydro-cephalic child who had shunt revision the day before and after 24 hours the child started deteriorating. There is a large blood clot in the right lateral ventricle surrounding the catheter. The ventricles are dilated. Presumably, during removal of the previous catheter there was tear of the choroid plexus, which was attached on the catheter. This caused hemorrhage, which in turn encased and occluded the new catheter.

catheter in bowel, scrotum, or subcutaneous tissue due to body lengthening), and hemorrhage from the choroid plexus, especially in shunt revision (Fig. 12).

2. Overdrainage. Early, manifested as subdural hematomas (Fig. 13) in the first few weeks from implantation, and late, manifested as slit ventricle syndrome (Fig. 14) or secondary craniosynostosis.

3. Infection.

4. Psychological side effects secondary to repeat hospitalizations and reoperations for shunt revisions.

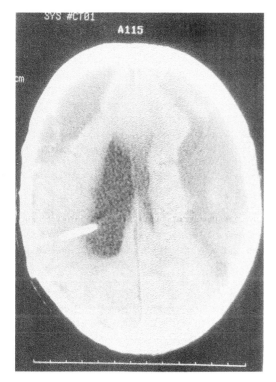

Figure 13 CT scan of the head of a 72-year-old man with normal pressure hydrocephalus, who three days before had shunt insertion. There are extensive large bilateral subdural hematomas as a result of collapse of the cortex in response to shunting.

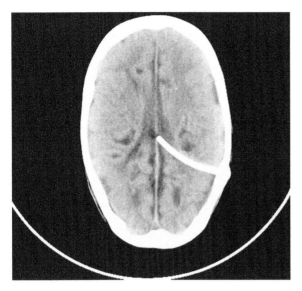

Figure 14 CT scan of the head of a hydro-cephalic 4-year-old girl, who was shunted the first few months of life and who is complaining of persistent headaches. The ventricles are slit, the cranium is comparatively thick for the patient's age and the shape of the head is oblong-scaphocephaly. The patient has slit ventricle syndrome and a mild secondary sagittal synostosis.

Mechanical obstruction is the most common complication following shunt implantation (34). The ventricular catheter is the most common site of obstruction usually from choroid plexus which ingrows due to flow of CSF drawing the choroid plexus in the ventricular catheter, followed by glial tissue from astrocyte proliferation (38) (Fig. 9). Also, it can be blocked by connective tissue, clotted blood, material degradation (necrotic brain tissue, fibers, proteins), ependymal cells, lymphocytes, multinucleated giant cells, and neutrophils (15). Obstruction of other parts of shunt such as valve, accessories (connectors), anti-siphon devices, and the distal shunt catheter can occur. Shunt valves create areas of flow restriction and dead space, which predispose to accumulation of debris and tissue colonization leading to obstruction of valve (35,39). Obstructive material can be a clot, debris or parenchymal tissue, bacterial proliferation, cellular immune reaction causing early or late shunt malfunction, or obstruction since the time of shunt insertion (37,39,40). Distal catheter obstructions can be due to progressive debris accumulation in the dead space beneath the slits of the slit catheters. The debris can be due to fibrin clumps, macrophages, mesothelial cells, lymphocytes, and fibroblasts. The risk of this type of obstruction does not exist with open-ended distal tubes. Partial distal obstruction can be due to reduced absorption capacity of peritoneum secondary to ascites or formation of pseudocyst around of distal tip end.

CONTROVERSIES ON SHUNT VALVES

After five decades of shunt design evolution, laboratory and clinical studies, and considerable scientific debate in countless meetings, the issues of superiority of shunt valve design remain unresolved. This by implication signifies the difficulties with the development of human implantable medical devices, as well as the economy of scales that affects medical devices in comparison to commercial electronic goods, for example, which incorporate infinitely more complicated technology than shunt valves and are sold for a fraction of the price, while they offer only enjoyment, and sometime they endanger life, rather than save it! At the same time, it has been rather striking how polarized neurosurgeons' views are on choice of shunts, while no conclusive scientific evidence exists, which implies that significant factors in the choice of a shunt play the history of education of each individual surgeon. Most surgeons choose valves that their mentors were using when they were training, in a parallel to the known assertion in commerce that most drivers will choose the same make of car when they change, provided they had no major problems with the previous one. The ability of the industry to penetrate in the local environment of neurosurgeons using the usual market techniques (advertisement, personal contacts, social trends, etc) also influences medical trends.

Several in vitro studies have examined the hydrodynamic properties of shunt valves, with particular reference to anti-siphon action (12,17). Two major valve-testing facilities exist: in

Cambridge, U.K. and in Heidelberg, Germany, in the respective Departments of Neurosurgery. Both these testing facilities have consistently shown that most shunt valves do not counteract effectively the overdrainage phenomenon in the erect position, despite manufacturers' claims (11,22,41). The standard differential pressure valves have major susceptibilities to overdrainage, the Codman Hakim programmable valve cannot counteract overdrainage in the erect position even in its higher setting, and the dome-designed anti-siphon devices (e.g., Delta chamber, Medtronic PS Medical) are susceptible to the subcutaneous pressure (42). This has been shown to render them inactive with time, as the subcutaneous tissue encases them in fibrous scar tissue and they lose their reference to atmospheric pressure, which deactivates the whole mechanism of increase of resistance to CSF flow.

Considerable controversy still exists on whether flow-regulated valves offer a superior clinical long-term outcome than the pressure-regulated valves. Several clinical studies and a randomized clinical trial have not answered this question conclusively yet (18,19), and it seems that although in the laboratory flow-regulated valves are better than differential pressure valves in counteracting the siphoning effect and maintaining normal ICP, in actual clinical practice the overall "shunt survival time" (time from shunt implantation to its first revision due to some complication, commonly obstruction) is not substantially different between the two shunt types, and the only difference is the type of complication that affects the two types of shunts (18,19). The differential pressure valves are associated with higher proximal obstruction rate, whereas the flow control valves are associated with higher valve obstruction rate. The differential pressure valves are associated with higher incidence of radiological appearance of slit ventricles, but only a minority of these patients develop the clinical features of the syndrome.

Cost comparison studies, performed mainly for the realities of the developing world, have shown no difference in clinical outcome in D.P. valves costing $60 and $600, demonstrating clearly the tremendous differences of performing neurosurgery in the developing and the developed world, and by implication the overpricing and inflationary effect of the medicolegal and commercially driven environment, that doctors practice in the western world.

For most hydrocephalic children older than 2 years and most adults, a medium pressure valve with an anti-siphon device offers good long-term results. Adult patients are not particularly susceptible to overdrainage, so even valves without anti-siphon offer good results. Neonates, young infants, and children in the first two years of life probably benefit most by a flow-control valve, as they are the most likely to develop slit ventricle syndrome. Children with established slit ventricle syndrome can be difficult to manage, often require several valve trials, and different neurosurgeons have different preferences on which valve to choose. They are most likely to need change from a differential pressure to flow control valve and can benefit often by adjustable valves if they have developed poor compliance and are very sensitive to small changes of pressure. Young infants with very big ventricles and small cortical mantle are particularly susceptible to overdrainage, collapse of the cortical parenchyma, and development of subdural hematomas; hence they should have high-resistance valves (high pressure + anti-siphon or flow control or adjustable set at high pressure).

REFERENCES

1. Laurence KM, Coates S. The natural history of hydrocephalus. Detailed analysis of 182 unoperated cases. Arch Dis Child 1962; 37:345–362.
2. Sgouros S, Malluci CL, Walsh AR, et al. Long term complications of hydrocephalus. Pediat Neurosurg 1995; 23:127–132.
3. Aschoff A, Kremer P, Hashemi B, et al. The scientific history of hydrocephalus and its treatment. Neurosurg Rev 1999; 22:67–93.
4. Davidoff LE. Treatment of hydrocephalus. Arch Surg 1929; 18:1737–1762.
5. Fisher RG. Surgery of the congenital anomalies. In: Walker EA, ed. A history of neurological surgery. Baltimore, MD: Williams & Wilkins, 1951:334–347.
6. Drake JM, Sainte-Rose C. The Shunt Book. Cambridge, MA: Blackwell Science, 1995.
7. Nulsen FE, Spitz EB. Treatment of hydrocephalus by direct shunt from ventricle to jugular vein. Surg Forum 1952; 2:399–403.
8. Aschoff A, John D. Holter and his century valve. Cerebrospinal Fluid Res 2004; 1:S1–S13.
9. Pudenz RH, Russel FE, Hurd AH, et al. Ventriculo-auriculostomy. A technique for shunting cerebrospinal fluid into the right auricle. J Neurosurg 1957; 14:171–179.

10. Ames RH. Ventriculoperitoneal shunts in the management of hydrocephalus. J Neurosurg 1967; 27:525–529.

11. Czosnyka M, Czosnyka Z, Whitehouse H, et al. Hydrodynamic properties of hydrocephalus shunts: United Kingdom Shunt Evaluation Laboratory. J Neurol Neurosurg Psychiatry 1997; 62:43–50.

12. Kadowaki A, Hara M, Numoto M, et al. Factors affecting cerebrospinal fluid flow in a shunt. Br J Neurosurg 1987; 1:467–475.

13. Portnoy HD. Hydrodynamics of shunts. Monogr Neural Sci 1982; 8:179–183.

14. Saint-Rose C, Hooven MD, Hirsch JF. A new approach in the treatment of hydrocephalus. J Neurosurg 1987; 66:213–226.

15. Ginsberg HJ, Drake JM. Physiology of cerebrospinal fluid shunt devices. In: Winn HR, ed. Youmans Neurological Surgery, 5th ed. Philadelphia, PA: Saunders, 2004.

16. Magram G, Liakos AM. Cerebrospinal fluid flow through an implanted shunt. Neurol Res 2000; 22:43–50.

17. Magnaes B. Body position and cerebrospinal fluid pressure. Part 2: Clinical studies on orthostatic pressure and the hydrostatic indifferent point. J Neurosurg 1976; 44:698–705.

18. Drake JM, Kestle JR, Milner R, et al. Randomized trial of cerebrospinal fluid shunt valve design in pediatric hydrocephalus. Neurosurgery 1998; 43:294–305.

19. Pollack IF, Albright AL, Adelson PD; the Hakim-Medos Investigator Group. A randomized, controlled study of a programmable shunt versus a conventional valve for patients with hydrocephalus. Neurosurgery 1999; 45:1399–1411.

20. Portnoy HD, Schulte RR, Fox JL, et al. Anti-siphon and reversible occlusion valves for shunting in hydrocephalus and preventing post-shunt subdural haematomas. J Neurosurg 1973; 38:729–738.

21. Allin DM, Czosnyka ZH, Czosnyka M, et al. In vitro hydrodynamic properties of the Miethke ProGAV hydrocephalus shunt. Cerebrospinal Fluid Res 2006; 3:9.

22. Aschoff A, Kremer P, Benesch C, et al. Overdrainage and shunt technology. A critical comparison of programmable, hydrostatic and variable-resistance valves and flow-reducing devices. Childs Nerv Syst 1995; 11:193–202.

23. Hamid NA, Sgouros S. The use of an adjustable valve to treat over-drainage of a cyst-peritoneal shunt in a child with a large sylvian fissure arachnoid cyst. Childs Nerv Syst 2005; 21:991–994.

24. Reinprecht A, Dietrich W, Bertalanffy A, et al. The Medos Hakim programmable valve in the treatment of pediatric hydrocephalus. Childs Nerv Syst 1997; 13:588–594.

25. Sindou M, Guyotat-Pelissou I, Chidiac A, et al. Transcutaneous pressure adjustable valve for the treatment of hydrocephalus and arachnoid cysts in adults. Experiences with 75 cases. Acta Neurochir 1993; 121(3–4):135–139.

26. Zemack G, Bellner J, Siesjo P, et al. Clinical experience with the use of a shunt with an adjustable valve in children with hydrocephalus. J Neurosurg 2003; 98:471–476.

27. Zemack G, Romner B. Adjustable valves in normal-pressure hydrocephalus: A retrospective study of 218 patients. Neurosurgery 2002; 51:1392–1400.

28. Zemack G, Romner B. Do adjustable shunt valves pressure our budget? A retrospective analysis of 541 implanted Codman Hakim programmable valves. Br J Neurosurg 2001; 15:221–227.

29. Zemack G, Romner B. Seven years of clinical experience with the programmable Codman Hakim valve: A retrospective study of 583 patients. J Neurosurg 2000; 92:941–948.

30. Kondageski C, Thompson D, Reynolds M, et al. Experience with the Strata valve in the management of shunt overdrainage. J Neurosurg. 2007; 106(2 suppl):95–102.

31. Blount JP, Campbell JA, Haines SJ. Complications in ventricular cerebrospinal fluid shunting. Neurosurg Clin N Am 1993; 4:633–656.

32. Boch A-L, Hermelin E, Sainte-Rose C, et al. Mechanical dysfunction of ventriculoperitoneal shunt due to calcification of the silicone rubber catheter. J Neurosurg 1998; 88:975–982.

33. Sainte-Rose C, Hoffman HJ, Hirsch JF. Shunt failure. Concepts Pediatr Neurosurg 1989; 9:7–20.

34. Sainte-Rose C, Piatt JH, Renier D, et al. Mechanical complications of shunts. Pediatr Neurosurg 1991–1992; 17:2–9.

35. Sainte-Rose C. Shunt obstruction: A preventable complication? Pediatr Neurosurg 1993; 19:156–164.

36. Walsh AR, Kombogiorgas D. Coiled ventricular-peritoneal shunt within the scrotum. Pediatr Neurosurg 2004; 40(5):257–258.

37. Walters BC, Hoffman HJ, Hendrick EB, et al. Cerebrospinal fluid infections. J Neurosurg 1984; 60:1014–1021.

38. Collins P, Hockley AD, Woollam DHM. Surface ultrastructure of tissues occluding ventricular catheters. J Neurosurg 1978; 48:609–613.

39. Sgouros S, Dipple SJ. An investigation of structural degradation of cerebrospinal fluid shunt valves performed using scanning electron microscopy and energy-dispersive x-ray microanalysis. J Neurosurg 2004; 100:534–540.

40. Gower DJ, Lewis JC, Kelly DL. Sterile shunt malfunction. A scanning microscopic perspective. J Neurosurg 1984; 61:1079–1084.
41. Czosnyka Z, Czosnyka M, Richards HK, et al. Posture-related overdrainage: Comparison of the performance of 10 hydrocephalus shunts in vitro. Neurosurgery 1998; 42:327–334.
42. da Silva MC, Drake JM. Effect of subcutaneous implantation of anti-siphon devices on CSF shunt function. Pediatr Neurosurg 1990–1991; 16(4–5):197–202.

Surgical Technique: Shunt Implantation

Yusuf Erşahin

Division of Pediatric Neurosurgery, Ege University Faculty of Medicine, Izmir, Turkey

CRANIAL END

The patient bathes or showers and shampoos with antiseptic soap the night before and the morning of the operation. The procedure is performed under general endotracheal anesthesia. In the operating room, along with the scrub of the rest of the field, the surgeon shampoos the entire head once again; the entire field is painted with antiseptic solution. The patient is positioned supine on the operating table and in a horizontal level plane to facilitate the subcutaneous tunneling, and the head is turned sharply to the side opposite the insertion. The solution dries while the surgeon scrubs, and then the field is draped with towels and iodine-impregnated adhesive plastic. The ventricular catheter may be placed into the frontal or occipital horn of the lateral ventricle depending on the preference of the surgeon and the individual patient's ventricular anatomy. Most surgeons prefer to fashion a small scalp flap. Some surgeons perform a linear skin incision. A small cruciate periosteal incision is performed and a burr hole is drilled. The burr hole site can be either posterior (4–6 cm above the inion and 2.5–3 cm off the midline) (Fig. 1) or frontal (1 cm anterior to coronal suture and 2.5–3 cm off the midline). If a linear skin incision has been performed, the burr hole is placed asymmetrically to one side of the incision to avoid the shunt reservoir ending directly under the skin incision, which could lead to unintended damage during a later shunt revision. The dura is coagulated with bipolar forceps and a dural opening sufficient for ventricular catheter is done. The arachnoid and pia mater are coagulated and incised. When using a flat bottom valve, an appropriate pocket must be created along the distal path before the shunt passer is withdrawn.

VENTRICULOPERITONEAL SHUNT

A midline paraumbilical incision is made and deepened to the level of the fascia. The peritoneal catheter is subcutaneously passed by using a shunt passer. A tunneling device is introduced from the scalp incision site to the abdominal incision site or vice versa. The abdominal portion is placed into the peritoneal cavity by either trocar technique or minilaparotomy. If the patient has undergone previous abdominal surgeries or had previous abdominal infections, the minilaparotomy should be used. Otherwise, the trocar method is preferred. Before inserting the trocar, the fascia is grasped with toothed forceps and opened with curved scissors. A Valsalva maneuver is performed to tighten the abdominal wall. The trocar is placed and advanced through the rectus musculature and the peritoneum with one smooth and controlled motion. An audible "pop" will often signal entrance into the peritoneum. The stylet is removed and the peritoneal catheter is then passed through the trocar (1–3).

VENTRICULOATRIAL SHUNT

A transverse skin crease incision along the anterior border of the sternocleidomastoid muscle at 2 or 3 cm below the angle of the mandible is made. The platysma is incised, and the common facial vein is identified and traced to its entry into the internal jugular vein. The atrial catheter is filled with saline and clamped. Vessel loops are placed proximally and distally, and the facial vein is tied proximally. A venotomy is performed. A vein pick is used to keep the venotomy open, and the atrial catheter is passed into the right atrium. Radiographically, the distal end of the atrial catheter should stay between T4 and T7. The proximal end of the catheter is subcutaneously tunneled to the cranial incision and connected to the valve. Fluoroscopy is extremely helpful in verifying the correct position of the catheter tip (1–3).

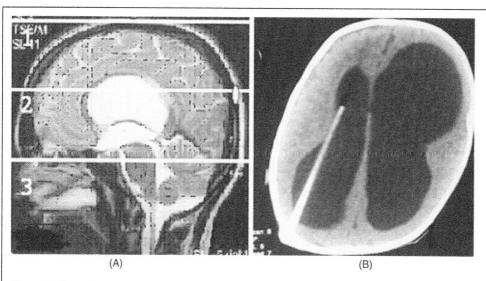

Figure 1 Posterior parietal ventriculostomy. (**A**) The burr hole is located half the distance (plane 2) between plane 1 and 3. Plane 1 is the plane along the vertex and plane 3 is the plane along the inion. (**B**) The burr hole is also located at the midpupillary line, and the ventricular catheter is aimed at the medial epicanthus of the ipsilateral eye.

VENTRICULOPLEURAL SHUNT

Ventriculopleural shunt should be avoided in children younger than 5 years of age because of insufficient CSF resorption capacity of pleural space. The patient is placed in a lateral position with arms swung directly forward and outstretched. An incision for entry into the pleural space is made between anterior and posterior axillary line at the fourth and fifth rib levels. The pectoralis major muscle is split and the intercostal muscles are exposed and the passer is subcutaneously tunneled to pass the distal catheter from the chest incision to the cranium. The distal catheter is trimmed to allow for the catheter to extend approximately to the level of the diaphragm. The ventricular catheter and the distal catheter are connected to the valve. The intercostal muscles at the superior aspect of the rib are separated using bland dissection. The lungs are then expanded with a Valsalva maneuver so that no air will be sucked into the pleural space. The abdominal trocar is used to penetrate the pleural cavity. The trocar should not be inserted into the pleural space by no more than 1 cm. The stylet is removed and the shunt catheter is inserted into the pleural space and then the layers are closed. A chest X-ray is obtained to verify the catheter position and to look for pneumothorax (3,4).

LUMBOPERITONEAL SHUNT

Lumboperitoneal shunt can be used in communicating hydrocephalus and pseudotumor cerebri. The patient is placed in lateral decubitus position. A 1-cm incision is made between L4 and L5 spinous processes (Fig. 2). A 14-Gauge Touhy needle is then passed into the lumbar subarachnoid space and the stylet is removed. The bevel of the Touhy needle is directed cephalad. A 5-cm to 10-cm catheter is threaded into the spinal subarachnoid space and secured in the lumbar fascia with plastic clips. A small incision is placed at the entry point of the catheter, and the shunt system is tunneled around to the abdomen. A small jump incision may be necessary sometimes.

The peritoneal catheter is introduced into the peritoneal cavity via either trocar or minilaparotomy (3,5).

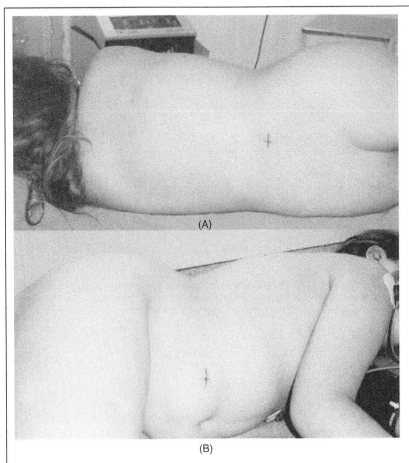

(A)

(B)

Figure 2   (**A**) The patient in lateral decubitus position for LP shunting and note the lumbar skin incision, and (**B**) operative photograph showing the abdominal incision site.

REFERENCES

1. Iantooca MR, Drake JM. Cerebrospinal fluid shunts. In: Albright AL, Pollack IF, Adelson PD, eds Operative Techniques in Pediatric Neurosurgery. New York: Thieme, 2001: 3–14.
2. Marlin AE. Shunting. In: Cheek WR, ed. Atlas of Pediatric Neurosurgery. Philadelphia, PA: WB Saunders Company, 1996:65–77.
3. Ruge HR, McLone DG. Cerebrospinal fluid diversion procedures. In: Apuzzo MLJ, ed. Brain Surgery: Complication Avoidance and Management. New York: Churchill Livingstone Inc, 1993:1463–1494.
4. Gaskill SJ, Marlin AE. Shunting techniques: Ventriculopleural shunts. Tech Neurosurg 2002; 17: 206–207.
5. Moss SD. Shunting techniques: Lumboperitoneal shunts. Tech Neurosurg 2002; 17:216–218.

Image-Guided Shunt Placement

Conor Mallucci

Department of Neurosurgery, The Walton Centre for Neurology and Neurosurgery, Liverpool, U.K.

Both frame-based and frameless neuronavigation systems have been used to guide the placement of ventricular catheters. However, most image guidance systems require rigid head fixation with pins. This has limited the application of neuronavigation in shunt surgery due to the added invasiveness, increased operating time and costs, and the particular risk of pin fixation in infants. Most reports of stereotactic placement of shunts are in the setting of slit ventricles, idiopathic intracranial hypertension, or disordered anatomy, where accurate cannulation of the ventricle is difficult freehand.

However, the potential advantages for routine shunt surgery have not been elucidated. The rate of shunt malfunction is 4% to 5% per year with up to 40% failure rate in children at one year (1,2). The majority of episodes of mechanical shunt failure are due to proximal catheter obstruction (3). Furthermore, in blind catheter placement, up to 5% of catheters are misplaced outside the ventricle. Therefore, optimal proximal catheter positioning under direct vision or real-time accurate navigation, particularly away from the choroid plexus, would seem to be the ultimate goal. Initial interest in placement of the ventricular catheter under direct vision dissipated following the endoscopic shunt placement trial (4), during which 393 children were randomized to shunt insertion either with an endoscope or without an endoscope. All children had ventriculomegaly, the endoscope was used down the lumen of the ventricular catheter to guide placement away from the choroids plexus. The primary outcome measure was time to shunt failure and there was no significant difference demonstrated between the endoscopic and nonendoscopic group. In addition, the secondary outcome measure of placement of the catheter away from the choroid plexus, as seen on the first postoperative CT imaging, again failed to show a difference between each group, with 67% sited away from choroid in the endoscopically placed group and 61% in the nonendoscopic group. The authors concluded that there was little to recommend endoscopic shunt placement.

Electromagnetic technology (Medtronic AXIEM™, Louisville, CO) enables frameless, pinless image guidance with real-time navigation at depth, as a direct line of sight between transmitter and receiver coil are not required. The introduction of stick-on reference frames further reduces the invasiveness of the guidance system, as a separate incision is not required (Fig. 1). Electromagnetic neuronavigation utilizes a low-frequency magnetic field for spatial localization. This has many advantages over standard optical navigation. Rigid head fixation is not required as the reference frame is attached to the skull and the head can be repositioned at any point after registration. The optimal entry point, target point, trajectory, and catheter length are planned preoperatively (Fig. 2). The electromagnetic stylet can then be used as an introducer inside ventricular catheters. This device uniquely is actively tracked at the tip, rather than a derived value common to other spacial localizing techniques; therefore, accurately directing catheter placement to a pre-planned target in real time (Fig. 3). Optimal placement at the target point is then confirmed on postoperative imaging. In our institution, we have performed to date over 120 cranial neurosurgical procedures using electromagnetic image guidance. Over 60% of these cases are for CSF diversion, including shunt placement idiopathic intracranial hypertension, slit ventricles, Ommaya reservoir placement for drug administration, and external ventricular drain placement in traumatic brain injury. In addition, we have been increasingly placing routine shunts with ventriculomegaly using electromagnetic image guidance and have experienced no proximal shunt failures in this group.

Our early experience with electromagnetic-guided shunt placement demonstrates accuracy of placement with minimal addition to operative time. The absolute indications for image-guided shunt placement are IIH and slit ventricles; however, expanding these

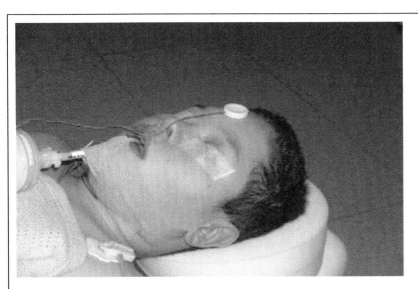

Figure 1 The stick-on reference electrode of the Axiem system obviates the need for pin fixation of the head and use of any screw-on reference instruments

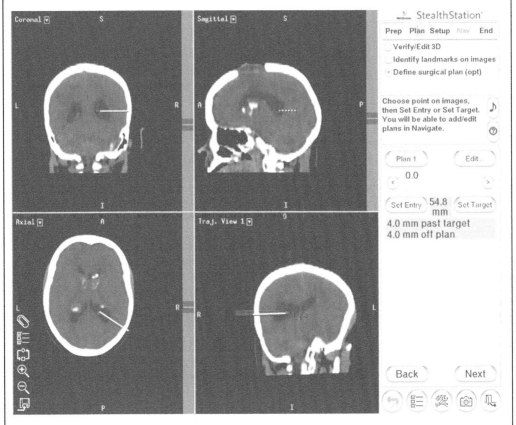

Figure 2 The use of image analysis software enables the clinician to plan the trajectory of shunt placement preoperatively.

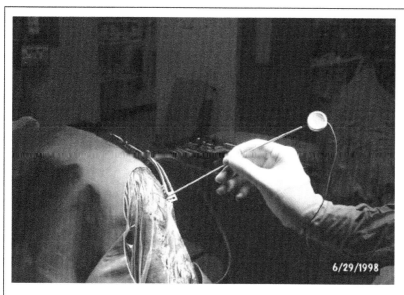

Figure 3 The electromagnetic stylet of the Medtronic Axiem system is used inside the shunt catheter, instead of an introducer, and guides shunt placement.

applications to all routine shunt surgery is possible with the noninvasive electromagnetic system. Long-term outcome in terms of shunt survival and the associated overall reduction in cost of multiple revision surgery is yet to be determined. A multicenter randomized trial of image-guided shunt placement versus blind placement would be required to demonstrate any reduction in the overall incidence of proximal shunt failure.

REFERENCES

1. Drake JM, Kestle JR, Milner R, et al. Randomized trial of cerebrospinal fluid shunt valve design in pediatric hydrocephalus. Neurosurgery 1998; 43:294–303; discussion 303–295.
2. Kestle J, Drake J, Milner R, et al. Long-term follow-up data from the Shunt Design Trial. Pediatr Neurosurg 2000; 33:230–236.
3. Sainte-Rose C, Piatt JH, Renier D, et al. Mechanical complications in shunts. Pediatr Neurosurg 1991; 17:2–9.
4. Kestle JR, Drake JM, Cochrane DD, et al. Lack of benefit of endoscopic ventriculoperitoneal shunt insertion: A multicenter randomized trial. J Neurosurg 2003; 98:284–290.

25 Shunt Complications

Patrick W. Hanlo† and R. G. J. Bloemen

Rudolf Magnus Institute of Neuroscience, Department of Neurosurgery, University Medical Center, Utrecht, The Netherlands

W. Peter Vandertop

Department of Neurosurgery, Neurosurgical Center Amsterdam, Amsterdam, The Netherlands

INTRODUCTION

Implantation of a CSF shunt is frequently used for the treatment of hydrocephalus. The functional survival time of a CSF shunt, however, is often limited by complications such as infection and mechanical failure. Shunt survival has improved over the last decades but still remains far from satisfactory. Shunt survival rates of 71% and 62% at one and five years, respectively, have recently been reported (1). Shunt complications not only carry a substantial risk of mortality and morbidity, but also necessitate multiple shunt revision surgeries in hydrocephalus patients. Because these shunt complications generate considerable health care costs, prevention of these complications is an important research field in shunt development. Rapid recognition, diagnosis, and treatment of shunt complications are paramount in minimizing the damaging effects of these shunt complications. However, there are no generally accepted guidelines in diagnosing and treating shunt complications. This chapter reviews recent literature on this subject and proposes recommendations for the diagnosis, clinical management, and prevention of shunt complications.

SHUNT INFECTION

Cerebrospinal fluid (CSF) shunt infection is a common complication in patients with hydrocephalus. Reported incidences vary substantially in recent studies and range from 0.57% to 27.3% (2–16). This may reflect not only actual variations between the different settings and populations, but may also, in part, be explained by different methods for calculating the incidence of shunt infection. Infection rates can be calculated as the number of infections per patient or per procedure. Infection rates per patient will be higher than infection rates per procedure, as many patients will have multiple procedures and therefore can experience multiple episodes of shunt infection. In addition, differences in the definition of shunt infection influences infection rates.

Shunt infection remains an important complication of shunt therapy in hydrocephalus patients, as it is associated with substantial risks of morbidity and mortality (15,17). The number of shunt infections has been found to be an independent predictor of death in pediatric patients requiring CSF shunts [hazard ratio (HR): 1.66, 95% CI: 1.02–2.72] (18).

The management of CSF shunt infections is not standardized and there is no consensus on optimal diagnostic and therapeutic strategies.

Pathogenesis

Table 1 shows the pathogens identified in 100 CSF cultures in patients with infected shunts compiled from six different studies (7,13,19–22). Although this may not represent the exact distribution of pathogens due to differences in the studied populations, it does show that most infections are caused by organisms that normally inhabit the skin, such as *Staphylococci*. This has led to the assumption that most shunt infections are caused by colonization during surgery (23,24). The fact that most infections occur within about four months following shunt insertion (7–11,25) reinforces this hypothesis. The source of the contamination is often thought to be the patient's own skin flora, although other sources, such as surgical personnel via breached gloves, have also been implicated (9).

---

†Deceased.

Table 1 Pathogens in 100 Positive CSF Cultures in Shunt Infection

Pathogen	No. of samples						
	Schuhman et al. (26)	Enger et al. (6)	Kanev et al. (8)	McClinton et al. (27)	Turgut et al. (25)	Lan et al. (10)	Total
Staphylococcus epidermidis	18	7	5	4	6		40
Staphylococcus aureus	7	1	1	4	6	1	20
Coagulase-negative *Staphylococcus*	2			1	3	6	12
Pseudomonas aeruginosa	1				3	1	5
Haemophilus influenzae			1	3			4
Candida albicans		2			1	1	4
Enterococcus faecalis	3						3
Propionibacterium acnes	2			1			3
Enterobacter cloacae					1	1	2
Streptococcus Group D						1	1
Escherichia coli						1	1
Neisseria meningitidis	1						1
Streptococcus Group B					1		1
Klebsiella pneumonia					1		1
Corynebacterium diphtheriae	1						1
Acinetobacter baumannii						1	1
Total number of positive cultures	35	10	7	13	22	13	100

Other less-common causes include shunt infection secondary to peritonitis (e.g., appendicitis), hematogenous contamination of a distant bacterial focus (e.g., otitis media), and gastrointestinal perforation of the distal catheter (24,28,29). These mechanisms are seen more frequently in late shunt infections and are usually caused by different pathogens, such as *Enterobacteriaceae*, *Streptococci*, and *Haemophilus influenzae* (15,29).

Many of the pathogens associated with shunt infections, especially coagulase negative *Staphylococci*, form biofilms, that is, organized communities of bacteria embedded in a slime-like matrix. This enables bacteria to adhere strongly to surfaces, including CSF shunts and provides high resistance against antimicrobial therapy (30,31,32). Furthermore, irregularities on the shunt surface may act as sites for bacterial adherence (21). Removal of the shunt system is often the only effective treatment option.

Risk Factors

Various risk factors for shunt infection have been identified in recent studies (Table 2). Young age at initial shunt placement, previous shunt infection, and the need for an initial shunt to be placed (as apposed to a shunt revision) appear to be preoperative risk factors for CSF shunt infections (3,6,7,9,10,15,16,33). Possible intraoperative risk factors include exposure of the shunt to breached surgical gloves, intraoperative use of neuroendoscope, and limited experience of the surgeon (5,9,11), although recent literature has been contradictory on the latter two (6,8). Finally, postoperative CSF leakage appears to be a major risk factor for shunt infection (9).

Therefore great care should be taken to minimize manual contact with the shunt system during surgery as well as to avoid a postoperative CSF leak, especially in high-risk patients, that is, young children and patients with prior shunt infection. Further studies should examine whether limiting the use of neuroendoscopes for technically difficult shunt implantations results in a reduction of shunt infections.

Table 2 Risk Factors for Shunt Infections

Risk factor	Hazard ratio	95% CI	References
Patient prematurity (<40 weeks' gestation)	4.72	1.71–13.06	(9)
Premature birth	4.81	2.19–10.87	(11)
Decreasing age in years	1.04	1.01–1.08	(11)
Age under 4 months	1.81	1.16–2.84	(15)
Antenatal diagnosis	2.23	1.13–4.4	(15)
Myelomeningocele[a]	2.14	1.37–3.36	(15)
Posthemorrhagic[a]	1.98	1.29–3.06	(15)
Previous shunt infection	3.83	2.40–6.13	(11)
Intraoperative use of a neuroendoscope	1.58	1.01–2.50	(11)
Exposure to breached surgical gloves	1.07	1.02–1.12	(9)
Postoperative CSF leak	19.16	6.96–52.91	(9)
Experience of surgeon	na	na	(5)

[a]Refers to the rate of infection for the total number of shunt operations. Although myelomeningocele and posthemorrhagic hydrocephalus were not significantly associated with infection after the first shunt insertion, these were very significantly associated with the overall risk of infection because of an increased risk during shunt revisions.

Diagnosis of Shunt Infection

Recognizing a shunt infection may be difficult for it can manifest itself in a variety of ways, ranging from only a mild fever (34,35) to severe sepsis and sudden death (25). Diagnosing a shunt infection is further complicated by the lack of generally accepted diagnostic criteria, which also makes it hard to compare the literature on this subject. Most authors consider positive CSF cultures to be the gold standard for shunt infection (10,26,27,36); however, false positive (contamination), false negative (previous antimicrobial therapy), and late positive cultures (so-called low-grade infections) do occur (36,37).

Other authors have included pyrexia, abdominal or neurological symptoms (4), CSF pleocytosis (6,11,16,25), surgical wound infection, bacteremia (in ventriculoatrial shunts), or peritoneal infection (in ventriculoperitoneal shunts) (9) to be diagnostic for shunt infections. Only one study has differentiated between internal and external shunt infections, indicating whether infection occurred at the luminal or adluminal surface of the shunt (7).

Clinical Features

Patients can present with a variety of signs and symptoms depending on the location of the infection and the type of shunt being used. Clinical features can be divided into acute and chronic signs. Acute shunt infection may present itself with signs of wound infection, meningitis, ventriculitis, or peritonitis (less common). Chronic (or late) shunt infection may present with signs of peritonitis, abdominal pseudocysts, or septicemia.

Wound infections usually cause fever and reddening of the incision site and/or shunt tract. With progression, discharge of pus from the incision and exposure of the shunt may be seen as the wound breaks down. Patients with meningitis or ventriculitis often present with fever, headache, irritability, neck stiffness, or nuchal rigidity. Peritonitis manifests itself with fever, anorexia, vomiting, and abdominal tenderness. Pseudocysts sometimes present as an abdominal mass only. Signs of shunt obstruction/increased intracranial pressure, such as headache, nausea, vomiting, bulging fontanelle, papilledema, or lethargy, can be present. In addition, infected ventriculoatrial shunt can cause septicemia, endocarditis, shunt nephritis, or other manifestations of immune complex disease, for example, arthralgia or rash (23).

Nonetheless, shunt infection can be hard to recognize as it can present itself with subtle or nonspecific signs. Fever is seen most frequently (Table 3) (10,25,27), but can initially be mild. (35) However, progression can be fulminant (34). Therefore, physicians must be highly suspicious of shunt infection to avoid unnecessary delays.

Blood Tests

Shunt infections can be insidious and present only with mildly raised or normal white blood cell (WBC) counts (24,35), whereas serum CRP (C-reactive protein) levels do seem to be sensitive in

Table 3 Clinical Presentations of Shunt Infection in 35 Children

Symptoms	Number of patients (%)
Fever	27 (77.1)
Vomiting	24 (68.5)
Seizure	15 (42.8)
Headache	4 (11.4)
Fever and vomiting	19 (54.2)
Vomiting and seizure	11 (31.4)
Fever and seizure	6 (17.1)
Fever, vomiting, and seizure	9 (25.7)
Fever, vomiting, seizure, and headache	2 (5.7)
Hyperemia of the shunt tract	4 (11.4)
Specific physical examination findings:	
Meningeal irritation signs	7 (20)
Abdominal distension	2 (5.7)
Fontanel distension	7 (20)
Septic appearance	1 (2.8)

Source: Adapted from Ref. (25).

shunt infection. Schuhman et al. (26) compared WBC counts and CRP levels of 84 investigations in 59 patients suspected of harboring infected shunts and 38 control patients. Although the mean WBC count was slightly higher in the infected shunt group (patients with suspected shunt infection, with a positive CSF culture), the data ranges overlapped too much to allow for diagnostic separation. A serum CRP level of more than 7 mg/L, however, was highly sensitive in determining the presence of an infected shunt with a sensitivity of 97.1%, a specificity of 73.5%, a positive predictive value of 72.3%, and a negative predictive value of 97.3%. If cases were excluded in which there was an obvious reason for CRP elevation other than shunt infection, the specificity and positive predictive value were 87.8% and 87.2%, respectively. The probability of missing a shunt infection in patients with a CRP level less than 7 mg/L was only 2.7%. The authors suggested that evaluating serum CRP levels before the shunt is tapped could reduce the number of shunt taps by approximately 45%.

Lan et al. (10) also found a significant difference in CRP levels between patients with shunt infection and patients with shunt malfunction or no shunt pathology. Using a serum CRP threshold of more than 100 mg/L, they found much lower sensitivity and positive predictive values of 40% and 36%, respectively. Specificity and negative predictive value were both 95%. Differences in selection criteria, cohort sizes, applied CRP thresholds, and study design may explain these somewhat contradictory results.

Blood cultures can be positive in shunt infection (25), especially in ventriculoatrial shunt infections (38). However, interpretation of positive blood cultures can be hard in the absence of obvious signs of CSF infection, as common contaminants are indistinguishable from the causative bacteria (23). Alternatively, anti-*Staphylococcus epidermidis* titre (ASET) can be used to diagnose ventriculoatrial (VA) shunt infection caused by this pathogen. Finally, immune complex disease may be confirmed by low complement fractions, indicating complement consumption.

A number of studies have evaluated the value of clinical signs and laboratory findings in diagnosing shunt infection (10,26,27). Although limited in number and cohort sizes, these studies identified several predictors of shunt infection (Table 4).

CSF Examination

McClinton et al. (27) have investigated the relationship between clinical features, CSF variables, and shunt infection or malfunction. CSF eosinophils of 5% or more had a positive and negative predictive value of 96% and 15%, respectively, for shunt pathology (either infection or malfunction). A CSF WBC count of more than $100/mm^3$, CSF neutrophils of more than 10%, and a history of fever were all predictive of shunt infection. However, positive predictive values

Table 4 Predictors of Shunt Infection

Variable(s)	Sensitivity (%)	Specificity (%)	Positive predictive value (%)	Negative predictive value (%)	References
History of fever	75	87	45	96	(27)
History of fever	60	85	24	96	(10)
History of seizure attack	40	87	19	95	(10)
Serum CRP >7 mg/L	97.1	73.5	72.3	97.3	(26)
Serum CRP >10 mg/dL	40	95	36	95	(10)
CSF WBC >100/mm^3	55	91	46	93	(27)
CSF WBC >100/mm^3	60	96	55	97	(10)
CSF neutrophils >10%	83	85	45	97	(27)
CSF neutrophils >10%	90	85	33	99	(10)
CSF protein >50 mg/dL	80	84	42	98	(10)
CSF glucose <40 mg/dL	60	93	40	97	(10)
CSF WBC > 100/mm^3 and CSF neutrophils >10%	55	97	75	93	(27)
History of fever and CSF neutrophils >10%	64	99	93	95	(27)

were quite low, although combining these predictors improved their positive predictive values somewhat (Table 4).

In a similar study, CSF leukocytosis, CSF neutrophilia, and a history of fever were identified as predictors of shunt infection, as well as CSF protein levels of more than 50 mg/dL, CSF glucose levels of less than 40 mg/dL, and a history of seizure(s) (Table 4) (20).

Schuhman et al. (26), on the other hand, failed to find a single CSF parameter with a diagnostic potential for shunt infection. Mean counts of nucleated cells did differ significantly between the different patient groups, but there was an enormous overlap and no threshold could be defined that would have allowed separation between groups. Glucose, protein, and CSF-CRP levels all did not differ between the patient groups suspected of having shunt infection (positive CSF culture group versus negative CSF culture group). Gram stains were only positive in 54.3% of shunt infection cases, but were 100% specific.

Cultures

Positive CSF culture is often considered the definitive proof of shunt infection (10,26,27,36). In addition, positive cultures from sites related to the shunt, such as the surgical wound (external shunt infection), blood, or peritoneal fluid, are also considered by some to be diagnostic for shunt infection (7,9). Often the infecting organism can be identified and its antibiotic susceptibility determined. In some cases, culture results may assist in identifying an underlying cause for the infection; for example, the finding of bacterial flora should raise suspicion of a gastrointestinal perforation of the distal catheter (24). However, using cultures as a diagnostic tool to guide therapy presents difficulties that principally arise from the delay for results. In one study (26), 40% of CSF cultures took longer than one day to become positive and 20% did not turn positive until Day 4. Certain pathogens (such as anaerobic bacteria including *Propionibacterium* sp.) are notorious for delayed growth in culture and late positive results (24,36). Furthermore, as these organisms are common contaminants, positive (broth) cultures may not reflect a true shunt infection and repeated CSF culturing may be necessary (37). Also, the culturing of biofilm bacteria has proven to be difficult and can result in massive underestimates or a false diagnosis of sterility (31). To overcome these problems, polymerase chain reaction might be an attractive, highly sensitive, and rapid modality for the detection of shunt infection in the future (36).

Imaging

Imaging is of limited use in diagnosing shunt infection. Head CT or MRI may show signs of ventriculitis, meningitis, or shunt obstruction (39). Abdominal imaging may reveal a pseudocyst, most commonly seen in low-grade shunt infections, or gastrointestinal perforation (28,38).

To summarize, patients with shunt infections are more likely to have raised serum WBC counts and CRP levels. Subsequent CSF examination will often reveal high WBC levels, a high percentage of neutrophils, high protein levels, and low glucose levels (10,26,27). A positive Gram stain is seen in about 50% of shunt infection cases (7,26). These findings can assist physicians in clinical decision making, when culture results are unreliable or delayed.

In addition, CSF examination appears to be of little or no benefit in patients with low serum CRP levels. By evaluating serum CRP levels before performing CSF examination, unnecessary shunt taps may be avoided (26).

Treatment of Shunt Infection

Treatment generally consists of intravenous antibiotics and removal of the shunt, followed by a period of external ventricular drainage (EVD) (3,8,11,24–26,36), but there have been very few trials comparing different treatment regimes.

Antibiotic Treatment

Empirical antibiotic therapy should consist of an agent that is able to reach adequate CSF concentrations and is effective against most common pathogens. Vancomycin, third-generation cephalosporins, and rifampin are often used (3,8,11,25,38). Owing to its lipophilicity, rifampin is able to achieve substantial CSF concentration (CSF/serum ratio of up to 56%) even in the absence of inflammation. In contrast, CSF penetration of cephalosporins and vancomycin, both hydrophilic agents, is greatly dependent on the state of the blood–brain barrier (40), with reported CSF/serum ratios for vancomycin of 48% and 18% in patients with and without meningitis, respectively (41).

While some consider intraventricular administration of antibiotics to be controversial (38), because of concerns about possible toxicity, others (42) consider it necessary to reach adequate antibiotic concentrations in the CSF. However, CSF antibiotic concentrations vary quite a lot between patients after intraventricular administration and are dependent on the volume of the CSF compartment and the rate of CSF drainage. These factors should be considered to ensure a safe and effective CSF antibiotic concentration (42).

Pfausler et al. (43) compared intravenous and intraventricular administration of vancomycin for drain-related ventriculitis in adult patients with temporary EVDs. Intraventricular administration of a single dose of 10 mg vancomycin per day resulted in CSF concentrations well over the recommended minimum inhibitory concentration level of 5 μg/mL for most part of the day. Maximum CSF levels were 565.58 ± 168.71 μg/mL, 1 hour after intraventricular administration, minimum levels were 3.74 ± 0.66 μg/mL, 21 hours after intraventricular administration. CSF concentrations in the group receiving 500 mg vancomycin intravenously four times a day rarely reached the recommended minimum inhibitory concentration (the highest mean CSF concentrations were 1.73 ± 0.4 μg/mL).

The authors suggested that the inflammation of the meninges and ventricular ependyma is usually mild to moderate in *staphylococcal* ventriculitis; CSF penetration of vancomycin after intravenous administration was therefore substantially less than the 48% reported previously in patients with meningitis (41). Nevertheless, both methods were effective in achieving CSF sterility and no toxicity was observed. However, concerns were expressed about the extremely low serum levels of vancomycin after intraventricular administration of 10 mg, which may increase the risk of vancomycin-resistance development. The authors concluded that intraventricular administration of vancomycin may be of particular value in patients in whom intravenous administration is relatively contraindicated (e.g., those with renal insufficiency or multiorgan dysfunction). Finally, using a daily dosage of 10 mg (10 mg once per day intraventricularly) instead of 2000 mg (4 times 500 mg a day intravenously) also has considerable economic advantages.

After the causative microorganism is identified, antibiotic therapy may be altered according to its susceptibility.

Surgical Treatment

In a thorough decision analysis, three treatment approaches have been compared with regard to cure rate, morbidity, and mortality (18). The analysis included 17 studies (publication dates:

1967–1995) that reported at least one of the following treatment modalities: intravenous antibiotics with or without intrashunt antibiotics with removal of the shunt and EVD; intravenous antibiotics with or without intrashunt antibiotics with removal of the shunt and immediate shunt replacement; and intravenous antibiotics with or without intrashunt antibiotics. The combined cure rates were 87.7% for the EVD strategy, 64.4% for the immediate replacement strategy, and 33.5% for the antibiotics only strategy. The analysis confirmed that the EVD strategy was the superior strategy, as long as the complication rate for EVD placement was less than 35.8%. As this complication rate is exceedingly high, the authors concluded that the EVD strategy should be considered the standard treatment for CSF shunt infections. In cases in which an EVD complication rate of more than 35.8% is anticipated or the EVD strategy is not feasible, shunt removal and immediate replacement should be attempted. The antibiotic only strategy should only be considered as a last resort in patients who are unfit for surgery.

However, it has been suggested that community-acquired meningitis caused by *Streptococcus pneumoniae*, *H. influenzae*, or *Neisseria meningitidis* can be treated without shunt removal (23,38). However, no recent studies were found that confirmed this, though the limited number of available patients would make any such study hard to conduct.

Duration of Treatment
The duration of antibiotic treatment and period of EVD vary substantially in recent studies. Some authors report reinserting the shunt after CSF has been sterile for a certain period of time (ranging from 3 to 21 days) (3,8,26,38). However, the duration of antibiotic treatment after CSF sterility that has been achieved does not appear to be related with the incidence of reinfection (44). Conversely, failure to achieve CSF sterility after a substantial period of treatment (e.g., 10 days) may indicate infection of the extraventricular drain, in which case the drain should be replaced.

As cultures can be unreliable during antibiotic treatment, resolution of CSF pleocytosis has been used as a criterion for reinserting a shunt (11,23,28). Also, serum CRP has been suggested as an indicator of clearance of a shunt infection, as patients with an elevated serum CRP level of more than 7 mg/L at the time of shunt reinsertion show a reinfection rate of 43% compared to 11.5% in patients with serum CRP levels of less than 7 mg/L at the time of shunt reinsertion (26). These results, however, did not reach statistical significance due to the limited number of patients involved.

The duration of antibiotic treatment and EVD must be long enough to minimize the risk of a recurrent infection of the new shunt, although secondary infections from a drain that is kept in place longer than necessary must also be avoided (23,45).

Abdominal Pseudocysts
A rare complication of peritoneal shunting is the formation of a collection of CSF that persists in the peritoneal cavity at the distal catheter tip. These abdominal pseudocysts (APC) can be difficult to treat. A recurrence rate of 50% was found in a series of 36 patients (with 64 APCs). The rate of infection was 23% for all APCs (28). However, APCs are also seen in so-called low-grade infection, in which CSF cultures are often negative. Therefore, a high suspicion of low-grade shunt infection must be maintained in the case of APC, even when cultures appear to be negative.

Treatment of noninfected APCs with immediate repositioning of the distal catheter led to high immediate recurrences, suggesting an inability of the peritoneum to accommodate CSF drainage in about 50% of those who present with APC for an unknown period of time. When adhesions prevent the surgeon from finding a suitable position for repositioning of the distal catheter, or when the patient has a recurrent APC, it is recommended that the distal catheter is placed in either the pleural space, the atrium, or the gallbladder. Infection will first have to be treated by removal of the entire shunt and a period of EVD, as stated above, before assessing the suitability of the abdomen (28,46).

Prevention of Shunt Infection
Careful planning and timing of shunt procedures, the use of antibiotic impregnated shunts, and strict perioperative measures (such as thorough antiseptic preparation, the use of prophylactic

antibiotics, minimizing theater traffic, double gloving, minimizing manual contact with the shunt, separating skin/nonskin instruments) and appropriate wound care may all contribute in minimizing shunt infections (2–4,7,8,12,13,17,21,47,48).

However, the most effective way to prevent shunt infection is to not have a shunt. Alternative surgical procedures, such as third ventriculostomy, must be considered whenever possible.

Recommendations

The following recommendations are based on both the literature discussed above and the expert opinions of the authors (see Appendix A for diagnostic and treatment algorithm for suspected shunt infection):

- A generally accepted definition and diagnostic criteria of CSF shunt infection must be developed, as this is of great value in both clinical and research settings. We propose to use the following definition: "A shunt infection is an infection of the shunt system (both intra- and extra-luminal) causing symptoms of possible shunt infection (see above), raised serum CRP (>7 mg/L) combined with either positive CSF gram stains, CSF pleocytosis (CSF WBC > 100/mm^3) or erythema over the track of the peritoneal catheter."
- Symptoms of CSF shunt infections are often subtle or unspecific. Physicians should be highly suspicious of shunt infection in all shunted patients presenting with unexplained general complaints. A low threshold for further blood testing should be maintained, particularly in premature infants and young children, who have had a shunt implanted recently or have experienced previous episodes of shunt infection.
- CSF evaluation should be considered in "symptomatic" patients, especially when CRP levels are raised.
- When cultures are delayed or unreliable, positive Gram stains, high WBC counts with a high percentage of neutrophils in CSF examination indicate shunt infection.
- Shunt infection should be treated with appropriate intravenous and/or intraventricular antibiotics, removal of the shunt, and EVD.
- Cultures may be unreliable during antibiotic treatment. Treatment should, therefore, persist until CSF sterility is achieved and the inflammatory response appears to be settling (normalization of serum CRP and CSF WBC levels).
- Failure to achieve CSF sterility after 10 days of treatment may indicate infection of the extraventricular drain, in which case the drain should be replaced.
- Careful planning and timing of shunt procedures, the use of antibiotic impregnated shunts, and strict perioperative measures, such as thorough antiseptic preparation, the use of prophylactic antibiotics, minimizing theatre traffic, double gloving, minimizing manual contact with the shunt, separating skin/nonskin instruments, and appropriate wound care all contribute in minimizing shunt infections.

SHUNT DYSFUNCTION

Shunt dysfunction remains a large problem in the treatment of hydrocephalus with one-year failure rates ranging from 15% to 48% (1,49–52). As alternative treatment such as a third ventriculostomy is not always possible for the treatment of hydrocephalus, many patients with a CSF shunt require multiple shunt operations throughout their lives. Swift diagnosis and treatment are imperative to reduce mortality and morbidity in this patient group. Moreover, effective strategies for preventing shunt dysfunction will reduce the need for medical care and improve quality of life.

Pathogenesis

Shunt malfunction can have many causes, which can be classified anatomically and functionally (Table 5) (53,54). A main cause of shunt malfunction (about 60%) is obstruction of the ventricular catheter (55). This can result from obstruction by choroid plexus, brain parenchyma, deposition of blood, debris (Fig. 1), or bacterial colonization, which will cause underdrainage. CSF leakage at the proximal catheter may cause secondary CSF cysts to form in an intracranial or extracranial compartment causing subdural, subgaleal, or subcutaneous perishunt compensatory CSF loculation.

Table 5   Classification of Shunt Malfunction

Type	Cause	Common time of presentation
Obstruction	Ventricular catheter obstruction	Any
	Shunt valve obstruction	Any
	Distal catheter obstruction	Any
Mechanical shunt failure	Fracture	Late
	Disconnection	Early
	Migration	Early
	Misplacement of ventricular or distal catheter	Early
Overdrainage	Extraaxial fluid collections	Early
	Slit ventricle syndrome	Late
Loculation		Late
Abdominal complications	Ascites	Any
	Pseudocyst	Late
	Perforation	Late

Sources: Based on Browd et al. (53,54).

Valve failure may result from mechanical failure; the valve's performance may be impaired by deposition of blood, sodium chloride crystals, debris, subcutaneous fibrous adhesions or bacteria (56). Choosing an inappropriate valve for the patient's intracranial dynamic properties can obviously result in over- or underdrainage as well. The protein content of CSF, however, appears to have little effect on valve function (57).

Distal failure is the second most common cause of shunt malfunction (20–25%) (55); it can be caused by obstruction by omentum, peritoneum, or distal adhesions. In addition, misplacement or migration of catheter tubing to sites that do not allow for CSF flow [e.g., preperitoneally (Fig. 2), intestine, or scrotum] and the formation of abdominal pseudocysts may interfere with CSF dispersion. Furthermore, fracture, disconnection (Fig. 3), kinking, and even the formation of knots in the catheter tubing may impair the functionality and patency of the catheter and cause underdrainage (58,59).

Overdrainage may cause a rapid decrease in ventricular volume resulting in subdural hemorrhage (Fig. 4), especially in the elderly. Prolonged overdrainage predisposes patients to develop slit ventricles, frequently resulting in a slit ventricle syndrome (Fig. 5). Similarly,

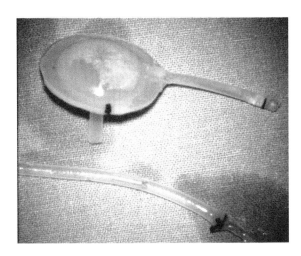

Figure 1   Occlusion of the valve chamber and distal catheter by deposition of debris. *Source*: Courtesy of A. Aschoff, Heidelberg, Germany.

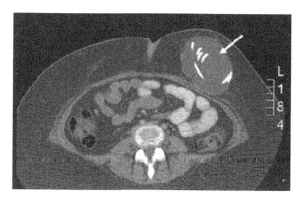

Figure 2 Axial abdominal computed tomogram illustrating shunt tubing coiled preperitoneally with associated cerebrospinal fluid collection in the subcutaneous tissues. *Source*: From Ref. 54.

craniosynostosis secondary to the placement of a CSF shunt is another complication associated with overdrainage and slit ventricles, particularly in infants (55).

In addition, immunological responses may be involved in shunt malfunctions, as higher rates of protein deposition around the shunt tubing and the formation of antibodies against these autologous proteins appear to be related to shunt malfunction (60).

An allergic reaction to the silicone, used in most shunt systems, can be a rare cause of sterile shunt dysfunction. These cases often present with multiple episodes of shunt dysfunction or other complications before the etiology becomes clear and a hypoallergic shunt system is inserted (20,48). Possible clues to an allergic cause of shunt dysfunction include an increased number of peripheral eosinophils, serum immunoglobulin E, and histological infiltration of eosinophils in tissues around the shunt tubing (e.g., in pseudocysts) (20).

In addition to the mechanisms described in Table 5, ventriculoatrial shunts may cause specific complications such as thrombophlebitis, thrombosis, thromboembolisms (pulmonary embolisms), pulmonary hypertension, and shunt nephritis (61–64).

Risk Factors

Various studies have been conducted in recent years to identify factors that predispose patients to develop shunt dysfunction. Risk factors that have been identified include young age at initial shunt placement, the time interval since previous surgical revision, the cause of the hydrocephalus (IVH-related, postmeningitic, and tumor-related), and the use of a shunt system either without a valve or with a low-pressure valve (Table 6) (52,65–67).

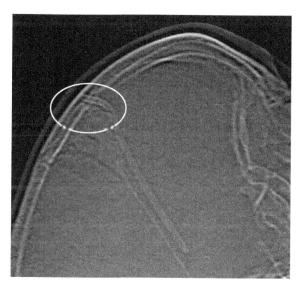

Figure 3 Proximal disconnection in a ventriculoperitoneal shunt.

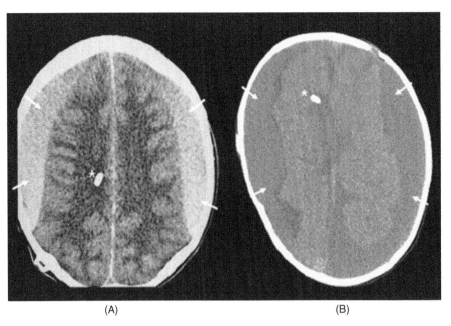

(A)   (B)

Figure 4   Axial noncontrast head computed tomograms depicting examples of shunt overdrainage with subsequent development of extra axial fluid collections. (**A**) Bilateral frontoparietal hyperdense extraaxial fluid collections (*arrows*) consistent with acute subdural hematoma. Asterisk (*) denotes ventricular catheter. (**B**) Bilateral hemispheric hypodense fluid collections consistent with either cerebrospinal fluid or chronic subdural hematoma. Asterisk (*) denotes ventricular catheter. *Source*: From Ref. (31).

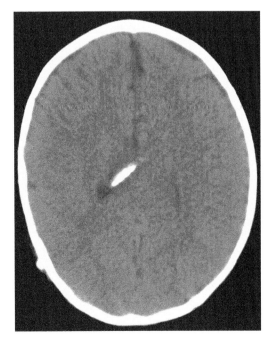

Figure 5   Slit ventricle syndrome as a complication of shunt therapy.

Table 6 Hazard Ratios, Confidence Intervals, and Probability Values Obtained in the First Three Failure Levels of Shunt Failure

Risk factor	Level 1[a]			Level 2[a]			Level 3[a]		
	HR	95% CI	p Value	HR	95% CI	p Value	HR	95% CI	p Value
Gap time of previous failure				1.72	1.28–2.30	<0.001	1.50	1.05–2.16	0.027
Age[b]									
<40 wk gestation	2.49	1.68–3.68	<0.001	1.59	0.93–2.74	0.096	1.71	1.05–2.79	0.032
40 wk gestation–1 yr	1.77	1.29–2.44	<0.001	1.33	0.84–2.11	0.22	0.90	0.57–1.42	0.65
Cause of hydrocephalus[c]									
Aquaductal stenosis	1.83	1.13–2.96	0.01	0.77	0.36–1.64	0.50		NS	
IVH	1.78	1.18–2.68	0.006	1.85	1.03–3.33	0.039			
Postmeningitis	2.08	1.26–3.44	0.004	2.32	1.19–4.54	0.014			
Myelomeningocele	1.95	1.34–2.85	<0.001	1.10	0.63–1.92	0.74			
Posttraumatic origin	2.80	1.39–5.64	0.004	1.86	0.67–5.18	0.23			
Tumor	2.33	1.48–3.68	<0.001	2.34	1.22–4.48	0.01			
Other	1.56	1.03–2.35	0.03	1.31	0.72–2.39	0.38			
VP compared with other shunt type	0.69	0.50–0.95	0.02		NS			NS	
Concurrent surgery	1.44	1.06–1.94	0.02		NS		1.89	1.01–3.53	0.047

[a] Shunt failure level = number of episodes of shunt failure experienced, level 1 = 1 episode of shunt infection experienced, level 2 = 2 episodes of shunt infection experienced, level 3 = 3 episodes of shunt infection experienced.

[b] Corrected for gestation, an age older than 1 year was chosen as the reference category.

[c] A congenital cause of hydrocephalus was the reference category.

Abbreviations: NS, not significant.

Source: From Ref. (67).

Diagnosis of Shunt Dysfunction

Clinical Features

Impaired function of a CSF shunt often results in the (re)appearance of symptoms of raised ICP such as headache, irritability, nausea, vomiting, progressive lethargy, and seizures. Physical examination may reveal ophthalmic abnormalities such as papillary edema and visual field disturbances, fluid accumulation over the ventricular insertion site or along the shunt tubing tract, discontinuities upon palpating the shunt tract or, in young children, a bulging fontanel, dilation of the veins on the surface of the cranium, separated sutures, increased head circumference, and downward shift in gaze (sunset eyes).

Shunt malfunction can also develop insidiously with only subtle signs such as changes in behavior or declining school performance. The clinical picture appears to be related to age. The characteristic features of hydrocephalus described above are seen more often in young children, whereas in young and middle-aged adults hydrocephalus often causes different complaints such as gait disturbances, headaches, urinary urgency, and cognitive dysfunction. Physical examination usually shows only minor signs such as minor gait changes and mildly abnormal Mini Mental State. This clinical picture and the discrepancy between symptoms and the subtlety of clinical signs are characteristic of the syndrome of hydrocephalus in young and middle-aged adults (SHYMA) (19). In adults who are shunted for normal pressure hydrocephalus (NPH) (Fig. 6), reappearance of the original symptoms of gait impairment, cognitive decline, and urinary incontinence or the appearance of "new" symptoms such as headache or delirium may indicate shunt malfunction (68,69).

More extensive oculomotor dysfunction is seen in the sylvian aqueduct syndrome, which is caused by existence of a pressure gradient across the periaqueductal gray matter and ventral tegmentum. It can be associated with more complex features such as parkinsonian syndrome, akinetic mutism, memory disturbances, staring gaze as a consequence of paralysis of the reflexes of fixation and pursuit, pyramidal signs, and coma. This clinical entity, also known as global rostral midbrain dysfunction, can be explained by the progressive involvement of anatomical structures located in upper midbrain (70). These symptoms can be seen in obstructive hydrocephalus due to aqueductal stenosis (preferably treated with third ventriculostomy), but appear more frequently in shunt malfunction than at the initial diagnosis of hydrocephalus because of the more rapid onset of ICP changes and consequent distortion of brain parenchyma (70).

In summary, shunt dysfunction may present itself with a variety of signs and symptoms, none however appear to be reliable predictors of raised ICP (71–73). Therefore, shunt dysfunction should be considered in any patient with a CSF shunt who presents with unexplained symptoms.

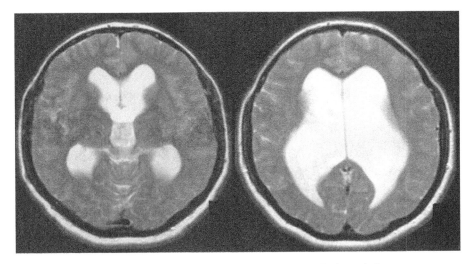

Figure 6   T2-weighted MRI scan of a patient with normal pressure hydrocephalus.

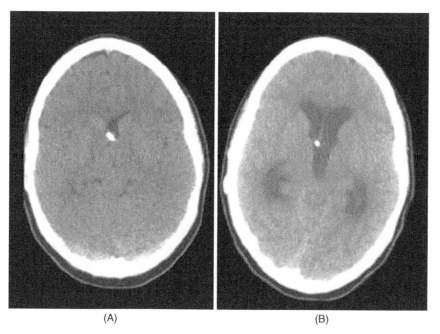

(A)   (B)

Figure 7 Axial noncontrast head computed tomograms revealing interval increase in the size of the ventricles from a baseline "well" scan (**A**) to a scan during a shunt failure (**B**). *Source*: From Ref. (54).

Imaging
CT imaging of the brain is an effective noninvasive way of detecting changes in ventricle size, provided baseline scans are available for comparison (Fig. 7) (71,74,75). Shunt dysfunction is rarely present in the absence of change in ventricle size (Table 7). CT scanning does, however, expose the patient to a considerable amount of radiation. Alternatively, rapid-sequence MRI can be used in elective evaluation of hydrocephalus. It produces images of good quality without exposing the patient to high levels of radiation (76).

In order to detect subtle changes in ventricular size, linear measurements of the ventricle relative to the brain, such as the bicaudate index, the Evans, fronto-occipital (FO) and ventricle-skull ratios (VSR), and the diagonal ventricular dimension (DVD) are often used. Of these linear measurements the VSR and DVD appear to be the most accurate indicators of increased CSF volume and raised ICP (73,74).

However, as computer programs, which are able to accurately determine the CSF volume from a series of two-dimensional CT or MRI studies, continue to improve and become more widely available, the linear measurements discussed above may become obsolete soon (77,78).

When brain imaging raises suspicion of shunt dysfunction, plain films of the shunt (shunt series) must be performed to exclude fractures or discontinuities of the shunt system (54).

Table 7 Accuracy of CT-Imaging and Shunt Series in Suspected Shunt Malfunction

Test	Sensitivity	Specificity	Positive predictive value	Negative predictive value	References
Head CT	83	76	55	93	(75)
Shunt series	20	98	75	78	(75)
Head CT or shunt series	88	74	55	95	(75)
Head CT	84	100	na	na	(71)

Demonstration of CSF Flow

In order to asses whether a shunt system is patent by determining if CSF is actually flowing through it, radionucleotide shuntograms can be made. By injection of radionucleotide into the reservoir, the patency of both the proximal (ventricular reflux or the ability to withdraw CSF freely) and distal shunt catheters can be investigated (assuming that the reservoir lies proximal to the shunt valve) (79,80). However, the actual shunt function is not completely assessed by demonstrating flow through the shunt system. In an attempt to evaluate shunt function further, dynamic shuntograms may be able to differentiate between slit ventricle syndrome and the syndrome of overdrainage and low intracranial pressure by measurements of the radionucleotide transit times (normal or low transit times indicating preexisting slit ventricles, rapid transit times indicating overdrainage). However, sensitivity, specificity, and predictive values of this method have not been stated (80).

Cooling CSF and using thermosensors or infrared cameras to detect flow of the cooled CSF was developed as a noninvasive, cheap, and fast method of assessing shunt function that is not connected to radiation (81). Despite these potential benefits, there have been very few studies on its accuracy in differentiating a functional from a nonfunctional shunt, leaving the accuracy of thermography to demonstrate CSF flow or to identify shunt obstruction (absent or reduced CSF flow) unclear.

Invasive ICP Measurements

The level of ICP is obviously an important parameter in diagnosing shunt dysfunction. Direct pressure measurement of the pressure of the CSF compartment by tapping the shunt, therefore, can be a useful diagnostic tool. However, many surgeons are reluctant to perform shunt taps because of the risk of causing a shunt infection. In addition, CSF pressure, measured at the shunt reservoir, may not always correspond with the true ICP or functionality of the shunt system. And as it provides only a "snapshot" of the level of ICP, normal values do not rule out the existence of abnormal ICP levels at different times.

Patients with shunt malfunction can be only minimally symptomatic or even asymptomatic. Accordingly, ICP may be normal in patients with shunt malfunction. Possible explanations for this are arrested hydrocephalus or compensatory CSF drainage to other extracranial sites, such as the subcutaneous tissue over the craniotomy site or through a functional subcutaneous fibrous tract around the shunt tubing (82). ICP monitoring, particularly during symptomatic episodes may show episodes of raised ICP in persistent hydrocephalus. Radionucleotide shuntograms may demonstrate a patent subcutaneous fibrous tract necessitating shunt revision (83).

In addition, pressure measurements using a shunt tap may be falsely low and may not correlate with the ICP in the presence of a partial proximal obstruction. Implantation of a separate reservoir, not in line with the shunt, provides a convenient access point to the CSF compartment that can be used for diagnostic (pressure measurements, CSF sampling) and therapeutic (emergency CSF drainage, intraventricular antibiotic administration) purposes. This strategy does not appear to affect the survival of the shunt and can provide accurate diagnostic information (84,85), although it is not universally popular as it necessitates a separate operation to the shunt insertion.

Infusion Tests

By infusion of artificial CSF into the patient's CSF compartment at a constant rate and measuring the subsequent changes in intracranial pressure, information can be gathered on the resistance of the CSF outflow system consisting of the shunt system and any remaining physiological CSF absorption capacity or compensatory mechanisms. Laboratory studies have shown that the end-equilibrium pressure in response to infusion at a constant rate correlates with the resistance of the shunt and therefore is a reliable indicator of shunt function (86). During infusion testing, pressure should not increase above the value given by the equation: *maximum end-equilibrium pressure < shunt operating pressure + {resistance of shunt × infusion rate} + 5 mm Hg* (the 5 mm Hg is a safety factor). Higher end-equilibrium pressure values indicate increased resistance of the shunt (i.e., shunt dysfunction).

Alternatively, CSF outflow resistance can be determined by infusing artificial CSF at increasing pressure levels and measuring the corresponding flow rates. CSF outflow resistance in shunted patients is mainly determined by the resistance of the shunt system and the intra-abdominal pressure. Resistances higher or lower than predicted are suggestive of shunt dysfunction (under- and overdrainage, respectively) (87,88).

Noninvasive Measurements of ICP

Measurement of anterior fontanelle pressure can be used in young children to accurately estimate the ICP. Direct measurement of anterior fontanelle pressure using the Rotterdam Teletransducer correlates well with invasively measured intraventricular pressure ($R = 0.96$–0.98) (89).

Several transcranial Doppler ultrasonography indices, such as the resistivity index (RI) and pulsatility index (PI), have been used to estimate ICP (90). However, the correlation between these indices and ICP is generally poor (91). Therefore, using a hydrodynamic model of the (cerebral) vascular system, a new Doppler index, the trans systolic time (TST), was defined (92). The trans systolic time is the width of the flow-curve halfway between the peak systolic blood flow velocity and the end-diastolic blood flow velocity. It is solely related to the relative changes in the flow velocity during the cardiac cycle, primarily a function of intracranial physical properties. Whereas the PI and RI are composed of actual values of the flow velocity, which are the result of both extra- and intracranial hemodynamic factors. The trans systolic time reflects changes in anterior fontanelle pressure after shunt implantation more accurately then PI and RI (92).

A more complex method of noninvasive ICP estimation has been developed recently, using arterial blood pressure, blood flow velocity, and several transcranial Doppler indices (trans systolic time, pulsatility index, and diastolic blood flow velocity) (93). This method was evaluated in head injured patients and found to correlate well with real ICP values (94).

In the near future, MRI-based estimates of ICP may provide an accurate alternative 22,95).

Treatment of Shunt Dysfunction

Treatment of shunt dysfunction should generally consist of replacement of the shunt system or parts of it, according to individual circumstances. Comatose patients, however, should be treated with EVD (to allow rapid and controlled correction of the ICP), before inserting a new shunt system. Reutilization of the proximal catheter can be considered if the shunt was recently implanted and if, on preoperative examination, dysfunction appears to be solely due to distal failure (96). Conversely, revision of only the proximal catheter can be considered if the distal parts have remained functional. Connectors should be placed above the level of the mastoid bone to avoid excessive stress by movements of the neck.

The use of programmable valves could theoretically prevent the necessity for a shunt revision in certain cases (e.g., overdrainage). However, a large randomized controlled study did not show any beneficial effect on shunt survival with the use of programmable valve systems (97).

The possible benefits or drawbacks of treating patients with asymptomatic or mildly symptomatic shunt failure, identified in routine outpatient screening, remain unclear (98). The decision whether or not to treat patients therefore is still based on the patients clinical presentation.

Prevention of Shunt Dysfunction

At this time a wide variety of valve systems and surgical methods are employed in the treatment of hydrocephalus. However, comparing the effectiveness of these systems and methods to prevent shunt dysfunction is impossible because most systems are evaluated in noncomparative observational studies (1,49,51). In one of the few multicenter randomized clinical trials on this subject, the use of a neuroendoscope to ensure correct placement of the proximal catheter was not found to improve shunt survival (50,99).

Other Shunt Complications

In addition to shunt infection and dysfunction, difficulties in placing the ventricular catheter may result in intraparenchymal or intraventricular hemorrhage. Intraparenchymal hemorrhage may cause neurological deficits, whereas intraventricular hemorrhage can result in impaired valve function. These complications may not be noticed until after surgery and removal of the shunt system with additional external drainage will be necessary. Furthermore, tunneling of the distal part of the shunt may cause several other complications depending of the type of shunt that is used (VP, VA, or ventriculopleural shunt): vascular lesions (especially in the neck region), perforation of the pleural cavity (implanting a ventriculoperitoneal shunt), lung perforation (implanting a ventriculopleural shunt), bowel perforation (especially when using a Portnoy trocard). These complications should be recognized promptly and treated surgically if necessary.

Recommendations

The following recommendations are based on both the literature discussed above and the expert opinions of the authors (see Appendix A for diagnostic and treatment algorithm for suspected shunt dysfunction).

- Shunt dysfunction should be considered in any patient with a CSF shunt who presents with unexplained symptoms.
- CT imaging of the brain is an effective noninvasive way of detecting changes in ventricle size, that is, changes in ICP due to shunt dysfunction, provided baseline scans are available. In pediatric patients, rapid sequence MRI can be used to limit radiation exposure.
- When brain imaging raises suspicion of shunt dysfunction, plain films of the shunt (shunt series) must be performed to exclude fractures or discontinuities of the shunt system (54).
- When brain imaging is unavailable or inconclusive and clinical sings are not as apparent, ICP measurement should be considered.
- If the functionality of the shunt is unclear, "radio-opaque shuntograms" can be used to assess patency and the existence of any CSF leakage.
- Infusion tests can be considered to assess the function of the entire CSF outflow system (consisting of the shunt system and any remaining physiological CSF absorption capacity or compensatory mechanisms).
- Treatment of shunt dysfunction should consist of restoring ventricular CSF outflow either by revision of the shunt system or, when applicable, with third ventriculostomy.
- The use of programmable valve systems should not be considered a first choice treatment in patients with hydrocephalus, as possible benefits of programmable valve systems have yet to be confirmed by proper comparative studies.

REFERENCES

1. Hanlo PW, Cinalli G, Vandertop WP, et al. Treatment of hydrocephalus determined by the european Orbis Sigma Valve II survey: A multicenter prospective 5-year shunt survival study in children and adults in whom a flow-regulating shunt was used. J Neurosurg 2003; 99:52–57.
2. Aryan HE, Meltzer HS, Park MS, et al. Initial experience with antibiotic-impregnated silicone catheters for shunting of cerebrospinal fluid in children. Childs Nerv Syst 2005; 21:56–61.
3. Bruinsma N, Stobberingh EE, Herpers MJHM, et al. Subcutaneous ventricular catheter reservoir and ventriculoperitoneal drain-related infections in preterm infants and young children. Clin Microbiol Infect 2000; 6:202–206.
4. Choksey MS, Malik IA. Zero tolerance to shunt infections: Can it be achieved? J Neurol Neurosurg Psychiatry 2004; 75:87–91.
5. Cochrane DD, Kestle J. Ventricular shunting for hydrocephalus in children: Patients, procedures, surgeons and institutions in English Canada, 1989–2001. Eur J Pediatr Surg 2002; 12:S6–S11.
6. Enger PØ, Svendsen F, Wester K. CSF shunt infections in children: Experiences from a population-based study. Acta Neurochir 2003; 145:243–248.
7. Govender ST, Nathoo N, van Dellen JR. Evaluation of an antibiotic-impregnated shunt system for the treatment of hydrocephalus. J Neurosurg 2003; 99:831–839.
8. Kanev PM, Sheehan JM. Reflections on shunt infection. Pediatr Neurosurg 2003; 39:285–290.
9. Kulkarni AV, Drake JM, Lamberti-Pasculli M. Cerebrospinal fluid shunt infection: A prospective study of risk factors. J Neurosurg 2001; 94:195–201.
10. Lan CC, Wong TT, Chen SJ, et al. Early diagnosis of ventriculoperitoneal shunt infections and malfunctions in children with hydrocephalus. J Microbiol Immunol Infect 2003; 36:47–50.
11. McGirt MJ, Zaas A, Fuchs HE, et al. Risk factors for pediatric ventriculoperitoneal shunt infection and predictors of infectious pathogens. Clin Infect Dis 2003; 36:858–862.
12. Mottolese C, Grando J, Convert J, et al. Zero rate of shunt infection in the first postoperative year in children—Dream or reality? Childs Nerv Syst 2000; 16:210–212.
13. Sciubba DM, Stuart RM, McGirt MJ, et al. Effect of antibiotic-impregnated shunt catheters in decreasing the incidence of shunt infections in the treatment of hydrocephalus. J Neurosurg 2005; 103:131–136.

14. Tuli S, Tuli J, Drake J, et al. Predictors of death in pediatric patients requiring cerebrospinal fluid shunts. J Neurosurg 2004; 100(5 suppl Pediatrics):442–446.
15. Vinchon M, Dhellemmes P. Cerebrospinal fluid shunt infection: Risk factors and long-term follow-up. Childs Nerv Syst 2006; 22:692–697.
16. Wang KW, Chang WN, Shih TY, et al. Infection of cerebrospinal fluid shunts: Causative pathogens, clinical features, and outcomes. Jpn J Infect Dis 2004; 57:44–48.
17. Taylor AG, Peter JC. Advantages of delayed VP shunting in post-haemorrhagic hydrocephalus seen in low-birth-weight infants. Childs Nerv Syst 2001; 17:328–333.
18. Schreffler RT, Schreffler AJ, Wittler RR. Treatment of cerebrospinal fluid shunt infections: A decision analysis. Pediatr Infect Dis J 2002; 21:632–636.
19. Cowan JA, McGirt MJ, Woodworth G, et al. The syndrome of hydrocephalus in young and middle-aged adults. Neurol Res 2005; 27:540–547.
20. Hashimoto M, Yokota A, Urasaki E, et al. A case of abdominal CSF pseudocyst associated with silicone allergy. Childs Nerv Syst 2004; 20:761–764.
21. Kockro RA, Hampl JA, Jansen B, et al. Use of scanning electron microscopy to investigate the prophylactic efficacy of rifampin-impregnated CSF shunt catheters. J Med Microbiol 2000; 49:441–450.
22. Raksin PB, Alperin NJ, Sivaramakrishnan A, et al. Noninvasive intracranial compliance and pressure based on dynamic magnetic resonance imaging of blood flow and cerebrospinal fluid flow: Review of principles, impementation, and other noninvasive approaches. Neurosurg Focus 2003; 14:1–8.
23. Bayston R. Epidemiology, diagnosis, treatment, and prevention of cerebrospinal fluid shunt infections. Neurosurg Clin N Am 2001; 36:703–708.
24. Brook I. Meningitis and shunt infection caused by anaerobic bacteria in children. Pediatr Neurol 2002; 26:99–105.
25. Turgut M, Alabaz D, Erbey F, et al. Cerebrospinal fluid shunt infections in children. Pediatr Neurosurg 2005; 41:131–136.
26. Schuhman MU, Ostrowski KR, Draper EJ, et al. The value of C-reactive protein in the management of shunt infections. J Neurosurg 2005; 103(3 suppl):223–230.
27. McClinton D, Carraccio C, Englander R. Predictors of ventriculoperitoneal shunt pathology. Pediatr Infect Dis J 2001; 20:593–597.
28. Mobley LW, Doran SE, Hellbusch LC. Abdominal pseudocyst: Predisposing factors and treatment algorithm. Pediatr Neurosurg 2005; 41:77–83.
29. Vinchon M, Lemaitre MP, Vallee L, et al. Late shunt infections: Incidence, pathogenesis, and therapeutic implications. Neuropediatrics 2002; 33:169–173.
30. Bayston R, Ashraf W, Barker-Davies R, et al. Biofilm formation by propionibacterium acnes on biomaterials in vitro and in vivo: Impact on diagnosis and treatment. J Biomed Mater Res A 2007; 81(3):705–709.
31. Braxton EE Jr., Ehrlich GD, Hall-Stoodley L, et al. Role of biofilms in neurosurgical device-related infections. Neurosurg Rev 2005; 26:249–255.
32. Livni G, Yuhas Y, Ashkenazi S, et al. In vitro bacterial adherence to ventriculoperitoneal shunts. Pediatr Neurosurg 2004; 40:64–69.
33. McGirt MJ, Leveque JC, Wellons JC, et al. Cerebrospinal fluid shunt survival and etiology of failures: A seven-year institutional experience. Pediatr Neurosurg 2002; 36:248–255.
34. Byard RW, Koszyca B, Qiao M. Unexpected childhood death due to a rare complication of ventriculoperitoneal shunting. Am J Forensic Med Pathol 2001; 22:207–210.
35. Murphy K, Bradley J, James HE. The treatment of *Candida albicans* shunt infections. Childs Nerv Syst 2000; 16:4–7.
36. Banks JT, Bharara S, Tubbs RS, et al. Polymerase chain reaction for the rapid detection of cerebrospinal fluid shunt or ventriculostomy infections. Neurosurgery 2005; 57:1237–1243.
37. Meredith FT, Phillips HK, Reller LB. Clinical utility of broth cultures of cerebrospinal fluid from patients at risk for shunt infections. J Clin Mirobiol 1997; 35:3109–3111.
38. Anderson EJ, Yogev R. A rational approach to the management of ventricular shunt infections. Pediatr Infect Dis J 2005; 24:557–558.
39. Goeser CD, McLeary MS, Young LW. Diagnostic imaging of ventriculoperitoneal shunt malfunctions and complications. Radiographics 1998; 18:635–651.
40. Lutsar I, McCracken GH Jr., Friedland IR. Antibiotic pharmacodynamics in cerebrospinal fluid. Clin Infect Dis 1998; 27:1117–1129.
41. Albanèse J, Léone M, Bruguerolle B, et al. Cerebrospinal fluid penetration and pharmacokinetics of vancomycin administered by continuous infusion to mechanically ventilated patients in an intensive care unit. Antimicrob Agents Chemother 2000; 44:1356–1358.
42. Bafeltowska JJ, Buszman E, Mandat KM, et al. Therapeutic vancomycin monitoring in children with hydrocephalus during treatment of shunt infections. Surg Neurol 2004; 62:142–150.

43. Pfausler B, Spiss H, Beer R, et al. Treatment of stapylococcal ventriculitis associated with external cere-brospinal fluid drains: A prospective randomized trial of intravenous compared with intraventricular vancomycin therapy. J Neurosurg 2003; 98:1040–1044.

44. Kestle JRW, Garton HJL, Whitehead WE, et al. Management of shunt infections: A multicenter pilot study. J Neurosurg 2006; 105(3 suppl):177–181.

45. Arthur AS, Whitehead WE, Kestle JRW. Duration of antibiotic therapy for the treatment of shunt infection: A surgeon and patient survey. Pediatr Neurosurg 2002; 36:256–259.

46. Santos de Oliveira R, Barbosa A, Avalloni de Moraes Villela de Andrade Vicente Y, Machado HR. An alternative approach for management of abdominal cerebrospinal fluid pseudocysts in children. Childs Nerv Syst 2007; 23(1):85–90. Epub 2006 Aug 30.

47. Hampl JA, Weitzel A, Bonk C, et al. Rifampin-impregnated silicone catheters: A potential tool for prevention and treatment of CSF shunt infections. Infection 2003; 31:109–111.

48. Tulipan N, Cleves M. Effect of an intraoperative double-gloving strategy on the incidence of cere-brospinal fluid shunt infection. J Neurosurg 2006; 104(1 suppl):5–8.

49. Kehler U, Klöhn A, Heese O, et al. Hydrocephalus therapy: Reduction of shunt occlusions using a peel-away sheath. Clin Neurol Neurosurg 2003; 105:253–255.

50. Kestle JRW, Drake JM, Cochrane DD, et al. Lack of benefit of endoscopic ventriculoperitoneal shunt insertion: A multicenter randomized trial. J Neurosurg 2003; 98:284–290.

51. Meling TR, Egge A, Tønnessen BD. The gravity-assisted Paedi-Gav valve in the treatment of pediatric hydrocephalus. Pediatr Neurosurg 2005; 41:8–14.

52. Robinson S, Kaufman BA, Park TS. Outcome analysis of initial neonatal shunts: Does the valve make a difference? Pediatr Neurosurg 2002; 37:287–294.

53. Browd SR, Gottfried ON, Ragel BT, et al. Failure of cerebrospinal fluid shunts: Part II: Overdrainage, loculation, and abdominal complications. Pediatr Neurol 2006; 34:171–176.

54. Browd SR, Ragel BT, Gottfried ON, et al. Failure of cerebrospinal fluid shunts: Part I: Obstruction and mechanical failure. Pediatr Neurol 2006; 34:83–92.

55. Di Rocco C, Massimi L, Tamburrini C. Shunts vs endoscopic third ventriculostomy in infants: Are there different types and/or rates of complications? : A review. Childs Nerv Syst 2006; 22:1573–1589.

56. Sgouros S, Dipple SJ. An investigation of structural degradation of cerebrospinal fluid shunt valves performed using scanning electron microscopy and energy-dispersive x-ray microanalysis. J Neuro-surg 2004; 100:534–540.

57. Baird C, Farner S, Mohr C, et al. The effects of protein, red blood cells and whole blood on ps valve function. Pediatr Neurosurg 2002; 37:186–193.

58. Gilkes CE, Steers AJW, Minns RA. A classification of CSF shunt malfunction. Eur J Pediatr Surg 1999; 9(S1):19–22.

59. Woerdeman PA, Hanlo PW. Ventriculoperitoneal shunt occlusion due to spontaneous intraabdominal knot formation in the catheter. J Neurosurg 2006; 105(3 suppl):231–232.

60. VandeVord PJ, Gupta N, Wilson RB, et al. Immune reactions associated with silicone-based ventriculo-peritoneal shunt malfunctions in children. Biomaterials 2004; 25:3853–3860.

61. Bruinsma GJBB, Janssen EWL, Meijburg HWJ, et al. Complications of a ventriculoatrial shunt neces-sitating thoracic surgery. J Neurosurg 1996; 84.709.

62. Milton C, Sanders P, Steele PM. Late cardiopulmonary complication of ventriculo-atrial shunt. Lancet 2001; 358:1608.

63. Vernet O, Rilliet B. Late complications of ventriculoatrial or ventriculoperitoneal shunts. Lancet 2001; 358:1569–1570.

64. Yurtseven T, Ersahin Y, Ömer K, et al. Thrombosis and thrombophilebitis of the internal jugular vein as a very rare complication of the ventriculoatrial shunt. Clin Neurol Neurosurg 2005; 107: 144–146.

65. Dickerman RD, McConathy WJ, Morgan J, et al. Failure rate of frontal versus parietal approaches for proximal catheter placement in ventriculoperitioneal shunts: Revisited. J Clin Neuroscience 2005; 12:781–783.

66. Lazareff JA, Peacock W, Holly L, et al. Multiple shunt failures: An analysis of relevant factors. Childs Nerv Syst 1998; 14:271–275.

67. Tuli S, Drake J, Lawless J, et al. Risk factors for repeated cerebrospinal shunt failures in pediatric patients with hydrocephalus. J Neurosurg 2000; 92:31–38.

68. Factora R. When do common symptoms indicate normal pressure hydrocephalus? Cleve Clin J Med 2006; 73:447–457.

69. Gallia GL, Rigamonti D, Williams MA. The diagnosis and treatment of idiopathic normal pressure hydrocephalus. Nat Clin Pract Neurol 2006; 2:375–381.

70. Cinalli G, Sainte-Rose C, Simon I, et al. Sylvian aqueduct syndrome and global rostral midbrain dysfunction associated with shunt malfunction. J Neurosurg 1999; 90:227–236.

71. Barnes NP, Jones SJ, Hayward RD, et al. Ventriculoperitoneal shunt block: What are the best predictive clinical indicators? Arch Dis Child 2002; 87:198–201.

72. Hanlo PW, Gooskens RHJM, Faber JAJ, et al. Relationship between anterior fontanelle pressure measurements and clinical signs in infantile hydrocephalus. Childs Nerv Syst 1996; 12:200–209.

73. van der Knaap MS, Bakker CJ, Faber JAJ, et al. Comparison of skull circumference and linear measurements with CSF volume MR measurements in hydrocephalus. J Comput Assist Tomogr 1992; 16:737–743.

74. Mesiwala AH, Avellino AM, Ellenbogen RG. The diagonal ventricular dimension: A method for predicting shunt malfunction on the basis of changes in ventricular size. Neurosurgery 2002; 50:1246–1252.

75. Zorc JJ, Krugman SD, Ogborn J, et al. Radiographic evaluation for suspected cerebrospinal fluid shunt obstruction. Pediatr Emerg Care 2002; 18:337–340.

76. Ashley WW Jr., McKinstry RC, Leonard JR, et al. Use of rapid-sequence magnetic resonance imaging for evaluation of hydrocephalus in children. J Neurosurg 2005; 103(2 suppl):124–130.

77. Drake JM. Comment on: The diagonal ventricular dimension: A method for predicting shunt malfunction on the basis of changes in ventricular size. Neurosurgery 2002; 50:1252.

78. Xenos C, Sgouros S, Natarajan K, et al. Influence of shunt type on ventricular volume changes in children with hydrocephalus. J Neurosurg 2003; 98:277–283.

79. Bartynski WS, Valliappan S, Uselman JH, et al. The adult radiographic shuntogram. Am J Neuroradiol 2000; 21:721–726.

80. O'Brien DF, Taylor M, Park TS, et al. A critical analysis of 'normal' radionucleotide shuntograms in patients subsequently requiring surgery. Childs Nerv Syst 2003; 19:337–341.

81. Goetz C, Foertsch D, Schoenberger J, et al. Thermography—a valuable tool to test hydrocephalus shunt patency. Acta Neurochir 2005; 147:1167–1173.

82. Gilkes CE, Steers AJW, Minns RA. Pressure compensation in shunt-dependent hydrocephalus with CSF shunt malfunction. Childs Nerv Syst 2001; 17:52–57.

83. Kazan S, Açikbas C, Rahat Ö, et al. Proof of the patent subcutaneous fibrous tract in children with V-P shunt malfunction. Childs Nerv Syst 2000; 16:351–356.

84. Lo TYM, Myles LM, Minns RA. Long-term risks and benefits of a separate CSF acces device with ventriculoperitoneal shunting in childhood hydrocephalus. Dev Med Child Neurol 2003; 45:28–33.

85. Sood S, Canady AI, Ham SD. Evaluation of shunt malfunction using shunt site reservoir. Pediatr Neurosurg 2000; 32:180–186.

86. Taylor R, Czosnyka Z, Czosnyka M, et al. A laboratory model of testing shunt performance after implantation. Br J Neurosurg 2002; 16:30–35.

87. Eklund A, Lundkvist B, Koskinen L-OD, et al. Infusion technique can be used to distinguish between dysfunction of a hydrocephalus shunt system and a progressive dementia. Med Biol Eng Comput 2004; 42:644–649.

88. Malm J, Lundkvist B, Eklund A, et al. CSF outflow resistance as predictor of shunt function. A long-term study. Acta Neurol Scand 2004; 110:156–160.

89. Peters RJA, Hanlo PW, Gooskens RHJM, et al. Non-invasive ICP monitoring in infants: The Rotterdam teletransducer revisited. Childs Nerv Syst 1995; 11:207–213.

90. Santos de Oliveira R, Machado HR. Transcranial color-coded Doppler ultrasonography for evaluation of children with hydrocephalus. Neurosurg Focus 2003; 15:1–7.

91. Hanlo PW, Gooskens RHJM, Nijhuis IJM, et al. Value of transcranial Doppler indices in predicting raised ICP in infantile hydrocephalus. Childs Nerv Syst 1995; 11:595–603.

92. Hanlo PW, Peters RJA, Gooskens RHJM, et al. Monitoring intracranial dynamics by transcranial Doppler—A new Doppler index: Trans systolic time. Ultrasound Med Biol 1995; 21:613–621.

93. Schmidt B, Czosnyka M, Schwarze JJ, et al. Evaluation of a method for noninvasive intracranial pressure assessment during infusion studies in patients with hydrocephalus. J Neurosurg 2000; 92:793–800.

94. Schmidt B, Klingelhöfer J. Clinical applications of a non-invasive ICP monitoring method. Eur J Ultrasound 2002; 16:37–45.

95. Alperin NJ, Lee SH, Loth F, et al. MR-intracranial pressure (ICP): A method to measure intracranial elastance and pressure noninvasevely. Radiology 2000; 217:877–885.

96. McGirt MJ, Wellons JC, Nimjee SM, et al. Comparison of total versus partial revision of initial ventriculoperitoneal shunt failures. Pediatr Neurosurg 2003; 38:34–40.

97. Pollack IF, Albright AL, Adelson PD. A randomized, controlled study of a programmable shunt valve versus a conventional valve for patients with hydrocephalus. Neurosurgery 1999; 45:1399–1408.

98. Vinchon M, Fichten A, Delestret I, et al. Shunt revision for asymptomatic failure: Surgical and clinical results. Neurosurgery 2003; 52:347–356.

99. Villavicencio AT, Leveque JC, McGirt MJ, et al. Comparison of revision rates following endoscopically versus nonendoscopically placed ventricular shunt catheters. Surg Neurol 2003; 59:375–380.

APPENDIX A

Diagnostic and Treatment Algorithm for Suspected Shunt Infection

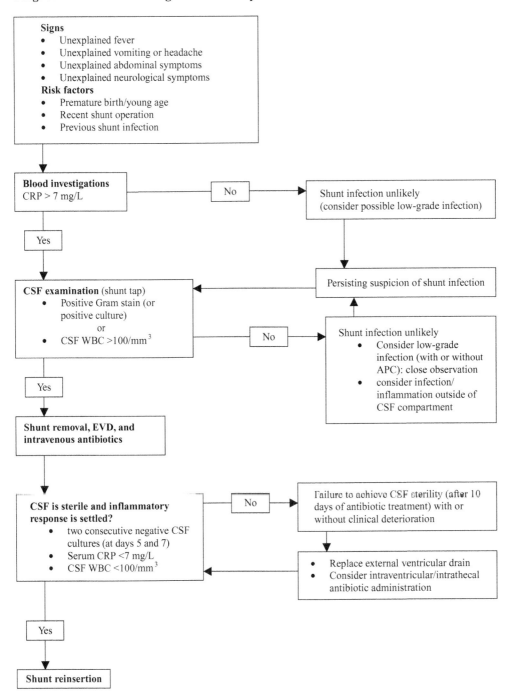

Signs
- Unexplained fever
- Unexplained vomiting or headache
- Unexplained abdominal symptoms
- Unexplained neurological symptoms

Risk factors
- Premature birth/young age
- Recent shunt operation
- Previous shunt infection

Blood investigations
CRP > 7 mg/L

No → Shunt infection unlikely (consider possible low-grade infection)

Yes

Persisting suspicion of shunt infection

CSF examination (shunt tap)
- Positive Gram stain (or positive culture)
  or
- CSF WBC >100/mm^3

No → Shunt infection unlikely
- Consider low-grade infection (with or without APC): close observation
- consider infection/ inflammation outside of CSF compartment

Yes

Shunt removal, EVD, and intravenous antibiotics

CSF is sterile and inflammatory response is settled?
- two consecutive negative CSF cultures (at days 5 and 7)
- Serum CRP <7 mg/L
- CSF WBC <100/mm^3

No → Failure to achieve CSF sterility (after 10 days of antibiotic treatment) with or without clinical deterioration

- Replace external ventricular drain
- Consider intraventricular/intrathecal antibiotic administration

Yes

Shunt reinsertion

Diagnostic and Treatment Algorithm for Suspected Shunt Dysfunction

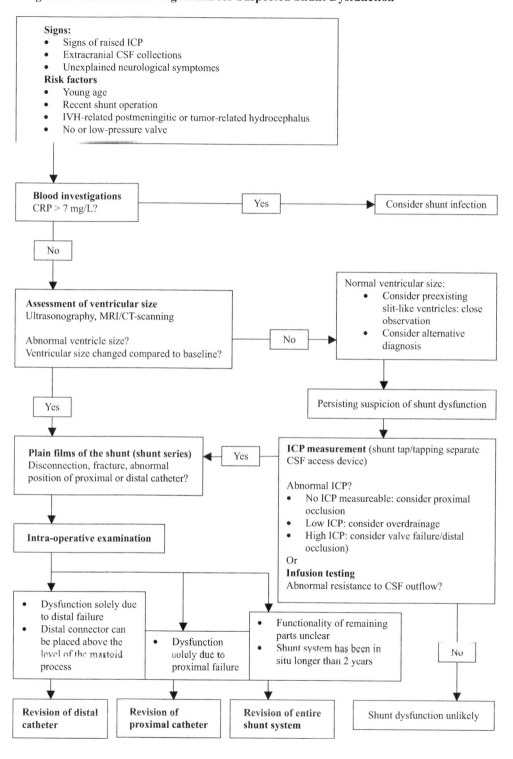

The Role of Antibiotic Impregnated Catheters in Preventing Shunt Infection

Caroline Hayhurst

Department of Neurosurgery, The Walton Centre for Neurology and Neurosurgery, Liverpool, U.K.

The majority of shunt infections (90%) are caused by Staphylococcal species, predominantly coagulase negative *Staphylococci*, implanted at the time of surgery. Most shunt infections manifest within two months of surgery. Impregnation of silicone shunt catheters with antibiotics has been shown in vitro to provide sustained bacteriocidal activity. Initial in vitro studies of antibiotic impregnated catheters (AIS) challenged with five staphylococcal species, including *S. epidermidis*, *S. aureus*, *S. haemolyticus*, and *S. hominis*, showed no colonization of processed catheters at 28 days (1). Antibiotic impregnation of the shunt catheter does not prevent bacterial adherence, but kills bacteria that become adherent. Therefore in principle a relatively high bacterial load introduced at the time of shunt implantation can be eliminated. However, antimicrobial activity reduces over time, with in vitro studies showing effective bacteriocidal activity up to 56 days (1).

The Bactiseal™ shunt catheter (Codman®, Johnson & Johnson, Raynham, MA, U.S.A.) is impregnated with 0.15% clindamycin and 0.054% rifampicin, a combination aimed at eliminating colonization with Gram positive organisms, without conferring additional morbidity due to toxicity. In addition, the combination of antibiotics has shown a clear advantage over single agents alone and reduces the potential risk of resistance.

To date there is no Class 1 evidence of the efficacy of AIS in reducing the incidence of shunt infection. Several reports of single institutional data appear to have conflicting results (2–8). A single prospective randomized study of the Bactiseal™ AIS in both children and adults reports a per procedure infection rate of 13.3% in the control group and 5% in the AIS group (2). These results were not statistically significant, as the study was underpowered. In this study, 69.2% of infections occurred in patients aged one year or younger. A retrospective cohort study of Bactiseal™ AIS catheters in a pediatric population (not including those below one year of age) by Sciubba et al. (6) show a 2.4-fold decreased likelihood of shunt infection in the AIS group, based on 6-month follow-up. Aryan et al. (8), in a cohort study of children aged 6 months to 17 years with a historical control group, reported a reduction in the infection rate from 15.2% to 3.1% following the introduction of antibiotic-impregnated catheters. Published data from our institution failed to demonstrate a significant difference between the overall shunt infection rate in children (including neonates), with a risk reduction of only 0.6% (from 10.4% to 9.8%), in a retrospective cohort study (5). This is the only study to report a subgroup analysis of shunt infections, demonstrating a reduction in shunt infection from 17% to 8.5% in de novo AIS shunts and a 16.3% reduction in infection rates in neonatal de novo shunts. However, no reduction in infection rates reached statistical significance. It should be noted that in each of these studies demonstrating a large risk reduction, the baseline infection rate in the non-AIS group is high.

Pattavilakom et al. (4) reported a significant reduction in infection rates with AIS catheters from 6.5% to 1.2% ($p = 0.0015$), comparing a prospective cohort against historical data. Kan and Kestle (3) report a reduction of infection rates from 8.8% to 5.0%, using a similar methodology, demonstrating that shunt infection was 2.83 times more likely to occur in the control group than the AIS group. However, this result did not achieve statistical significance. Ritz et al. (7) did not show any change in infection rates in a prospective cohort study, with an infection rate of 5.18% in both cohorts of a predominantly adult series.

The majority of studies continue to demonstrate the predominance of staphylococcal species in infective episodes and there is no overall increase in the time to development of infection. Only one study has reported bacterial sensitivities in cases of shunt infection with AIS catheters, with one of five staphylococcal infections demonstrating resistance to both clindamycin and rifampicin (7). Concerns regarding the emergence of indolent, atypical infections, remain unfounded at present.

Overall, there appears to be an advantage to using AIS catheters particularly in infants, where most shunt infections occur, although the magnitude of the effect in reducing shunt infection is uncertain. Only an adequately powered randomized trial would provide the definitive answer.

REFERENCES

1. Bayston R, Lambert E. Duration of protective activity of cerebrospinal fluid shunt catheters impregnated with antimicrobial agents to prevent bacterial catheter-related infection. J Neurosurg 1997; 87(2):247–251.
2. Govender ST, Nathoo N, van Dellen JR. Evaluation of an antibiotic-impregnated shunt system for the treatment of hydrocephalus. J Neurosurg 2003; 99(5):831–839.
3. Kan P, Kestle J. Lack of efficacy of antibiotic-impregnated shunt systems in preventing shunt infections in children. Childs Nerv Syst 2007; 23(7):773–777.
4. Pattavilakom A, Xenos C, Bradfield O, et al. Reduction in shunt infection using antibiotic impregnated CSF shunt catheters: An Australian prospective study. J Clin Neurosci 2007; 14(6):526–531.
5. Hayhurst C, Cooke R, Williams D, et al. The impact of antibiotic-impregnated catheters on shunt infection in children and neonates. Childs Nerv Syst 2008; 24(5):557–562.
6. Sciubba DM, Stuart RM, McGirt MJ, et al. Effect of antibiotic-impregnated shunt catheters in decreasing the incidence of shunt infection in the treatment of hydrocephalus. J Neurosurg 2005; 103(2 suppl):131–136.
7. Ritz R, Roser F, Morgalla M, et al. Do antibiotic-impregnated shunts in hydrocephalus therapy reduce the risk of infection? An observational study in 258 patients. BMC Infect Dis 2007; 7:38.
8. Aryan HE, Meltzer HS, Park MS, et al. Initial experience with antibiotic-impregnated silicone catheters for shunting of cerebrospinal fluid in children. Childs Nerv Syst 2005; 21(1):56–61.

Multiloculated Hydrocephalus

Toba Niazi and Marion L. Walker

*Department of Neurosurgery, Primary Children's Medical Center, University of Utah,
Salt Lake City, Utah, U.S.A.*

INTRODUCTION

Multiloculated hydrocephalus is a rare form of hydrocephalus defined by septations or obstructions within the ventricular system that allow cerebrospinal fluid (CSF) to accumulate in isolated compartments. These compartments gradually enlarge and exert mass effect on the surrounding structures with resultant elevation in intracranial pressure (1–7). Multiloculated hydrocephalus has also been variously termed "compartmentalized hydrocephalus," "ventricular compartmentalization," "intraventricular septations," and "polycystic brain disease" (4). It is important to distinguish between multiloculated hydrocephalus and other forms of hydrocephalus because of the marked differences in their pathogenesis, treatment, and prognosis (3–7). Improved imaging modalities over the last two decades, namely, computerized tomography (CT) and magnetic resonance imaging (MRI), have enabled improved diagnosis of this condition and have allowed for the earlier recognition of the disease process (3,4,7). Nevertheless, multiloculated hydrocephalus still offers a formidable challenge in the realm of neurosurgical management. This chapter discusses the causes and pathogenesis of multiloculated hydrocephalus as well as the treatment options available, most notably neuroendoscopic management.

CAUSES AND PATHOGENESIS

Although its cause is not entirely understood, multiloculated hydrocephalus is most commonly attributed to damage occurring during the neonatal period, with most cases associated with intraventricular hemorrhage and/or intracranial infection (1,3-11). Other cases of multiloculated hydrocephalus have been associated with shunt-related infection, shunt overdrainage, direct ependymal trauma during catheter insertion, and intracranial injury (3,4,7). In 1970, Salmon (10) was the first to describe a case of multiloculated hydrocephalus resulting from neonatal meningitis, and this relationship has since been well developed. The damage incurred within the ventricular system, from either an inflammatory or a chemical process, promotes a subependymal gliotic process forming tufts upon which exudate and debris collect, encouraging the formation of septations within the ventricular system. When these septations interrupt the normal flow of CSF by obstructing key structures responsible for adequate flow, such as the interventricular foramina of Monro, cerebral aqueduct, and foramina of Luschka and Magendie, elevations in intracranial pressure ensue (4,5,7,11). Inflammation of the ependyma tends to be of a chronic nature in most cases, with the appearance of new septa and new obstructions over time (4,5,7,11). For this reason, multiloculated hydrocephalus has often been considered a progressive disease process (4,5,7,11).

DIAGNOSIS

When a patient presents with symptoms suggestive of hydrocephalus, CT and MRI are performed. Early in the disease process, CT is less effective at confirming the diagnosis of multiloculated hydrocephalus because the loculations have a consistency similar to that of CSF (1,3,5–7,11). Protein concentrations have not yet had the chance to accumulate within the cysts, and the septations are thin and not well visualized by CT. In more advanced stages of the disease process, the loculations increase in their protein concentration, and septations become more pronounced and increased in number, thereby altering the normal ventricular anatomy. At this point, detecting multiloculated hydrocephalus via CT becomes easier (1–4,7,11). High-resolution MRI using T1- and T2-weighted imaging or with CISS (constructive interference of steady state) and DRIVE (driven equilibrium radiofrequency reset pulse)

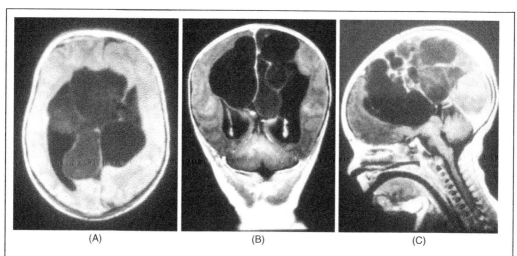

Figure 1 T1 MRI in axial (**A**), coronal (**B**), and sagittal (**C**) images showing multiloculated cysts with the lateral ventricles.

sequences can provide greater anatomical details of the anomalies than are visible on CT imaging and allow detection of septations at an earlier stage (1–4,7,11). Multiplanar imaging allows for greater anatomical delineation of the cyst walls (Fig. 1). Despite the details that can be seen by MRI, contrast CT ventriculography is still in use because it can verify the lack of communication between the ventricular system and the cyst cavity (3,7). This modality enables the visualization of the anatomy of the ventricular cavity, allowing for improved operative planning for the ideal neuroendoscopic path to the cyst (3,7). In those children that have preexisting shunt systems in place, plain films of the shunt system are of paramount importance to exclude a disconnection, kinking, or breakage of the system (3,4,7).

TREATMENT

Multiloculated hydrocephalus is a difficult disease process to treat. Despite the various therapeutic options available, no treatment has proven to be entirely curative (1–14). For this reason, there is no one set paradigm for treating this disease process and all the options available remain controversial. However, the treatment modalities have similar goals in common: to relieve the elevated intracranial pressure, to simplify any necessary shunt systems, and to minimize operative morbidity (3,4,7).

Treatment options include placement of cystoperitoneal shunts with the use of multiperforated catheters, stereotactic cyst aspiration, craniotomy for fenestration of intraventricular septations, and neuroendoscopic cyst fenestration (3,4,7). The traditional surgical treatment, placement of multiple shunts, is associated with a high rate of complications (3–7,12–15). Shunt failure caused by the collapse of the shunt-treated compartment, shunt infections, and scarring is frequent and can lead to the need for multiple shunt revisions (3–7,12–15). Nida and Haines (4) retrospectively reported a shunt revision rate in their series as high as 2.75 shunt revisions per year. Shunt infections are not only associated with a need to remove all hardware and establish external drainage, but recurrent shunt infections also establish a cycle of ependymal inflammation, often leading to further septations (3,4,7).

Stereotactic aspiration is usually a safe alternative; however, the cysts may be mobile or resistant to stereotactic perforation because of very thick walls. Because the cysts are not widely devascularized or fenestrated (<1 cm), the septations are likely to recur (3,4,7).

Craniotomy with transcallosal fenestration of intraventricular septations was first described by Rhoton and Gomez in 1972 (9). Use of this procedure has resulted in lower shunt revision rates, as seen in Nida and Haines's series (4), where the shunt revision rate went from a median of 2.75 per year to 0.25 per year. Direct visualization enables the removal of the septations and creation of a single communicating cavity that can be drained by a single cystoperitoneal shunt system (1,3,4,6,7,9). This reduces the complications associated with multiple shunt systems but has its own set of risks. The risks associated with craniotomy are associated with the trajectory involved with gaining access into the ventricular system. These include, but are not limited to, venous and arterial injuries (injury to bridging veins and pericallosal artery), disconnection syndromes (damage to the corpus callosum), and damage to the fornices and subcortical nuclei (1,3,4,6,7,9). In addition, the transcallosal approach may also lead to subdural collections secondary to the thin overlying cortical mantle (3,4,6,7,9).

The evolution of neuroendoscopy since its first use in the 1970s has made a less invasive alternative to microsurgical ablation of septations available to patients with multiloculated hydrocephalus (3,5,7,12,14,16,17). With technical improvements in optics, miniaturization, and instrumentation, the anatomy of the ventricular system can be analyzed more easily (3,5,7,12,14,16,17). Endoscopic fenestration of the intraventricular septa creates a wide communication (>1 cm) between the intraventricular cavities, thereby allowing one shunt to drain the entire ventricular system (3,5,7,12,14,16,17). In conjunction with frameless stereotactic neuronavigation, improved intraoperative spatial orientation in the axial, sagittal, and coronal planes assists with neuroendoscopic navigation (16). Intraoperative ultrasound in conjunction with neuroendoscopy can be used before leaving the operative suite to assess the communication between the different cavities to confirm that one shunt system will be effective in draining the entire system (3). Lewis et al. (3) demonstrated that the symptoms of hydrocephalus were controlled with neuroendoscopy and that the shunt revision rate was reduced from 3.04 to 0.25 per year, similar to the results obtained from transcallosal craniotomy for treatment of loculations. In a retrospective analysis of series of 30 patients with multiloculated hydrocephalus treated endoscopically, Spennato et al. (7) also found that the shunt revision rate decreased from 2.07 to 0.35 per year in patients with preexisting shunt systems after neuroendoscopic fenestration. Despite the decrease in shunt revision rate, patients may still require endoscopic reoperations (3,5,7,12,14,16,17), yet this approach still offers a revision rate superior to the multiple shunt revision rate before the availability of neuroendoscopy as a form of treatment (7).

An ideal neuroendoscopic candidate is one who has been diagnosed early and can be treated early in the disease process (5,7). Spennato et al. (7) demonstrated that of seven patients with no preexisting shunt systems who were diagnosed early in the process of their loculations, three required no shunts, three required only one shunt, and only one patient required two shunts. In patients who are diagnosed early in the disease process, there is less architectural distortion of the ventricular anatomy, allowing safer and easier navigation within the ventricular system (3,5,7,12,14,16,17). The success of neuroendoscopy in treating multiloculated hydrocephalus can also be attributed to its flexibility (17). Several procedures, such as the fenestration of the septum pellucidum and opening of intraventricular cysts, can be accomplished during the same surgical procedure (7). The minimally invasive nature of this treatment allows for a shorter patient recovery period with decreased operative morbidity (3,7).

Despite the benefits of neuroendoscopic ablation, the complication rate is not trivial even in patients treated by surgeons with extensive experience (12). To achieve optimal results, prudent patient selection based on preoperative imaging studies and comprehensive training in neuroendoscopic technique is required (12). Neuroendoscopy should be considered as the initial treatment in eligible patients before pursuing alternative treatments for multiloculated hydrocephalus (3,5,7,12,14,16,17). This is in an effort to minimize the complexity of the shunt system, relieve intracranial hypertension, as well as to reduce the high rate of shunt revision and the comorbidities associated with shunting as the primary treatment.

REFERENCES

1. Albanese V, Tomasello F, Sampaolo S. Multiloculated hydrocephalus in infants. Neurosurgery 1981; 8:641–646.
2. Albanese V, Tomasello F, Sampaolo S, et al. Neuroradiological findings in multiloculated hydrocephalus. Acta Neurochir (Wien) 1982; 60:297–311.

3. Lewis AI, Keiper GL Jr, Crone KR. Endoscopic treatment of loculated hydrocephalus. J Neurosurg 1995; 82:780–785.
4. Nida TY, Haines SJ. Multiloculated hydrocephalus: Craniotomy and fenestration of intraventricular septations. J Neurosurg 1993; 78:70–76.
5. Oi S, Abbott R. Loculated ventricles and isolated compartments in hydrocephalus: Their pathophysiology and the efficacy of neuroendoscopic surgery. Neurosurg Clin N Am 2004; 15:77–87.
6. Sandberg DI, McComb JG, Krieger MD. Craniotomy for fenestration of multiloculated hydrocephalus in pediatric patients. Neurosurgery 2005; 57:100–106; discussion 100–106.
7. Spennato P, Cinalli G, Ruggiero C, et al. Neuroendoscopic treatment of multiloculated hydrocephalus in children. J Neurosurg 2007; 106:29–35.
8. Kalsbeck JE, DeSousa AL, Kleiman MB, et al. Compartmentalization of the cerebral ventricles as a sequela of neonatal meningitis. J Neurosurg 1980; 52:547–552.
9. Rhoton AL Jr, Gomez MR. Conversion of multilocular hydrocephalus to unilocular. Case report. J Neurosurg 1972; 36:348–350.
10. Salmon JH. Isolated unilateral hydrocephalus following ventriculoatrial shunt. J Neurosurg 1970; 32:219–226.
11. Schultz P, Leeds NE. Intraventricular septations complicating neonatal meningitis. J Neurosurg 1973; 38:620–626.
12. Cinalli G, Spennato P, Ruggiero C, et al. Complications following endoscopic intracranial procedures in children. Childs Nerv Syst 2007; 23:633–644.
13. Cipri S, Gambardella G. Neuroendoscopic approach to complex hydrocephalus. Personal experience and preliminary report. J Neurosurg Sci 2001; 45:92–96.
14. Gangemi M, Maiuri F, Donati P, et al. Neuroendoscopy. Personal experience, indications and limits. J Neurosurg Sci 1998; 42:1–10.
15. Lam CH, Horrigan M, Lovick DS. The Seldinger technique for insertion of difficult to place ventricular catheters. Pediatr Neurosurg 2003; 38:90–93.
16. Mangano FT, Limbrick DD Jr, Leonard JR, et al. Simultaneous image-guided and endoscopic navigation without rigid cranial fixation: Application in infants: Technical case report. Neurosurgery 2006; 58:ONS-E377; discussion ONS-E377.
17. Wagner W, Gaab MR, Schroeder HW, et al. Experiences with cranial neuronavigation in pediatric neurosurgery. Pediatr Neurosurg 1999; 31:231–236.

26 | Clinical Trials in Hydrocephalus: What Have We Learned?

John Kestle

Division of Pediatric Neurosurgery, University of Utah, Salt Lake City, Utah, U.S.A

Clinical research has contributed a great deal of information to the understanding of hydrocephalus and its management. In a few areas, prospective clinical studies have been performed to address specific questions. In order to review these, a "clinical trial" has been defined as a study with (a) prospective multicenter data collection, (b) a specific outcome of interest, and (c) in children.

1. There isn't one "best shunt".
    In the late 1990s, a randomized clinical trial was completed, comparing the initial management of hydrocephalus with a Delta valve, a differential pressure valve or the original Sigma valve (1,2). Patients younger than 18 years of age were randomized to one of these three valves and followed for a minimum of one year. There were 10 centers participating from Canada, United States, and Europe. Three hundred forty-four patients were randomized and 177 patients had shunt failure. The one-year shunt survival was 62% and the infection rate was 8.4%. Overall there was no significant difference in the time to first shunt failure (Fig. 1).
2. The valves fail in different ways.
    In the Shunt Design Trial, the type of shunt failure was assessed based on the clinical presentation and operative findings. Shunt obstruction was a common problem with all three designs, and infection did not seem to differ among these three groups. Although overdrainage was rare, it did appear to be slightly different. There were 10 cases of overdrainage with the Delta valve, 3 with the differential pressure valve and none at all with the Orbis Sigma valve. The incidence of obstruction of the valve itself (as opposed to the ventricular catheter or distal tubing) was higher with the Sigma valve (Fig. 2).
3. A baseline scan after shunting is required one to two years postop.
    The ventricle size was measured in the Shunt Design Trial using a ventricular volume index. The ventricle size of functioning shunts is demonstrated in Figure 3. The ventricle size decreased considerably from baseline to the 3-month follow up scan and then continued to decrease until 12 months of age. Between 12 months of age and 24 months of age, the ventricle size did not change. Based on this, it seems reasonable to obtain a late scan one year after shunt insertion as a basis for subsequent follow-up. The rate of change in ventricle size was not the same for all valves (Fig. 4). The Delta valve and differential pressure valve resulted in a similar decrease in ventricle size over time, but the ventricles appeared to decrease in size more slowly with the Sigma valve.
4. Shunt infection and overdrainage can occur very late.
    The timing of the different shunt failure endpoints is demonstrated in Figure 5. Obstruction is a common problem, which can occur at any time in the life of a shunt. There were 13 cases of overdrainage in the Shunt Design Trial, 12 of which were acute subdural collections. The majority of these occur in the first year, but three cases occurred almost two years after shunt insertion. Infection usually occurs early as well, but there were two cases of infection that occurred at almost two years, and one a little beyond three years, again without any intervening surgical procedures on the shunt.
5. Failure of adjustable valves is similar to nonadjustable valves.
    The Strata valve was evaluated in a nonrandomized prospective cohort study (3). All patients received the valve. There were two study cohorts: (*i*) patients undergoing their first shunt insertion, and (*ii*) patients undergoing shunt revision. Shunt insertion patients were eligible based on criteria that were the same as those used previously in published

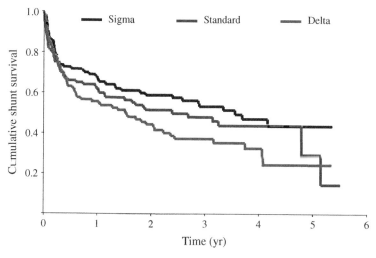

Figure 1 Time to first failure after initial shunt placement in children.

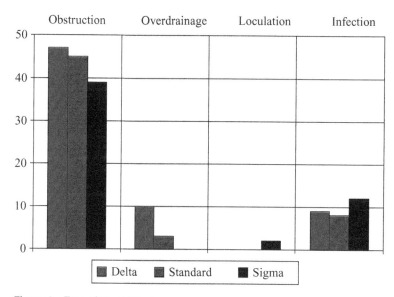

Figure 2 Type of shunt failure.

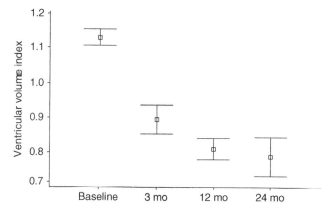

Figure 3 Ventricle size after shunt insertion.

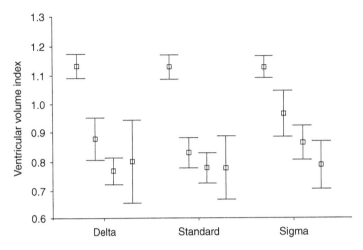

Figure 4   Valve specific ventricle size after shunt insertion.

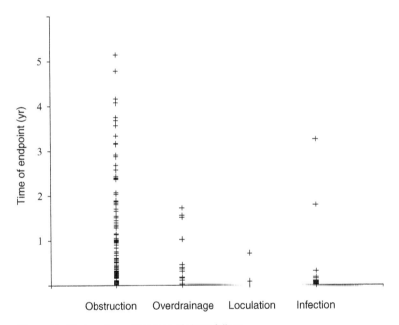

Figure 5   Timing of specific types of shunt failure.

hydrocephalus trials (4,5). There were 201 patients in this group and they were followed at least one year or until they underwent shunt revision surgery. The overall shunt survival is demonstrated in Figure 6 along with point estimates from the published literature of other valve survivals. The one-year survival was 67%. When the one-year survival was compared to other clinical trials, this was very similar and if 95% confidence intervals are applied to the one-year Strata survival and that of each of the SDT valves, they all overlap.

A randomized trial of adjustable Hakim-Medos valves compared to differential pressure valves was reported by Pollack (6). This study included children and adults and patients who were having first shunt placement and shunt revision. In both these groups, there was no detectable difference in the time to first shunt failure.

In the Strata study, the valves that were adjusted were compared to the valves that were not adjusted. Although the curves separate a little bit in the first few months, the shunt survival at one year for these two groups was identical. This suggests that adjusting the valve may have delayed shunt failure a little bit, but not avoided it.

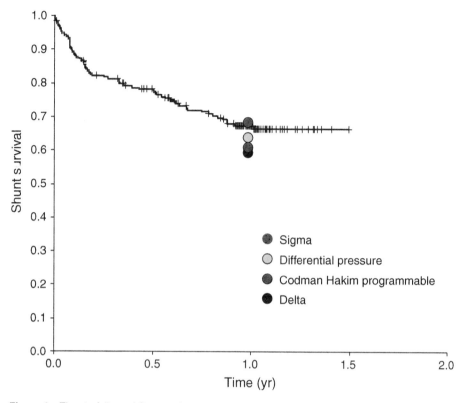

Figure 6   Time to failure of Strata valve.

6. Adjustment of the valve may improve symptoms. This is apparent within 24 hours.
   In the Strata valve study (3), patients' symptoms were self-reported after valve adjustments. Patients were asked if their presenting symptoms had completely resolved, improved, but not resolved, stayed the same, or worsened. Follow-up was available after 236 of 256 adjustments. Symptom improvement or resolution occurred in 149 of 236 (63%) patients. Sixty-one (26%) had complete symptom resolution and 88 (37%) had symptom improvement, but not resolution. When symptoms improved or resolved, they did so within 24 hours in 132 of 149 (89%) patients. Repeated adjustment of the valve beyond the first day or two without obvious improvement is therefore probably not warranted. The potential placebo effect of valve adjustment was not evaluated in this study.

7. Adjustable valves can change on their own. Twenty-two of 315 patients had an unexplained change in their valve setting at follow-up. Seventeen of these patients were asymptomatic at the time and 12/17 had their valve reset to the original level. There were five patients who had symptoms when their unexplained valve change was identified; in three of them the symptoms were thought to be related to the change and the valve was reset. Changes in valve setting have been reported with exposure to magnets (7).

8. The endoscope does not help for first time shunt insertion.
   A randomized clinical trial including 393 children being treated with a shunt for the first time randomized them to ventricular catheter placement, with and without the endoscope. The minimum follow-up was one year and the outcome was time to shunt failure. In this study (5), the overall shunt survival in the endoscope group was no better than in the non-endoscope group (Fig. 7). In the secondary analysis, based on postoperative imaging, it appears that the ventricular catheter tip position may be important. The survival curve looks favorable when the catheter tip ends up away from the choroid plexus. Positioning the catheter tip away from the choroid plexus seems like a reasonable goal, but based on the primary analysis this was not accomplished with the endoscope.

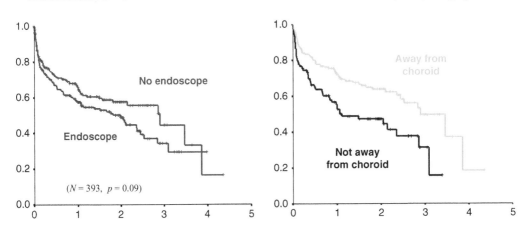

Figure 7 RCT of endoscopic ventricular catheter insertion.

9. Shunt infections come back.
    In a multicenter pilot study on the management of shunt infection, 70 patients were
    observed and the methods of treatment for their shunt infection were recorded (8). Rein-
    fection after treatment occurred in 18 of 70 (26%) patients. Twelve of these were with the
    same organism and six of them were with a different organism. Thirteen of the 70 patients
    had shunt infection in the past. If the shunt infection occurred in the preceding six months,
    there was 43% recurrence rate, and if the shunt infection occurred prior to six months
    previously, the recurrence rate was 24%. The management of shunt infection in this study
    was quite variable. The duration of therapy was recorded and the average treatment time
    after the CSF was clean was 13 days, but ranged from 3 to 46 days. There did not appear to
    be a difference in reinfection rate, based on the duration of treatment. Reinfection occurred
    in 20% of patients who were treated for less than or equal to seven days and in 28% of
    patients who were treated for more than seven days. When the analysis was limited to
    Staphylococcus epidermidis alone, there were 34 patients and the reinfection rate was 10 of
    34 (29%). There was marked variation again in the total treatment time with an average of
    12.5 days, but ranging from 3 to 39 days. *Staphylococcus epidermidis* patients who were
    treated for seven days or less had a reinfection rate of 27% and patients treated for more
    than seven days had a reinfection rate of 28%. It therefore appeared that the duration of
    therapy and recurrence of infection were not strongly correlated and further research in this
    area seems appropriate. The alarmingly high recurrence rate of 26% overall after treatment
    of shunt infection certainly justifies further investigation as well.
10. Experience does matter.
    The possibility of a "July effect" has been investigated in a number of areas in surgery and
    critical care medical (9–11,12). In two recent analyses, contradictory results were obtained
    with regard to hydrocephalus and shunt surgery (13,14). Barker used the National Inpatient
    Database with outcomes of death and neurologic deficit and could not demonstrate worse
    results in the summer.
        Based on pooling clinical trials data, Kestle et al. demonstrated a decreased shunt
    survival, an increased infection rate, and an increased wound dehiscence rate for patients
    treated with shunt surgery in July and August compared to the rest of the year.

    Both basic and clinical research are essential if we are to advance the care of patients with
hydrocephalus. Coordinated clinical trials have the potential to directly impact patient care. The
majority of clinical research questions require a multicenter approach, and further development
of cooperative groups of neurosurgeons, biostatisticians, data managers, and study coordinators
should be supported.

REFERENCES

1. Drake JM, Kestle JR, Milner R, et al. Randomized trial of cerebrospinal fluid shunt valve design in pediatric hydrocephalus. Neurosurgery 1998; 43:294–305.
2. Kestle J, Drake J, Milner R, et al. Long-term follow-up data from the Shunt Design Trial. Ped Neurosurg 2000; 33:230–236.
3. Kestle JRW, Walker ML; for the Strata Investigators. A multicenter prospective cohort study of the Strata valve for the management of hydrocephalus in pediatric patients. J Neurosurg 2005; 102(2 suppl):141–145.
4. Drake J, Kestle J. Rationale and methodology of the multicenter pediatric cerebrospinal fluid shunt design trial. Childs Nerv Syst 1996; 12:434–447.
5. Kestle J, Drake J, Cochrane D, et al. Lack of benefit of endoscopic ventriculoperitoneal shunt insertion: A multicenter randomized trial. J Neurosurg 2003, 90.284–290.
6. Pollack I, Albright A, Adelson P, et al.; Hakim-Medos Investigator Group. A randomized, controlled study of a programmable shunt valve versus a conventional valve for patients with hydrocephalus. Neurosurgery 2000; 45:1399–1408; discussion 1408–1411.
7. Anderson R, Walker M, Kestle J. Adjustment and malfunction of a programmable valve after exposure to toy magnets. J Neurosurg 2004; 101:222–225.
8. Kestle J, Garton H, Whitehead W, et al. Management of shunt infections: A multicenter pilot study. J Neurosurg Pediatr 2006; 105:177–181.
9. Barry W, Rosenthal G. Is there a July phenomenon? The effect of July admission on intensive care mortality and LOS in teaching hospitals. J Gen Intern Med 2003; 18:639–645.
10. Borenstein SH, Choi M, Gerstle JT, et al. Errors and adverse outcomes on a surgical service: What is the role of residents? J Surg Res 2004; 122:162–166.
11. Claridge JA, Schulman AM, Sawyer RG, et al. The "July phenomenon" and the care of the severely injured patient: Fact or fiction? Surgery 2001; 130:346–353.
12. Finkielman JD, Morales IJ, Peters SG, et al. Mortality rate and length of stay of patients admitted to the intensive care unit in July. Crit Care Med 2004; 32:1161–1165.
13. Kestle J, Cochrane D, Drake J. Shunt insertion in the summer: Is it safe? J Neurosurg 2006; 105(3 Suppl Pediatr):165–168.
14. Smith E, Butler W, Barker F. Is there a "July phenomenon" in pediatric neurosurgery at teaching hospitals? J Neurosurg 2006; 105(3 suppl):169–176.

The U.K. Shunt Registry

Hugh Richards

Cambridge Shunt Registry, Cambridge, U.K.

The U.K. Shunt Registry has been set up in Cambridge to collect and analyze data from shunt operations performed in the United Kingdom and Ireland per year. This registry has the support of the Council of the Society of British Neurological Surgeons, the Executive Committee of the British Association of Paediatric Surgeons, the United Kingdom Hydrocephalus Group, and ASBAH (Association for Spina Bifida and Hydrocephalus).

Data are collected from theater staff by means of a simple form (one sheet of A4 size). The simplicity of data collection is designed to maintain a high reporting rate. Although analysis is performed anonymously, patient name and address are required so that patients can be tracked if they are treated at different hospitals. The only other demographic data collected are age and gender. Clinical diagnosis is requested, as are date, time, technical aspects of the procedure, surgeon, and the details (including catalogue and serial numbers) for any hardware used. If the procedure is a shunt revision, the reason for revision is also requested. If we collect several forms for a single patient, this gives us information on procedures that are subsequently revised for a known reason. Using a Kaplan–Meier statistical model, we are able to calculate cumulative revision rates.

Between May 1995 and April 2006, we have received data on 36,649 shunt-related surgical procedures. From auditing during this period, we estimate our reporting rate to be 85%, so these figures represent 3000 to 3500 operations per year, with approximately 2700 new valves used each year.

There are currently 15 to 20 valves commonly used in the United Kingdom and Ireland. The pattern of valve usage is constantly changing as new designs are introduced onto the market and older designs are discarded. An interesting trend is the increased use of adjustable (programmable) valves. Our data show that the proportion of adjustable valves has steadily increased from 4.6% in 2000 to 22.8% in 2006. The proportion appears to be higher in older patients.

Patients undergoing CSF shunting represent a heterogeneous population, both in terms of age and pathology. The reasons for shunting are illustrated in Figure 1. In both adults and children, 65% of shunts are inserted for hydrocephalus secondary to existing pathology.

Our data indicate that 30.3% of shunts in adults fail within five years. In children the failure rate is 46.9%. The reasons for revision are given in Figure 2. In both age groups, underdrainage is the most commonly given reason for revision, representing 40.7% of all revisions (39.5% in adults and 42.1% in children), with involvement of the proximal catheter occurring approximately twice as often as the distal catheter. Overdrainage is the reported cause of revision in 7.3% of patients older than 70 years of age, but only 4.0% in patients younger than 70 years.

Fifteen percent of shunt revisions are reported to be due to infection. In children younger than one year of age, the proportion is 34.6%. These figures represent data from 1995 to 2005, but in recent years antimicrobial catheters have been developed, which may substantially reduce shunt infection. Data collected by the Registry suggest these catheters may reduce shunt infections by one-half (1).

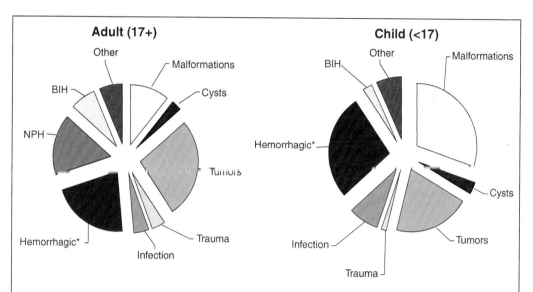

*Note – In adults, subarachnoid Hemorrhage accounts for 18% of shunts and in children perinatal IVH for 25%

Figure 1 Reasons for shunting.

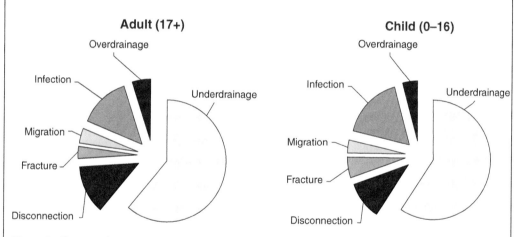

Figure 2 Reasons for revision.

REFERENCE

1. Hugh Richards, Helen Seeley, John Pickard. Do antibiotic-impregnated shunt catheters reduce shunt infection? Data from the UK Shunt Registry. http://www.cerebrospinalfluidresearch.com/content/3/S1/S55.

27 | Endoscopy for Hydrocephalus—General Aspects

J. André Grotenhuis
Department of Neurosurgery, Radboud University Nijmegen Medical Center, Nijmegen, The Netherlands

Sherif Mohammed Al-Sayed Al-Kheshen
Department of Neurosurgery, Faculty of Medicine, Tanta University, Tanta, Egypt

Khaled Elsayed Mohammed
Department of Neurosurgery, Faculty of Medicine, Suez Canal University, Ismailia, Egypt

INTRODUCTION

Neuroendoscopy has enjoyed a renewed interest in the last decade. Although it is not new as a technique—Walter Dandy and other pioneers have used it as early as the beginning of the 20th century—technological advancements have made it safer and easier, making endoscopic treatment of hydrocephalus feasible even in neonates and newborns. Neuroendoscopy has now gained a widespread acceptance, particularly among neurosurgeons who deal with the pediatric population and even after the initial enthusiasm and renewed interest has settled and consolidated endoscopic third ventriculostomy (ETV) for treatment of obstructive hydrocephalus is generally considered nowadays as first tier in the management of many patients (1–14).

Because the use of neuroendoscopes and instruments is inherently different from classic microneurosurgical techniques, careful planning and preparation are very important to avoid complications and poor outcomes.

INDICATIONS FOR THE USE OF ENDOSCOPES FOR HYDROCEPHALUS

The cause for hydrocephalus can be manifold. The current indications to use neuroendoscopy include (*i*) treatment of obstructive hydrocephalus by fenestrating the floor of the third ventricle, (*ii*) dilating or stenting an obstructed aqueduct, (*iii*) direct positioning of a proximal shunt catheter, (*iv*) fenestration of intraventricular membranes, (*v*) opening of the septum pellucidum in unilateral obstruction of the foramen of Monro, (*vi*) biopsy or excision of intraventricular tumors, (*vii*) fenestration of intra- and paraventricular arachnoid cysts and marsupialization of neuroepithelial cysts. But certainly the indications are still evolving (7,8,15).

PREOPERATIVE WORKUP

Magnetic resonance (MR) imaging is the diagnostic modality of choice as it gives exact anatomical details in three planes, which greatly enhances preoperative planning. Sometimes, for example, for multiloculated hydrocephalus, a CT scan with intraventricular contrast is better for demonstrating the communicating and noncommunicating parts of the ventricular system.

For precise placement of the burr hole and calculation of the appropriate, often angled trajectory and guidance of the neuroendoscopes towards the target, the neuroendoscope can be used in conjunction with frame-based or frameless stereotaxy, and the development of electromagnetic (EM) navigation made its use much easier because rigid fixation of the head during the procedure is no longer necessary and this makes it also applicable for the very young patients (7,8).

EQUIPMENT

Neuroendoscopes

Two types of endoscopes are commonly employed for neuroendoscopy: lenscope-based endoscopes, which are rigid shaft instruments, and fiberoptic-based endoscopes, which can be either build into a rigid shaft or come as flexible endoscopes. The lenscope provides the best image clarity, resolution, and illumination. Its straight design makes it easy to introduce and also allows easy orientation. Hence, it is the best type of endoscope to start with and to master basic neuroendoscopic skills. However, the disadvantage of rigid lenscopes is the comparatively large diameter of the endoscope.

Nowadays, many different rigid neuroendoscopes are available, like the 6-mm Caemaert cerebral endoscope by Wolf; the 6-mm Gaab neuroendoscope by Storz, with an angled eyepiece and a straight operating sheath and the MINOP system by Aesculap with trocars; and an 2.7-mm angled neuroendoscope, which can also be used for endoscope-assisted microneurosurgery. The rigid fiberscope, like the Workscope by Medtronic, is as easy in handling as the lenscopes. Its weight is much less than that of lenscopes, but its particular advantage is the small size of the optical fibers, which permits a much larger instrument channel relative to the total endoscope diameter of 4 mm. The image quality, however, is inferior to that of a lenscope, although incorporation of 30,000 fibers has improved much of the image quality.

The main advantage of the flexible fiberscope is the deflection and therefore the moving capability of the working tip, enabling both looking and working "around the corner." Because the shaft of the endoscope is flexible, the endoscopic image will rotate during deflection of the tip and this pairs a more challenging anatomical orientation with an inferior image quality. In addition, as its working channel is quite small, the flexible instruments for these endoscopes are also very small. This makes them more difficult to manipulate precisely because they exhibit delay or rotation on actuation. Flexible and steerable neuroendoscopes are available, for example, with an outer diameter of 4 mm and a steerable tip that can be rotated 100/160 degrees, one working channel of 1 mm, and a flexible working length of 38 cm with 10 cm markings.

A fiberscope, mainly used for placement of the proximal shunt catheter, is the Stylet or the 1.2-mm Neuroview Neuroendoscope, which is a semi-rigid fiberscope that can be introduced into the ventricular catheter during a shunting procedure. It also has a flushing channel and it can be used for other procedures like diagnostic ventriculoscopy and some neurosurgeons also use it for third ventriculostomy. About the same size is the Neuroguide, but it has no flushing channel. The Neuroguide is only used in shunting procedures.

Next to endoscopes, one will need a light source, a camera and video system, an irrigation device, a device for fixation of the endoscope, and an array of instruments for neuroendoscopy, like grasping and biopsy forceps, scissors, laser equipment, Radio Frequency Dissector, bipolar coagulation electrode, puncturing needle, and balloon catheter.

ENDOSCOPIC TREATMENT OF HYDROCEPHALUS: THE TECHNIQUE

In general, endoscopic procedures within the ventricular system will be performed through one burr hole, also referred to as a monoportal procedure compared to a biportal procedure in which two different approaches are used. In some instances, like procedures for ventricular tumors, this can be advantageous because it broadens the possibilities of manipulation and it gives the possibility to control the shaft of each endoscope by the other. One should keep in mind that using trajectories for two 4-mm endoscopes (together a cross-sectional area of 25 mm^2) is still less invasive than one trajectory for a 6-mm endoscope (cross-sectional area of 28 mm^2) (6,7,16).

The preferred treatment for symptomatic *communicating* hydrocephalus is ventriculoperitoneal shunting, although sometimes lumboperitoneal shunting can suffice. One key to long-term success of a shunt probably is the correct placement of the ventricular catheter. The use of an endoscope allows precise positioning of the proximal catheter away from the choroid plexus. We advise anyone to rehearse catheter placement as often as possible on a teaching-head because, although it sounds quite simple, there is a steep learning curve for successful performance of this procedure (as is for all endoscopic procedures). In what is called the direct method, a very small stylet-like endoscope is placed directly through the ventricular catheter, so there is no need for additional passage of a cannula through the brain.

Obstructive hydrocephalus can be treated effectively with an endoscopic procedure, which will avoid the insertion of a shunt, ETV, fenestration of obstructive cysts, or balloon dilatation of aqueductal stenosis with or without stenting is now the primary treatment options for patients with an obstructive hydrocephalus. ETV has proven to be effective and safe if some

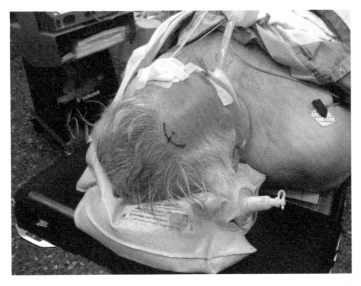

Figure 1   Position of skin incision and burr hole; just precoronal, paramedian, in the midpupillary line.

precautions are taken. The procedure is performed in cases of obstructive hydrocephalus with patent subarachnoid spaces and a dilated third ventricle (6,7,16).

Making a connection between the subarachnoid space (interpeduncular cistern) and the third ventricle through its floor can reestablish normal CSF flow and eliminate the need for a shunt. Crucial for the success of this treatment is proper patient selection. Mandatory is a preoperative MRI, revealing large ventricles, ballooning of the third ventricle, thinning of its floor, and a confirmation of the site of CSF obstruction. Cine-MRI, showing the lack of a CSF flow void signal in the aqueduct, is desirable (6,7,16).

The endoscope is introduced through a burr hole at or slightly in front of the coronal suture and about 2.5 cm paramedian, which mostly equals the midpupillary line (Figs. 1–5). After entering the anterior horn one should identify the choroid plexus or a vein, which is followed towards the foramen of Monro where the choroid plexus enters the third ventricle, and the septal vein and thalamostriate vein coalesce. The foramen should be large enough

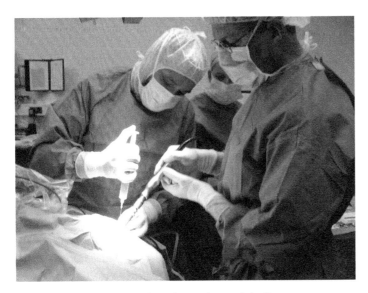

Figure 2   Drilling the burr hole under continuous irrigation.

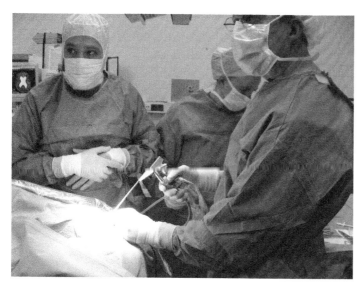

Figure 3 Introduction of the endoscope.

(which is usually the case in obstructive hydrocephalus) to allow entrance of the endoscope without touching the fornix.

Within the third ventricle, the mamillary bodies are rapidly recognized (although they can be less prominent in infants, but then they are recognizable by their vascular pattern). In front of the mamillary bodies, the thinned-out, translucent floor of the third ventricle and the basilar artery beneath it are often visible. Somewhat more frontally the hypervascularized area of the infundibular recess is a well-recognizable landmark (6,7,16).

By staying exactly in the midline and within the anterior third of a line from the anterior border of the mamillary bodies to the infundibular recess, opening of the floor should be safe. There are many techniques to perforate the floor of the third ventricle. As blunt perforation can be hazardous, especially when vital structures are obscured, several methods and instruments have been described and used. A gentle thrust of the endoscope itself is simplest, but not without

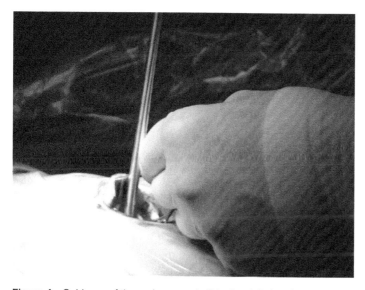

Figure 4 Guidance of the endoscope shaft by the right-handed surgeon's left hand.

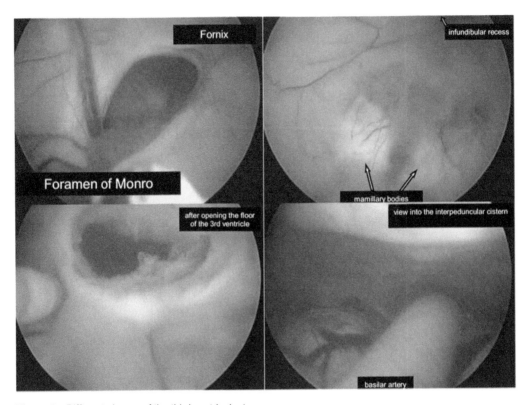

Figure 5   Different phases of the third ventriculostomy.

danger. A puncturing device can be adequate, allowing the introduction of a balloon catheter to dilate the orifice of a ventriculostomy (6,7,16).

Besides monopolar coagulation wires and radio frequency dissectors, laser assistance has also proven to be valuable. However, conventional laser-tips require large amounts of energy for ablation of the floor of the third ventricle with considerable risk to underlying, vital structures such as the basilar artery and its branches. A special laser catheter with an atraumatic ball-tip, pre-treated with a layer of carbon particles, which absorbs approximately 90% of the energy, has been developed by Vandertop for the purpose of perforating membranes safely. As the heat is generated in this very thin layer of carbon coating, only a few Watts of energy are necessary for a fraction of a second in order to reach ablative temperatures instantly at the tip with virtually no heat effect on surrounding tissues or deeper structures. The precoated tip enables the surgeon to predict the depth of ablation and the extent of coagulation. At the moment of perforation, the light emitted from the fiber is minimal and highly scattered so that no temperature increase can be created in distal structures. This combination of low energy and high absorption makes the application safe and controlled (6,7,16).

A new technique, using suction for the initial opening of the floor and spreading to enlarge this opening, has been developed in 1998 by the first author. The tip of the probe, which resembles a corneal trephine, is placed against the floor of the 3rd ventricle, and by pushing a trumpet valve the suction is applied to the floor, which will be fixed to the tip of the probe. By a gentle turning and withdrawing action, the floor is lifted up a little and a small round opening is made in the floor with the exact diameter of the tip of the probe. Then a second, forceps-like instrument is used which is placed in the opening. It is made in two designs, one standard size and one neonatal size. The small rounded hooks at its tip will hold the edges of the opening, the floor is then lifted up and the spreading action of the instrument will then gently enlarge the opening to the desired size. The standard size instrument will spread to 8.5 mm; the neonatal size to 4.65 mm. Because no instrument will enter the interpeduncular cistern, the structures inside, for example, basilar artery with its branches and both oculomotor nerves, are not at risk. So the combined use of a suction-perforator and a dilator greatly reduces the risk of ETV. Experience over many years and hundreds of cases have shown that the use of the "Grotenhuis Endoscopic Perforator™" and the "Grotenhuis Dilator™" is an extremely safe technique for ETV (6,7,8,16).

ENDOSCOPIC TREATMENT OF HYDROCEPHALUS: THE CONTROVERSIES

ETV in Patients Younger Than Two Years

In the literature, the vast majority of authors reporting their experience and results with ETV mention a low success rate in patients younger than two years (4,9,10,17). This has even led to recommendations by some authors not to perform ETV in patients younger than two years at all. By contrast, a few others indicate that there is no difference in success rate in the very young patients compared to the older age group or that it is only slightly lower and still useful to try (13,14,18–21).

In an own but already older study from 1991 to 1999 of a series of 48 patients younger than two years (out of a total group of 179 patients), of which 41 patients were younger than one year and only 7 between one and two years old, 27 patients had a successful outcome, defined as being symptom-free and without a shunt (7,8).

This is a success rate of 56.3%, which was much lower than in the total cohort of patients. So, at first sight, it seems that this confirmed the gloomy outlook for ETV in this age group. But on analysis of the result in more detail we have looked at the different types of hydrocephalus, and we found that the success rate in the primary and secondary aqueductal stenosis group, although small in this age group, is as excellent as in older patients. In conclusion, based upon those data there has been no reason for us to withhold ETV in patients below the age of two years. As it is in every age group, the success mainly depends on the etiology of the hydrocephalus. But since this remains to be an unsolved question to date, a prospective study has been initiated and started in 2006.

ETV in Postinfectious and Posthemorrhagic Hydrocephalus

ETV in patients with a history of subarachnoid hemorrhage or intraventricular hemorrhage (IVH) and/or cerebrospinal fluid (CSF) infection has always been a matter of debate. Because ETV should need an open subarachnoid space to be effective and because hydrocephalus as a consequence of hemorrhage and/or infection is thought to be due to a blocked subarachnoid space, the application of ETV in such cases was generally thought to be ineffective. However, the safety and efficacy have been investigated in a multicenter study (22) and they found interesting facts: A higher rate of treatment failure was associated with three factors— classification in the combined infection/hemorrhage group, premature birth in the posthemorrhage group, and younger age in the postinfection group. A higher success rate was associated with a history of ventriculoperitoneal (VP) shunt placement before ETV in the posthemorrhage group, even among those who had been born prematurely, who were otherwise more prone to treatment failure. As a conclusion, they found that patients with obstructive hydrocephalus and a history of either hemorrhage or infection might be good candidates for ETV, with safety and success rates comparable with those in more general series of patients. Patients who have sustained both hemorrhage and infection are poor candidates for ETV, except in selected cases and as a treatment of last resort. In patients who have previously undergone shunt placement posthemorrhage, ETV is highly successful. It is also highly successful in patients with primary aqueductal stenosis, even in those with a history of hemorrhage or CSF infection.

ETV in Patients with Myelomeningocele

Spinal dysraphism is associated with hydrocephalus in very high percentage. In a number of patients, the hydrocephalus is already overt at birth but mostly it becomes apparent within one or two weeks after repair of the myelomeningocele. Hydrocephalus in these cases is considered to be of an obstructive type due to the associated Chiari malformation and the often-concurrent aqueductal deformity.

So, from a theoretical standpoint, ETV could be a good alternative treatment to the standard shunt implantation, especially because in spina bifida patient, the chance of shunt infection and shunt malfunction is quite high. The literature on ETV in patients with myelomeningocele is rather sparse (7,8,18,21,23–25).

Teo and Jones have reported their rather large experience with 69 patients with hydrocephalus and myelomeningocele in which ETV was performed between 1978 and 1995 (25). In 14 of their patients, ETV had been the initial treatment; the others had been previously shunted. They described an overall success rate of 72%, although selecting only patients who have been previously shunted or who were older than six months at the time of endoscopy increased this to 80%.

Our own results in a group of 20 patients divulge a striking discrepancy between those patients with previous shunting and those without. From our data one can see that in the 11 patients with ETV as initial treatment, there had been a success rate of 27.3% (3 patients), while in those 9 patients who had been previously shunted, the success rate was 77.8% (7 patients) (7,26).

So, in conclusion, these results indicate that ETV is a safe and effective means of treating hydrocephalus, especially in the older myelomeningocele population that have been shunted previously. But as an initial treatment it is certainly less effective and one can argue to postpone the option of ETV and choose shunting as a first treatment, especially because ETV in the very young myelomeningocele patient is also challenging from an anatomical standpoint because of the dysraphic changes inside the ventricular system. However, if MRI shows a favorable anatomical situation and even considering the low success rate of around 25%, it maybe can offer the hope of a shunt-independent life later in life.

ETV in Normal Pressure Hydrocephalus

Normal pressure hydrocephalus (NPH) is a condition that still is not well understood but generally has been considered a form of communicating hydrocephalus and hence ETV did not seem to be a logical choice. But nevertheless, in smaller series, a group of older patient with NPH has been reported with good results after ETV and this triggered reevaluation. The concept has been developed by a functional aqueductal stenosis caused by atrophy of the brain and thus changing the anatomical situation in such a way that the CSF cannot flow freely from the foramen of Monro and the third ventricle through the aqueduct because the angle between the entrance of the aqueduct and the fourth ventricle had changed. Indeed, on MRI scan, turbulent flow and stasis of CSF near the entrance have been described. So, in a limited number of patients with NPH there could be an indication for ETV (7,8,27,28).

Do Benefits Outweigh (Possible) Complications?

Every surgical intervention contains the risk of a complication. Serious, even fatal adverse events that can occur during ETV include intraoperative hemorrhage, traumatic aneurysms, intracerebral hematoma, cardiac dysrhythmias, cranial nerve palsies, neurological deficits, subdural effusions, cerebrospinal fluid leaks, hypothalamic imbalance, epilepsy, and infection. Rates of complications for neuroendoscopy in general and ETV in particular, reported in the literature, vary from 6% to 20% (1,4,7,8,10,13,29,30). But the same is of course true for insertion of a ventriculoatrial or ventriculoperitoneal shunt. The procedure itself harbors relatively low risks (rarely hemorrhage, more frequently misplacement of the ventricular catheter), but long-term complications are manifold and more frequent.

Although ETV harbors clearly a one-time surgical risk during the procedure, there are hardly any long-term problems (maybe with the exception of the reclosure of the stoma and the need to perform the ETV a second time), while the long-term success rate remains as high as the initial success rate. So, in conclusion, one can clearly state that the benefits of ETV for obstructive hydrocephalus indeed outweigh the possible complications of the procedure.

REFERENCES

1. Brockmeyer D, Abtin K, Carey L, et al. Endoscopic third ventriculostomy: An outcome analysis. Pediatr Neurosurg 1998; 28:236–240.
2. Cinalli G. Alternatives to shunting. Childs Nerv Syst 1999; 15:718–731.
3. Cinalli G, Sainte-Rose C, Chumas P, et al. Failure of third ventriculostomy in the treatment of aqueductal stenosis in children. J Neurosurg 1999; 90:448–454.
4. Cohen AR. Endoscopic ventricular surgery. Pediatr Neurosurg 1994; 19:127–134
5. Genitori L, Peretta P, Mussa F, et al. Endoscopic third ventriculostomy in children: Are age and etiology of hydrocephalus predictive factors influencing the outcome in primary and secondary treated patients? A series of 254 patients and 276 procedures. Childs Nerv Syst 2003; 19: 618.
6. Grotenhuis JA. Third ventriculocisternostomy. In: Grotenhuis JA, ed. Manual of Endoscopic Procedures in Neurosurgery. Nijmegen, The Netherlands: Uitgeverij Machaon, 1995:98–104.
7. Grotenhuis JA. Endoscopic third ventriculostomy in the treatment of hydrocephalus [Thesis]. Nijmegen, The Netherlands: University of Nijmegen, 2000:1–248.
8. Hellwig D, Grotenhuis JA, Tirakotai W, et al. Endoscopic third ventriculostomy for obstructive hydrocephalus. Neurosurg Rev 2005; 28(1):1–34; discussion 35–38.
9. Jones RF, Kwok BC, Stening WA, et al. The current status of endoscopic third ventriculostomy in the management of non-communicating hydrocephalus. Minim Invas Neurosurg 1994; 37:28–36.
10. Kunz U, Goldmann A, Bader C, et al. Endoscopic fenestration of the 3rd ventricular floor in aqueductal stenosis. Minim Invas Neurosurg 1994; 37:42–47.
11. Mallucci C, Vloeberghs M, Punt J. Should shunts be revised when neuroendoscopic third ventriculostomy is available? Br J Neurosurg 1997; 11:473.
12. Osman-Farah J, Javadpour M, Buxton N, et al. Endoscopic ventricular fenestration and ETV for the treatment of multicompartmental neonatal hydrocephalus. Childs Nerv Syst 2003; 19:702–703.
13. Sainte-Rose C, Chumas P. Endoscopic third ventriculostomy. Tech Neurosurg 1996; 1:176–184.
14. Teo C. Third ventriculostomy in the treatment of hydrocephalus: Experience with more than 120 cases. In: Hellwig D, Bauer BL, eds. Minimally Invasive Techniques for Neurosurgery. Berlin, Germany: Springer Verlag, 1998:73–76.
15. Murshid WR. Endoscopic third ventriculostomy: Towards more indications for the treatment of non-communicating hydrocephalus. Minim Invasive Neurosurg 2000; 43:75–82.
16. Grotenhuis JA. General principles of neuroendoscopy. In: Grotenhuis JA, ed. Manual of Endoscopic Procedures in Neurosurgery. Nijmegen, The Netherlands: Machaon, 1995:12–35.
17. Fritsch MJ, Medhorn HM. Indication and controversies for endoscopic third ventriculostomy in children. Childs Nerv Syst 2003; 19:706–707.
18. Alvarez JA, Cohen AR. Neonatal applications of neuroendoscopy. Neurosurg Clin N Am 1998; 9: 405–413.
19. Beems T, Grotenhuis JA. Is the success rate of endoscopic third ventriculostomy age-dependent? An analysis of the results of endoscopic third ventriculostomy in young children. Childs Nerv Syst 2002; 18:605–608.
20. Burn SC, Saxena A, Tyagi A, et al. Endoscopic third ventriculostomy in children during the first year of life. Childs Nerv Syst 2003; 19:618–619.
21. Buxton N, Macarthur D, Mallucci C, et al. Neuroendoscopic third ventriculostomy in patients less than 1 year old. Pediatr Neurosurg 1998; 29:73–76.
22. Siomin V, Cinalli G, Grotenhuis A, et al. Endoscopic third ventriculostomy in patients with cerebrospinal fluid infection and/or hemorrhage. J Neurosurg 2002; 97:519–524.
23. Buxton N, Macarthur D, Mallucci C, et al. Neuroendoscopy in the premature population. Childs Nerv Syst 1998; 14:649–652.
24. Jones RF, Kwok BC, Stening WA, et al. Third ventriculostomy for hydrocephalus associated with spinal dysraphism: Indications and contraindications. Eur J Pediatr Surg 1996; 6(suppl 1):5–6.
25. Teo C, Jones R. Management of hydrocephalus by endoscopic third ventriculostomy in patients with myelomeningocele. Pediatr Neurosurg 1996; 25:57–63.
26. Grotenhuis JA, Beems T. The role of endoscopic third ventriculostomy in the treatment of hydrocephalus associated with myelomeningocele. Minim Invasive Neurosurg 1999; 42:161–162.
27. Meier U, Zeilinger FS, Schonherr B. Endoscopic ventriculostomy versus shunt operation in normal pressure hydrocephalus: Diagnostics and indication. Minim Invasive Neurosurg 2000, 43, 87–90.

28. Mitchell P, Mathew B. Third ventriculostomy in normal pressure hydrocephalus. Br J Neurosurg 1999; 13:382–385.
29. Grotenhuis JA. Complications of neuroendoscopy. In: Grotenhuis JA, ed. Manual of Endoscopic Procedures in Neurosurgery. Nijmegen, The Netherlands: Machaon, 1995:57–63.
30. Teo C, Rahman S, Boop FA, et al. Complications of endoscopic neurosurgery. Childs Nerv Syst 1996; 12:248–253.

ETV Techniques and Complications

Wolfgang Wagner and Dorothee Koch-Wiewrodt

Neurochirurgische Klinik und Poliklinik, Bereich Pädiatrische Neurochirurgie, Johannes Gutenberg-Universität Mainz, Germany

Technical aspects of ETV encompass several points to be considered when choosing appropriate surgical steps and instruments.

- Location of the burr hole (relation to the coronal suture; distance from the midline),
- Types of endoscope (rigid, semi-rigid, flexible; lens scope, fiber scope; outer diameter; use of a peel-away sheath),
- Technique of perforation of the ventricular floor (sharp, blunt; using endoscope tip, deflated balloon catheter, bipolar or monopolar coagulation, forceps, contact laser with specially coated tip, water jet, "No-through-perforator" suction device),
- Technique of widening the stoma (using inflatable balloon catheter, endoscope, forceps, coagulation),
- Inspection of the basal cisterns (with the option of detecting and perforating a "second membrane"),
- Optional use of ultrasound or neuronavigation (in order to define the approach trajectory or to localize the basilar tip before perforating the ventricular floor),
- Optional insertion of a ventricular access device (with the possibility of CSF taps or ICP measurement when ETV failure is suspected), etc. (1–3).

In the context of intraoperative complications and their prevention, the most critical step in performing an ETV is the way to open a stoma in the floor of the third ventricle.

Complications of ETV may occur during surgery or in the postoperative course. These include vascular injury (hemorrhage, infarction), circulatory compromise (bradycardia, asystole), damage to neural structures (fornices, hypothalamus, etc.) resulting in neurologic deficit (cranial nerve injury, hemiparesis, hyperthermia, seizure, confusion, drowsiness), hormonal disorders (e.g., diabetes insipidus, hyponatremia), infection (meningitis, ventriculitis), disturbed wound healing (dehiscence, CSF fistula), subdural hygroma, or hematoma. If even minor and transient complications are taken into account, there is a reported overall incidence of up to 20% of procedures (3–11). The frequency of serious complications (mortality or permanent morbidity) in several large clinical series, however, was far lower (0–1.6%) (4,7–10). The clearly most dangerous and frightening complication is injury to arterial vessels in the basal cisterns (basilar artery or its branches) when perforating the floor of the third ventricle (7,8,12–16).

Based on prospectively collected data of 193 ETV in 188 patients and on a thorough review of the literature, Schroeder and coworkers published an extensive and systematic study on ETV complications (10). Misplacement of the fenestration at the floor of the third ventricle was found to be the main reason for severe complications like basilar (or perforating) artery injury or oculomotor nerve palsy. The use of a laser [at least without specially coated fiber tips (17)] for the perforation of the floor of the third ventricle was reported to be potentially hazardous because of the risk of injury to the basilar artery (15). However, an analysis of the techniques used to open the ventricular floor (as far as they are published in the literature in case reports or clinical series on ETV complications) yields no direct impact on the occurrence of vascular or neural injury, as the distribution of the perforating instruments (mostly endoscope tip, forceps, balloon catheter, and monopolar or bipolar coagulation) used in cases with complications did not differ from those without complications. In the seven published cases with injury to the basilar artery or its branches during ETV, the perforating tools were endoscope (7,8,12), coagulation (13,14), balloon catheter (16), and laser (plus endoscope) (15).

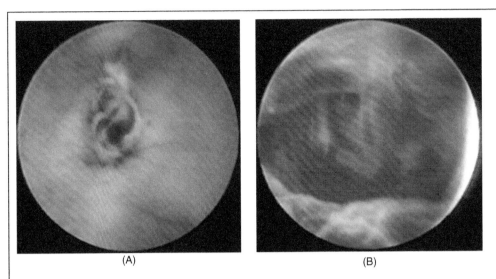

(A)   (B)

Figure 1 (**A**) ETV in a six-month-old boy with aqueductal stenosis. The floor of the third ventricle is not transparent; clear anatomical landmarks are hardly visible. The stoma was intended to be opened in the midline, behind the clivus and in front of the basilar artery. (**B**) A close-up view through the widened stoma shows the upper dorsal aspect of the basilar artery bifurcation and the ventral aspect of the pons with perforators. The position of this ventriculostoma is clearly too far posterior. Fortunately, no vascular or other complication occurred in this case.

Most authors conclude from their experience that the perforation of the floor should be made halfway between the infundibular recess and the mammillary bodies (or just dorsal to the dorsum sellae) in the midline, using a blunt instrument (1–3,8,10,11). By observing these important rules, "keep to the midline" and "perforate anteriorly to the basilar tip," "use a blunt instrument," and "abandon the procedure if it cannot be done safely," the risk of vascular or neural injury is minimized (Fig. 1).

Relationships between other complications and particular procedural steps in performing an ETV have been reported as well. Increase in local pressure (by brisk and prolonged inflation of the balloon catheter) or intracranial pressure (by excessive irrigation, especially when outflow from the endoscope is obstructed) or mechanical manipulation of the hypothalamus (by exerting strong forces on a thick and tough ventricular floor) may all lead to intra- or postoperative circulatory disorders or signs of hypothalamic dysfunction. It is mandatory for the neurosurgeon to hear the cardiac monitor throughout the whole operation; prompt reaction to, for example, bradycardia may prevent serious complications. Monopolar or bipolar coagulation, if applied at all, should be set at a very low current level and not used for complete perforation but only to create a "notch" in the floor to weaken the tissue and facilitating and guiding the perforation by the Fogarty or hourglass balloon catheter. Optimal planning of the trajectory from the burr hole through the foramen of Monroe to the ventricular floor may avoid damage to the fornix; this is particularly important when—in addition to ETV—a biopsy of, for example, a pineal region tumor is planned in the same procedure. It is generally recommended to gently reexpand the ventricles by rinsing before removing the endoscope and to plug the parenchymal corridor with gelfoam after withdrawing the instrument in order to avoid subdural hygromas or hematomas (11). The frequency of this complication may be influenced by the use of large diameter (6 mm or more) "adult" endoscopes versus small diameter (3 mm or less) "pediatric" endoscopes, but this has not been systematically studied in larger series (18). So-called water-tight wound closure is deemed essential to prevent a CSF fistula; however, the postoperative leakage of CSF should cast suspicion on a continuing high ICP, possibly (not necessarily) indicating ETV failure.

Another important aspect of ETV complications and their avoidance is surgical experience. As with other surgical procedures, the incidence of ETV complications decreases with the absolute number and the frequency of endoscopic operations done by the single surgeon or by the institution as a whole, respectively. The relationship between an increase in practice and experience and a decrease in complications over years has been shown in several clinical series (7,8,10).

In conclusion, the overall safety of ETV is high. When the procedure is carefully done by an experienced neurosurgeon, avoiding methods and techniques known to be potentially dangerous, the rate of serious complications is very low.

REFERENCES

1. Brockmeyer D. Techniques of endoscopic third ventriculostomy. Neurosurg Clin N Am 2004; 15(1):51–59.
2. Cinalli G. Endoscopic third ventriculostomy. In: Cinalli G, Maixner WJ, Sainte-Rose C, eds. Pediatric Hydrocephalus. Milano, Italy: Springer, 2004:361–388.
3. Hellwig D, Grotenhuis JA, Tirakotai W, et al. Endoscopic third ventriculostomy for obstructive hydrocephalus. Neurosurg Rev 2005; 28(1):1–34.
4. Beems T, Grotenhuis JA. Long-term complications and definition of failure of neuroendoscopic procedures. Childs Nerv Syst 2004; 20(11–12):868–877.
5. Buxton N, Ho KJ, Macarthur D, et al. Neuroendoscopic third ventriculostomy for hydrocephalus in adults: Report of a single unit's experience with 63 cases. Surg Neurol 2001; 55(2):74–78.
6. Di Rocco C, Massimi L, Tamburrini G. Shunts versus endoscopic third ventriculostomy in infants: Are there different types and/or rates of complications? A review. Childs Nerv Syst 2006; 22(12):1573–1589.
7. Kadrian D, van Gelder J, Florida D, et al. Long-term reliability of endoscopic third ventriculostomy. Neurosurgery 2005; 56(6):1271–1278.
8. Navarro R, Gil-Parra R, Reitman AJ, et al. Endoscopic third ventriculostomy in children: Early and late complications and their avoidance. Childs Nerv Syst 2006; 22(5):506–513.
9. Peretta P, Ragazzi P, Galarza M, et al. Complications and pitfalls of neuroendoscopic surgery in children. J Neurosurg 2006; 105(3 suppl):187–193.
10. Schroeder HW, Niendorf WR, Gaab MR. Complications of endoscopic third ventriculostomy. J Neurosurg 2002; 96 (6):1032–1040.
11. Teo C. Complications of endoscopic third ventriculostomy. In: Cinalli G, Maixner WJ, Sainte-Rose C, eds. Pediatric Hydrocephalus. Milano, Italy: Springer, 2004:411–420.
12. Abtin K, Thompson BG, Walker ML. Basilar artery perforation as a complication of endoscopic third ventriculostomy. Pediatr Neurosurg 1998; 28(1):35–41.
13. Cinalli G, Salazar C, Mallucci C, et al. The role of endoscopic third ventriculostomy in the management of shunt malfunction. Neurosurgery 1998; 43(6):1323–1329.
14. Horowitz M, Albright AL, Jungreis C, et al. Endovascular management of a basilar artery false aneurysm secondary to endoscopic third ventriculostomy: case report. Neurosurgery 2001; 49(6):1461–1465.
15. McLaughlin MR, Wahlig JB, Kaufmann AM, et al. Traumatic basilar aneurysm after endoscopic third ventriculostomy: Case report. Neurosurgery 1997; 41(6):1400–1403.
16. Schroeder HW, Warzok RW, Assaf JA, et al. Fatal subarachnoid hemorrhage after endoscopic third ventriculostomy. Case report. J Neurosurg 1999; 90(1):153–155.
17. Vandertop WP, Verdaasdonk RM, van Swol CF. Laser-assisted neuroendoscopy using a neodymium-yttrium aluminum garnet or diode contact laser with pretreated fiber tips. J Neurosurg 1998; 88(1):82–92.
18. Wiewrodt D, Schumacher R, Wagner W. Hygromas after endoscopic third ventriculostomy in the first year of life: Incidence, management and outcome in a series of 34 patients. Childs Nerv Syst 2008; 24.57–63.

28 | Endoscopic Management of Specific Disease Entities

Daniel J. Guillaume
Department of Neurosurgery, Oregon Health & Science University, Portland, Oregon, U.S.A.

Charles Teo
The Centre for Minimally Invasive Neurosurgery, Prince of Wales Private Hospital, Randwick, New South Wales, Australia

INTRODUCTION

With technological advances and enhancements in the design and development of endoscopy equipment, applications are growing. In parallel with this progress have been the training, experience, and familiarity with endoscopy of both practicing neurosurgeons and residents. The modern neuroendoscope in the hands of a properly trained neurosurgeon becomes a valuable tool with many uses. Neuroendoscopy also fits in with a growing trend toward minimal invasiveness with access and visualization through the smallest opening possible, greatest action at the point of interest, and minimal retraction and disruption of normal brain tissue.

Neuroendoscopy has been most useful, and gained most attention, in the treatment of noncommunicating and complex hydrocephalus. Other types of intraventricular pathology are now successfully treated using neuroendoscopy including intraventricular tumors and cysts. In many cases, shunts can be avoided or removed. Craniotomies can also be avoided with less pain, shorter hospital stays, and in many cases improved cosmetic result. Endoscopic endonasal transsphenoidal surgery gives access to pathology located in the sellar, parasellar, suprasellar, subfrontal, cavernous sinus, petrous apex, and clival regions with the advantage of improved vision of the surgical field and a minimally traumatic approach.

General aspects concerning endoscopic management of hydrocephalus including endoscopic third ventriculostomy (ETV) in general with its indications, technique, and results are covered in the preceding chapter. This chapter focuses on endoscopic applications for specific etiologies including complex hydrocephalus and tumor management and not on ETV for obstructive hydrocephalus. We hope to present the rationale behind endoscopic management of these specific pathologies, technique, and evidence supporting their use.

COMPLEX HYDROCEPHALUS

Aqueductal Stenosis, Isolated Fourth Ventricle, and Dandy–Walker Syndrome

Aqueductal stenosis is responsible for more than 50% of cases of hydrocephalus presenting within the first year of life (1). Initial attempts to bypass this obstruction began in the 1920s when Dandy tried to communicate the third ventricle with the chiasmatic cistern using a subfrontal approach (2). Because early ventriculostomies were associated with unacceptable morbidity and mortality (3,4), implanted cerebrospinal fluid shunts became the standard treatment of nearly all forms of hydrocephalus (3,5). With continued complications of shunts (6–12), and significant technological improvements in neuroendoscopy, ETV has become the primary management strategy for obstructive hydrocephalus caused by aqueductal stenosis (4,5,13–19), with success rates of 80% and better (13,15–17,20–24).

Often, anatomic variations can make ETV a dangerous or impossible option. Cerebral aqueductoplasty has gained popularity as an effective treatment for membranous and short-segment stenosis of the cerebral aqueduct (25–27). This procedure can be performed via a pre-coronal approach (burr hole placed 8 cm from nasion and 3 cm lateral to midline), passing through the lateral ventricle, foramen of Monro, and third ventricle into the aqueduct (28), or via a suboccipital foramen magnum trans-fourth ventricle approach (26,29). Transient vertical diplopia or upgaze weakness has been reported as a complication of this technique (26,30).

To address the benefit of an intra-aqueductal stent to ensure continued patency of the aqueduct following this procedure, Cinalli and colleagues conducted a retrospective evaluation of the effectiveness of endoscopic aqueductoplasty performed alone or accompanied by placement of a stent in the treatment of isolated fourth ventricle in seven patients with supratentorial shunts and loculated hydrocephalus (31). They found placement of a stent to be more effective in preventing the repeated occlusion of the aqueduct compared to aqueductoplasty alone.

The decision to treat aqueductal stenosis by ETV versus aqueductoplasty depends on the anatomy of the individual patient and the experience and comfort of the endoscopist. Miki and colleagues analyzed 110 patients who presented with obstructive hydrocephalus due to aqueductal stenosis and found only 6 (5.5%) to be suitable for endoscopic aqueductoplasty on the basis of the MRI features of the aqueduct and intraoperative neuroendoscopic findings. Indications included obstructive triventricular hydrocephalus with increased ICP, translucent membranous stenosis or aqueduct obstruction, and prestenotic dilatation of the aqueduct. In this study, the remaining 104 patients were treated with ETV (32). A foramen magnum trans-fourth ventricular approach may offer advantages compared to the more traditional anterior approach. The fourth ventricular approach does not traverse brain tissue, does not depend on ventricular dilatation, and is a straight approach with no pressure on foramen of Monro structures (26,27).

Treatment for hydrocephalus associated with Dandy–Walker syndrome (DWS) can be complex. In the past, patients have often required combinations of shunting systems to effectively drain both the supratentorial and infratentorial compartments. Endoscopy offers a useful way to simplify this. DWS has been successfully treated using various innovative techniques including image-guided transtentorial endoscopic ventriculocystostomy followed by placement of a cystoventricular catheter connected to a peritoneal shunt (33), a frontally placed single-catheter system draining the supratentorial and infratentorial compartments (34), and ETV with placement of a stent from the third ventricle to the posterior fossa cyst (35).

Isolated Lateral Ventricle and Multiloculated Hydrocephalus

Neuroendoscopic management is now becoming an effective treatment for complex multi- and uniloculated hydrocephalus, which has more traditionally been treated with multiple shunts, cystoperitoneal shunts, multiperforated catheters, stereotactic aspiration or shunt placement, and craniotomy and lysis of intraventricular septations (36–38). Multiple shunts are often unsuccessful due to increased risk of infection, obstruction, and hemorrhage associated with their removal (38).

Neuroendoscopy is extremely valuable in treating loculated ventricles and isolated compartments (Fig. 1). The goal is communication of all CSF spaces. Procedures include foramen of Monro reconstruction, septum pellucidotomy (39), septal wall removal, cyst wall fenestration, ETV, stenting between lateral and third ventricles (40), fourth ventriculostomy, and endoscopic shunt placement (41).

In an attempt to simplify cases of complex hydrocephalus using minimally invasive endoscopic techniques, we studied 114 patients treated endoscopically with either more than one shunt and/or multiloculated hydrocephalus (47 patients), isolated lateral ventricle (25 patients), isolated fourth ventricle (20 patients), arachnoid cyst (15 patients), slit ventricle syndrome (4 patients), or cysticercosis (3 patients). The endoscopic procedures performed included cyst or membrane fenestration, septum pellucidotomy, ETV, aqueductal plasty with or without stent, endoscopic shunt placement, and retrieval and removal of cysticercotic cysts. Reduction to one shunt was possible in 72%, shunt independence in 28%, and only 11% required shunt revisions long-term (98).

There are numerous benefits to this approach. Multiloculated hydrocephalus is most commonly secondary to infection. Establishing CSF flow and removal of shunts may be beneficial. With just one shunt, there are fewer opportunities for obstruction, malfunction, disconnection, and infection. Moreover, in patients with multiloculated hydrocephalus, it is easier to identify the source of shunt malfunction, compared to multiple shunts.

Endoscopic management of loculated CSF spaces appears to be effective in children less than one year of age. Fritsch et al. retrospectively reviewed 15 infants who underwent

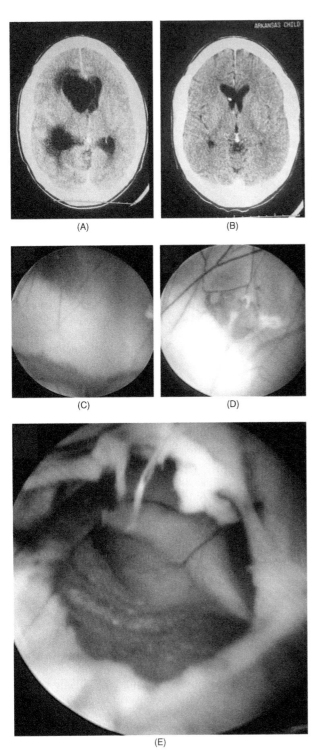

Figure 1 Septum pellucidotomy. This young boy presented with an isolated right lateral ventricle. Noncontrast head CT (**A**) shows bulging of the septum pellucidum to the left and evidence of transependymal flow. Intraoperative endoscopic view (**C**) showed bulging of the septum pellucidum. The septum was coagulated (**D**) and a large opening created. Contralateral choroid plexus (**E**) is visualized following the fenestration. The postoperative CT scan (**B**) shows excellent decompression of the lateral ventricle and communication of CSF spaces. The catheter tip noted in the right lateral ventricle is connected to a reservoir, and this patient did not require CSF diversion.

neuroendoscopic treatment of CSF space loculation and hydrocephalus with procedures including ETV, arachnoid cyst fenestration, aqueductoplasty, septostomy, and endoscopic fenestration of isolated ventricular compartments with good results (42).

The following principles should direct surgical approach. (*i*) The burr hole should be made in a position to make the cortical passage as short as possible, the endoscope will enter the largest cavity and the trajectory will take the endoscope to the membrane that separates the two cavities that need to be joined. (*ii*) If there is a preexisting ventricular catheter that does not drain an isolated portion of the ventricle, then its tract can be used to enter the ventricle. (*iii*) The trajectory should try to communicate as many cavities as possible. (*iv*) As many fenestrations as possible should be made using a sharp technique (98).

ENDOSCOPIC MANAGEMENT OF INTRAVENTRICULAR TUMORS

Neuroendoscopy plays several roles in the surgical management of brain tumors (43,44). It plays an important role in diagnosis, both in terms of visualization with ventriculoscopy and with pathological diagnosis after endoscopic tumor biopsy (Fig. 2). The advantages include improved

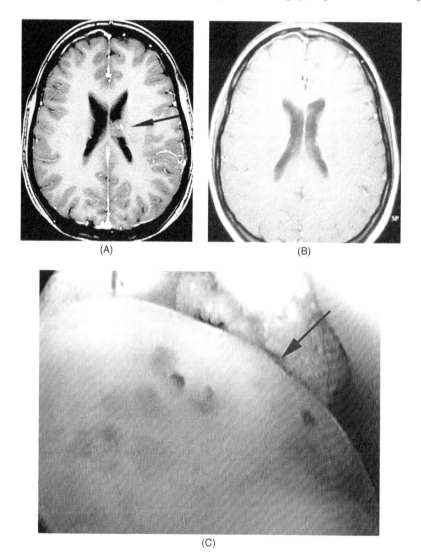

(A)   (B)

(C)

Figure 2 Intraventricular tumor resection. This patient presented with a tumor localized within the left lateral ventricle (*arrow* in part **A**). The tumor was easily visualized (**C**) and completely resected endoscopically. Postoperative CT scan confirms complete resection (**B**).

visualization, safer and more accurate biopsies, minimally invasive removal of intraventricular tumors, and adjuncts to traditional tumor management with the ability to "look around corners."

Colloid cysts, benign lesions that arise from the velum interpositum or choroid plexus of the third ventricle can produce hydrocephalus by obstruction of the foramina of Monro. They represent the ideal tumor for purely endoscopic excision (small with minimal vascularity). Charalampaki and colleagues reported 28 procedures over a 10-year period that used a key-hole approach with total removal of the cyst in 100% with no recurrent cysts and clinical improvement in 96% (45). Along these same lines, purely endoscopic removal of cisternal neurocysticercal cysts has been reported (46).

In addition to biopsy and resection of cystic tumors, resection of solid intraventricular tumors can be performed using a purely endoscopic technique. An aqueductal ependymoma causing obstructive hydrocephalus (47) and a posterior third ventricular ependymoma (48) were successfully resected with endoscopic surgery.

The absence of ventriculomegaly in those with an intraventricular tumor is not a contraindication to endoscopic tumor biopsy or resection. Souweidane analyzed 80 patients who underwent endoscopic management of intraventricular brain tumors, and of those, 15 did not have hydrocephalus. In all patients without hydrocephalus, the ventricular compartment was successfully cannulated and the intended goal (biopsy vs. resection) was accomplished (49). Moreover, newly developed models of neurofiberscopes with a small outer diameter can be effectively used in patients without ventriculomegaly. The case of a successful neurofiberscopic biopsy of a third ventricular anaplastic astrocytoma in a shunted patient without hydrocephalus was reported (50). In the case of small or slit ventricles, neuronavigation can be considered.

Neuroendoscopy can also be used to refine the staging evaluation of pineal region germinomas. Current treatment strategies for CNS germinoma include reducing the volume and dose of radiation by adding pre-irradiation chemotherapy, and accurate staging is needed to accomplish this. Reddy and colleagues reported eight patients with pineal germinoma who underwent endoscopic biopsy, ETV if needed, and direct visualization of the third ventricular region. All six patients had tumor studding of the third ventricular floor on endoscopic visualization, while only four had MRI evidence of disease in that region (51). Direct endoscopic visualization of the third ventricle may be more sensitive than MRI in evaluating the presence of suprasellar disease and may be added to the staging evaluation when feasible.

Treatment of cystic craniopharyngiomas using neuroendoscopy to drain the cystic component and/or to remove the solid component and to fenestrate the interposed septa to create a single communicating cavity, followed by placement of a single catheter and Ommaya reservoir system for subsequent aspiration and bleomycin injection was shown to be effective and safe as an alternative to microsurgery in patients with regrowing and recurrent cystic craniopharyngiomas (52).

Often, tumor mass leads to symptomatic secondary phenomena such as hydrocephalus and cystic compartmentalization that needs to be promptly addressed in addition to obtaining tissue diagnosis. Endoscopic biopsy with or without additional endoscopic procedures can be performed at the same session (53–57).

ARACHNOID CYST

Optimal treatment of arachnoid cysts remains controversial. Options include no treatment, craniotomy with resection of cyst wall, shunting, stereotactic cyst fenestration, and endoscopic management. When cyst wall fenestration into the basal cisterns is contemplated, neuroendoscopy is valuable due to its better visualization, magnification, angled perspective, and ability to maintain cyst distention during the procedure (Fig. 3). Neuroendoscopic management of arachnoid cysts has been extensively reported (21,50,58–64).

Greenfield et al. recently analyzed a prospectively generated database of 33 patients who underwent endoscopic fenestration of arachnoid cysts. Fenestration was successful as judged by cyst decompression and symptom resolution in 97%, with only one failure that was successful after repeated endoscopic fenestration (60).

Suprasellar cysts, which represent less than 10% of all intracranial arachnoid cysts, can also be successfully treated endoscopically with good clinical outcome and low surgical morbidity (58,65–67). Ventriculocystocisternostomy should be attempted, but when the communication

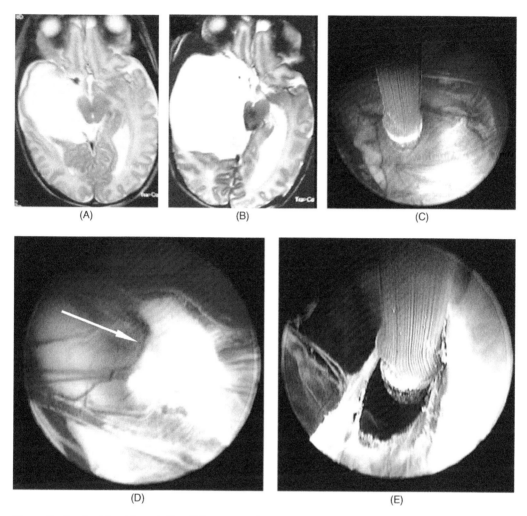

Figure 3 Arachnoid cyst fenestration. This young patient presented with a large type III right middle cranial fossa arachnoid cyst, with displacement of the brainstem to the left (**A**). Using an endoscopic technique, the thickened medial cyst wall was identified (**C**), coagulated (**D**), and fenestrated into the basilar cisterns (**E**). The postoperative T2-weighted MRI shows significantly decreased size of the cyst, with less compression and displacement of the brainstem (**B**).

between the cyst and the cistern is considered too dangerous, ventriculocystostomy is acceptable.

Successful endoscopic treatment of quadrigeminal cistern arachnoid cysts (61,68) and posterior fossa arachnoid cysts (69–71) has also been reported. The endoscopic management of temporal arachnoid cysts may not be as successful as cysts in other locations, despite adequate communication with the basal cisterns (98).

CHIARI MALFORMATION

Chiari malformations are a group of conditions with different etiologies that are similar in that they involve abnormalities in the posterior fossa and craniovertebral junction and are often associated with abnormalities in cerebrospinal fluid (CSF) flow at the level of the craniovertebral junction. In Chiari malformation type I (CM I), hydrocephalus occurs in 6% to 11% of cases, with most of these patients also presenting with syringomyelia (72,73). At least part of the etiology of hydrocephalus formation is explained by fourth ventricular outlet stenosis (28,74–77), resulting in increased compression of the cisterna magna by the herniated cerebellar tonsils.

ETV successfully treats obstructive hydrocephalus associated with CM I secondary to foramen of Magendie obstruction with aqueductal patency (16,28,78,79) and has also been shown to be effective treatment for the associated communicating syringomyelia (80,81).

In contrast to CM I, approximately 90% of those with Chiari malformation type II (CM II) and myelomeningocele will develop hydrocephalus requiring diversion (82–84). ETV has only a 30% success rate in these patients (5,85). However, when used in shunted children returning with shunt malfunction, the success rate range increases to 50% to 80% (5,16,85), possibly because many of these children have developed aqueductal stenosis, which may be more treatable by ETV and because many of these children are older.

OTHER APPLICATIONS FOR NEUROENDOSCOPY

Applications for endoscopy are numerous and depend only on the experience and imagination of the surgeon. There are likely many very innovative applications that have not been reported. Management of patients with tuberculous meningitis with hydrocephalus can be accomplished with such neuroendoscopic techniques as ETV, septostomy, monroplasty, tuberculoma decompression and biopsy, and abscess drainage (86,87). Acute obstructive triventricular hydrocephalus secondary to hypertensive caudate hemorrhage into the ventricular system was successfully treated with endoscopic removal of the third ventricular hematoma (88). Endoscopic management of patients with spontaneous primary or secondary tetraventricular intraventricular hemorrhage compares favorably with more conventional treatments (89). An endoscopic technique using stereotactic guidance has been described for evacuating thalamic hematomas (90).

INTRACRANIAL NEURONAVIGATION

The combination of neuronavigation with neuroendoscopy can greatly aid with things such as tumor biopsy, tumor resection, third ventriculostomy, cyst wall fenestration, and simply to access small or slit ventricles. The usefulness of neuronavigation in intracranial endoscopy has been extensively studied (91–94). It can be used to plan the correct entry point and trajectory, minimizing the potential for damage to the foramen of Monro and other brain tissue by reducing back-and-forth and side-to-side motion of the endoscope. The technique can be performed using a simple rigid endoscope through predetermined entry points and trajectories. Navigational tracking is most helpful in entering small ventricles, in approaching the posterior third ventricle when the foramen of Monro is narrow, and in selecting the best approach to colloid cysts. It is essential in some cystic lesions lacking clear landmarks such as intraparenchymal cysts or multiloculated hydrocephalus (93).

Selden and colleagues reported testing and preliminary clinical use of a device for the direct cranial fixation and point-to-point neuronavigation of a rigid ventricular endoscope (92). This may be especially helpful in cases of small ventricles, ambiguous intraventricular landmarks, and in children too young for a head-holder.

COMPLICATIONS

Although neuroendoscopy has revolutionized the treatment of hydrocephalus, specific complications occur due to risks inherent in the procedure and sometimes inexperience, and attempts should be made to avoid these problems. These complications have been reviewed extensively with suggestions for their avoidance (95).

Complications specific to ETV include bradycardia and asystole during manipulation of the third ventricular floor, damage to fornices with scope manipulation or poorly placed burr holes, hypothalamic damage, vascular damage, cranial neuropathies, and subdural hygromata or hematomata (96,97). As a general rule, the endoscope should not be used to find the ventricle. Even though the ventricle may be grossly dilated, inaccurate placement of an endoscope, unlike a fine brain needle, is not well tolerated. Similarly, side-to-side movements of the scope can tear bridging veins or stretched neural structures and should be minimized. CSF should be drained from cysts and ventricles slowly, and once the procedure has been accomplished, the cavities should be refilled in order to minimize the risk of subdural collections. Another important maneuver is the placement of a piece of Gelfoam in the cortical tract to lessen the egress of CSF into the subdural space.

CONCLUSIONS

In general, the neuroendoscope should be thought of as a tool that provides superior magnification and illumination, as well as the ability to "see around corners" with angled scopes. Their usefulness depends on the availability of endoscopes at the institution, and on the experience, training and innovativeness of the surgeon.

REFERENCES

1. Hirsch JF, et al. Stenosis of the aqueduct of Sylvius. Etiology and treatment. J Neurosurg Sci 1986; 30(1–2):29–39.
2. Dandy W. An operative approach for hydrocephalus. Bull Johns Hopkins Hosp 1922, 33:189–190.
3. Bauer D, Hellwig D. Current Endoneurosurgery. Adv Neurosurg 1994; 22:113–120.
4. Grant JA, et al. Third ventriculostomy: A review. Surg Neurol 1997; 47(3):210–212.
5. Teo C, et al. Management of hydrocephalus by endoscopic third ventriculostomy in patients with myelomeningocele. Pediatr Neurosurg 1996; 25(2):57–63; discussion 63.
6. Abu-Dalu K, et al. Colonic complications of ventriculoperitoneal shunts. Neurosurg Clin N Am 1983; 13:167–169.
7. Choudhury A. Avoidable factors that contribute to the complications of ventriculoperitoneal shunt in childhood hydrocephalus. Childs Nerv Syst 1990; 6:346–349.
8. Piatt JJ, Carlson C. A search for determinants of cerebrospinal fluid shunt survival: Retrospective analysis of a 14-year institutional experience. Pediatr Neurosurg 1993; 19:233–242.
9. Pudenz RH, et al. Hydrocephalus: Overdrainage by ventricular shunts. A review and recommendations. Surg Neurol 1991; 35(3):200–212.
10. Raimondi AJ, et al. Suprasellar cysts: surgical treatment and results. Childs Brain 1980; 7(2):57–72.
11. Sainte-Rose C, et al. Mechanical complications in shunts. Pediatr Neurosurg 1991; 17(1):2–9.
12. Sekhar LN, et al. Malfunctioning ventriculoperitoneal shunts. Clinical and pathological features. J Neurosurg 1982; 56(3):411–416.
13. Drake J. Ventriculostomy for treatment of hydrocephalus. Neurosurg Clin N Am 1993; 4:657–666.
14. Grunnert P, Perneczky A, Resch K. Endoscopic procedures through the foramen interventriculare of Monro under stereotactic conditions. Minim Invasive Neurosurg 1994; 37:2–8.
15. Hoffman H, Harwood-nash D, Gilday D. Percutaneous third ventriculostomy in the management of noncommunicating hydrocephalus. Neurosurgery 1980; 7:313–321.
16. Jones RF, et al. Endoscopic third ventriculostomy. Neurosurgery 1990; 26(1):86–91; discussion 91–92.
17. Jones RF, et al. The current status of endoscopic third ventriculostomy in the management of non-communicating hydrocephalus. Minim Invasive Neurosurg 1994; 37(1):28–36.
18. Kunz U, et al. Endoscopic fenestration of the 3rd ventricular floor in aqueductal stenosis. Minim Invasive Neurosurg 1994; 37(2):42–47.
19. Teo C. Third ventriculostomy in the treatment of hydrocephalus: Experience with more than 120 cases. In: Hellwig D, Bauer B, eds. Minimally Invasive Techniques for Neurosurgery. Heidelberg, Berlin, Germany: Springer Verlag, 1998:73–76.
20. Buxton N, et al. Neuroendoscopic third ventriculostomy for hydrocephalus in adults: Report of a single unit's experience with 63 cases. Surg Neurol 2001; 55(2):74–78.
21. Choi JU, et al. Endoscopic surgery for obstructive hydrocephalus. Yonsei Med J 1999; 40(6): 600–607.
22. Dalrymple S, PJ Kelly. Computer-assisted stereotactic third ventriculostomy in the management of noncommunicating hydrocephalus. Stereotact Funct Neurosurg 1992; 54:105–110.
23. Gangemi M, et al. Endoscopic third ventriculostomy for hydrocephalus. Minim Invasive Neurosurg 1999; 42(3):128–132.
24. Kadrian D, et al. Long-term reliability of endoscopic third ventriculostomy. Neurosurgery 2005; 56(6):1271–1278; discussion 1278.
25. Rekate HL, Rekate HL. Endoscopic fourth ventricular aqueductoplasty. J Neurosurg 2005; 103 (5 suppl):385–386; discussion 386–387.
26. Sansone JM, et al. Endoscopic cerebral aqueductoplasty: A trans-fourth ventricle approach. J Neurosurg 2005; 103(5 suppl):388–392.
27. Gawish I, et al. Endoscopic aqueductoplasty through a tailored craniocervical approach. J Neurosurg 2005; 103(5):778–782.
28. Suehiro T, et al. Successful neuroendoscopic third ventriculostomy for hydrocephalus and syringomyelia associated with fourth ventricle outlet obstruction. Case report. J Neurosurg 2000; 93(2):326–329.
29. Toyota S, et al. A neuroendoscopic approach to the aqueduct via the fourth ventricle combined with suboccipital craniectomy. Minim Invasive Neurosurg 2004; 47(5):312–315.

30. Teo C, Young R II. Endoscopic management of hydrocephalus secondary to tumors of the posterior third ventricle. Neurosurg Focus 1999; 7(4):e2.

31. Cinalli G, et al. Endoscopic aqueductoplasty and placement of a stent in the cerebral aqueduct in the management of isolated fourth ventricle in children. J Neurosurg 2006; 104(1 suppl):21–27.

32. Miki T, et al. Indications for neuroendoscopic aqueductoplasty without stenting for obstructive hydrocephalus due to aqueductal stenosis. Minim Invasive Neurosurg 2005; 48(3):136–141.

33. Weinzierl MR, et al. Endoscopic transtentorial ventriculocystostomy and cystoventriculoperitoneal shunt in a neonate with Dandy–Walker malformation and associated aqueductal obstruction. Pediatr Neurosurg 2005; 41(5):272–277.

34. Sikorski CW, et al. Endoscopic, single-catheter treatment of Dandy–Walker syndrome hydrocephalus: Technical case report and review of treatment options. Pediatr Neurosurg 2005; 41(5):264–268.

35. Mohanty A. Endoscopic third ventriculostomy with cystoventricular stent placement in the management of Dandy–Walker malformation: Technical case report of three patients. Neurosurgery 2003; 53(5):1223–1228; discussion 1228–1229.

36. Eller T, Pasternak J. Isolated ventricles following intraventricular haemorrhage. J Neurosurg 1985; 62:357–362.

37. Kalsbeck JE, et al. Compartmentalization of the cerebral ventricles as a sequela of neonatal meningitis. J Neurosurg 1980; 52(4):547–552.

38. Lewis AI, et al. Endoscopic treatment of loculated hydrocephalus. J Neurosurg 1995; 82(5):780–785.

39. Aldana PR, et al. Results of endoscopic septal fenestration in the treatment of isolated ventricular hydrocephalus. Pediatr Neurosurg 2003; 38(6):286–294.

40. Tirakotai W, et al. Neuroendoscopic stent procedure in obstructive hydrocephalus due to both foramina of Monro occluding craniopharyngioma: Technical note. Surg Neurol 2004; 61(3):293–296; discussion 296.

41. Oi S, et al. Loculated ventricles and isolated compartments in hydrocephalus: Their pathophysiology and the efficacy of neuroendoscopic surgery. Neurosurg Clin N Am 2004; 15(1):77–87.

42. Fritsch MJ, et al. Endoscopic intraventricular surgery for treatment of hydrocephalus and loculated CSF space in children less than one year of age. Pediatr Neurosurg 2002; 36(4):183–188.

43. Teo C, et al. Neuro-oncologic applications of endoscopy. Neurosurg Clin N Am 2004; 15(1): 89–103.

44. Teo C, et al. Application of endoscopy to third ventricular tumors. Clin Neurosurg 2005; 52:24–28.

45. Charalampaki P, et al. Endoscope-assisted removal of colloid cysts of the third ventricle. Neurosurg Rev 2006; 29(1):72–79.

46. Gravori T, et al. Endoscopic removal of cisternal neurocysticercal cysts. Technical note. Neurosurg Focus 2002; 12(6):e7.

47. Terasaki M, et al. Minimally invasive management of ependymoma of the aqueduct of Sylvius: Therapeutic considerations and management. Minim Invasive Neurosurg 2005; 48(6):322–324.

48. Luther N, et al. Neuroendoscopic resection of posterior third ventricular ependymoma. Case report. Neurosurg Focus 2005; 18(6A):E3.

49. Souweidane MM. Endoscopic surgery for intraventricular brain tumors in patients without hydrocephalus. Neurosurgery 2005; 57(4 suppl):312 318; discussion 312–318.

50. Chernov M, et al. Minimally invasive management of the third ventricle glioma in a patient without hydrocephalus: Neurofiberscopic biopsy followed by gamma knife radiosurgery. Minim Invasive Neurosurg 2004; 47(4):238–241.

51. Reddy AT, et al. Refining the staging evaluation of pineal region germinoma using neuroendoscopy and the presence of preoperative diabetes insipidus. Neuro Oncol 2004; 6(2):127–133.

52. Nicolato A, et al. Multimodality stereotactic approach to the treatment of cystic craniopharyngiomas. Minim Invasive Neurosurg 2004; 47(1):32–40.

53. Yurtseven T, et al. Neuroendoscopic biopsy for intraventricular tumors. Minim Invasive Neurosurg 2003; 46(5):293–299.

54. Nishikawa T, et al. Application of endoscopy for a midbrain tumor. Minim Invasive Neurosurg 2003; 46(3):182–185.

55. Mizoguchi M, et al. Neuroendoscopic biopsy of tectal glioma: A case report. Minim Invasive Neurosurg 2000; 43(1):53–55.

56. Robinson S, et al. The role of neuroendoscopy in the treatment of pineal region tumors. Surg Neurol 1997; 48(4):360–365; discussion 365–367.

57. Veto F, et al. Biportal endoscopic management of third ventricle tumors in patients with occlusive hydrocephalus: Technical note. Neurosurg 1997; 40(4):871–875; discussion 875–877.

58. Van Beijnum J, et al. Navigated laser-assisted endoscopic fenestration of a suprasellar arachnoid cyst in a 2-year-old child with bobble-head doll syndrome. Case report. J Neurosurg 2006; 104(5 suppl):348–351.

59. Nowoslawska E, et al. Neuroendoscopic techniques in the treatment of arachnoid cysts in children and comparison with other operative methods. Childs Nerv Syst 2006; 22(6):599–604.

60. Greenfield JP, et al. Endoscopic management of intracranial cysts. Neurosurg Focus 2005; 19(6):E7.

61. Gangemi M, et al. Endoscopic treatment of quadrigeminal cistern arachnoid cysts. Minim Invasive Neurosurg 2005; 48(5):289–292.

62. Abbott R. The endoscopic management of arachnoidal cysts. Neurosurg Clin N Am 2004; 15(1):9–17.

63. Schroeder HW, Gaab MR. Intracranial endoscopy. Neurosurg Focus 1999; 6(4):e1.

64. Kim MH. The role of endoscopic fenestration procedures for cerebral arachnoid cysts. J Korean Med Sci 1999; 14(4):443–447.

65. Charalampaki P, et al. Endoscopic and endoscope-assisted neurosurgical treatment of suprasellar arachnoidal cysts (Mickey Mouse cysts). Minim Invasive Neurosurg 2005; 48(5):283–288.

66. Sood, S, et al. Endoscopic fenestration and coagulation shrinkage of suprasellar arachnoid cysts. Technical note. J Neurosurg 2005; 102(1 suppl):127–133.

67. Fioravanti A, et al. Bobble-head doll syndrome due to a suprasellar arachnoid cyst: Endoscopic treatment in two cases. Childs Nerv Syst 2004; 20(10):770–773.

68. Inamasu J, et al. Endoscopic ventriculo-cystomy for non-communicating hydrocephalus secondary to quadrigeminal cistern arachnoid cyst. Acta Neurol Scand 2003; 107(1):67–71.

69. Nomura S, et al. Endoscopic fenestration of posterior fossa arachnoid cyst for the treatment of presyrinx myelopathy—Case report. Neurol Med Chir (Tokyo) 2002; 42(10):452–454.

70. Gangemi M, et al. Cyst of the velum interpositum treated by endoscopic fenestration. Surg Neurol 1997; 47(2):134–136; discussion 136–137.

71. Hayashi N, et al. Endoscopic ventriculocystocisternostomy of a quadrigeminal cistern arachnoid cyst. Case report. J Neurosurg 1999; 90(6):1125–1128.

72. Tubbs RS, McGirt MJ, Oakes WJ. Surgical experience in 130 pediatric patients with Chiari I malformations. J Neurosurg 2003; 99(2):291–296.

73. Milhorat TH, et al. Chiari I malformation redefined: Clinical and radiographic findings for 364 symptomatic patients. Neurosurgery 1999; 44(5):1005–1017.

74. Amacher AL, Page LK. Hydrocephalus due to membranous obstruction of the fourth ventricle. J Neurosurg 1971; 35(6):672–676.

75. Barr M. Observations on the foramen of Magendie in a series of human brains. Brain Dev 1948; 71:281–289.

76. Dandy W. The diagnosis and treatment of hydrocephalus due to occlusions of the foramen of Magendie and Luschka. Surg Gynecol Obstet 1921; 32:112–124.

77. Oldfield EH, et al. Pathophysiology of syringomyelia associated with Chiari I malformation of the cerebellar tonsils. Implications for diagnosis and treatment. J Neurosurg 1994; 80(1):3–15.

78. Cinalli G, et al. Failure of third ventriculostomy in the treatment of aqueductal stenosis in children. Neurosurg Focus 1999; 6(4):e3.

79. Mohanty A, et al. Neuroendoscopic third ventriculostomy in the management of fourth ventricular outlet obstruction. Minim Invasive Neurosurg 1999; 42(1):18–21.

80. Decq P, et al. Chiari I malformation: a rare cause of noncommunicating hydrocephalus treated by third ventriculostomy. J Neurosurg 2001; 95(5):783–790.

81. Nishihara T, et al. Third ventriculostomy for symptomatic syringomyelia using flexible endoscope: Case report. Minim Invasive Neurosurg 1996; 39(4):130–132.

82. el Gammal T, et al. MR imaging of Chiari II malformation. AJR Am J Roentgenol 1988; 150(1):163–170.

83. McLone DG, Dias MS. The Chiari II malformation: Cause and impact. Childs Nerv Syst 2003; 19(7–8):540–550.

84. Oakes WJ, Tubbs RS. Chiari malformations. In: Winn H, ed. Youman's Neurological Surgery, 2005:3347–3361.

85. Jones RF, et al. Third ventriculostomy for hydrocephalus associated with spinal dysraphism: Indications and contraindications. Eur J Pediatr Surg 1996, 6(suppl 1):5–6.

86. Husain M, et al. Role of neuroendoscopy in the management of patients with tuberculous meningitis hydrocephalus. Neurosurg Rev 2005; 28(4):278–283.

87. Singh D, et al. Endoscopic third ventriculostomy in post-tubercular meningitic hydrocephalus: A preliminary report. Minim Invasive Neurosurg 2005; 48(1):47–52.

88. Barbagallo GM, et al. Long-term resolution of acute, obstructive, triventricular hydrocephalus by endoscopic removal of a third ventricular hematoma without third ventriculostomy. Case report and review of the literature. J Neurosurg 2005; 102(5):930–934.

89. Longatti PL, et al. Neuroendoscopic management of intraventricular hemorrhage. Stroke 2004; 35(2):e35–e38.

90. Hsieh PC, Hsieh PC. Endoscopic removal of thalamic hematoma: A technical note. Minim Invasive Neurosurg 2003; 46(6):369–371.

91. Kim IY, et al. Neuronavigation-guided endoscopic surgery for pineal tumors with hydrocephalus. Minim Invasive Neurosurg 2004; 47(6):365–368.
92. Selden NR, et al. Intracranial navigation using a novel device for endoscope fixation and targeting: Technical innovation. Pediatr Neurosurg 2005; 41(5):233–236.
93. Schroeder HW, et al. Frameless neuronavigation in intracranial endoscopic neurosurgery. J Neurosurg 2001; 94(1):72–79.
94. Broggi G, et al. Image guided neuroendoscopy for third ventriculostomy. Acta Neurochir (Wien) 2000; 142(8):893–898; discussion 898–899.
95. Teo C, et al. Complications of endoscopic neurosurgery. Childs Nerv Syst 1996; 12(5):248–253; discussion 253.
96. Teo C. Complications of endoscopic third ventriculostomy. In: Cinalli G, Maixner W, Sainte Rose C, eds. Pediatric Hydrocephalus. Milano, Italy: Springer-Verlag, 2004:411–420.
97. Schroeder HW, et al. Incidence of complications in neuroendoscopic surgery. Childs Nerv Syst 2004; 20(11–12):878–883.
98. Kadrian, Teo. In press.

ETV in Shunt Malfunction

Jothy Kandaswamy and Conor Mallucci

Department of Neurosurgery, The Walton Centre for Neurology and Neurosurgery, Liverpool, U.K.

The use of ETV in the treatment of shunt malfunction is gaining popularity, with proven outcome data. The risk of VP shunt malfunction is between 25% and 40% in the first year after shunt placement, and it remains at 4% to 5% per year thereafter (1–3,5–9). Indeed, shunt failure remains almost an inevitability during a patient's life, with 81% of shunts requiring revision after 12 years (6).

In a multicenter study, Siomin et al. addressed the success of ETV in patients with CSF infection and/or hemorrhage (9). The authors detailed high success rates (100%) for primary ETV in the aqueductal stenosis groups and also for secondary ETV in cases of IVH-induced hydrocephalus, that is, in patients in whom a VP shunt was initially placed and who subsequently underwent ETV at the time of shunt malfunction. This series had poor success rates for primary ETV in patients with premature birth and IVH-induced hydrocephalus (0%). Within a subgroup of 101 patients from this seven-center series who had undergone ETVs after both infection and hemorrhage, there was a mean success rate of 57.4%. As in other series, a wide variation in successful outcomes between centers occurred in this subgroup, from 41.7% to 100%. This variation may reflect the severity of individual cases in terms of both the infection and the hemorrhage. The question of whether practice differences between centers influence ETV outcomes remains unanswered. By documenting a high ETV failure rate in patients with a history of hemorrhage and premature birth, and in those with both hemorrhage and infection, this study demonstrated that the preferred initial mode of treatment for these types of hydrocephalus is VP shunt placement. Our own data are in line with that of this multicenter series in demonstrating poor success for a primary ETV in treating IVH-induced hydrocephalus (4). We also confirm the success of secondary ETV in IVH-induced patients with hydrocephalus who present with VP shunt malfunction (4). This pattern of ETV success (poor primary and good secondary) was also seen in the infection-related hydrocephalus groups in our series (4). The high success rate for secondary ETV in cases of IVH is confirmed by data from Nottingham and Paris (4) (Table 1). However, our success with secondary ETV in cases caused by infection is not maintained in their series, which probably reflects the fact that there are a small number of such cases at all three institutions (Table 1). When comparing the overall effect of original etiology and success of ETV, whereas in primary ETV etiology was found to be a significant variable, this significance disappeared for secondary ETV implying etiology after a period with a shunt is no longer an important predictor of success of ETV (4).

The success of secondary ETV in cases with infection and hemorrhage as a cause for the original hydrocephalus is possibly explained by the following hypothesis: whereas these patients initially present with a "communicating" hydrocephalus due to obstruction of the subarachnoid spaces and arachnoid granulations rather than the intravetricular pathways, the placement of a VP shunt, by diverting CSF to the abdominal cavity for a period of time allows the subarachnoid spaces to reestablish themselves and the inflammation from the original insult of infection/hemorrhage to disband. The extracranial diversion may also induce an acquired aqueductal stenosis, which together with reestablishment of the subarachnoid spaces makes the likelihood of an ETV being successful greater at a later date when a shunt malfunction occurs.

The successful outcomes observed in patients with aqueductal stenosis in the primary ETV series were also evident in the secondary series. Patients with midline and posterior fossa arachnoid cysts who underwent primary and secondary ETV enjoyed maximal success (4). In the spina bifida cases, the high success rates in the primary series (older patients) were not present in the secondary series. Patients with tumors also had a high

Table 1 Comparison of the Liverpool, Nottingham, and Paris Series in Which an ETV was Performed After a Shunt Malfunction[a]

| Original cause of hydrocephalus | No. of cases (% success) | | | |
	Paris: 8-yr FU	Nottingham: 1-yr FU	Liverpool: 4-yr FU	Total
Aqueductal stenosis	10 (90)	9 (78)	19 (68)	38 (76)
Spina bifida	—	4 (100)	20 (55)	24 (64)
IVH	4 (100)	10 (60)	7 (71)	21 (71)
Meningitis	5 (40)	6 (50)	4 (75)	15 (53)
Tumor	7 (71)	—	6 (83)	13 (77)
Other	4 (75)	6 (83)	7 (86)	17 (82)
Total	30 (77)	35 (74)	63 (70)	128 (75)

[a]The number of ETV cases performed in each origin group with shunt malfunction as well as the percentage of successful outcome cases in each is given. The rationale for selecting these three series was that the senior author (C. L. M.) worked in all three institutions and that the endoscopic practices are similar in each.
Abbreviations: FU, follow-up; —, not applicable.

rate of success in both the primary and the secondary ETV series. The delayed death in our secondary series (4) makes the point that sudden deterioration can occur following ETV, as in hydrocephalus, which is managed with shunt placement. This possibility makes follow-up and patient/family counseling regarding symptoms of raised ICP an imperative. One can never assume that hydrocephalus is cured after an ETV and removal of a malfunctioning shunt (4).

A VP shunt infection does not usually lead to communicating hydrocephalus, as neonatal meningitis tends to do. The preexistence for some time of a functioning shunt in patients with shunt infections can also lead to secondary aqueductal stenosis, which would make the likelihood of ETV success greater after removal of the infected shunt. Occurrences of shunt infection are probably most frequent after shunt revision for shunt malfunction and infection; therefore an ETV may offer a lower rate of infection than does shunt revision. With ETV we have had success in addressing the nightmare scenario of multiple shunt revisions/infections, in which it sometimes seems that there are few treatment options left and that expectations of success are low.

An ETV is a safe procedure with few complications and with a high success rate in the shunt malfunction group. Unlike primary ETV cases, successes in shunt malfunction cases are not particularly origin-specific. A bonus is the success of ETV in addressing the problem of infected shunts. Most failures will be evident early, but long-term follow-up is vital. Both ETV and shunt surgery are complementary techniques to be tailored to selected patients.

REFERENCES

1. Aquilina K, Edwards RJ, Pople IK. Routine placement of a ventricular reservoir at endoscopic third ventriculostomy. Neurosurgery 2003; 53:91–97.
2. Bierbrauer KS, Storrs BB, McLone DG, et al. A prospective, randomised study of shunt function and infections as a function of shunt placement. Pediatr Neurosurg 1990–1991; 16: 287–291.
3. Drake JM, Kestle J, Milner R, et al. Randomized trial of cerebrospinal fluid shunt valve design in pediatric hydrocephalus. Neurosurgery 1998; 43:294–305.
4. O'Brien DF, Javadpour M, Collins DR, et al. Endoscopic third ventriculostomy: An outcome analysis of primary cases and procedures performed after ventriculoperitoneal shunt malfunction. J Neurosurg 2005; 103(5 suppl):393–400.
5. Piatt JH Jr, Carlson CV. A search for determinants of cerebrospinal fluid shunt survival: Retrospective analysis of a 14-year institutional experience. Pediatr Neurosurg 1993; 19: 233–242.

6. Quigley M, Reigel D, Kortyna R. Cerebrospinal fluid shunt infections. Report of 41 cases and a critical review of the literature. Pediatr Neurosci 1989; 15:111–120.

7. Sainte-Rose C, Piatt JH, Renier D, et al. Mechanical complications in shunts. Pediatr Neurosurg 1991; 17:2–9.

8. Schroeder HW, Niendorf WR, Gaab MR. Complications of endoscopic third ventriculostomy. J Neurosurg 2002; 96:1032–1040.

9. Siomin V, Cinalli G, Grotenhuis A, et al. Endoscopic third ventriculostomy in patients with cerebrospinal fluid infection and/or hemorrhage. J Neurosurg 2002; 97: 519–524.

Repeat Endoscopic Third Ventriculostomy

Vit Siomin and Shlomi Constantini

Department of Pediatric Neurosurgery, Tel Aviv Medical Center, Dana Children's Hospital, Tel Aviv, Israel

INTRODUCTION

Treatment of obstructive hydrocephalus (HCP) has been revolutionized with the advent of neuroendoscopic techniques. The initial enthusiasm of neurosurgeons after years of using shunts as the only treatment of all types of HCP has been fading away despite numerous studies and technological "breakthroughs" to improve shunt technology. The reality is that the overall survival of shunts and the complication rate of shunting have improved only modestly in the last 10 to 20 years. Endoscopic third ventriculostomy (ETV) may help to avoid placement of and reliance upon hardware. This procedure is a safe and effective alternative to establish a "natural" pathway for CSF flow in patients with triventricular hydrocephalus. If successful, it might eliminate a need for a shunt in 50% to 90% of patients in this group, depending on the specific pathology (1–5).

While primary ETV has been shown to be effective and rather safe, repeat ETV procedures have been less thoroughly studied. Therefore, the current mainstream approach to ETV failure is shunting rather than to attempt another endoscopic procedure. Only a few authors have described their experience with repeat ETV (3,6,7). This chapter will focus on some of the key aspects of repeat ETV.

TYPES OF ETV FAILURES

Although ETV is a conceptually attractive and technically feasible procedure, 20% to 50% of patients undergoing ETV will fail in the first six months following surgery. Failures fall into the following two categories:

1. *Early* postoperative failure: These usually occur due to technical problem during surgery, obliteration of the orifice during the immediate postoperative period, or poor absorption mechanism of the CSF (3).
2. *Delayed* failure: These patients benefit from the primary ETV for various periods of time. Most delayed failures, however, happen within the first two years after the procedure. Obliteration of the stoma by scar tissue is probably the most common cause of failure (7).

   Radiographically, obliteration of the orifice may be demonstrated by the absence of flow-void phenomenon or cine flow on MRI; increase in ventricular size, particularly of the third ventricle; and down-bulging of the floor of the third ventricle.

COMPARISON OF PRIMARY AND REPEAT ETV

Safety

It appears that repeat ETV is as safe as the first ETV. The complication rate of 5% is similar in both primary and repeat ETV series and compares favorably to cumulative complication rates for shunting (5,7,8). In one clinical series (7), the surgeons in series did not observe any additional intraoperative difficulties and felt that the repeat procedures were technically similar to the primary surgeries.

Outcome

Successful outcome following an ETV should be defined as resolution of symptoms caused by increased ICP secondary to CSF flow obstruction. Additionally, the surgeon should view both primary and repeat ETV as a process of weaning the patient off of a shunt.

The available literature indicates that the success rate of the primary and repeat ETV is similar and falls somewhere between 60% and 70%. Decrease in ventricular size should not be considered a final goal after either primary or repeat ETV, because changes in the ventricular size are hard to evaluate, particularly in long-standing hydrocephalus, unless volumetric techniques are applied.

PATIENT SELECTION

The selection of patients for a repeat ETV should essentially be based on the same criteria that are used to recommend primary ETV (7).

In other words, endoscopic exploration is indicated in patients with triventricular HCP with no evidence of CSF flow (i.e., closed stoma) on midsagittal MR. Conversely, patients with a patent stoma on MR should be offered a shunt

THE DEFINITION OF POSTOPERATIVE FAILURE

Temporary CSF diversion and a "no rush approach" may play a key role in care of patients after repeat ETV. If the patient's preoperative condition is not stable, the surgeon may choose to leave a tunneled EVD (external ventricular drain) at the end of surgery. In our opinion, however, the most "physiological" way of temporary CSF diversion is lumbar drain placement, as it helps not only remove the CSF excess, but also challenge the stoma from below, by encouraging the CSF flow through it in the desired physiological direction. Perioperative placement of an ICP bolt might be helpful as well by providing valuable information regarding ICP either while the CSF is drained or after the drain is removed. A patient is considered a failure only if the symptoms persist after a few attempts of CSF drainage, preferably through the lumbar drain.

CONCLUSIONS

1. Failure of an ETV in most cases is due to obstruction of the stoma, which changes pathophysiology of HCP back to obstructive.
2. Repeat ETV in selected patients is as safe and effective as the primary procedure and may be preferable to placement of a shunt.
3. A patient is considered a failure only if symptoms persist after a few attempts of CSF drainage, preferably through the lumbar drain.

REFERENCES

1. Brockmeyer D, Abtin K, Carey L, et al. Endoscopic third ventriculostomy: An outcome analysis. Pediatr Neurosurg 1998; 28:236–240.
2. Cinalli G. Alternatives to shunting. Childs Nerv Syst 1999; 15:718–731.
3. Cinalli G, Sainte-Rose C, Chumas P, et al. Failure of third ventriculostomy in the treatment of aqueductal stenosis in children. J Neurosurg 1999; 90:448–254,227–236.
4. Cinalli G, Salazar C, Mallucci C, et al. The role of endoscopic third ventriculostomy in the management of shunt malfunction. Neurosurgery 1998; 43:1323–1327; discussion 1327–1329.
5. Hopf NJ, Grunert P, Fries G, et al. Endoscopic third ventriculostomy: Outcome analysis of 100 consecutive procedures. Neurosurgery 1999; 44:795–804; discussion 804–806.
6. Mohanty A, Vasudev MK, Sampath S, et al. Failed endoscopic third ventriculostomy in children: management options. Pediatr Neurosurg 2002; 37(6):304–309.
7. Siomin V, Weiner H, Wisoff J, et al. Repeat endoscopic third ventriculostomy: Is it worth trying? Childs Nerv Syst 2001; 17(9):551–555.
8. Abtin K, Thompson BG, Walker MT. Basilar artery perforation as a complication of endoscopic third ventriculostomy. Pediatr Neurosurg 1998; 28:35–41.

ETV in Children Younger Than Two Years

Abhaya V. Kulkarni

Department of Neurosurgery, Hospital for Sick Children, Toronto, Ontario, Canada

Several studies have assessed the role of age, and in particular young age, as a predictor of success of ETV. The data have not been consistent, with some studies suggesting poor results in infants irrespective of etiology, while others suggesting that ETV can be performed with reasonable success in infants with specific etiologies of hydrocephalus.

For example, in a series of 18 children all younger than one year of age, Fritsch et al. found good success for ETV in the 4 children with obstructive hydrocephalus, but much poorer results in the 14 with myelomeningocele or communicating hydrocephalus (1). Etus and Ceylan reported similar results in 25 children younger than two years of age (2). Even amongst the most favorable group of infants with aqueductal stenosis, Koch and Wagner found a success rate of only 57% (4 out of 7), but this was substantially better than those infants with other forms of hydrocephalus (3). Kadrian et al. found a progressive increase in the success rate of ETV with advancing age, even within the infant age range, that is, those at 6 to 24 months of age faired better than those younger than 6 months (4).

It is not clear physiologically why ETV success rates in infants are, in general, worse than for older children. It has usually been thought that the CSF reabsorptive capacities of infants are poorer. However, in a series of infants undergoing repeat endoscopic exploration following failed ETV, Wagner and Koch reported a high incidence of scarring, stenosis, or closure at the ETV site. They postulated that infants have greater tendency toward arachnoidal scarring, thus explaining their higher ETV failure rate (5).

Despite the seemingly overall poorer results in infants, there is legitimate on-going interest in the usefulness of ETV in this population. Infants with hydrocephalus represent a difficult group to manage, regardless of whether CSF shunting or ETV is used. They are more prone to acute overdrainage, wound complications, and infection. The question of whether ETV is truly preferable in this age group has yet to be answered. It is for this reason that the International Infant Hydrocephalus Study (IIHS) was initiated under the aegis of the International Study Group for Neuroendoscopy and the International Society for Pediatric Neurosurgery (6). The IIHS will be a truly international, multicenter study with participants from North America, South America, Europe, and Asia. It will look specifically at infants younger than two years of age with defined aqueductal stenosis and triventricular hydrocephalus. These infants will be randomized to receive either ETV or CSF shunting. It is recognized, however, that when comparing two such different surgeries, parental preference for one over the other might be strong. Therefore, while randomization will be encouraged, the IIHS will use what is called a comprehensive cohort design, to allow for parental choice in the treatment decision. An important feature of the IIHS is that it will look beyond simple mechanical failure outcomes: the children will be followed into early childhood, with the primary study outcome being quality of life at five years of age. This will be the first randomized trial of any type comparing ETV to CSF shunting, but also the first trial in pediatric hydrocephalus to use quality of life as the primary outcome.

REFERENCES

1. Fritsch MJ, Kienke S, Ankermann T, et al. Endoscopic third ventriculostomy in infants. J Neurosurg 2005; 103:50–53.
2. Etus V, Ceylan S. Success of endoscopic third ventriculostomy in children less than 2 years of age. Neurosurg Rev 2005; 28:284–288.
3. Koch D, Wagner W. Endoscopic third ventriculostomy in infants of less than 1 year of age: Which factors influence the outcome? Childs Nerv Syst 2004; 20:405–411.

4. Kadrian D, van Gelder J, Florida D, et al. Long-term reliability of endoscopic third ventriculostomy. Neurosurgery 2005; 56:1271–1278; discussion 1278.
5. Wagner W, Koch D. Mechanisms of failure after endoscopic third ventriculostomy in young infants. J Neurosurg 2005; 103:43–49.
6. Sgouros S, Kulkarni AV, Constantini S. The International Infant Hydrocephalus Study: Concept and rationale. Childs Nerv Syst 2006; 22:338–345.

Predicting Success of ETV in Children with Hydrocephalus

Abhaya V. Kulkarni
Department of Neurosurgery, Hospital for Sick Children, Toronto, Ontario, Canada

The role for endoscopic third ventriculostomy (ETV) for pediatric hydrocephalus appears to be expanding. In weighing the option of CSF shunting versus ETV for a given child, there are usually many factors that one needs to take into account to determine the preferred option. One of the main issues comes down to predicting what the expected chances of successful ETV are for a child. It is often difficult, however, to easily obtain this answer from the literature. While the ETV literature is expanding and approaching a certain level of maturity, many studies have obvious statistical limitations. Most, for example, have modest sample size (usually hailing from single centers). Many also tend to analyze success using several different subgroup analyses (e.g., the success rate was "X"% for infants under 12 months and "Y"% for children with aqueductal stenosis and previous shunt) or, in a more sophisticated way, they might report relative risk estimates for a specific factor (e.g., infants younger than 12 months were "X" times as likely to fail ETV and those with aqueductal stenosis were "Y" times less likely). While these types of analyses are important in helping us scientifically determine the important factors that determine a successful ETV, they do not allow us to accurately determine the expected chance of ETV success in, for example, a 4 year old with tectal glioma and a previous shunt. This type of accurate prediction requires specific statistical analyses involving the development of a predictive equation based on a logistic regression model that is then tested for validity. To be successful, this process requires a very large sample of patients—several hundred at a minimum. One then randomly selects only some of these (usually around 70%) who are then used to develop the logistic regression model. This model analyses patient factors known or thought to be related to ETV success (e.g., patient age or etiology of hydrocephalus). One can then create a probability equation using the regression coefficients from the model. Then, one needs to test how well the model actually predicts success using a sample of patients different from the one in which the model was developed. This is done by utilizing the remaining patients from the large initial sample (i.e., the approximately 30%) who were not randomly selected for model development. For each patient in this sample (frequently called the validation sample), the probability equation will provide the predicted chance that the ETV will succeed. This can then be compared to whether the patient's ETV actually did succeed or not. Numerous statistical tests can be performed that measure the predictive abilities of a model.

Recently, an analysis of this nature was performed by a multicenter, international collaboration consisting of 12 pediatric neurosurgical institutions from Canada, Israel, and the United Kingdom (*Kulkarni, Drake, Mallucci, Sgouros, Roth, Constantini,* and *the Canadian Pediatric Neurosurgery Study Group—unpublished data, currently under peer-review*). These centers ranged from those who had only performed a few ETVs to those performing over 100. In total, 618 patients were represented. Following the methodology described above, 455 patients (approximately 70%) were randomly chosen for the development of a logistic regression model. This included the following predictors: patient age (which was, by far, the strongest predictor of ETV success), etiology of hydrocephalus, and presence of a previous shunt. Age was categorized as <1 month, 1 to <6 months, 6 to <12 months, 1 to <10 years, and ≥10 years. Etiology of hydrocephalus was categorized as aqueductal stenosis, postinfectious, myelomeningocele, post-intraventricular hemorrhage, tectal tumor, other brain tumors (nontectal), and other. The volume of ETV's performed at a center did not appear to influence the results and was not retained in the final model. The model yielded the following equation that can be used to calculate the expected probability of ETV success or failure. To calculate this first, the linear predictor, X, is calculated based on the presence (1) or absence (0) of the following patient variables:

$$X = 1.888 + 0.283 \times \text{(aqueductal stenosis)} - 1.092 \times \text{(postinfectious)}$$
$$- 0.104 \times \text{(myelomeningocele)} - 0.426 \times \text{(intraventricular hemorrhage)}$$
$$+ 0.177 \times \text{(tectal tumor)} - 0.558 \times \text{(nontectal tumor)} + 0 \times \text{(other etiology)}$$
$$- 2.275 \times \text{(age} < 1 \text{ month)} - 1.960 \times \text{(age } 1 - 6 \text{ months)}$$
$$- 1.012 \text{(age } 6 - 12 \text{ months)} - 0.750 \times \text{(age } 1 - 10 \text{ years)} + 0 \times \text{(age} > 10 \text{ years)}$$
$$- 0.580 \times \text{(previous shunt)}$$

The predicted probability of ETV success or failure is then given by (where e is the base of the natural logarithm)

$$\text{Probability of ETV success} = \frac{e^X}{1 + e^X}$$

$$\text{Probability of ETV failure} = 1 - \frac{e^X}{1 + e^X}$$

For example, the linear predictor for a 12 years old with aqueductal stenosis and no previous shunt would be $X = 1.888 + 0.283 = 2.17$. The probability of ETV success is then

$$\text{Probability of ETV success} = \frac{e^{2.17}}{1 + e^{2.17}} = 0.90$$

Therefore, there is 90% chance of success in this child. Similarly, one could calculate the chance for success in a 3 months old with intraventricular hemorrhage about 38%. A computerized calculator (Excel-based) is available that performs these calculations automatically.

Although the statistics show that the predictive properties of this model are good, there is still more work that will need to be done. The number of patients in the sample with myelomeningocele and postinfectious hydrocephalus was quite small, leading to potentially inaccurate predictions. Also, this model will need to be validated on a group of patients treated at other centers in other countries to see if its predictions remain accurate. Finally, predicting mechanical or physiological success of a procedure addresses only part of the issue in deciding between ETV and shunt; the other outcomes that will need to be studied in greater detail will be long-term cognition and quality of life following these procedures.

29 | Hydrocephalus and Epilepsy

Argirios Dinopoulos
3rd Pediatric Department of the University of Athens, "Attikon" University Hospital, Athens, Greece

Epilepsy and hydrocephalus are common pediatric neurological problems. The prevalence of epilepsy is 5–10 cases per 1000 children, while the prevalence of hydrocephalus is 1–3 per 1000 children in the population. The etiologies of both situations are diverse, a fact that complicates the context of epilepsy and shunt surgery. Since the introduction of shunting therapy for hydrocephalic patients, controversies have developed between the likelihood of epileptic seizures developing as a result of the shunting itself and its complications or the epileptic seizure being the result of the underlying brain pathology. Several authors have reported an increased risk of epileptic seizures after shunt placement, but true mechanisms are still controversial. A review of these controversies is elaborated eloquently by Sato et al. (1). Complexities arise because there are several mechanisms that may play a role on generation of epilepsy including

- the underlying brain pathology, regardless of the procedure;
- the CSF dynamics of hydrocephalus;
- the insult to the brain at the time of ventricular catheter insertion;
- the presence of the shunt tube itself as a foreign body; and
- the burr-hole location.

There are also several factors such as the presence of mental retardation, the infection as a complication, the number of shunt revisions after malfunction that may precipitate or even facilitate the presence of seizures and indirectly increase the risk for epilepsy. Although ventricular shunts have been the standard treatment for hydrocephalus for decades, the long-term morbidity, including postshunt epileptic seizures, has to be taken seriously. The use of neuroendoscopic techniques when indicated may ameliorate this problem a great deal in the future. This chapter tries to answer some key questions that arise in clinical setting in the management of this group of patients.

DO SHUNTED HYDROCEPHALIC PATIENTS HAVE A HIGHER RISK OF DEVELOPING SEIZURES?

The issue of prevalence of epilepsy in hydrocephalic patients, especially in shunted subjects, is complicated because many factors are implicated. There is agreement that patients with hydrocephalus are at a higher risk of having or developing a seizure disorder than the general population. The majority of the papers in the literature suggest that overall there is an increased risk of seizures in patients with shunted hydrocephalus ranging from 17% to 38%. The paper by Bourgeois et al. gives one of the most well-documented evaluations of the correlation between hydrocephalus and epilepsy. According to this paper, seizures were recorded in 32% of the 802 children and the frequency was much lower (~29%) in the preshunted group than in postshunted group (~71%). Regarding the seizure type, generalized seizures were common in the preshunted group and partial epilepsy, a common seizure in the postshunted seizure group, was observed in 50% of them (2).

It is not always easy to define the criteria of epilepsy (seizures are not always epilepsy), and Piatt and Carlson aimed to describe an association of epilepsy with hydrocephalus as depicted by the initiation of antiepileptic drug (AED) treatment. The date of onset of epilepsy was taken as the date of initiation of therapy. The prevalence of AED treatment at diagnosis of hydrocephalus was 12% but by 10 years after diagnosis 33% of patients had been treated with epilepsy and no trend towards diminishing annual risk was observed. There was no age difference at the initial prevalence of AED treatment (3). With respect to the time-course after shunting, the paper by Johnson et al. (4) gives us some information by reviewing a cohort of 817 shunted hydrocephalic children. It was found that 38% of the patients had seizures, with the first seizure occurring at a median 1.6 years after the original shunt insertion and only 12% had their first seizure during the first week after shunt surgery (4). Another study states that the peak for the onset of seizures was within months following shunt placement (5). The age at initial shunt insertion seems to also influence the occurrence of the epileptogenic scar, and the younger the patient at the date of surgery, the greater the chance of epileptogenesis during the second year after surgery (6).

DOES THE ETIOLOGY OF HYDROCEPHALUS PLAY ROLE IN THE INCIDENCE OF EPILEPSY?

The etiology of hydrocephalus reflects in a way the underlying brain pathology and hence plays a significant role on the risk of developing a seizure both in shunted and nonshunted hydrocephalic individuals. It is well documented that patients with meningomyelocele experience a significantly lower incidence compared with those with other central nervous system malformations. In studies with a high number of patients with meningomyelocele, an overall lower incidence of seizures in shunted individuals is observed (7). There is some agreement in that birth injury is a significant risk factor for the development of seizures, and the incidence of epilepsy is elevated among children who suffered hemorrhage, infection, or anoxia during the neonatal period (3–5). Those with prenatal hydrocephalus demonstrated a prevalence of 38% of developing seizures and those with meningitis and postinfective hydrocephalus carried a high risk of epilepsy in the order of 50%. A high incidence is documented in the groups in which causes were abscess, intracranial hemorrhage, trauma, and prematurity but relatively low in the group with spina bifida.

DOES MENTAL RETARDATION INCREASE THE RISK OF DEVELOPING EPILEPSY?

Mental retardation aggravates the risk of having or developing seizures in hydrocephalic patients. Keene and Ventureyra, in a retrospective study of 197 shunted hydrocephalic children, reported that the group with seizures tends to be more severely mentally retarded and to have more abnormalities seen on imaging studies. Hydrocephalic children without epilepsy showed normal intelligence in 66% of cases, while when hydrocephalus was associated with epilepsy normal intelligence was observed in 24% only (7). Another study reports that only 13% of the children with hydrocephalus and epilepsy had an IQ above 90, and children with IQ scores 70 or below were more likely to experience seizures than were children with normal intelligence (8). Overall there is a strong indication about the close correlation between epilepsy and poor psychointellectual outcome. It is clear that the underlying brain abnormalities (macroscopic or microscopic) and particularly those located in the cortex are responsible for the susceptibility for seizures after shunt placement.

DOES SHUNT MALFUNCTION INCREASE THE RISK FOR SEIZURES?

A shunt malfunction is not an uncommon complication and it is a matter of concern and preoccupation for neurosurgeons. A higher incidence of epilepsy has been reported among patients with shunt malfunction and the average number of shunt revisions was significantly higher in children with seizures than in those who did not develop seizures. Without revision the incidence of epilepsy was only 20%, while it was 52% in the patients in whom more than three revisions were done. The incidence is even higher when the malfunction is combined with infection. The seizures as the presenting symptom of acute shunt dysfunction occurred in only 8.6% of patients (2). There is evidence that the need for more frequent valve revisions increases the tendency for epilepsy as, in a study by Dan and Wade, only 5.9% of those who did not have shunt revision developed epilepsy, compared with 24.5% of those with two or more shunt revisions (9). The onset of a first time seizure in a shunted patient should alert one to shunt obstruction, although the seizure as the only symptom of shunt malfunction is not a common feature. Among 1831 revisions only 2.6% of the shunted children who were brought to the emergency department because of a seizure were found to have shunt malfunction requiring shunt revision (4). On the other side, there are studies that do not support that notion: Keene and Ventureyra found no correlation between the number of shunt revisions and seizure occurrence, but in this study the overall incidence of seizures is the lowest observed, and Klepper et al. report that the risk of epilepsy based on AED treatment was not influenced by the number of shunt revisions (5,7). Although shunt malfunction, especially when combined with infection, and the number of shunt revisions seem to increase the risk of developing epilepsy, a seizure as the only presenting symptom of shunt malfunction is not a common phenomenon.

DOES BURR HOLE SITE PLAY A ROLE IN SEIZURE OCCURRENCE?

Correlation between subsequent risk of seizure occurrence and location placement or burr hole site is another debatable issue. According to Dan and Wade, among patients with parietal ventricular catheterization site only 6.6% had convulsions, in contrast to 54.5% of those with a frontal site (9). Buchhalter and Dichter support the view that the majority of focal interictal EEG abnormalities in patients were lateralized to the site of shunt placement, and frontal shunt placement was associated with a significantly higher incidence of seizures than a posterior location (10). Piatt and Carlson found that burr hole site had no detectable effect on the prevalence of AED treatment and hence epilepsy. A trend toward slightly less AED treatment in the parietal burr hole group was seen, compared with frontal burr hole group especially in those subjects that were shunted as neonates. Regarding multiple burr hole sites, patients with meningomyelocele who had CSF shunts inserted at both frontal and parietal burr hole sites required more AED treatment than patients with shunts at only one site (3). In another study that was limited exclusively to patients with meningomyelocele, the location of the shunt catheter was not predictive of seizures (8). By summarizing the above debating evidence it seems that shunt placement does cause local epileptogenic irritation, but the underlying brain abnormality is more important in determining whether or not a patient will develop epilepsy.

DOES THE EEG PATTERN CHANGE IN SHUNTED HYDROCEPHALUS?

Partial and partial with secondary generalization are the most frequent types of seizures associated with shunted patients, and they usually originate from the shunted hemisphere. EEG abnormalities described in these patients include focal slow-wave activity accompanied by focal spikes and sharp waves. There is a higher incidence of abnormal EEG traces in the shunted group (95%) than in the nonshunted group (47%), and focal interictal EEG abnormalities are localized to the site of shunt placement (10). On the study by Bourgeois et al., preshunted EEGs disclose lower incidence of a single epileptic focus than postshunted EEGs (27% vs. 50%). In addition, a direct relationship was found between the side of radiological abnormalities and the site of the EEG focus (2).

Nevertheless, on other studies it has been shown that the frequency of various EEG abnormalities is similar in the shunted and nonshunted group, but the frequency of epileptiform activity is higher in the shunted group. Hydrocephalus in children is associated with generalized or focal EEG abnormalities and shunting may cause more specific epileptiform activity.

Occasionally, hypsarrhythmia and even continuous spike and waves during sleep may occur (2,3). An important observation is the presence of an epileptic encephalopathy with continuous spikes and waves during sleep (CSWS) in children with shunted hydrocephalus. The phenomenon was first described by Veggiotti et al. in six patients with ventriculoperitoneal shunt placement during the first year of life. All patients with CSWS experienced epileptic seizures as well (11). CSWS is more frequently associated with shunted hydrocephalus of early onset than in general population. It is worth noting that in congenital hydrocephalus patients with seizures, language, and behavioral problems CSWS should be suspected. The early identification of this particular electroclinical picture is crucial because early treatment may change the outcome. The finding of EEG abnormalities, and especially dramatic ones in form of CSWS, in shunted hydrocephalic children is highly suggestive that shunt implantation is a factor in the causation of electrical changes and ultimately in the development of seizures (12).

CONCLUSIONS

There is agreement that patients with hydrocephalus are at a higher risk of having or developing a seizure disorder than the general population and shunting increase that risk. The age at initial shunt insertion seems to influence the occurrence of the epileptogenic scar, and the younger the patient at the date of surgery, the greater the chance of epileptogenesis during the second year after surgery. The etiology of hydrocephalus does play a role in the frequency of epilepsy with the higher incidence observed in patients with infection, intracranial hemorrhage, birth asphyxia, and prematurity, and the lower incidence in the group with spina bifida and meningomyelo-cele. Mental retardation aggravates the risk of having or developing seizures in hydrocephalic patients. Shunt malfunction, especially when combined with infection and the number of shunt revisions, may increase the risk of developing a seizure but the underlying brain abnormality is more important in determining whether or not a patient will develop epilepsy. The seizure as the only presenting symptom of shunt malfunction is not a common phenomenon. Multiple burr hole sites and possible frontal shunt placement carry a higher risk of developing epilepsy. Hydrocephalus in children is associated with generalized or focal nonspecific EEG abnormalities, but shunting may cause more specific and lateralizing epileptiform activity. In patients with congenital hydrocephalus with seizures and language and behavioral problems, an epileptic encephalopathy with continuous spike and wave activity during sleep should be suspected.

REFERENCES

1. Sato O, Yamguchi T, Kittaka M, et al. Hydrocephalus and epilepsy. Childs Nerv Syst 2001; 17:76–86.
2. Bourgeois M, Sainte-Rose C, Cinalli G, et al. Epilepsy in children with shunted hydrocephalus. J Neurosurg 1999; 90:274–281.
3. Piatt JH Jr, Carlson CV. Hydrocephalus and epilepsy: An actuarial analysis. Neurosurgery 1996; 39:722–727; discussion 727–728.
4. Johnson DL, Conry J, O'Donnell R. Epileptic seizure as a sign of cerebrospinal fluid shunt malfunction. Pediatr Neurosurg 1996; 24:223–7; discussion 227–228.
5. Klepper J, Busse M, Strassburg HM, et al. Epilepsy in shunt-treated hydrocephalus. Dev Med Child Neurol 1998; 40:731–736.
6. Varfis G, Berney J, Beaumanoir A. Electro-clinical follow-up of shunted hydrocephalic children. Childs Brain 1977; 3:129–139.
7. Keene DL, Ventureyra EC. Hydrocephalus and epileptic seizures. Childs Nerv Syst 1999; 15:158–162.
8. Noetzel MJ, Blake JN. Seizures in children with congenital hydrocephalus: Long-term outcome. Neurology 1992; 42:1277–1281.
9. Dan NG, Wade MJ. The incidence of epilepsy after ventricular shunting procedures. J Neurosurg 1986; 65:19–21.
10. Buchhalter JR, Dichter MA. Migraine/epilepsy syndrome mimicking shunt malfunction in a child with shunted hydrocephalus. J Child Neurol 1990; 5:69–71.
11. Veggiotti P, Beccaria F, Papalia G, et al. Continuous spikes and waves during sleep in children with shunted hydrocephalus. Childs Nerv Syst 1998; 14:188–194.
12. Caraballo RH, Bongiorni L, Cersosimo R, et al. Epileptic encephalopathy with continuous spikes and waves during sleep in children with shunted hydrocephalus: A study of nine cases. Epilepsia 2008; 49:1520–1527.

30 | Fetal Surgery for Spina Bifida

Carys M. Bannister
Department of Neuroscience, University of Manchester, Manchester, U.K.

THEORETICAL BACKGROUND

The rationale for fetal repair of the back lesion in spina bifida was outlined by Heffez and associates in 1990 in a paper titled "The paralysis associated with myelomeningocele: Clinical and experimental data implicating a preventable spinal cord injury" (1). They exposed the spinal cord of fetal rats to amniotic fluid and found that the rats were born with severe weakness of the hind limbs and tail. Histology of the affected spinal cords showed necrosis and erosion of the neural tissue, which they thought looked similar to that seen in the myelomeningoceles of children with spina bifida. The authors thought that the paralysis in these children was due not only to the myelodysplasia but also to intrauterine injury, a hypothesis which they called the "two hit" theory. They went further to suggest that "... intrauterine protection of the exposed spinal cord might prevent some or all of the paralysis." Fetal surgery for the repair of the back lesion in spina bifida in human fetuses was proposed by Joe Brunner and his colleagues at Vanderbilt Medical Center, Nashville, in the 1990s (2). As a preliminary they created a model of spina bifida in sheep and showed that it was possible to endoscopically cover the exposed spinal cord with skin grafts. The rationale for the procedure was based on the hypothesis proposed by Meuli and associates who agreed with Heffez's contention that "... the neurologic deficit associated with open spina bifida is not directly caused by the primary defect but rather is due to chronic mechanical and chemical trauma since the unprotected neural tissue is exposed to the intrauterine environment" (3). In support of this proposition, Meuli showed that the spinal cord of normal midterm fetal sheep exposed to the amniotic fluid in the cavity of the uterus was progressively destroyed during pregnancy unless it was covered by a skin graft, in which case its form and function were largely preserved. While the fetal rat and sheep models clearly did not closely resemblance the spinal cord malformed by a myelomeningocele, it was thought the findings were relevant if it was accepted that early in fetal developmental significant neurological function was present in the human spinal cord deformed by a myelomeningocele and that this function was lost by exposure to the amniotic fluid.

EARLY REPORTS OF PROCEDURES AND OUTCOME OF FETAL SURGERY FOR MYELOMENINGOCELES

The first intrauterine procedures carried out on human fetuses with spina bifida were reported in 1998 (4). Three 28-week-old fetuses diagnosed ultrasonically as having spina bifida underwent a standard repair of the back lesion exposed by hysterotomy. The three infants were delivered by caesarian section at between 33 and 36 weeks of gestation; postnatally all of them were reported to have neurological defects appropriate for the anatomical level of their back lesions. Subsequently two of the infants were recorded as not needing cerebrospinal fluid (CSF) diversion. Following this early report of successful intrauterine closure, there was a veritable explosion of reports of cases operated on mainly in three centers in the United States; Vanderbilt Medical Center in Nashville, the Fetal Treatment Center of the University of California in San Francisco, and the Children's Hospital of Philadelphia, with by far the greatest number of cases being performed in Nashville.

Only the Nashville center has reported carrying out a technique other than a standard repair of the back lesion exposed by hysterotomy; in four cases at between 22 and 24 weeks of gestation, using endoscopy, the back lesion was covered with a split-skin graft taken from the mother; the outcome was compared with four fetuses undergoing a standard neurosurgical closure at 28 or 29 weeks of gestation (5). The outcome for the fetuses treated with split-skin graft was disastrous; two of the fetuses died, one as the result of chorioamnionitis and the other following placental abruption; both the survivors required a standard neurosurgical closure of their back lesions postnatally following absorption of the skin grafts in utero. The four fetuses treated by conventional neurosurgical closure survived to be delivered at between 33 and 36 weeks of gestation, all had healed scars on their backs. Not surprisingly, no further cases of repair with skin grafts have been reported. However, in a significant number of cases [13 out of 56 in one series (6)] on exposure of the myelomeningocele, the fetuses were found to have back lesions that were classified as myeloschisis and in them there was insufficient skin available to perform a primary skin closure. In these cases, bipedicular skin flaps were used to close the lesions. Although it was reported that adequate coverage of the dural sac was achieved at the time of operation, postnatally the cosmetic results were judged to be suboptimal.

NEUROLOGICAL DEFICITS FOLLOWING INTRAUTERINE REPAIR

The expectation that fetal repair of a myelomeningocele would result in children born with significantly fewer neurological deficits in their lower limbs and with improved bladder and bowel function compared to children repaired postnatally has not been realized. Following initial anecdotal reports of individuals having better than expected leg function taking into account the vertebral level of the back lesion, postnatal studies of larger numbers of patients have indisputably not supported the previously hoped for outcome that intrauterine surgery would result in all cases having minimal or even normal neurological function in the lower limbs, and that bladder and bowel continence would be achieved (7–10).

HINDBRAIN HERNIATION AND SHUNT INSERTION RATES

It was observed that fetuses who underwent magnetic resonance (MR) scans of their brains before and after intrauterine repair of their back lesions appeared to show regression of the tonsillar herniation component of their Chiari II malformation and that this was accompanied by the appearance of a cisterna magna that had not previously been seen (9,11). Sutton and his colleagues suggested that these changes were due to alteration in the fluid dynamics of the CSF that could no longer escape from the CSF pathways following closure of the back lesion and that the resultant change in the fluid dynamics prevented downward displacement of the cerebellar tonsils through the foramen magnum. In addition, follow up studies of the fetuses postnatally seemed to show that intrauterine repair lead to a reduced incidence of shunt-dependent hydrocephalus. Johnson and his colleagues (12) retrospectively reviewed 50 fetuses who had been repaired in utero; all of them were operated on at less than 26 weeks gestation for back lesions that ranged in level from the thorax to S1, at the time of operation none had talipes or ventriculomegaly of greater than 17 mm, all had normal karyotypes and none had additional abnormalities. The mean age of delivery of the group was 34 weeks. Postnatally all of the patients were demonstrated to have reversal of their hindbrain herniation. At the time of review, there were 47 survivors of whom 55% had had CSF diversion compared to 85% of a historic cohort of 297 controls operated on pastnatally. From this early experience of fetal repair of myelomeningoceles, it was concluded that there was a decreased need for ventriculoperitoneal shunting, that arrest or slowing of progressive ventriculomegaly occurred, and that there was consistent resolution of hind-brain herniation, although it was conceded that longer term follow-up was needed to evaluate other aspects of outcome such as neurodevelopment and bladder and bowel function. Tulipan and colleagues (13) also reported a reduced incidence of shunt-dependent hydrocephalus following intrauterine repair. They followed-up 104 patients aged one year old or older who had undergone surgery as fetuses either at Vanderbilt University or in the Children's Hospital in Philadelphia and compared their outcome with 189 postnatally treated controls. The results showed that there was a statistically significant reduction in the incidence of shunt-dependent hydrocephalus in those children who had had a repair for a lesion below the L2 level. The incidence of hydrocephalus also correlated with the age at which the repair had been carried out; it was significant if performed at or before 25 weeks of gestation but not if carried out later. The conclusion drawn from this study was that fetuses with lesions above L3 operated on after 25 weeks of gestation were not statistically less likely to need shunt insertion for hydrocephalus that those treated postnatally. Brunner and colleagues in

Vanderbilt carried out a further study at one year after birth of 116 out of 178 fetuses who had had an intrauterine repair carried out to see if they could identify factors that would allow them to predict which patients postnatally would be shunt-independent (14). Their conclusions were not unexpectedly in keeping with those of the combined study carried out by the teams in Vanderbilt and the Children's Hospital in Philadelphia; 61 (54%) of the 116 fetuses in the study required a shunt before the age of 12 months. The likelihood for the need for a shunt was significantly increased if the back lesion was at or above L4 [38 of the 48 patients (79%) compared to 25 of 68 (37%) with lesions below L4], if the operation was performed after 25 weeks of gestation [37 (71%) of the 52 patients operated on after 25 weeks of gestation were shunted compared to 37 (61%) of the 61 operated on or before 25 weeks of gestation] and if at the time of the repair the ventriculomegaly measured 14 mm or more. In the best possible cases where the back lesion was below L4, the operation was carried out at or before 25 weeks of gestation and the ventriculomegaly was less than 14 mm, only 8 out of 35 (23%) were shunted in the first year of life. Danzer and colleagues investigated the impact of fetal myelomeningocele repair on the head biometry by carrying out fetal ultrasound measurements taken before operation and for eight weeks postoperatively (15); the head circumference, ventricular diameter, and the Cortical Index were recorded at each examination. As has been noted previously (16), the head circumferences of fetuses with a myelomeningocele are demonstrably smaller than those of controls; however, eight weeks after repair, the difference was found to have largely resolved. There was also a 20% increase in the Cortical Index measurements compared to 51% in the controls. However, it was also found that there was an average increase in the ventricular diameter of 3.9 mm. Danzer and colleagues concluded that there are noteworthy alterations in the head biometry following intrauterine repair of a myelomeningocele and that these were not due to the effects of hydrocephalus alone. Few would disagree with this view; nevertheless, it is debatable to what extent the changes recorded are significantly different than those seen in fetuses who have not undergone intrauterine surgery.

The conclusion from the above studies suggests that the need for insertion of a shunt for hydrocephalus in infancy may be reduced if a fetus with a myelomeningocele is operated on at or before 25 weeks of gestation, has a favorable back lesion (one that can be repaired by primary skin closure and it at or below L4), and has ventriculomegaly of less than 14 mm. However, it needs to be asked what price was paid by the fetus and its mother to achieve this in terms of morbidity and mortality rates. It also remains to be seen whether the reduced shunt rate in these patients treated as fetuses compared to those treated in the postnatal period persists when longer term follow up studies are carried out.

MATERNAL AND FETAL COMPLICATIONS OF INTRAUTERINE REPAIR OF MYELOMENINGOCELES

It is not easy to get a complete picture of the incidence and nature of all the complications associated with intrauterine repair of myelomeningoceles experienced by both the fetuses and their mothers from a reading of the published literature. In an Editorial in the British Medical Journal, Farmer in 2003 stated that "... fetal surgery for this disorder has been associated with serious maternal and fetal complications, including uterine rupture, maternal bleeding, fetal death, and prematurity" (17). It is of interest that the website *fetal-surgery.com—Fetal Surgery for Spina Bifida* under the heading Risks of Fetal Surgery informs potential patients that the mother may have blood loss leading to transfusion, gestational diabetes, and weight gain as a result of prolonged bed rest; the latter presumably being necessary if the mother has to be given tocolytic agents to try to prevent a prematurely contracting uterus from expelling a recently repaired fetus. The website also informs the mother that she must assume that all future pregnancies will end in delivery by caesarian section, which means that if she elects to have further children her uterus will be subjected to at least a further operative procedure in addition to the hysterotomy needed to perform the fetal surgery and the caesarian section that will be carried out to deliver the operated fetus. There is no mention in the website of other complications that may beset the mother, for instance, wound infection, amniotic leaks due to premature rupture of the membranes and chorioamnionitis that has reportedly occurred in at least two patients (5).

The complications experienced by the fetuses are, if anything, even more formidable than those suffered by the mothers. The numbers of babies born prematurely after intrauterine repair of their back lesions is extremely high and is such a common event that there seems general acceptance in the literature that it is the norm not only for fetuses operated on for a myelomeningocele but also for the nonoperated ones as well which is not the case for the latter, the majority of whom are born at full term. The risks of prematurity are well known and include the need for prolonged ventilation, respiratory distress syndrome, chronic lung disease, and intraventricular hemorrhage, leading in a number of cases to brain damage and hydrocephalus. In one study of 100 infants who had undergone an intrauterine repair, 44 were born at less than 34 weeks of gestation and these were compared with 74 matched controls born prematurely for other reasons; complete data was only available for 37 of the operated cases, of these 11 developed respiratory distress syndrome and 6 chronic lung disease. There was no significant difference in the incidence of these conditions and intraventricular hemorrhage between the two groups (18). The unit at Vanderbilt reported that their overall risk of extreme prematurity, that is infants born at less than 30 weeks gestation, was 11% (19). There had been concern that fetuses operated on early (at a mean age of 23 weeks) would be likely to be born more prematurely than those operated on later (at a mean age of 26 weeks), but the average age of delivery for both groups was 34 weeks (20). In a series of 177 repairs, the operative fetal death rate was stated to be 4%, the 7 deaths being directly attributed to the surgery; 5 infants died from extreme prematurity, presumably because they were delivered immediately after operation, 1 fetus died in utero following surgery, and 1 infant died from pulmonary hypoplasia (19).

NEURODEVELOPMENT OF CHILDREN UNDERGOING INTRAUTERINE REPAIR OF MYELOMENINGOCELE

The results of only a few neurodevelopmental studies have been published. Brunner and associates studied a small group of 29 cases in 1999. The age of the infants at the time of assessment ranged from 2 to 18 months. The tool used to make the assessment was the Bayley Scale of Infant Development. The infants aged corrected for prematurity had a mean score of 100, with a range of 80 to 118 (21). In a more recent paper published in 2006 by Johnson and colleagues, 30 children of the 51 fetuses operated on for repair of the back lesions in the Center for Fetal Diagnosis and Treatment in Philadelphia returned to the center for neurodevelopmental assessment when they were two years old (22). Forty-three percent of the children had had a shunt inserted for treatment of hydrocephalus. These children were also tested using the Bayley Scale of Infant Development and in addition they were assessed with the Preschool Language Scales. Sixty-seven percent had cognitive language and personal–social skills within the normal range, 20% were mildly delayed, and 13% were significantly delayed. The children with shunts scored lower than those without shunts. The authors concluded that the children who had been operated in utero did not appear to have been worsened by the fetal surgery and some may have benefited by not having shunt dependent hydrocephalus.

MANAGEMENT OF MYELOMENINGOCELE STUDY (MOMS)

There are number of controversial issues concerning several aspects of the intrauterine repair of myelomeningoceles that in the past and currently remain unresolved (23). Collection of data about children operated on in a number of centers has been fragmentary, making it difficult to correlate the findings so that a meaningful comparison could be made with postnatally treated historical controls. Recognizing the importance of providing answers to questions posed by many convinced critics of the procedure, three maternal–fetal units in the United States (the University of California in San Francisco, the Children's Hospital of Philadelphia, and Vanderbilt University) funded by the National Institute of Child Health and Human Development decided to carry out a randomized controlled trial. The Management of Myelomeningocele Study or MOMS trial begun in 2003 is currently underway and, for its duration, the three participating units have agreed not to perform fetal back repairs outside of the trial. If recruitment rate of entry proceeds as expected, 200 pregnant women with fetuses diagnosed with a myelomeningocele in the third trimester of pregnancy divided equally into operated and nonoperated groups should have been recruited by the year 2008. The two principal questions addressed by the trial are does intrauterine repair of a fetal myelomeningocele at 19 to 25 weeks of gestation using a multilayered closure of the back lesion (*i*) improve the outcome compared to a standard postnatal repair as measured by death or the need for a ventricular shunting during the first year of life and (*ii*) improve neurodevelopment function at 30 months of age (corrected for weeks of prematurity) as measured by a combined rank score on the Bayley Scales of Infant Mental Development Index and improvement in lower limb function as measured by the difference between the motor and vertebral level of the back lesion. The follow up studies will be carried out by an independent team of examiners.

COMMENT

The literature does not wholly address the disquiet felt by some about the robustness of the theoretical justification for performing an intrauterine repair of a myelomeningocele. In the majority of patients with a myelomeningocele abnormalities can be detected in the entire neuraxis, which in all probability represent embryological maldevelopment. A number of theories have been put forwards to explain the abnormal development of the brain and the spinal cord in the condition; they include developmental arrest, tissue overgrowth, effects of abnormal cerebrospinal fluid hydrodynamics, and bursting open of the previously closed neural tube. The developmental arrest theory proposes that part of the neural tube destined to become the spinal cord fails to roll up and fuse leaving a flattened plaque of undeveloped neural tissue on the dorsal surface of the embryo. The observation that myelomeningoceles commonly arise in the lower lumbar and sacral regions suggests that abnormal closure of the neural tube's posterior neuropore is implicated in the etiology (24). A myelomeningocele is almost inevitably accompanied by the Chiari II malformation, a complex abnormality involving far more than the cerebellar tonsils; beaking of the tectum, kinking and caudal displacement of the pons, medulla and cervicomedullary junction, absence of the cisterna magna, and small, sometimes very small cerebellar hemispheres are nearly always present. The arrest theory accounts for Chiari II development by suggesting that it is failure of the pons to flex that leads to the pons, medulla, and the adjacent part of the fourth ventricle being forced into the upper cervical spinal canal. When related parts of the cerebellar vermis and choroid plexus begin to develop at about 12 weeks of gestation, they do so in the upper cervical spinal canal as do the cerebellar tonsils when they grow later in gestation. The overgrowth theory is similar; Cleland in 1883 (25) suggested that excessive growth of the edges of the neural plate prevents its inverting and fusing, and overgrowth of the cerebellum and the brainstem lead to their downward displacement and the development of the Chiari II malformation. The hydrodynamic theory suggested by a number of authors, but refined by Gardner (26) proposes that prior to the eighth or ninth week of gestation, when the foramina of Luschka and Magendie open in the roof of the fourth ventricle allowing CSF to escape from the ventricular system, a state of physiological hydrocephalus exists and causes distension of the central canal of the lower end of the neural tube. If perforation of the roof of the fourth ventricle does not occur at the correct time, further production of CSF leads to the cerebellar tonsils and part of the fourth ventricle being displaced downwards into the upper cervical spinal canal. At the same time, the myelomeningocele is formed by the bursting open of the central canal of the lower end of the distended neural tube. Padget (27) also believed that the primary deficit in spina bifida was the bursting open of the closed neural tube. She thought that fluid from the central canal raised a bleb in the mesoderm beneath the ectoderm, which later ruptured to form the myelomeningocele. The Chiari II malformation arose as a secondary response to the escape of fluid from the neural tube and also accounted for microcephaly and a small posterior fossa.

Irrespective of how the abnormalities in the spinal cord and the brain are thought to arise, it cannot be disputed that they are identifiable in the human embryo from as early as the eighth week of gestation and are established in the fetus by the 12th week. In addition, the above theories support the view that from its embryonic inception a myelomeningocele is composed of abnormal and deformed neural tissue that is unlikely to be capable of undergoing the complex maturation and differentiation of the normal spinal cord. Accompanying the anatomical abnormalities is the probability that there is severe functional compromise making it unlikely that the deformed cord would ever be capable of fulfilling many, if any, of the intricate roles performed by a normal spinal cord.

The overall development of the cerebral hemispheres in spina bifida is almost always abnormal; apart from the frontal lobes being narrow and small (accounting for the front of the well-known lemon-shape of the skull), there are numerous other abnormalities present including polymicrogyria, cortical heterotopia, an enlarged massa intermedia, and ventriculomegaly.

The spectrum of abnormalities throughout the neuraxis, the time of their development, their severity and whether the neuroplaque is or was ever capable of functioning normally are crucially important as to whether it is possible to achieve a successful outcome by an intrauterine repair of myelomeningocele. The "two hit" theory is irrelevant if the neuroplaque has no and never has had any useful function; the anatomical changes thought to be induced by exposure to the amniotic fluid are equally irrelevant for the same reason. Changes in CSF hydrodynamic following a repair, alteration in the position of the cerebellar tonsils, and even a reduction in the incidence of shunt-dependent hydrocephalus may not be sufficient to compensate for the profound abnormalities present elsewhere in the brain, which may play an important causative role in the poor short-term memory, poor concentration, and myriads of other problems that have been identified in the older spina bifida patient, and which have been shown to interfere profoundly with education, employment, and independent living.

It is hoped that the MOMS trial will play a decisive role in answering some of the outstanding concerns about intrauterine repair of myelomeningoceles, but it will only do so if it is continued for a sufficient length of time. Neurodevelopment cannot be assessed with certainty even at the age of 5; many learning skills are not developed by a child until the age of 10 and extend even beyond that age. Bladder and bowel functions are difficult to evaluate before the age of 1, and ambulation is known to deteriorate in late childhood in some patients with spina bifida. It is also to be hoped that the MOMS trial will indicate the extent to which prematurity plays a part in the overall outcome. Being born prematurely is extremely serious and is accompanied by complications involving many organ systems including the brain.

In the final assessment, the risks to the mother and fetus must be off set against the benefits experienced by the patient. It can be argued that these risks are only justifiable if the end product is a normal or near normal child (23). The introduction of new techniques such as robotic-assisted endoscopic repair (28) may offer some advantages but unless it improves fundamentally the outcome it is unlikely to prove to be the ultimate solution to the problem. That may lie not in the treatment of the fetus but in the embryo as exemplified by the use of folic acid; although in the end best management strategies may come from preconception treatment of the condition following identification of the genetic and molecular biological underlying the abnormalities.

REFERENCES

1. Heffez DS, Aryanpur J, Hutchins GM, et al. The paralysis associated with myelomeningocele: Clinical and experimental data implicating a preventable spinal cord injury. Neurosurgery 1990; 26:987–992.
2. Copeland ML, Brunner JP, Richards WO, et al. A model for in utero endoscopic treatment of myelomeningocele. Neurosurgery 1993; 33:542–544.
3. Meuli M, Meuli-Simmen C, Hutchins GM, et al. In utero surgery rescues neurological function at birth in sheep with spina bifida. Nat Med 1995; 1:342–247.
4. Tulipan N, Brunner JP. Myelomeningocele repair in utero: A report of three cases. Pediatr Neurosurg 1998; 28:177–180.
5. Brunner JP, Tulipan NB, Richards WO, et al. In utero repair of myelomeningocele: A comparison of endoscopy and hysterotomy. Fetal Diagn Ther 2000; 15:83–88.
6. Mangels KJ, Tulipan N, Brunner, JP, et al. Use of bipedicular advancement flaps for intrauterine closure of myeloschisis. Pediatr Neurosurg 2000; 32:52–56.
7. Cochrane DD, Irwin B, Chambers K. Clinical outcome that fetal surgery for myelomeningocele needs to achieve. Eur J Pediatr Surg 2001; 11:18–20.
8. Hirose S, Farmer DL, Albanese CT. Fetal surgery for myelomeningocele. Curr Opin Obstet Gynecol 2001; 13:215–222.
9. Sutton LA, Adzick NS, Bilaniuk LT, et al. Improvement in hindbrain herniation demonstrated by serial fetal magnetic resonance imaging following fetal surgery for myelomeningocele. JAMA 1999; 282:1826–1831.
10. Tubbs RS, Chambers MR, Smythe MD. Late gestational intrauterine myelomeningocele repair does not improve lower extremity function. Pediatr Neurosurg 2003; 38:128–132.

11. Brunner JP, Tulipan N. Fetal surgery for myelomeningoceles and the incidence for shunt-dependent hydrocephalus. JAMA 1999a; 282:1819–1825.
12. Johnson MP, Sutton LN, Rintout N, et al. Fetal myelomeningocele repair: Short term clinical outcomes. Am J Obstet Gynecol 2003; 189:482–487.
13. Tulipan N, Sutton LN, Brunner JP,et al. The effect of intrauterine myelomeningocele repair on the incidence of shunt-dependent hydrocephalus. Pediatr Neurosurg 2003; 38:27–33.
14. Brunner JP, Tulipan N, Reed G,et al. Intrauterine repair of spina bifida: Preoperative predictors of shunt-dependent hydrocephalus. Am J Obstet Gynecol 2004; 190:1305–1312.
15. Danzer E, Johnson MP, Wilson RD, et al. Fetal head biometry following in-utero repair of myelomeningocele. Ultrasound Obstet Gynecol 2004; 24:606–611.
16. Bannister, CM, Russell SA, Rimmer S. Pre-natal brain development in fetuses with a myelomeningocele. Eur J Pediatr Surg 1998; 8:15–17.
17. Farmer D. Editorial: Fetal surgery. BMJ 2003; 326:461–462.
18. Hamdan AH, Walsh W, Brunner JP, et al. Intrauterine myelomeningocele repair: Effect on short-term complications of prematurity. Fetal Diagn Ther 2004; 19:83–86.
19. Bennett KA, Davis GH, Tulipan N, et al. Fetal surgery for myelomeningocele. In: Wyszynski DF, ed. Neural Tube Defects: From Origin to Treatment. New York: Oxford University Press, 2006:227.
20. Hamdan AH, Walsh W, Heddings A. Gestational age at intrauterine myelomeningocele repair does not influence the risk of prematurity. Fetal Diagn Ther 2002; 17:66–68.
21. Brunner JP, Tulipan N, Paschall RL. Fetal surgery for myelomeningocele and the incidence of shunt-dependent hydrocephalus. JAMA 1999b; 282:1819–1825.
22. Johnson MP, Gerdes M, Rintoul N, et al. Maternal–fetal surgery for myelomeningocele: Neurodevelopmental outcomes at 2 years of age. Am J Obst Gynecol 2006; 194:1145–1150.
23. Bannister CM. The case for and against intrauterine surgery for myelomeningocele. Eur J Obstet Gynecol Repord Biol 2000; 92:109–113.
24. Copp AJ. Relationship between timing of the posterior neuropore closure and development of spinal neural tube defects in mutant (curly tail) and normal mice embryos in culture. J Embryol Exp Morphol 1985; 88:39–54.
25. Cleland J. Contributions to the study of spina bifida, encephalocele and anencephalus. J Anat Physiol 1883; 17:238–258.
26. Gardner WJ. The dysraphic states from syringomyelia to anencephaly. Amsterdam. The Netherlands: Exerpta Medica, 1973:1–201.
27. Padget DH. Spina bibidsa embryonic neuroschisis—A causal relationship. Definition of the postnatal conformations involving a bifid spine. Johns Hopkins Med J 1968; 128:233–241.
28. Aaronson OS, Tulipan N, Cywes R,et al. Robert-assisted endoscopic intrauterine myelomeningocele repair: A feasibility study. Pediatr Neurosurg 2002; 36:85–89.

31 | The Patient's Perspective—Support and Social Integration

Rosemary Batchelor

Association for Spina Bifida and Hydrocephalus, Peterborough, U.K.

Founded in 1966, the Association for Spina Bifida and Hydrocephalus (ASBAH) is there for everyone with spina bifida and hydrocephalus, helping them to get the most out of life and encouraging them to achieve their ambitions in a society full of opportunities for children, young people, and adults alike (1).

ASBAH should be regarded as a back up, reinforcing the information clinicians present to patients, supporting the extended families and giving the time not always available in clinic.

There are 15,000 families known to ASBAH with over 600 new contacts annually. Whereas in 1966 the majority of families supported by ASBAH were affected by spina bifida, today, due to advances in antenatal screening and termination of spina bifida pregnancies, most families are affected by hydrocephalus with a small proportion of those associated with spina bifida.

ASBAH operates a low call rate Helpline, which can be reached on 0845 450 7755 or by email helpline@asbah.org. The ASBAH website www.asbah.org is regularly visited worldwide by individuals, families, and professionals.

Neurosurgeons and other health professionals practising in the United Kingdom can—and should—refer their patients with hydrocephalus to the ASBAH, the leading charity for people with these conditions in the United Kingdom.

ASBAH SERVICES

In addition to the ASBAH National Helpline and website, ASBAH has a team of Area Advisers and Specialist Advisers.

ASBAH employs some 29 paid regional advisers, all with relevant professional backgrounds and each working with families in their designated areas covering most of England, Wales, and Northern Ireland.

The advisers' professions include physiotherapy, occupational therapy, nursing, teaching, psychology, social work, and those with experience in the law, welfare rights, mobility, and housing.

The regional adviser teams are supported by specialist medical and education advisers with access to high-quality, up-to-date information, who keep abreast of the latest research, and who work with a network of experts in all medical, educational, and social aspects of the disabilities.

WHO DOES ASBAH SUPPORT?

Individuals and families affected by spina bifida and/or hydrocephalus from point of diagnosis to death.

The initial approach is often by parents after the diagnosis of congenital hydrocephalus on ultrasound scan.

The Association gives advice on the condition, answers the parents' questions (and advise what questions they should be asking the medical staff), may suggest going to a pediatric neurosurgeon with their scan pictures, and will support them through whichever decision they make about the outcome of the pregnancy.

This decision—whether to progress or to terminate the pregnancy—is for the parents to make with information and advice from their medical team.

If the decision is to terminate the pregnancy, the parents know that there is someone at ASBAH that they can talk to. ASBAH will also offer information about their Book of

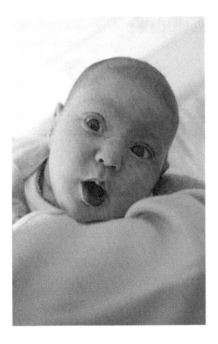

Figure 1 The news that our baby, Elisabeth, had spina bifida and hydrocephalus was a great shock, but the support of relatives, friends, and ASBAH helped us prepare for the new—and much wanted—addition to our family. (Sam Copeland)

Remembrance and the Forget-Me-Not fund, a practical way to commemorate the baby's life while helping to raise funds for ASBAH to continue its work.

For those who continue with the pregnancy, there will be lifelong contact with ASBAH, the opportunity to meet up with other families of children with hydrocephalus and support of ASBAH's specialist advisers.

At the beginning—especially when the baby with hydrocephalus is a sick baby—there will be a high level of involvement with ASBAH, reassuring the parents, explaining what hydrocephalus means, helping to claim state benefits, and preparing the family for life with a child with hydrocephalus.

These "new" families tend to "dip in and out" of ASBAH. There are times when they will be very needy, and long periods when life with a child with hydrocephalus is much easier.

The early days will inevitably and rightly include ASBAH working with the siblings and grandparents who are often left out of the information loop by health professionals, but who need the support as much as the parents do.

Once the initial period of surgery and hospitalization is over, the family tend to settle down with occasional calls, usually around times of illness ("Do you think it is his shunt?"), vaccination programs, lack of therapy, developmental delay, and queries about sports and holidays.

Interestingly, the same types of queries come from the professional responsible for some aspects of the baby's wellbeing—health visitors, GPs, nursery staff, social workers.

The next period of close contact is likely to be around the time of entry to nursery or school where ASBAH education advisers can be involved. Their roles will be around reassurance and advice to school staff naturally anxious about taking a child with a shunt or ETV into their care; there may be issues around challenging behavior and discussions about integrating the child into mainstream school or looking at specialist units.

Going to school may be the first time that the child with hydrocephalus has been parted from his parents for any length of time. The families will naturally be anxious that their child will settle into school and that there will be adequate and appropriate support in place. This may mean the school employing a Learning Support Assistant to help the child in lesson time and at break times; the child may need an adapted learning program. The families may have issues around the possibility of their "different" child being bullied and they may be worried about the possibility of shunt damage if their child joins in the sports and games that the rest of the class enjoy.

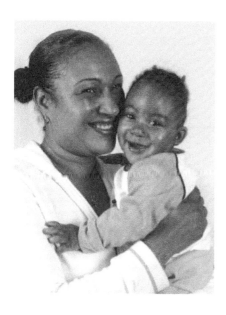

Figure 2 I have had valuable help and advice from my ASBAH adviser when dealing with Aidan's extra needs. (Anne Marie Bryan)

Later, there will be transition to college or university or into employment. This time may also coincide with transition from pediatric to adult medical services.

Both experiences can be traumatic for the young person with hydrocephalus, who resists change, cannot cope with change, and who often cannot understand why things should change.

ASBAH will be there to hopefully help smooth the path and with the adviser's role changing too—this time from offering generic family support to working more closely with the young person as client.

This work may involve visiting or giving information about colleges or universities or talking about hydrocephalus with prospective employers.

The Association's aim is always to encourage independence and to endeavor to ensure that their Services staff are furnished with the skills to give the professional advice and help to achieve this.

Young adulthood brings its own challenges—challenges that can be more difficult for someone with a disability.

ASBAH is used to rising to the challenge! They know that this age group will want information that is age and ability appropriate and that they will have anxieties around a variety of subjects.

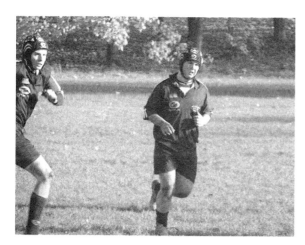

Figure 3 Our son, Josh, who loves sport to the extreme was rushed into hospital with what we thought was a head cold but after 36 hours he was eventually diagnosed with hydrocephalus. From feeling completely alone and bewildered ASBAH offered us so much help and advice plus information about different treatments which are available. Suddenly our nightmares faded. (Alan Pendlebury)

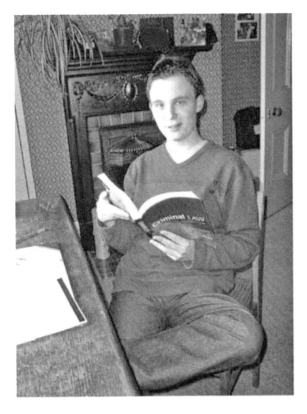

Figure 4 My goal is to become a very success-ful barrister, specialising in criminal law. Who knows. I could be the first hydrocephalic person to become a major cog in the Judiciary. (Ben Edwards)

Over the years, the ASBAH has developed professional expertise in advising on driving (2), relationships and sex, how to explain to friends and partners about the possible effects of hydrocephalus and how to encourage young adults to take responsibility for their condition including recognizing potential shunt malfunction. ASBAH can help draw up programs to help with time management, personal care, handling finances, and keeping "on track" when following educational courses.

Young people living away from home for the first time may need help adjusting to the responsibility of independent living, and parents need help to "let go."

Employers and employees need to be aware that the person with hydrocephalus may not respond to facial expressions or body language, may need prompting to stay motivated, may be very regimented in their work methods, and will not work well under pressure. But they may present as confident and capable.

ASBAH can work with employers to help them and people with the disability over these hurdles.

AND WHAT ABOUT LATER YEARS?

The hydrocephalic population is not only growing but also growing older with expectations, which may have seemed unlikely some years ago.

ASBAH continues to work closely with this older age group and are able to anticipate their likely difficulties.

Claiming state benefits means a plethora of complicated forms (3), which can be difficult for people who have always relied on parents to complete them.

Suitable housing, how to apply, and how to care for the home environment are important areas that adults who have always been cared for at the parental home will need help with.

Forming relationships can be difficult. Too many disabled people rely on Internet "chat rooms" for friendship and need to be made aware of the potential risks.

There is an ASBAH users' group, Your Voice, with over 300 members all with either spina bifida or hydrocephalus and aged 18 and over.

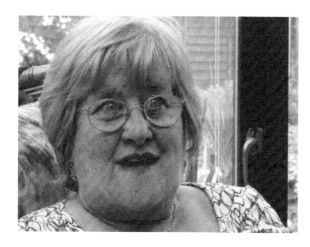

Figure 5 You're going about your normal day to day life and can't understand why crossing a road with a kerb is a problem. Its things like this that nobody tells you, there was no leaflets on Normal Pressure Hydrocephalus, so it was a relief when I contacted ASBAH—it took a weight off my mind I tell you. (Wendy Simons)

This group meets several times a year for residential weekends around a specific theme, that is, hydrocephalus and shunts, employment, sports, continence management but where there is also emphasis on the social aspects of the program and the chance to meet up with others with similar disabilities.

Pregnancy is another milestone that introduces new anxieties.

Obstetricians, midwives, and GPs are often unaware of how the CSF shunt may be affected by pregnancy and labor: the extended family and partner will have their own worries.

Both groups, professional and family, come to ASBAH for advice.

Families want to be assured that others with hydrocephalus have had successful pregnancies and appreciate contact with other mothers with shunts.

For the professionals, research in the United States has shown that any CSF shunt malfunctions around this time appear unlikely to be related to the pregnancy or delivery (4).

Normal pressure hydrocephalus (NPH), usually affecting people age 60 or over, brings its own very different needs.

The families of service users with NPH probably need more input than the service users themselves.

Some patients leave hospital postshunting with little advice about the shunt or about the minutiae of this "new life." Maybe health professionals feel they do not need to know or that they will not understand?

The family or partner will worry about shunt malfunction and how to recognize it. When to call the doctor? When to contact the hospital? How long before their relative is "back to normal"?

The patient with NPH is often more pragmatic. Will readjusting (programming) the shunt be painful? How often will it need doing? For how long will they have to continue visit the outpatients' department at the neurosurgical unit (often some distance away)? Can they perm/color/cut their hair?

This older age group is less likely to want to "bother the doctor" with mundane queries, they may not hear well and are embarrassed to say so in a busy clinic, so they rely heavily on ASBAH in the early months after surgery.

The ultimate aim of the ASBAH is to enable people with hydrocephalus to live fulfilled, independent lives through support, education, and practical advice, and many thousands of individuals are testimony to ASBAH's ability to do just that.

RESEARCH

ASBAH is a member of the Association of Medical Research Charities (AMRC) and has always supported research into spina bifida and hydrocephalus.

ASBAH's first Research Fellow, Dr. Roger Bayston (1976–1979), was able to progress his work on prevention of CSF shunt infections, which ultimately led to the invention of an antimicrobial impregnated shunt material now used world wide.

In the present financial climate, the Association's research fund has diminished and applications to trusts and funders on behalf of researchers now funds most ASBAH-backed research.

All researchers submit a protocol, which goes before the Medical Advisory Committee (MAC) or Education Advisory Committee (EAC) for approval. If necessary, the protocol will go for peer review before acceptance.

The MAC and EAC are made up of consultants and educationalists expert in the field of hydrocephalus.

CAMPAIGNING

ASBAH will campaign for changes to policy and legislation that will directly impact on the quality of life for service users with hydrocephalus and spina bifida.

This work includes actively lobbying government for inclusion and equality in education and for fortification of flour with folic acid to help prevent fetal neural tube defects.

The Association also takes part in consultations around better health provision for patients with neurological conditions and comments on the issues that affect people with spina bifida and hydrocephalus. This may be through the specialist medical, nursing, and educational press or through the general media.

EXPERT INFORMATION

The world of hydrocephalus is rapidly expanding and ASBAH has training programs to ensure that they are able to keep abreast of new developments.

Professional training is ongoing with attendance at seminars, study days, and clinics and with a yearly residential conference.

ASBAH belongs to the Society for Research into Hydrocephalus and Spina Bifida (SRHSB) (www.srhsb.org) and is represented on the SRHSB's executive committee.

PUBLICATIONS

The Association creates awareness and understanding by disseminating high-quality information through the website (www.asbah.org) and printed materials and by promoting their position as a source of expertise and support.

The information sheets on all aspects of hydrocephalus and spina bifida (downloadable from the website) are highly regarded and continually updated: All go before the Medical advisory committee and Education advisory committee for approval before being made available to the public.

Also available are the child friendly "Benny the Bear" books dealing with hydrocephalus, issues facing a young child going into hospital, on holiday, school, etc. (sponsored by Codman and now in six languages) for young children with hydrocephalus. Year 2006 saw the publication of four continence management books for young children with spina bifida and their families— the "Russell and Millie" books (sponsored by Hollister).

In 2006, with assistance from Codman U.K., an interactive CD-ROM about NPH was launched explaining the condition, its effects, and treatment and with input from both neurosurgeons and other clinicians and patients and their families.

CONFERENCES AND EVENTS

ASBAH has an ongoing national program of study days, mostly for parents but some for professionals, made possible by the generosity of neurosurgeons, neurologists, psychologists, and therapists who give up their time to speak.

Parents of children aged six years and under are given the opportunity to meet at the annual Family Weekend held at venues around the country.

Parents attend two days of lectures from professionals including a "user friendly" neurosurgeon and have time to ask all those questions they have never had the opportunity to ask before. The disabled children and their siblings are cared for and entertained by ASBAH staff.

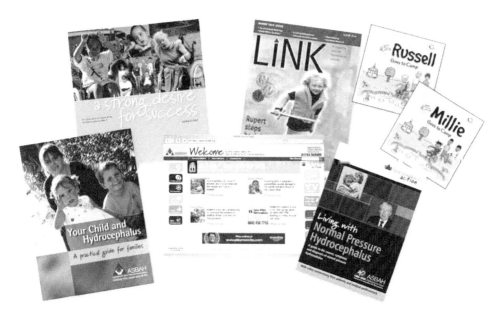

Figure 6 In 2004, ASBAH published "Your Child and Hydrocephalus," a guide for parents of children aged up to 11 years.

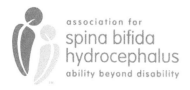

Figure 7 42 Park Road, Peterborough PE1 2UQ
Telephone: 01733 555988
Helpline: 0845 450 7755
Facsimile: 01733 555985
Email: info@asbah.org
www.asbah.org
(For Scotland, contact the Scottish Spina Bifida Association on 08459 111112, email familysupport@ssba.org.uk)

SIGNPOSTING

Neurosurgeons, pediatricians, neurologists, GPs, and Health Visitors should signpost their patients with hydrocephalus and spina bifida to ASBAH for the specialized support that they may not have the time and resources to give.

The ambition of the ASBAH is to be widely recognized and known as the leading source of information and expertise on hydrocephalus, providing this expertise to families, patients, and professionals in the United Kingdom.

All patients and their families affected by issues relating to spina bifida hydrocephalus, normal pressure hydrocephalus, or associated conditions can self-refer by contacting the ASBAH Helpline on 0845 450 7755 or through the ASBAH website www.asbah.org.

REFERENCES
1. Andrew Russell, Chief Executive, ASBAH. Annual report 2006.
2. Angela Lansley. Driving with Hydrocephalus, ASBAH 2005.
3. Disabled Living Allowance, Department of Work and Pensions.
4. Liakos AM, Bradley NK, McAllister JP, et al. Hydrocephalus and pregnancy: the medical implications of maternal shunt dependency. Eur J Pediatr Surg 1997; 7 Suppl 1:51–52.

Quantification of Outcome in Children with Hydrocephalus

Abhaya V. Kulkarni

Department of Neurosurgery, Hospital for Sick Children, Toronto, Ontario, Canada

Aside from the numerous mechanical complications associated with CSF shunts, children with treated hydrocephalus have variable long-term health outcome and quality of life (QOL). There are those children who, despite their condition, lead seemingly near-normal lives, while others are severely incapacitated and suffer from physical, cognitive, or social–emotional deficits. These aspects of health can be difficult to measure and quantify in a reproducible and valid manner. Attempts at such measurement have commonly relied on the use of very specific neuropsychological tests, yielding some important results. Cognitive functioning of many types is detrimentally affected by hydrocephalus. Academic progress is significantly affected by the demonstrated difficulties that children with hydrocephalus have with reading comprehension and with inferencing skills. Further, these difficulties are not due to deficits in word recognition or vocabulary, and they occur regardless of the child's cognitive level. In a selected group of children with hydrocephalus between 6 and 15 years of age, and all with IQs over 90, a significant deficit of reading comprehension was described compared to controls. This group also demonstrated impairment of oral comprehension and narrative discourse. Children with hydrocephalus have been shown to have poor math skills. Suggestions for possible causes for difficulties in math for these children include their relatively slow information processing skills and their visuospatial deficits. Hydrocephalic children have demonstrated lower scores on measures of fine motor, visual-motor, and spatial skills compared to controls. The evidence concerning memory performance in children with hydrocephalus is less clear. A comprehensive review article notes that there have been few studies concerning memory function in children with hydrocephalus, and these studies have shown inconsistent results. A review of a number of studies investigating executive function suggests that children with hydrocephalus may have done more poorly on some tests than control children mainly because they performed more slowly, although they were able to complete the tasks correctly. For example, they needed more trials to successfully complete a task or had motor or processing speed deficits that hindered their performance.

While useful for documenting specific areas of cognitive dysfunction, neuropsychological tests do not provide an overall picture of the child's health and frequently require special expertise for their administration and interpretation. Proper scientific assessment of broad QOL outcome requires the use of a questionnaire that is both consistently reproducible in repeated testing (i.e., it is reliable) and truly quantifies the health and QOL of the patient (i.e., it is valid). Questionnaires to assess health can be broadly categorized as *generic* (which can be used on a wide variety of childhood populations) or *disease-specific* (which are only meant to be used in a specific patient population). Generic measures attempt to broadly sample the spectrum of many domains of health status that apply to many different situations. Disease-specific measures (or in the case of hydrocephalus, *condition-specific*) are more limited in scope and are designed to measure health status only within a specific patient population, defined usually by a specific disease process and/or specific therapeutic intervention. Therefore, these measures may be perceived as more relevant to the patient population since they tend to address their concerns more specifically.

Several generic health measures exist (e.g., Pediatric Evaluation of Disability Inventory, Health Utilities Index, Functional Status II-R, etc.). However, a few of these have been used extensively in the pediatric hydrocephalus population, so their reliability and validity in this population is not yet firmly established. The Hydrocephalus Outcome Questionnaire

(HOQ) is so far the only disease-specific measure of outcome in the pediatric hydrocephalus population with proven reliability and validity. It is a 51-item questionnaire that takes about 10 to 15 minutes for parents to complete. There is also a child-completed version (cHOQ). The possible scores for the HOQ range from 0 (worse health) to 1.0 (better health). The HOQ provides a score of Overall Health, and the following subscores: Physical Health, Cognitive Health, and Social–Emotional Health. Reliability coefficients have been shown to be high (>0.80) with good evidence of construct validity.

Use of the HOQ in a typical pediatric population has quantified the spectrum of impairment in QOL that these children can suffer. The mean HOQ scores were as follows: Overall Health 0.66 [standard deviation (SD) 0.20], Physical Health 0.68 (SD 0.25), Cognitive Health 0.56 (SD 0.28), Social–Emotional Health 0.72 (SD 0.18). The distribution of HOQ Overall score is shown in Figure 1.

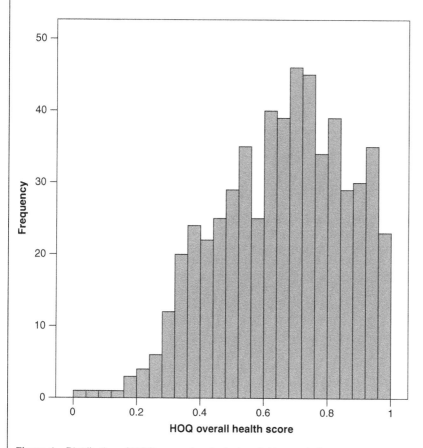

Figure 1 Distribution of HOQ scores in a typical pediatric population.

When quantifying outcome in pediatric hydrocephalus, one must recognize that the viewpoint of parents might differ from that of the child. Frequently, it is not an option to seek opinions from the child because they are either too young or, in some cases, are too cognitively impaired. However, we know that there is a substantial subgroup of older, higher-functioning children with hydrocephalus who are able to give their own assessment of outcome. Early work has highlighted the difference that frequently exists between their viewpoint and that of their parents. In general, in areas of cognitive and social–emotional outcome, in particular, the children tend to rate themselves as better off than their parents.

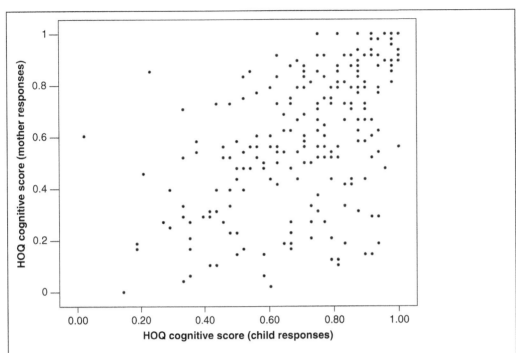

Figure 2 Comparison of mother and child HOQ scores.

This is shown in the scatterplot in Figure 2, which compares child versus mother assessment of HOQ Cognitive score.

It is clear that research into quantification of QOL in children with hydrocephalus is still in its early stages. Future work will need to deal more explicitly with the differences between parent and child viewpoints and deal with the limitations in assessing younger children.

32 | Ethical Considerations in the Treatment of CSF Disorders

Anthony D. Hockley[†]

Department of Neurosurgery, Birmingham Children's Hospital, Birmingham, U.K.

INTRODUCTION

Congenital anomalies of the central nervous system, notably CSF disorders that include hydrocephalus and spina bifida, are major causes of mortality and morbidity in children and adults. There is no real "cure" for many of these conditions, with repeated medical and surgical attention necessary. Survival is possible with handicap, needing special and expensive facilities. Problems may arise from a delay in their diagnosis and the recognition of complications, which may be part of the natural disease process, or due to inadequate surgical or medical care.

With increasing technological advances, ethical considerations remain important in virtually all medical decisions. The technological imperative *"if you can do something you must do it"* needs to be balanced by the ethical question *"What ought to be done?"* (1). While law concentrates on rights and tells us what we must do, ethics looks at values and tells us what we ought to do.

Medicine is as old as mankind, and ethics as old as medicine. It is of interest that the earliest ethical codes identified surgeons, not only for their skills and judgment, but also their personal risks of criticism and punishment.

The first ethical code dates back to 1750 BC in Babylon, when King Hammurabi (2) had the following engraved on a stone (which can be seen today in the Louvre Museum, Paris): *"If Surgeon preserves sight: 10 shekels of silver . . .. If sight destroyed: surgeon's hands cut off."* The Edwin Smith Papyrus (3) from Egyptian times in 1550 BC advised doctors on decision making, based on the patients' condition as follows: *"Treat with good prognosis. If hopeless, leave alone."* Hippocrates (460–377 BC) (4) introduced two new ethical principles: *"Primum non Nocere"* (first avoid injury), and a *"Duty of confidentiality"* by the doctor. These principles remain the basis and have been incorporated into modern medical ethics. A useful "Four Principles" approach was developed in the 1970s by the American philosophers, Beauchamp and Childress (5), summarized as follows:

1. Autonomy
2. Beneficence
3. Nonmaleficence
4. Justice

Autonomy, literally "self-rule," means the patient has responsibility in making a free and informed choice for treatment offered. Clearly, a young child (or older person with mental impairment) may be unable to do so.

Beneficence or "doing good" for one's patient is not always medically possible, but it implies a duty of care to patients. It raises the question of who should be the judge of what is best for the patient.

Nonmaleficence or the "avoidance of harm," from Hippocrates, is well established. However, medicine and surgery may involve doing harm, as a result of complications (hopefully temporary) from otherwise successful treatment, side effects of the therapy, or decisions made in difficult dilemmas such as the surgical separation of conjoined twins.

Justice or "acting fairly" covers several aspects. Most obvious is that patients should have equal access to health care, and the question of resources naturally has to be considered ("distributive justice"). Two other areas of justice apply to medical ethics, the respect for patients' rights ("rights based justice") and respect for morally acceptable laws ("legal justice").

[†]Deceased.

These four principles are the basis for every medical decision, but can conflict when a competent patient or parent chooses a course of action that is not in their or their children's best interests. A further conflict exists between our duties to individual patients and an obligation as a scientist to contribute to knowledge. Claude Bernard (6) in 1865 wrote: *"It is our duty and our right to perform an experiment on man whenever it can save his life, cure him or give him some personal benefit."*

The appalling experiments carried out by some Nazi doctors led in 1946 to the first internationally agreed guidelines on medical research involving humans, the "Nuremberg Code" (7). Its principles were incorporated into the "Helsinki Declaration" (8) of 1964 (last updated in 2004) that permits doctors to use a new treatment if it can save life or relieve suffering, providing the benefits and risks can be assessed against the best current methods.

DECISION MAKING FOR INFANTS WITH CONGENITAL ABNORMALITIES

With the improved technology, debate has continued concerning the treatment of infants with major developmental abnormalities. The first important question is whether all such babies should be treated? The second question concerns consent, and who should decide?

Where a fetal abnormality in utero has been recognized, mother may have a choice of termination. Inadequate or no counseling with parents not afforded the opportunity to consider an abortion may result in a "wrongful life" decision in law (9). Another fundamental question is when the fetus becomes a patient in its own right. There are religious differences concerning this moment in time. Hence, this issue becomes relevant when decisions need to be made concerning termination of pregnancy in the interests of the fetus or the mother, where in rare circumstances there may be a serious threat to maternal health. While the diagnostic and interventional techniques are now available, what is the role of intrauterine surgery? (discussed in Chap. 30).

After birth parents need to be given a realistic and experienced view of their child's problem, including its natural history and treatment possibilities. While it is the child who is at the disadvantage, it will be the parents who have the burden of care, and not surprisingly there is a high incidence of subsequent marital breakdown.

SACRIFICE OR NONTREATMENT

Sacrifice or the nontreatment of defective infants ("Infanticide") has been practiced in several cultures throughout history. Moreno (10) reminds us that infants have been put to death for a variety of reasons, including physical abnormalities, illegitimacy, population control, and undesirable sex. Infanticide is referred to in the Bible (11), and Plato in "The Republic" (12) supported the international exposure of sickly babies. Eskimos have only recently stopped this practice for economical reasons, but China and India have continued to practice infanticide, especially of female infants, for population control.

When an infant is born, particularly with an unexpected disability, it will often be the pediatrician who has to assume the leadership responsibility for decision making. Because of advances in neonatal medicine it is possible to prolong the lives of many sick infants, with an obvious conflict between the *"sanctity of life"* and the *"quality of life."* In an individual case, it is *"the best interest of the child"* which is usually adopted in clinical decision making, and also when difficulties arise that require resolution by legal authorities.

The term *"best interest"* supposes that all infants have interests, but for some the medical and physical problems of continued life can outweigh the benefits. Some authors have introduced other criteria using statistics. The aim has been to determine which infants are likely to benefit from treatment and only objective criteria are used in this approach. Such an *"objectivism"* approach (13) was advocated by John Lorber, a pediatrician in Sheffield, U.K., when advising a selective approach for the treatment of infants born with spina bifida.

It was in the late 1950s that effective surgical treatment for children with spina bifida became possible with the development of shunts for the associated hydrocephalus. Lorber (14) in 1971 published the results of the surgical treatment of 524 cases from Sheffield. He described so-called *"adverse criteria"* correlating handicap with more serious spina bifida cases. There then followed a trial of no treatment in 25 infants with these criteria. All but two died within six months, the remainder by nine months. This had a profound effect on medical management in the United Kingdom where "selection" for these infants became the standard policy. It was not really accepted by colleagues in North America. Later the issue was reopened, when several centers reported survivors in cases where the decision had been initially not to treat surgically. An important study in 1994 from Dublin (15) showed that among babies "selected" for nontreatment, fatalities were confined to the first three months. While a reduced incidence has been reported in many countries now, both real and from permitted termination of pregnancies following prenatal screening, the trend of management for surviving infants with spina bifida has returned towards active surgical and medical treatment.

A further ethical standard "personal interest" was proposed by Gostin (16), with criteria indicating there is "reasonable certainty that a competent individual would not chose to continue life in the circumstances presented." The specific criteria include the following:

1. The neonate is not conscious or sapient.
2. The potential for dealing with, and responding to, sensory information and experiencing thought is minimal.
3. The neonate is terminally ill and in the process of dying.

Expressed differently, the central question of decision making in these cases involves the infant's *"right to die."* A failure to respect the infant's right to die can result in the infant being deprived of the fundamental need not to suffer pain and not to be alienated from other human beings.

The nontreatment of defective newborns did not receive much attention until 1981 when in the United Kingdom a decision to let a newborn baby with Down's syndrome and multiple congenital anomalies die lead to a murder charge against the pediatrician (the "Arthur" case) (17). In the same year, parents refused surgery to their newborn infant with Down's syndrome and bowel obstruction. The Court of Appeal overruled the parents' wishes and ordered operative treatment (18) in the "best interests" of the child. In 1982, in the United States, there was an identical case (known as "Baby Doe") (19) where the parents and physicians refused surgery, and the Indiana Court supported their views. One year later a baby girl actually named Baby Jane Doe was born in New York with spina bifida. Again treatment was withheld while medical and legal disputes continued (20). Even though she survived, the delay in treatment was associated with infective complications that left her severely retarded. Political maneuvers to support the legal protection of disabled children reached Congress, which, in October 1984 (21), extended the definition of child abuse or neglected to include the denial of fluids, nutrition, and medical treatment for birth defects. These events and the subsequent major governmental attempts to supervise obstetrical practice in the United States were referred to as "Baby Doe" squads (22).

PROGNOSIS AND WITHDRAWAL OF TREATMENT

For treatment of any condition to be worthwhile, it should improve on the natural history of the disorder. Before the advent of shunts, the outcome for children with hydrocephalus was poor. There was an approximately 20% chance of reaching adulthood and a 50% chance of brain damage. With the introduction of shunts, the natural mortality of hydrocephalus was reduced by half after surgical treatment (23), and the number of educable survivors double in the operated as opposed to the nonoperated group (24). The present position is that now 70% to 80% of children with shunts survive long term. The majority attend normal school and can achieve social independence.

The differences in outcome depend on the cause of hydrocephalus. Children with aqueduct stenosis have an excellent prognosis. While there may be major physical deficits from other aspects of their condition, children with spina bifida have a better intellectual outcome than children whose hydrocephalus is the result of previous meningitis or neonatal intraventricular hemorrhage (25).

The difficult ethical problem is to know if and when to withdraw active treatment, once started, in patients with multiple or recurrent serious clinical problems who have a recognized limited prognosis. The neonate with intraventricular hemorrhage and multiple organ failure requiring prolonged intensive care is an example where such decisions have to be made. Usually parents and the family accept the position, but in some cases the final decision has to go to law.

There are two conditions related to CSF circulation which deserve special mention, "hydranencephaly" and "anencephaly."

Hydranencephaly

Hydranencephaly is a rare sporadic condition, where the greater part of the cerebral hemispheres is replaced by large membranous sacs filled with CSF (26). It may arise from inadequate blood flow from the internal carotid arteries in fetal life, although the mechanism is speculative. The structures supplied by the vertebral arteries, including the basal parts of the temporal and occipital lobes, basal ganglia, cerebellum, and brainstem, are usually preserved. The prognosis for development is hopeless and for survival very poor. Some infants may survive for several years, often without the correct diagnosis (27). The condition needs to be distinguished from congenital hydrocephalus, which carries a much better prognosis with treatment. The head may be large at birth or sometimes rapidly enlarge after birth probably as a result of secondary aqueduct obstruction, so that the ethical dilemma is whether to insert a shunt in such infants. Some would consider this justified as a palliative aid to nursing care, while others would regard the procedure as of no benefit. All would agree that parents need to be appropriately counseled to the implications of this diagnosis and be supported for the inevitable outcome.

Anencephaly

This lethal defect arises from failure of rostral neural tube closure between 18 and 25 days of gestation. The cranial vault is absent, and an angiomatous mass lies on the floor of the skull. The eyes are protuberant and there is variable involvement of the spinal cord. When identified by antenatal ultrasound, an increasing number of such pregnancies are terminated (28). In live-born anencephalic babies, the initial neurological examination may be "normal" if brainstem structures are intact, and seizures may occur despite the absent cerebral hemispheres. However, babies usually die within hours or days.

CONSENT

Having decided the appropriate treatment in an individual case, the next and important ethical consideration is consent, and from whom. Decision making depends on the age of the patient. If adults, consent is primarily their responsibility. Often patients are too small to make an autonomous decision, so parents or others act as proxy. Frequently, the clinical condition may require an early neonatal decision. Following are the ethical differences between babies and adults defined by Campbell (2000) (29):

1. Babies are incompetent. All decisions must be made by others on their behalf.
2. Decisions to provide or withhold treatment are made at the beginning of a potential life rather than towards the end of life.
3. Prognosis both for survival and the degree of impairment is usually less clear in babies than in adults of advanced age with terminal disease.
4. Decisions to treat babies with conditions causing severe life-long disabilities have a great impact on the lives of others—parents, siblings, and the community.

Who then should make the decision? Should it be parents, doctors, hospital ethical committees, the media, or the law? In each case, there is a possibility of a conflict of interest. Infants and children have their own fundamental rights in many countries, irrespective of parental wishes, actions, apathy, or religious beliefs. Between 1970 and 2000 many laws were introduced to protect children from inappropriate parental behavior, including, for example, the withholding of life-saving blood transfusions and antibiotics.

Many countries now legally protect the welfare and right to life of infants, illustrated by the "Baby Doe" events described above from the United States in 1982, in the United Kingdom by the Children Act (1989) (30), and internationally by the Human Rights Act (1998) (31), with disapproval of euthanasia even when suggested by parents or doctors. The reverse scenario also occurs, and there have been several well-publicized legal cases where parents may demand continuing treatment considered "futile" by the treating doctors. The debate has been referred to by some as the "right to live," but by others as the "right to die." For at least 25 years, U.K.

Courts have had to decide where doctors and parents disagree, about how to or not to treat a severely disabled child.

CONJOINED TWINS

The ethical issues of sacrifice and consent are well illustrated in the management of conjoined twins. In some cases, with specific anatomical arrangements, the sacrifice of one infant may be required so that the other may survive. In 1977 conjoined twins joined at the chest were born in Philadelphia (32). Their shared heart could only support one child, and parents accepted the medical advice of surgical separation with the necessary sacrifice of one infant. This is an example of what ethicists refer to as a "doctrine of double effect," which states *"an act which produces a bad effect is morally possible if the act is good in itself with the intent of producing a good effect"* (33). This became a major consideration in a well-publicized first U.K. legal case (34), where the Court ruled in favor of the doctors, as parents did not accept the proposed surgical separation.

When joined at the head ("craniopagus"), twins similarly may have complex shared vascular arrangements that makes operative separation an extremely high-risk procedure. In 2003, a fatal outcome due to intraoperative hemorrhage was reported in adult sisters, who were the first conjoined twins in history to give personal consent (35).

In relation to CSF disorders, it is not surprising that the surgical separation of craniopagus twins often can lead to a disruption of the CSF absorptive pathways (36).

In recent years, there have been several reports (37,38) concerning the successful surgical separation of infants, with one or both twins developing hydrocephalus at some point, requiring CSF diversion.

CONCLUSION

This chapter has examined ethical issues, which apply to all medicine, including the Management of CSF Disorders. While the law tells us what we must do, ethics is concerned with values and tells us what we ought to do. One of its ultimate criteria is *"Thou shall not kill."* Another is the respect for a patient with a limited and fatal prognosis. Most of us are aware of the rhyme, which covers both principles:

> *Thou shall not kill; but need not strive officiously to keep alive.*

The importance of ethical considerations in medical decision making has been increasingly recognized. There are special issues in looking after children. "Ethics" should continue to be part of medical and surgical training.

REFERENCES

1. Kennedy I. The Unmasking of Medicine. The Reith Lectures. London: Allen and Unwin, 1988.
2. Haeger K. The beginnings of medicine. In: Van Leuven J, ed. The Illustrated History of Surgery. London: Harold Starke, 1988:17–20.
3. Ellis H. The early years of written history Mesopotamia, Egypt, China and India. In: Ellis H, ed. A History of Surgery. London: Greenwich Medical Media Ltd, 2001:13–14.
4. Ellis H. Surgery in Ancient Greece and Rome. In: Ellis H, ed. A History of Surgery. London: Greenwich Medical Media Ltd, 2001:21–23.
5. Beauchamp TL, Childress JF. Principles of Biomedical Ethics, 5th ed. New York: Oxford University Press, 2001.
6. Bernard C. An Early Introduction to the Study of Experimental Medicine 1865 (First English Translation by Greene HC). New York: McMillan & Co. Ltd., 1927.
7. Mitscherlich A, Mielke F. Doctors of Infamy: The Story of Nazi Medical crimes. New York, NY: Schuman, 1949:xxiii–xv.
8. Declaration of Helsinki. 18th World Medical Assembly, Finland, 1964.
9. Teff H. The Action for "Wrongful Life" in England and The United States. Int Comp Law Q 1985; 34:423–441.
10. Moreno JD. Ethical and Legal Issues in the Care of the Impaired Newborn. Clin Perinatol 1987; 14:345–360.
11. The Bible "You Sacrifice Your Children in the Ravines . . . ." Isaiah 57.5.
12. Plato. The Republic Translated into English by Lee D Penguin Classics, 2003:175.

13. Rostain AR, Bhutani VK. Ethical dilemmas of neonatal perinatal surgery. Clin Perinatol 1989; 16: 275–302.
14. Lorber J. Results of treatment of myelomeningocele. Dev Med Child Neurol 1971; 13:279–303.
15. Guiney EG, Surana R. Selective treatment of spina bifida. Arch Dis Child 1994; 56:822–830.
16. Gostin L. A moment in human development: Legal protection, ethical standards and social policy on the selective nontreatment of handicapped neonates. Am J Law Med 1985; 11:31–78.
17. Editorial, Dr Leonard Arthur: His trial and its implications. Br Med J 1981; 283:1340–1341.
18. Re B (a minor). (Wardship: Medical treatment) [1981] 1 WLR 1421.
19. Wallis C. The Stormy Legacy of Baby Doe. Time Magazine 26th September, 1983.
20. Annas GJ. The case of Baby Jane Doe: Child abuse or unlawful federal intervention? Am J Pub Health 1984; 74(7):727–729.
21. Child Abuse Amendments (1984) Pub L. 98–457 Title 1, Part B, Section 121(3).
22. Dunea G. Squeal Rules in the Nursery. Br Med J 1983; 287:1203–1204.
23. Laurence KM, Coates S. The natural history of hydrocephalus. Arch Dis Child 1962; 37:345–362.
24. Milhorat TH. In: Hydrocephalus and the Cerebrospinal Fluid. Baltimore, MD: Williams and Wilkins, 1972.
25. Sgouros S, Mallucci C, Walsh AR, et al. Long term complications of hydrocephalus. Pediatr Neurosurg 1995; 23:127–132.
26. Becker LE, Takada K. Structural malformations of the cerebral hemispheres. In: Hoffmann HJ, Epstein F, eds. Disorders of the Developing Nervous System: Diagnosis and Treatment. Oxford, U.K.: Blackwell, 1986:211–213.
27. Brett EM, Harding BN. Hydrocephalus and congenital anomalies of the nervous system other than myelomeningocele. In: Brett EM, ed. Paediatric Neurology, 3rd ed. London: Churchill Livingstone, 1997:513.
28. Warkany J, Lemire RJ. Pathogenesis of neural tube defects. In: Hoffman HJ, Epstein F, eds. Disorders of the Developing Nervous System: Diagnosis and Treatment. Oxford, U.K.: Blackwell, 1986:22.
29. Campbell N. The impaired fetus and the newborn. In: Dooley B, Fearnside M, Gorton M, eds. Surgery, Ethics and the Law. Melbourne, VIC: Blackwell Asis, 2000.
30. Children Act 1989.
31. Human Rights Act 1988.
32. Drake D. The Twins Decision: One Must Die So One Can Live. The Philadelphia Inquirer October 16, 1977.
33. Saini P. The doctrine of double effect and the law of murder. Med Legal J 1999; 67:106–107.
34. Re A (children) (conjoined twins: medical treatment) [2000] 4 All ER 961, CA.
35. Hawkes N. Twins who Lived as One Go to Their Graves Alone. The Times 9th July 2003:3.
36. Goodrich JT, Staffenberg DA. Craniopagus Twins: Clinical and Surgical Management. Childs Nerv Syst 2004; 20:618–624.
37. Goh KYC. Separation surgery for total craniopagus twins. Chil Nerv Syst 2004; 20:567–575.
38. Campbell S. Separation of craniopagus twins: the Brisbane experience. Childs Nerv Syst 2004; 20:601–606.

33 | Treatment of Hydrocephalus in the Developing World

Benjamin C. Warf

Department of Neurosurgery, Children's Hospital Boston and Harvard Medical School, Boston, Massachusetts, U.S.A.

INTRODUCTION

Hydrocephalus is a common, underrecognized, and undertreated diagnosis among children in the developing world, where many challenges converge to impede its proper management. A dearth of centers with sufficient expertise is one obvious impediment. East and Central Africa, where I spent 6 years helping to develop a neurosurgical hospital for children (CURE Children's Hospital of Uganda), is representative. The ratio of trained neurosurgeons to total population at this writing is around 1 to 4 million in Kenya, 1 to 7 million in Uganda, and 1 to 18 million in Tanzania. In Congo, Rwanda, and Malawi, there are none. Given that more than half the population in this region is younger than the age of 15, it goes without saying that neurosurgical problems among children, hydrocephalus being the most common, are severely underserved. Obstacles to gaining access to one of the rare centers with competence to treat hydrocephalus only compound the problem. Poverty renders travel a costly enterprise for most families, while poor infrastructure and areas of insecurity make it time-consuming and dangerous. On arrival, a family may be confronted with prohibitive costs or an ill-equipped facility. For instance, a shunt may not be available or, if so, payment up-front for its cost may be required--a prohibitive proposition for most.

Cultural obstacles to treatment may also exist. In Uganda the nature of hydrocephalus was often not understood by the family, or sometimes even the local healthcare workers. Even when the condition was properly recognized, it was a prevalent notion that hydrocephalus could not be effectively treated, or at least that treatment was not available. It was a common belief that such children were cursed, which often resulted in the initial "treatment" being performed by a traditional healer (often referred to as a witch doctor). The typical practice of scarification by burning or cutting of the scalp often resulted in disfigurement (Fig. 1), and there was the further effect of draining the family's meager financial resources before care was sought elsewhere.

All of these conditions conspired to delay definitive treatment, such that many of our patients presented to us some months after the onset of noticeable macrocephaly. As a result, in our early experience, 63% of infants presented with a head circumference more than 2 cm above the 95th percentile, and in nearly 30%, this was exceeded by more than 6 cm. The preoperative mean cortical mantle thickness as gauged by cranial ultrasound was 1.64 cm, with 73% of infants presenting with mantle thickness less than 2 cm (1). Over time, however, we have noted a shift towards earlier presentation that we attribute to several years of public education through the media as well as developing an informed referral base and working in partnership with the Uganda Ministry of Health.

This chapter highlights the causes and prevalence of hydrocephalus in East Africa, describes the problems of treating these children in the context of a developing country, and explains strategies that have helped overcome these obstacles. Finally, a way forward in improving and expanding access to care for these children throughout the developing world will be suggested.

PREVALENCE AND CAUSES OF HYDROCEPHALUS

Hydrocephalus is common among infants and children in East Africa. CURE Children's Hospital of Uganda, alone, is currently presented with 300 to 500 new cases of hydrocephalus each year, about 80% of them being infants under the age of one year (1). Based on the demographics

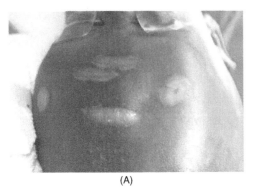
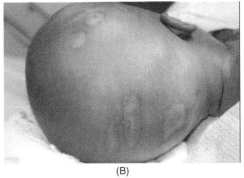

(A)   (B)

Figure 1 (**A**) Forehead and (**B**) occipital views of scalp scarification as treatment for macrocephaly in an infant with hydrocephalus.

of our own patient population, I estimated that each year in Uganda (population around 28 million) between 1000 and 2000 infants develop hydrocephalus in their first year of life.

In contrast to a previous report from Central Africa (2), as well as one from Saudi Arabia (3), the most common cause of hydrocephalus in our population was infection (meningitis/ventriculitis), with postinfectious hydrocephalus (PIH) accounting for 60% of cases (1). This has been subsequently confirmed in a review of our first 1000 children presenting for treatment of hydrocephalus (Fig. 2). In 76% of the cases, the infection had occurred in the first month of life, thus implicating neonatal sepsis as the primary cause. Risk factors for this may be tied to regional obstetrical practices. More than 60% of births in Uganda occur in a rural setting with no skilled attendant (4). This anticipates an increase in known risk factors for neonatal sepsis, including premature gestational age at delivery, premature rupture of the membranes, low Apgar score after one minute, and chorioamnionitis and/or funisitis (5). Other contributing factors may include practices such as cutting the umbilical cord with an unclean instrument and placing a cow dung poultice on the fresh umbilical stump (6). The reported in-hospital mortality of neonatal meningitis from one Central African country approached 50% (7). Thus, in addition to being the leading cause of infant hydrocephalus, it is also a major contributor to infant mortality, with those that survive to develop hydrocephalus representing only a fraction. There is no known association of malaria with hydrocephalus, but in malaria endemic areas such as Uganda the proper diagnosis and treatment of meningitis in children can be delayed because any febrile illness is often presumptively treated as malaria (1,7). We investigated whether there was any relationship between HIV status and the development of PIH, and found no correlation in our population (1).

Neonatal meningitis has been previously associated with ventriculitis, aqueductal obstruction, ventricular loculations, and cerebral infarction (8–10). These were all common findings in our patients presenting with PIH (Fig. 3), in which 2/3 presented with aqueductal obstruction confirmed at the time of ventriculoscopy (1) (Fig. 4). As discussed below, this suggested endoscopic third ventriculostomy (ETV) as a viable treatment option, because the majority had obstructive hydrocephalus.

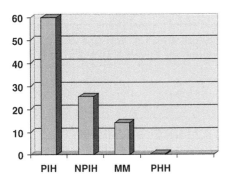

Figure 2 Causes of hydrocephalus in Uganda: 1000 consecutive children. *Abbreviations*: PIH, postinfectious hydrocephalus; NPIH, non-postinfectious hydrocephalus; MM, myelomeningocele; PHH, posthemorrhagic hydrocephalus.

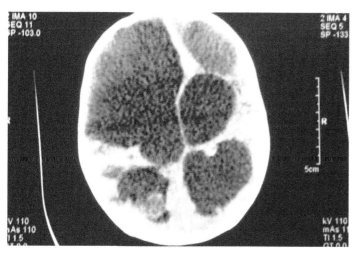

Figure 3 CT scan of infant with postinfectious hydrocephalus. Note loss of brain parenchyma and intraventricular deposits of pus.

In more than 1/4 of infants presenting with hydrocephalus, there was no history or clinical evidence of previous infection (non-postinfectious hydrocephalus, or NPIH) (1). This included those with congenital aqueduct stenosis, Dandy–Walker malformation, encephalocele, and all other instances of congenital hydrocephalus, and those few presenting with obstruction from a mass lesion. More than 10% of infants had hydrocephalus associated with spina bifida (myelomeningocele, or MM) (1). An important cause of infant hydrocephalus in the developed world, posthemorrhagic hydrocephalus of prematurity, was hardly ever seen because such infants do not survive in this environment.

It is reasonable to speculate that in other developing countries where much of the population lives in a poor rural setting, neonatal infection may be a leading cause of hydrocephalus as it is in Uganda. Anecdotally and from my own observation, this appears to be the case in other

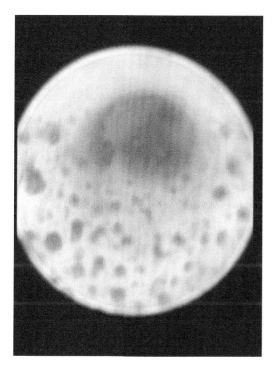

Figure 4 Endoscopic view of obstructed aqueduct in infant with postinfectious hydrocephalus. Note membrane obstructing the aqueduct ostium and punctuate inflammatory deposits. (The posterior commissure is at the top of the image.)

East and Central African countries. Thus, the burden of hydrocephalus in many developing countries may be a public health and preventative medicine issue rooted in their economic and political realities. It is arguable that around half of the cases of infant hydrocephalus in Uganda, and possibly other developing countries, could be prevented with improved access to basic obstetric and neonatal care to reduce the incidence of neonatal meningitis, and folic acid (either through provision of supplements to women of child bearing age or a national program of grain fortification) to reduce the incidence of neural tube defects.

MANAGEMENT OF HYDROCEPHALUS WITH SHUNTS

In 1952, Nulsen and Spitz first reported the use of a valved system to shunt CSF from the ventricle into the jugular vein (11). Over the subsequent half century, with the introduction of Silastic tubing, the ventriculoperitoneal shunt (VPS) became the procedure of choice for treating hydrocephalus. This involves placement of a proximal catheter into one of the lateral ventricles, connecting this to a subcutaneous one-way valve attached to distal subcutaneous tubing that terminates in the peritoneal cavity.

Shunt placement remains the primary method of treatment in the majority of children for the foreseeable future. Although not technically difficult to place, the usefulness of shunts in the context of a developing country is limited by two major difficulties: (*i*) cost and (*ii*) shunt failure. In addition, both malnutrition and severe macrocephaly can lead to thin skin and poor healing, which can add additional risk (Fig. 5).

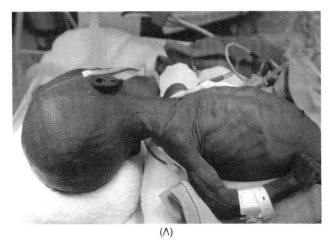

(A)

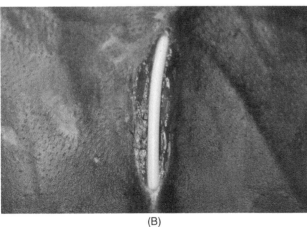

(B)

Figure 5   (**A**) Malnourished infant positioned for shunt placement; (**B**) patient with skin erosion over shunt tubing that had been exposed for two weeks prior to presentation.

Shunt systems typically utilized in developed countries can cost anywhere from US $500 to $3000. This represents an expense equal to several times the annual income for many families. Less-expensive alternatives have been reported, such as a locally made shunt that has been used in Zimbabwe and Malawi (2). This (the "Harare shunt") consists of a length of Silastic tubing tied off at its distal end with slit "valves" created just proximal to this. The inexpensive Chhabra shunt (G. Surgiwear Ltd., India) is in common use throughout India and Sub-Saharan Africa. This system, costing less than US $50, utilizes a simple slit-in-spring differential pressure valve.

Upon opening our hospital in Uganda, the Chhabra shunt was available to us without cost through the provision of the International Federation for Spina Bifida and Hydrocephalus. At the time, we also had a supply of 50 shunts from the United States, the Codman-Hakim Micro Precision shunt system [Medos S. A. (Johnson & Johnson Co.), Switzerland], which was approximately 20 times more expensive. We therefore had the opportunity to assess any difference in performance between the two systems by way of a randomized prospective trial (12). This was undertaken to investigate (i) whether shunts could be used in this context with failure and infection rates comparable to those in the developed world, and (ii) whether such an inexpensive shunt could be used just as effectively as a much more expensive, "sophisticated," type typically used in North America and Europe.

The result for 195 consecutive children, the majority of whom were younger than one year of age, in whom shunts were placed was studied prospectively. In one group of 90 patients, one of the two shunt systems (Chhabra or Codman) was selected at the time of surgery according to a randomization protocol. In these children, shunting had been nonselectively chosen as the primary treatment for their hydrocephalus because endoscopic management was not available at the time. The other group of patients was comprised of 105 children in whom ETV had either been unable to be performed at the time of surgery (technical failure) or in whom ETV had failed to adequately treat the hydrocephalus. The Chhabra shunt was used in all these patients by default because the supply of Codman shunts had come to an end ("randomization by availability"). The outcome at one year was assessed for all patients in regard to shunt malfunction (ventricular catheter, valve, or distal catheter obstruction), infection, shunt migration or disconnection, wound complication, and death. The results are presented in Table 1. This study demonstrated two important points. (i) There was no significant difference at one year in any outcome parameter between the two shunt systems. (ii) Our one-year results for treating infant hydrocephalus (80% were less than one year of age) with shunt placement in the context of an emerging country were quite comparable to those reported from North America and Europe (13–18). Thus, 20 patients could be treated for the cost of one "first world shunt," and just as safely and effectively.

So, it was confirmed that shunting could be performed with good results in developing countries using a very inexpensive shunt system, a very encouraging outcome indeed for those who labor in that setting to treat these children. But, creating shunt-dependence in children in developing countries presents a unique problem: maintenance of shunt function. Under the best

Table 1 Results at One Year for Chhabra and Codman Shunts

| | Number of patients (%) | | | |
	Chhabra	Codman	Total	p Value
No. of patients	152	43	195	
Lost at <1 yr	12	7	19	0.1410
Total followed	140 (92)	36 (84)	176 (90)	-
Dead at <1 mo	8 (5.3)	0	8 (4.1)	0.3631
No problems	75 (54)	21 (58)	96 (54.5)	1.0000
Dead by 1 yr	22 (15.7)	6 (17)	28 (15.9)	1.0000
Infection	13 (9.3)	4 (11)	17 (9.7)	1.0000
Wound complication	8 (5.7)	2 (5.6)	10 (5.7)	1.0000
Valve obstruction	6 (4.2)	0	6 (3.4)	0.3448
Proximal obstruction	4 (2.9)	1 (2.7)	5 (2.8)	1.0000
Distal obstruction	2 (1.4)	0	2 (1.1)	1.0000
Migration	8 (5.7)	3 (8.3)	11 (6.3)	0.6982

of circumstances, 20% to 40% of shunts can be expected to fail within a year of placement and more than half within two years (15–18). And, shunts continue to fail over time with a steady attrition rate, and often with multiple failures over the course of childhood (19,20). What's more, the risk of infection after implanting a shunt is around 10% (13,14). Therefore, shunt-dependence requires a reliable "safety net" that provides ready access to emergency treatment for shunt malfunction. The contrast is stark between developed and developing countries in this regard. Because of the obstacles to accessing neurosurgical care cited above, shunt-dependence is simply more dangerous for children in emerging countries.

AVOIDING SHUNT-DEPENDENCE THROUGH ENDOSCOPIC TREATMENT OF HYDROCEPHALUS

Endoscopic Third Ventriculostomy (ETV)

The danger of shunt-dependence in regions like East and Central Africa provided the impetus to aggressively explore other treatment options. CURE Children's Hospital of Uganda was fortunate to have obtained the necessary equipment for ventriculoscopy through a grant from the International Federation of Spina Bifida and Hydrocephalus. After initial success in selected cases, we purposed to pursue a prospective study in which we attempted ETV in every case. Third ventriculostomy is a minimally invasive endoscopic technique in which an opening is made in the floor of the third ventricle to create a passage for CSF directly from the third ventricle into the interpeduncular and prepontine cisterns below (Fig. 6). This bypasses any

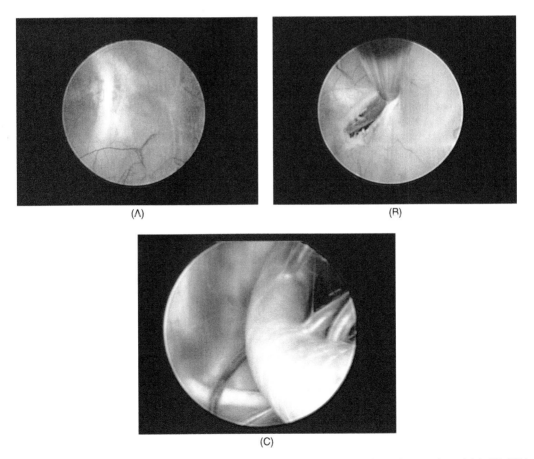

(A)   (B)

(C)

Figure 6   (**A**) Endoscopic view onto the floor of 3rd ventricle (pituitary is at left, basilar apex is at right); (**B**) ETV opening being made in floor with Bugby wire; and (**C**) view through ETV into prepontine cistern (basilar artery and branches on right, dura of clivus on left).

intraventricular obstruction at or distal to the aqueduct of Sylvius and allows for CSF to escape from the ventricles into the subarachnoid spaces where it can be absorbed physiologically. The first 300 cases in this series were very instructive (1). ETV was completed in more than 76%, with technical failures mostly occurring because of severe anatomic distortion or inadequate visibility secondary to turbid CSF among those with PIH. Among infants older than one year, the technique was very effective. Shunt-dependence was avoided in 81% of patients with PIH and in 90% of those with NPIH. (There were no patients with MM older than one year.) But, more than 80% of the patients were younger than one year. Among these, the result was successful in less than 50%, with the important exception of infants presenting with postinfectious aqueduct obstruction (comprising 2/3 of the PIH group, and the single largest subgroup of patients in the series). Among those, 70% were treated successfully with ETV. Overall, shunt-dependence was avoided in 59% of all children treated by ETV.

Endoscopic Third Ventriculostomy Combined with Choroid Plexus Cauterization (ETV/CPC)

Although the result for ETV was encouraging, another treatment option was sought to improve the outcome for the other infant subgroups (NPIH, MM, and PIH with an open aqueduct) (21). Others have reported age as an important determinant of outcome for ETV (22–24). Unique to the Ugandan experience, however, was the prevalence of postinfectious aqueduct obstruction, and this was the one group of infants in which ETV was reasonably successful (70%) (1). I thought this supported the hypothesis that ETV is less successful in obstructive hydrocephalus of infancy because of a concomitant "communicating" component of the hydrocephalus. This follows, because infants who were normal at birth and suffered an insult resulting in aqueduct obstruction would have previously developed competent CSF circulation and absorption mechanisms, whereas, those with congenital obstructive hydrocephalus would not. Thus, the new efflux of CSF from an ETV would likely be more successfully handled in the former situation than the latter.

Thus, if failure of ETV in infants was in some instances due to an imbalance between CSF production and absorption, it was speculated that even a temporary, partial reduction in the rate of CSF production at the time of the ETV operation might make the difference between success and failure for some infants. This notion was further supported by the moderate success that had been reported for CPC in children with "communicating" hydrocephalus (25,26). Furthermore, given the existence of obstructive hydrocephalus in cases where the aqueduct is open (27), such as obstruction of the 4th ventricle outlet foramina (e.g., in the Chiari II malformation) or in cases of posterior fossa scarring from infection or hemorrhage, it was not reasonable to restrict ETV only to those patients with demonstrable aqueduct obstruction. Thus, a model evolved in which infants were all considered to potentially harbor both obstructive and communicating components of hydrocephalus. This supported the ultimate decision to begin adding CPC to the ETV procedure (Fig. 7). The technical details of the combined ETV/CPC operation have been described and will not be reiterated here (21). It will be noted, however, that the technique entails a thorough cauterization of all choroid plexus from the foramen of Monro to the temporal horn in both lateral ventricles. This can be accomplished through a single right frontal approach along with the ETV, but only if a flexible endoscope is used.

The initial experience with the ETV/CPC performed in 266 patients was compared to that in 284 undergoing ETV alone. The results were very encouraging and were compatible with the hypothesis described above (Figs. 8 and 9) (21). On the whole, children older than one year did not benefit from the addition of CPC, whereas those younger than one year clearly did. The ones to benefit most significantly were those infants with congenital forms of hydrocephalus (NPIH and MM), with success increasing from 38% to 70% ($p = 0.0025$) and from 35% to 76% ($p = 0.0045$), respectively. The addition of CPC did not have a significant effect on outcome among infants with PIH, with success increasing from 52% to 62% ($p = 0.1607$). Infants with PIH and an open aqueduct seemed to benefit more (39–57%; $p = 0.1687$), whereas, there was no apparent benefit for those with aqueduct obstruction (61–65%; $p = 0.6203$). The mortality, morbidity, and infection rates for ETV/CPC were all 1% or less (21).

Further analysis of our data demonstrated that the presence of cisternal scarring at the time of ETV was a significant predictor of failure among infants with PIH, regardless of whether

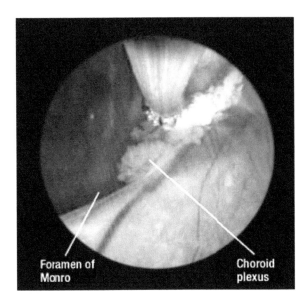

Figure 7 Cauterization of choroid plexus with the Bugby wire, beginning at the foramen of Monro (anterior on left).

CPC was performed (28). The success in these cases was less than 50%, and we have since adopted the practice of inserting a VP shunt at the time of the ETV when dense scarring of the interpeduncular and prepontine cisterns is present and cannot be dissected through into a clean CSF space. This subset of patients excluded, the success for ETV/CPC has been more than 70% among infants younger than one year with PIH and an open aqueduct, and the success of ETV alone when the aqueduct is obstructed has been more than 80%. The resulting treatment protocol and the expected success based on the initial results in each patient category are presented in Table 2.

As we have continued to follow the Ugandan patients over time, it is apparent that the success of ETV or ETV/CPC is durable. For instance, in the homogenous group of infants with hydrocephalus associated with myelomeningocele, the 20 that had been treated with ETV alone (follow up period 14–49 months, mean 32 months) have had a mean time to failure of 3.4 months, with 77% of failures presenting by two months postoperatively and no failures presenting after six months. Of 93 myelomeningocele infants treated with ETV/CPC (mean age at operation 3.0 months, mean follow-up 19.0 months), the rate of success was 76%, with 86% of failures presenting within six months of the operation (29). This should be contrasted with the long-term performance of shunts in the spina bifida population, where more than half of patients have a shunt failure in the first year, a third of patients go on to have two or more failures, and the attrition rate has been estimated at 10% per year after the second year (19,20). In addition, we have found no neurocognitive developmental advantage to shunting in this population compared to primary treatment by ETV/CPC (30).

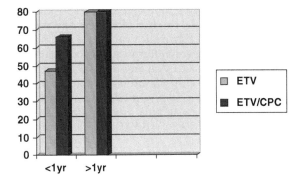

Figure 8 Percentage success for ETV alone versus ETV/CPC according to age (<1 year, $n = 423$, $p < 0.0001$; >1 year, $n = 100$, $p = 1.000$).

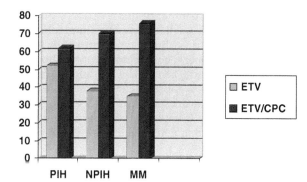

Figure 9 Percentage success for ETV alone versus ETV/CPC in infants <1 year old according to cause of hydrocephalus (PIH, $n = 251$, $p = 0.1607$; NPIH, $n = 101$, $p = 0.0025$; MM, $n = 65$, $p = 0.0045$).

HELPING CHILDREN WITH HYDROCEPHALUS IN THE DEVELOPING WORLD

I am convinced that avoiding shunt dependence in children who live outside the "safety net" alluded to above should be a high priority when considering treatment for hydrocephalus in this context. Furthermore, in those cases that require a shunt and in those situations where endoscopic management is not available, an inexpensive shunt is adequate and should be made available. Insisting upon the use of prohibitively expensive shunt systems, as we have encountered in some institutions, creates an unreasonable and completely unnecessary barrier to treatment.

The task of addressing the cultural, political, and economic factors that conspire to impede the treatment of these children is Herculean at best, but strategies that successfully help them despite their circumstances can be envisioned, and, indeed, already exist. For instance, the International Federation for Spina Bifida and Hydrocephalus (IF) has a growing number of projects with local partners (existing government facilities, NGOs, and mission organizations involved in healthcare) in developing countries that include the provision of inexpensive shunts without cost to the patient's family.

The goal of treating hydrocephalus in emerging countries while avoiding shunt dependence demands training and funding sufficient to create centers with the requisite cache of competencies and equipment. This is a formidable task that will require the commitment of many partners to make a serious difference. The Program to Advance the Treatment of Hydrocephalus (PATH) has developed as one model that works towards this goal. Briefly, this program provides an intensive period of training to neurosurgeons from selected institutions in emerging countries followed by the provision of the necessary equipment to the hospital along with training for the operating theater staff. We have now trained and equipped centers in Uganda, Nigeria, Tanzania, Zambia, Nepal, Vietnam, Bangladesh, and Ghana. A fundamental component of the project is to develop training centers in the developing world where, in contrast to centers in Europe and North America, the volume is high and the patient population and practice context are relevant.

CONCLUSIONS

Hydrocephalus is a major cause of suffering, death, and disability for the developing world's children. In East and Central Africa, and probably other impoverished regions of the world, the single most common cause is neonatal infection. When this is considered along with the association between hydrocephalus and neural tube defects, it is clear that simply improving

Table 2 CURE Children's Hospital of Uganda Treatment Protocol (% success)

	<1 yr/open	>1 yr/open	<1 yr/closed	>1 yr/closed
PIH (open cistern)	ETV/CPC (71%)	ETV/CPC (89%)	ETV (84%)	ETV/CPC (83%)
NPIH	ETV/CPC (63%)	ETV/CPC (86%)	ETV/CPC (78%)	ETV (90%)
MM	ETV/CPC (76%)	-	-	-

According to patients' age, aqueduct open or closed and cause of hydrocephalus. All MM patients were <1 yr and not categorized according to aqueduct status.

maternal and child healthcare could prevent many cases. Treatment with shunts in developing countries can be done cheaply and safely with efficacy equivalent to that seen when implanting expensive shunt systems in European and North American children, but the majority of shunts fail over time, making shunt dependence dangerous when emergency treatment for a shunt malfunction is difficult to obtain. Performing ETV, with the addition of CPC in infants, can successfully avoid shunt dependence in the majority without compromising neurocognitive development. Thus, pending the necessary and profound cultural, political, and economic changes necessary to the existence of the shunt maintenance "safety net," the development of centers in strategic areas that are capable of endoscopic treatment may be an important contribution to the well-being of these vulnerable young people.

REFERENCES

1. Warf BC. Hydrocephalus in Uganda: The predominance of infectious origin and primary management with endoscopic third ventriculostomy. J Neurosurg Pediatrics 2005; 102:1–15.
2. Adeloye A. Management of infantile hydrocephalus in Central Africa. Trop Doc 2001; 31:67–70.
3. el Awad ME. Infantile hydrocephalus in the south-western region of Saudi Arabia. Ann Trop Paediatr 1992; 12:335–338.
4. UNICEF: At a Glance: Uganda. http://unicef.org/infobycountry/uganda.html. Accessed October 9, 2007.
5. Martius JA, Roos T, Gora B, et al. Risk factors associated with early-onset sepsis in premature infants. Eur J Obstet Gynecol Reprod Biol 1999; 85(2):151–158.
6. Warf BC. Pediatric neurosurgery in the third world. In: Albright L, Pollack IF, Adelson PF, eds. Principles and Practice of Pediatric Neurosurgery, 2nd ed. New York, NY: Thieme. 2008:43–48.
7. Molyneux E, Walsh A, Phiri A, et al. Acute bacterial meningitis in children admitted to the Queen Elizabeth Central Hospital, Blantyre, Malawi in 1996–97. Trop Med Int Health 1998; 3:610–618.
8. Bortolussi R, Krishnan C, Armstrong D, et al. Prognosis for survival in neonatal meningitis: Clinical and pathologic review of 52 cases. Can Med Assoc J 1978; 118:165–168.
9. Kaul S, D'Cruz J, Rapkin R, et al. Ventriculitis, aqueductal stenosis and hydrocephalus in neonatal meningitis: Diagnosis and treatment. Infection 1978; 6:8–11.
10. Ment LR, Ehrenkranz RA, Duncan CC. Bacterial meningitis as an etiology of perinatal cerebral infarction. Pedatr Neurol 1986; 2:276–279.
11. Nulsen FE, Spitz EB. Treatment of hydrocephalus by direct shunt from ventricle to jugular vein. Surg Forum 1952; 2:399–403.
12. Warf BC. Comparison of 1-year outcomes for the Chhabra and Codman-Hakim micro precision shunt systems in Uganda: A prospective study in 195 children. J Neurosurg (Pediatrics 4) 2005; 102:358–362.
13. Haines SJ. Shunt infections. In: Albright AL, Pollack IF, Adelson PD, eds. Principles and Practice of Pediatric Neurosurgery. New York, NY: Thieme, 1999:91–106.
14. Pople IK, Bayston R, Hayward RD. Infection of cerebrospinal fluid shunts in infants: A study of etiological factors. J Neurosurg 1992; 77:29–36.
15. Albright AL, Haines SJ, Taylor FH. Function of parietal and frontal shunts in childhood hydrocephalus. J Neurosurg 1988; 69:883–886.
16. Blount JP, Campbell JA, Haines SJ. Complications in ventricular cerebrospinal fluid shunting. Neurosurg Clin N Am 1993; 4:633–656.
17. Drake JM, Kestle JR, Milner R, et al. Randomized trial of cerebrospinal fluid shunt valve design in pediatric hydrocephalus. Neurosurgery 1998; 43:294–305.
18. Sainte-Rose C, Hoffman HJ, Hirsch JF. Shunt failure. Concepts Pediatr Neurosurg 1989; 9:7–20.
19. Tuli S, Drake J, Lamberti-Pasculli M. Long-term outcome of hydrocephalus management in myelomeningoceles. Childs Nerv Syst 2003; 19:286–291.
20. Steinbok P, Irvine B, Cochrane DD, et al. Long-term outcome and complications of children born with meningomyelocele. Childs Nerv Syst 1992; 8:92–96.
21. Warf BC. Comparison of endoscopic third ventriculostomy alone and combined with choroid plexus cauterization in infants younger than 1 year of age: A prospective study in 550 African children. J Neurosurg 2005; 103(6 suppl Pediatrics):475–481.
22. Drake JM. Canadian Pediatric Neurosurgery Study Group: Endoscopic third ventriculostomy in pediatric patients: The Canadian experience. Neurosurgery 2007; 60:881–885.
23. Kadrian D, van Gelder J, Florida D, et al. Long-term reliability of endoscopic third ventriculostomy. Neurosurgery 2005; 56:1271–1278.
24. Koch D, Wagner W. Endoscopic third ventriculostomy in infants of less than 1 year of age: Which factors influence the outcome? Childs Nerv Syst 2004; 20:405–411.

25. Pople IK, Ettles D. The role of endoscopic choroid plexus coagulation in the management of hydrocephalus. Neurosurgery 1995; 36:698–702.
26. Scarff JE. The treatment of nonobstructive (communicating) hydrocephalus by endoscopic cauterization of the choroid plexuses. J Neurosurg 1970; 33:1–18.
27. Kehler U, Gliemroth J. Extraventricular intracisternal obstructive hydrocephalus—A hypothesis to explain successful 3rd ventriculostomy in communicating hydrocephalus. Pediatr Neurosurg 2003; 38:98–101.
28. Warf BC. Combined endoscopic third ventriculostomy and choroid plexus cauterization (ETV/CPC) for hydrocephalus in infants and children with special emphasis on the developing world. Tuttlingen, Germany: Endo-Press, 2006.
29. Warf BC, Campbell JW. Combined endoscopic third ventriculostomy and choroid plexus cauterization as primary treatment of hydrocephalus for infants with myelomeningocele. long-term results of a prospective intent-to-treat study in 115 East African infants. J Neurosurg Pediatrics 2008; 2:310–316.
30. Warf BC, Ondoma S, Kulkarni A, et al. Neurocognitive outcome and ventricular volume in myelomeningocele children treated for hydrocephalus in Uganda. J Neurosurg Pediatrics (in press).

Appendix

CHARITIES

Society for Research into Hydrocephalus and Spina Bifida (SRHSB)
Clinicians international research group meeting once a year, encompassing hydrocephalus, spina bifida, and syringomyelia within its interest areas http://www.srhsb.org

Association for Spina Bifida and Hydrocephalus (ASBAH)
An association of patients with spina bifida and hydrocephalus in the United Kingdom http://www.asbah.org

Arbeitsgemeinschaft Spina bifida und Hydrocephalus e.V. (ASbH e.V.)
An association of patients with spina bifida and hydrocephalus in Germany http://www.asbh.de

APAISER, Association Pour Aider et Informer les Syringomyéliques Européens Réunis
An association of patients with syringomyelia in France http://www.apaiser.asso.fr

Conquer Chiari
Also known as C&S Patient Education Foundation
An association of patients with Chiari malformation and syringomyelia in the United States. http://www.conquerchiari.org

The Ann Conroy Trust
An association of patients with Chiari malformation and syringomyelia in the United Kingdom http://www.theannconroytrust.org.uk

World Arnold Chiari Malformation Association
An association of patients with Chiari Malformation in New York, U.S.A. http://www.wacma.com

Eurordis, European Organisation for Rare Diseases
A patient driven alliance of patient organizations and individuals active in the field of rare diseases (e.g., achondroplasia) http://www.eurordis.org

Birth Defects Foundation (BDF)
A foundation for disabled children in United Kingdom http://www.bdfnewlife.co.uk

Hydrocephalus Association
An association of patients with hydrocephalus in the United States http://www.hydroassoc.org

Spina Bifida Association
An association of patients with spina bifida in the United States http://www.sbaa.org

ABBREVIATIONS

aFP	alpha Fetoprotein
ASD	Antisiphon device
BBB	Blood–brain barrier
CBF	Cerebral blood flow
CBV	Cerebral blood volume
CSF	Cerebrospinal fluid
CT	Computerized tomography
ECG	Electrocardiogram
EEG	Electroencephalogram
ETV	Endoscopic third ventriculostomy
EVD	External ventricular drain

hCG   Human chorionic gonadotrophin
ICP   Intracranial pressure
IQ   Intelligence quotient; PIQ: performance IQ ; VIQ: verbal IQ
IVH   Intraventricular hemorrhage
MR   Magnetic resonance
NPH   Normal pressure hydrocephalus
PET   Positron emission tomography
SAH   Subarachnoid hemorrhage
SDH   Subdural hematoma
SPECT   Single photon emission computerized tomography
SVS   Slit ventricle syndrome
TB   Tuberculosis; TBM: tuberculous meningitis

Index

Printed and bound by CPI Group (UK) Ltd, Croydon, CR0 4YY

23/10/2024

01778257-0006